W9-BJA-404

THE ART, SCIENCE AND SPIRIT OF NURSING

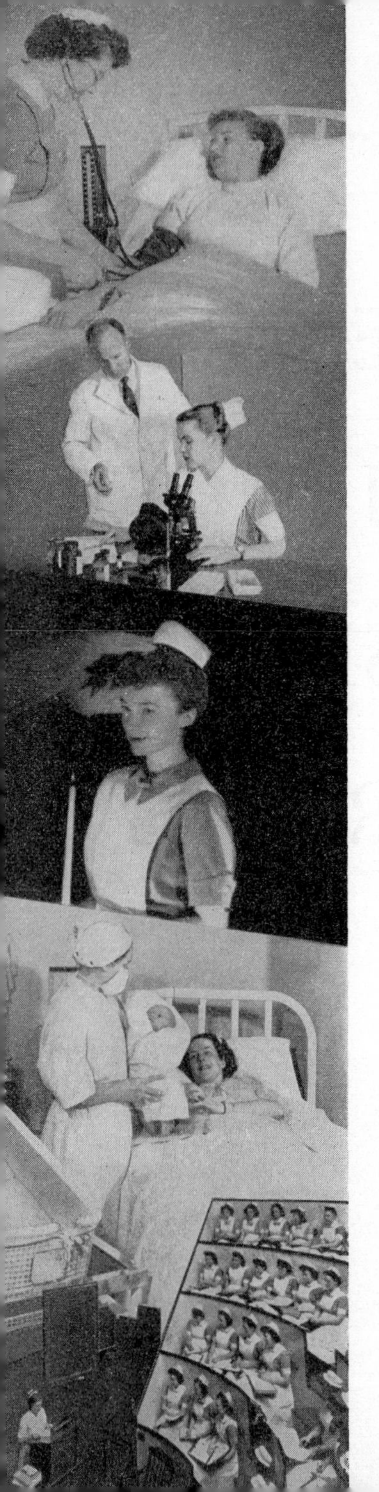

By

ALICE L. PRICE, R.N., M.A.

Formerly Counselor, School of Nursing,
Presbyterian Hospital, Chicago
Nurse Consultant, Hill-Rom Co., Inc.
Batesville, Ind.

ILLUSTRATED

W. B. SAUNDERS COMPANY

Philadelphia and London

THE ART, SCIENCE AND SPIRIT OF NURSING

REPRINTED SEPTEMBER, 1954, NOVEMBER, 1954, AUGUST, 1955,
MAY, 1956, AND APRIL, 1957

MADE IN THE UNITED STATES OF AMERICA

PRESS OF W. B. SAUNDERS COMPANY, PHILADELPHIA

LIBRARY OF CONGRESS CATALOG CARD NUMBER: 54-6091

TO

J. L.

WHO IS UNAWARE THAT MUCH OF THIS TEXT

WAS WRITTEN BY HIM

Preface

The nurse of today serves as the central figure in a corps of workers which includes physicians, laboratory specialists, psychologists, physiotherapists, social workers, dietitians, and others. Nursing service, because of its close relationship to the welfare of the patient, must coordinate the services of all the other various groups or specialties. The nurse of today must be concerned with such factors in patient care as early ambulation, shortened hospital stay for the surgical or obstetrical patient, rehabilitation for the disabled, and responsibilities in civil defense in event of wartime disaster. Textbooks in nursing must keep pace with these broadened concepts in the profession.

"The Art, Science and Spirit of Nursing," the newest textbook in the field of nursing arts, has been written to help familiarize beginning students of nursing with responsibilities which were unknown to the nurses of previous generations. It is based on results of a study made in 1951, while the author was a graduate student at the University of Wisconsin. Approximately 650 nursing arts instructors throughout the United States and 200 students of nursing were surveyed, to determine what factors they would choose for inclusion in a textbook of nursing arts. The answers they gave to a questionnaire have influenced the choice of content and manner of presentation for the text.

A topical outline introduces each chapter, because the students requested it. Scientific principles and situation type problems are presented at the request of the instructors. Suggested references have been limited to a few pertinent articles in current technical or popular magazines, as requested by most students and by many instructors.

Each chapter includes a summary of its important features and a listing of factors to teach the patient. No attempt has been made to instruct the student in step-by-step performance of various procedures, because instructors unanimously agreed that they preferred to teach techniques of nursing from their own hospital procedure books.

This text is new also in the utilization of illustrative material. The book is generously illustrated, with a total of 274 photographs contributed by many different schools of nursing and suppliers of various items of hospital equipment. The response of directors of schools of nursing in all parts of the country to a request for illustrative material was most gratifying. Some sent a substantial number of photographs;

others had pictures taken for specific use in the text, and many sent explanatory subject material along with the requested illustrations. The author is pleased to acknowledge the valuable contribution made to the text by these photographic illustrations.

Grateful acknowledgment is also given the Public Relations Department of Miami Valley Hospital, in Dayton, Ohio, for permission to use the attractive drawing which appears on the cover of the book.

Others who have given valuable and needed assistance include Miss Ruth Taff, recent graduate of the School of Nursing of Presbyterian Hospital in Chicago, who supplied the small sketches which appear at the head of each chapter; Mrs. C. R. Hinton who typed the entire manuscript, twice; and Miss Alice B. Morrissey, who graciously permitted reproduction of parts of the table of chronological events in the history of rehabilitation which appears in the first chapter of her book "Rehabilitation Nursing," published by G. P. Putnam's Sons, New York.

The author will feel amply rewarded, and the primary purpose of this text will have been accomplished, if "The Art, Science, and Spirit of Nursing" helps the student to understand and to meet all the needs of her patients.

ALICE L. PRICE

Chicago, Illinois

Contents

PART I. INTRODUCTION

PART II. THE HOSPITAL ENVIRONMENT

PART III. BASIC PROCEDURES FOR PRECLINICAL STUDY

PART VI PROCEDURES FOR ADVANCED CLINICAL STUDY

PART I

Introduction

CHAPTER 1

An Introduction to Nursing

TOPICAL OUTLINE

Nursing Defined
Profession Defined
The Professional Nurse
Development of Nursing
The Hospital
The School of Nursing
Students' Orientation to Nursing

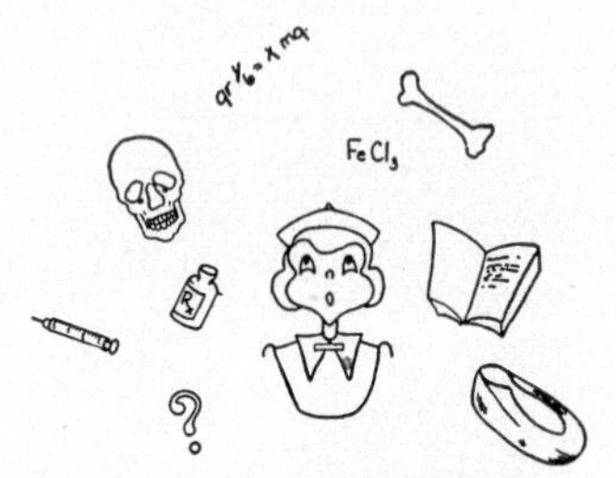

Some persons grow with responsibility—others merely swell.

Each student who takes her place as a new member in a school of nursing needs some knowledge of the growth and development of the organization or group which she has elected to join.

The following brief account of the development of hospitals, of nursing schools, and of nursing will serve to acquaint the student with activities of the group in the past and to help her understand the need for continued progress in the future.

NURSING DEFINED

Nursing has long been defined as a science and an art, not a pure science, not a true art, but a combination of the two. Nursing, as a profession, will embrace more than an art and a science; it will be a blending of three factors: of art and science and the spirit of unselfish devotion to a cause primarily concerned with helping those who are physically, mentally, or spiritually ill.

Nursing is an art, in that the nurse must develop skilled technique in the performance of the various procedures required for giving adequate care to the patient.

Nursing is a science, in that the underlying principles of nursing care depend on knowledge of the biological sciences, such as anatomy and physiology, microbiology, and chemistry. These sciences are fundamental to an understanding of the human body in its normal physical condition and in the abnormal condition that results when it is attacked by disease.

Nursing is possessed of a spiritual quality in that its primary aim is to serve humanity, not only by giving curative care to the bodies of the sick and injured, but by serving the needs of the mind and spirit as well.

Nursing, then, may be defined as a service to the individual which helps him to regain, or to keep, a normal state of body and mind; when it cannot accomplish this, it helps him gain relief from physical pain, mental anxiety, or spiritual discomfort.

Today there are many classifications of the term "nurse"; since this text is primarily concerned with the "registered" or "professional" nurse and the services required of her as a member of a "profession," it becomes necessary to define the terms "profession" and "professional nurse."

PROFESSION DEFINED

The term "profession" has been defined by Webster thus: "The occupation, if not purely commercial, mechanical, agricultural, or the like, to which one devotes oneself; a calling in which one professes to have acquired some special knowledge used by way either of instructing, guiding, or advising others or of serving them in some art; as, the profession of arms, of teaching, of chemist. The three professions, or learned professions, is a name often used for the professions of theology, law, and medicine. . . . Broadly, one's principal calling, vocation, or employment."

Criteria expressed by Flexner and generally accepted as denoting professional standing include a definite knowledge or training, and constant experimentation and research to enrich and enlarge that knowledge. All qualified members must spend a period of time in study in institutions of higher learning. The group's primary aim must be that of service; the nature of that service must be practical as well as theoretical. The group must be organized, self governing, and social in nature.

Full professional status will be accorded the nursing group when all criteria for professional standing can be met. In the meantime, the status of nursing changes, and as improvements are achieved recognition can be given the group. Its members may thus come closer to the "professional" standard to which they have subscribed.

THE PROFESSIONAL NURSE

The American Nurses' Association defines the professional or registered nurse as "One who has met all legal requirements for registration in a state, and who may practice nursing by virtue of her technical knowledge and practical ability." The professional nurse, then,

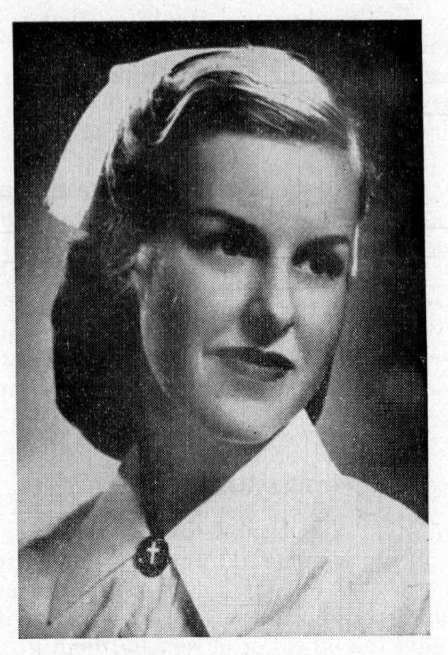

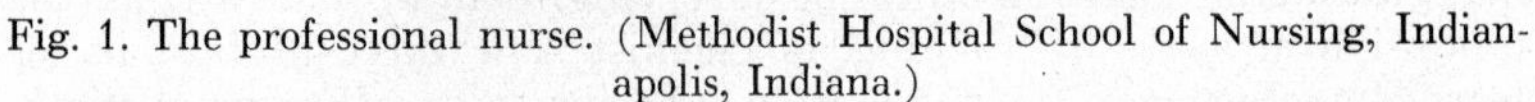

Fig. 1. The professional nurse. (Methodist Hospital School of Nursing, Indianapolis, Indiana.)

is the nurse who has received the maximum amount of education or training offered by recognized and accredited schools of nursing. Graduates of accredited schools may be licensed to practice nursing in schools, in industry, in private homes, in hospitals, and in other institutions.

THE DEVELOPMENT OF NURSING

Although nursing as an art and a science is relatively modern, nursing in actual practice (the spirit of nursing) has existed since the beginning of time. Women of nomadic tribes, in the early days of history, in ministering to the needs of the very young, the very old, and the infirm, were performing nursing duties of their time.

The impulse to serve is the basis on which the spirit of nursing has been fostered through the ages. As the needs of humanity have changed, during the progress of civilization, nursing has developed broader interests and functions. Now nursing means many things—it means to *nourish*, to *protect*, to *prevent* (illness), to *avoid* (injury), to *educate*, to *sustain*, and to *give*.

The word "nurse" comes from the Latin word *nutricius*, which means "that nourishes, fosters, and protects."

Many persons think of nurses only in connection with care given

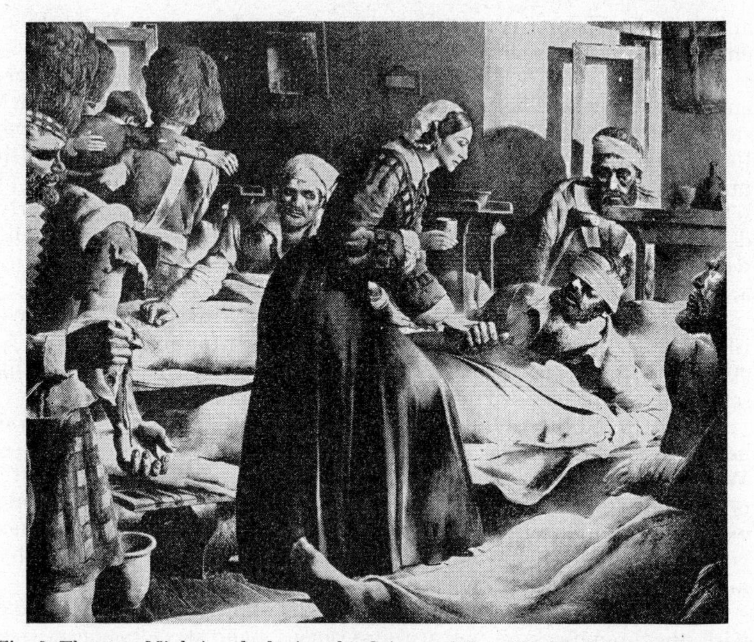

Fig. 2. Florence Nightingale during the Crimean War. (Parke, Davis & Company, Detroit, Michigan.)

the sick and injured because nurses, as well as doctors, have been chiefly concerned in the past with treatment and cure. In reality, nurses are active in the *prevention* of disease, as well as in its cure. They serve as teachers helping to educate the public in regard to health measures. They care for the mind, as well as the body, and are deeply interested in the normal as well as in the diseased or abnormal human organism.

Throughout the history of civilization, when the family was the unit of group living, it became the duty of the women of the family to care for the young and helpless and to look after the sick. For many years the only nursing that was done was carried on inside the family group.

The first "visiting nurses" were the untrained, untaught women workers known as *Deaconesses* and *Widows*. The desire to be of service to others was their only preparation for the duties of nursing which they performed.

The first instruction or training for nurses was instituted in Paris, France, in 1633 by St. Vincent de Paul, who organized the nursing order called "Sisters of Charity."

In the early part of the 19th century Theodor Fliedner and his wife, Frederika, opened a small hospital in Kaiserswerth, Germany, and gave instruction to women in the duties of nursing. There Florence Nightingale began her training in 1851.

Nursing as a profession had its beginning with the advent of Florence Nightingale. The reforms she instituted in the care of the sick still form the basis for nursing as it is practiced now. She firmly believed that the tasks of caring for the sick and teaching good health practices were sufficiently important to warrant establishment of schools and training of personnel to carry on the work. She bitterly denounced the accepted idea that nursing should be left to those who were disappointed in love or who were desperate for means of earning a livelihood.

In gratitude for her heroic work during the Crimean War, the British awarded Miss Nightingale 44,000 pounds (approximately $211,000.00) to use as she wished. With the funds she established a training school for nurses at St. Thomas Hospital in London.

In the United States the achievement of women workers in the war between the states in the 1860's led to improved hospital nursing care. With the founding of the United States Sanitary Commission and the organization of women interested in giving care to the sick and wounded of both armies, arrangements were made to select 100 women who would be given one month of nurses' training to prepare them for nursing duties in the army.

These volunteer army nurses had no rank and were constantly faced with the prejudices of the army surgeons against *petticoat nurses*. They were forced to perform the work of cook, chaplain, laundress, housekeeper, and social worker, as well as nurse. In some instances they were even required to serve as soldiers.

In 1873 nursing schools, patterned after the Nightingale school in London, were established in the United States. Three schools, established at almost the same time, have each had a profound influence on the development of modern nursing. They were the Bellevue Hospital school of nursing in New York, the Boston Training-School at the Massachusetts General Hospital in Boston, and the Connecticut Training-School at the New Haven Hospital.

The early schools gave approximately one year of training, but as medical research made advancement in medicine possible it became necessary to extend the course in nursing. A three-year course of study for nurses was generally accepted during the early part of the 20th century. Graduates from the early schools went to various parts of the United States to establish more schools. By the time three-year schools were well organized the total number of such schools was well over 400.

In the very early schools student nurses worked long hours and performed the duties of cook, dietitian, maid, trained attendant, and social worker. Formal classroom teaching was conspicuously absent, and students "learned to do by doing."

In 1896 a national society for nurses in the United States and

Canada was formed under the name "The Nurses' Alumnae of the United States and Canada." In 1911 the organization was changed, and the "American Nurses' Association" was formed in the United States. The Canadian nurses formed their own association.

In 1900 "The American Journal of Nursing" appeared as the official publication of the American Nurses' Association. For the first few years the Journal office was in a suitcase under the bed of Miss Sophia F. Palmer, its first editor. Now large offices are maintained at an imposing address in New York City.

About the time the Journal came into being the first course offering advanced training to the graduate nurse was put into effect at Teachers College, Columbia University. This course provided the means of improving the preparation of nurses who were to serve as instructors and as directors of nursing schools.

Public Health Nursing had its beginning as early as 1877, and by 1900 "visiting nurse" services were established throughout the country. Public Health nursing, furnishing nursing service for health, as well as for illness, is now a recognized part of the work of the nursing profession.

In 1914, at the time of World War I, there were only about 400 members of the Army Nurse Corps. In 1917, toward the closing months of the war, the number of nurses serving in the army was approximately 9,000. During the war years the importance of nursing was recognized, and definite steps were taken toward establishment of endowed university schools; more graduate nurses were employed in hospitals, and nursing schools which had given inadequate training were forced to close.

During World War II all programs for the education and training of nurses were accelerated. Students were admitted twice yearly and in greater numbers than ever before. To assist in preparing more nurses for army and navy service, inactive graduate nurses went back into civilian hospitals, federal aid was given for post-graduate study, refresher courses were set up, auxiliary workers (paid and volunteer) were recruited and given "on the job" training, and the nursing course for students was streamlined to fit the needs of the time.

From World War II nursing has emerged as a widely publicized and recognized community service. Today the nurse is found wherever people are found. She plays an important role in institutions, in homes, in industry, in schools, in transportation, and in the military services. She cares for the sick and injured, she aids in the fight against disease, and she teaches individuals, families, and communities the fundamentals of personal and public hygiene.

The opportunities in nursing today are practically without limit. Such positions as private duty nurse, public health nurse, general staff nurse, office nurse, industrial nurse, head nurse, supervisor, instructor, administrator, counselor, consultant, writer, and research worker are open to the young graduate nurse.

The spirit of nursing remains unchanged—applicants to schools of nursing today, questioned why they chose nursing as a career, indicate that they are interested in nursing because they like people and want to help them.

Recent advances in nursing have made it possible for the profession to offer young women opportunity for interesting work, independence, security, and the satisfaction of performing important and much-needed services for their fellow man. In the days ahead nursing should develop along sound educational lines and become even stronger and more widely recognized as an established and proud profession.

THE HOSPITAL

The hospital of today, with its modern facilities for the prevention and treatment of disease, only slightly resembles the hospital of early times which provided little more than makeshift shelter for the poor, the aged, and the sick. Like most community agencies, the hospital has developed according to the health needs of the community which it serves. At present it has become a community health center where the patient may receive medical and nursing care while ill, with assurance that further care will be provided after he has been dismissed from the institution and is convalescing at home.

The Growth and Development of Hospitals. Although little is known of the early beginning of hospitals, most historians believe that the earliest hospitals were the "guest houses" of Europe which furnished food and shelter for the traveler, provided some nursing care for the sick, and at times offered hospitality to the very poor.

Women entered hospital work with the coming of Christianity and helped to bring about improvement in the care and management of the so-called "Inn" hospitals. Early hospitals were often attached to churches or monasteries, since it was the duty of early Christians to provide charity for those in need of care and attention.

The first public hospital to be established for the primary purpose of serving the sick is thought to have been built in Rome as early as 380 A.D. During the middle ages the segregation of patients with leprosy was largely responsible for the beginning of preventive health work and also provided the impetus for additional hospital development.

At the time Florence Nightingale was instituting reforms in nursing, hospitals were being constructed, furnished, equipped, and managed to provide adequate care for the sick. Improvement in hospitals played a major role in the advancement of nursing and the beginning reforms in medical and surgical practices.

Among the first hospitals which were established in the United States and which still provide care for the sick and infirm are the Pennsylvania Hospital in Philadelphia, New York Hospital in New

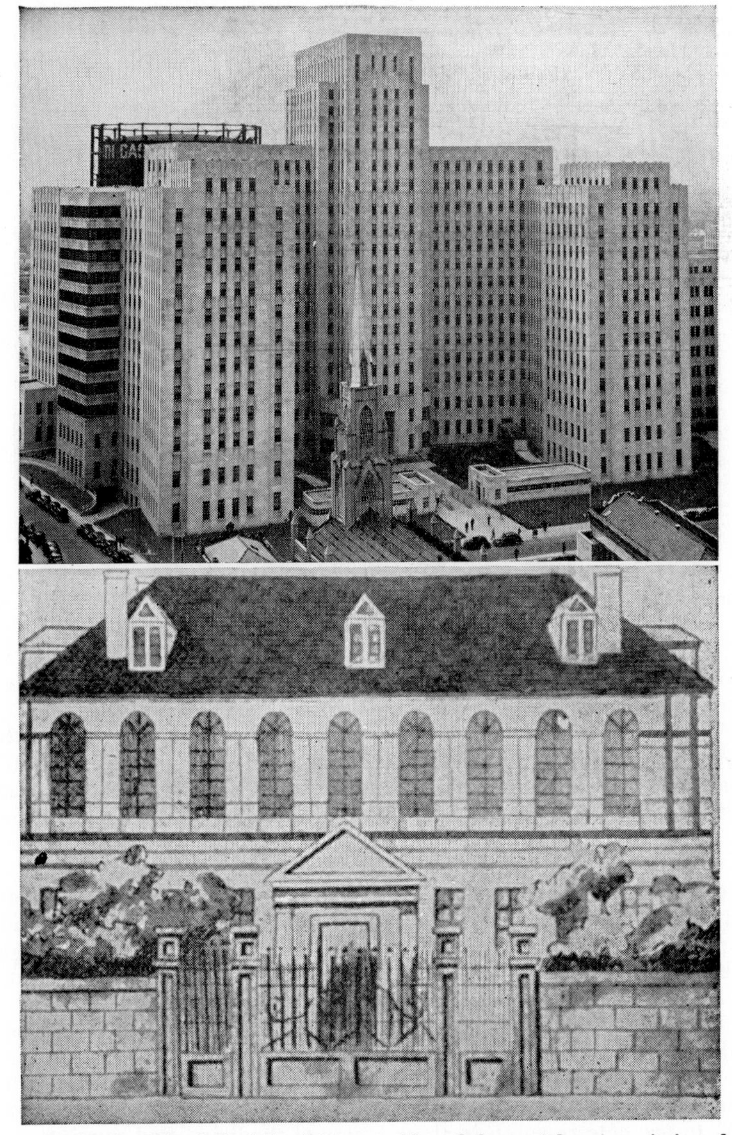

Fig. 3. Charity Hospital of Louisiana, at New Orleans (above) as it is today; (below) artist's drawing of the hospital, 1815–1832.

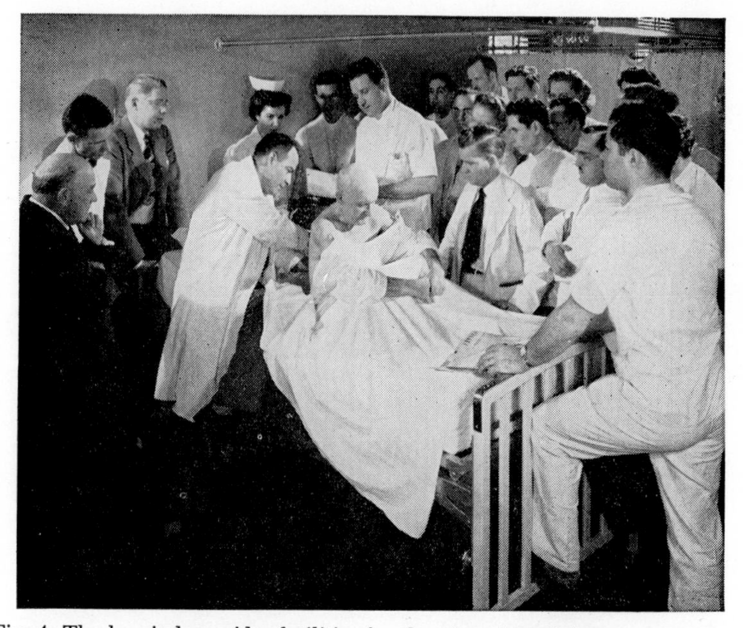

Fig. 4. The hospital provides facilities for the education of doctors, nurses, and other hospital personnel. (Presbyterian Hospital, Chicago, Illinois.)

York City, and Charity Hospital in New Orleans, Louisiana. The first mental hospital was founded in Williamsburg, Virginia, in 1772.

The rapid growth and development of hospitals throughout the country provided opportunity for improved patient care, for the training of nurses and doctors, and for addition of such valuable adjuncts as contagion wards, outpatient clinics, and dietary departments.

Today hospitals provide laboratory facilities for the teaching of all classifications of personnel from the skilled, professional, medical staff member to the untrained, non-professional workers found in all departments. In medical and university centers the hospital may provide for extensive research in medicine, nursing, and other health fields. The future promises further development of hospital facilities and even more usefulness to the community the hospital serves.

Functions. The five chief functions of the hospital are: (1) to provide care for the sick and injured; (2) to prevent disease; (3) to promote individual and community health; (4) to provide facilities for the education of doctors, nurses, and other hospital personnel; and (5) to promote research in the sciences of medicine and nursing.

The extent to which a hospital may serve these various functions is governed by the size and location of the building, the existence of necessary laboratory facilities, its accreditation as a nursing school or for the training of interns, the size and qualifications of its staff, and the financial status of the organization.

Classification. Hospitals may be classified (1) according to control and ownership, (2) the type of service rendered, and (3) the standards of service maintained.

According to Control. Governmental hospitals or "public" hospitals are those owned and controlled by the federal government, such as the Army or Navy hospitals and Veterans hospitals. The state, city, and county hospitals are government controlled on a local level.

Non-governmental hospitals or "private" hospitals are those owned and controlled by churches, fraternal orders, corporations, industries, groups, or individuals. Such hospitals are usually operated without profit and are supported by endowments, trust funds, earnings, and public subscriptions.

Proprietary hospitals are privately owned and operated to produce a profit for the owner.

According to Type of Service Rendered. General hospitals care for patients with various illnesses. They usually provide for a number of different clinical services and offer free care for some patients, although the majority of patients are expected to pay. *Special* hospitals are those treating only a specific kind of illness, as mental diseases, children's diseases, or communicable diseases.

According to Standard of Service Maintained. Hospitals are accredited by certain professional organizations, such as the American College of Surgeons, when the hospital buildings, equipment, administration, teaching facilities, and care given to patients meet the standards set by the organization.

Hospitals are classified by the American Medical Association as to suitability for the education and training of interns. The American Nurses' Association classifies hospitals as to educational and clinical facilities for maintaining an accredited school of nursing.

Plan and Location. Large numbers of hospital buildings are interesting and attractive in appearance, regardless of whether they were constructed in the early part of the 20th century when the one-story pavilion type hospital seemed preferable, or in more recent years when the tendency has been toward buildings of great height. Skyscraper hospitals form a part of the characteristic skyline silhouette of almost any large city. By building skyward a hospital in the most congested area of a large city may still offer its patients plenty of sunlight, a desirable view, and escape from city noises.

The advantage of taller, more compact hospital buildings is manifest, too, in better planning for centralized special services. One main kitchen, centrally located, may serve many more patient departments than could be served by the same kitchen attached to a rambling pavilion hospital. Transportation of patients in the taller hospitals may be done more rapidly and more efficiently, since it is largely accomplished by means of the elevator.

In recent years attempt has been made to provide a more comfortable and more attractive environment, not only for the patient, but for hospital personnel as well. In addition to sun rooms, enclosed porches, roof gardens, rooms with adjoining baths, recreation rooms, coffee shops, gift shops, and libraries for patients and their visitors, carefully planned institutions provide efficient and attractive offices for business and administration personnel.

On the various clinical departments, chart rooms are usually located near the nurses' station. Nursing personnel are provided with a lounge room and dressing room. A ward classroom on the department may be used for ward classes or for ward conferences between the student and the nurse in charge.

Elevators are automatic, doors are wide to permit beds to be moved readily. Wheelchairs, carts, etc., are equipped with rubber tires to lessen noise and to make transportation of the patient less difficult.

The hospital of today offers more adequate protection from fires through the use of fireproof materials in construction and of huge metal doors which can be closed to seal off an entire section of the building should fire occur.

Indirect lighting to reduce glare and thus make the patient more comfortable, modern heating systems which provide a uniform temperature throughout the building, and air conditioning units in special departments, as the operating room, or for the entire building, are all considered essential for the modern hospital. Should the community power plant fail during an emergency situation or in time of disaster, an independent lighting system for the hospital insures adequate and continuous care for the patients.

Clinical service departments (Fig. 5), providing for nursing care of patients, may differ somewhat in detail but are basically the same in regard to floor plan, furnishings, and equipment. Such departments usually consist of 20 to 40 patient units or rooms, the head nurse's station, a kitchen, utility room, linen room, storage room, flower room, a treatment and dressing room, and sufficient closet space for the storage and care of mops, brooms, and other cleaning equipment used by the housekeeping personnel for that particular department.

Each clinical service department is usually provided with a sun room that can be used as a waiting room for visitors as well as a pleasant and spacious place for recreational activities of patients permitted to be out of bed and out of their own room or unit.

All patient rooms on the clinical service department should have hot and cold running water and adequate nursing care facilities.

The semi-private rooms (two-bed rooms) and the wards should provide patient units that can be separated from adjoining units by heavy curtains which hang from rods fastened to the ceiling. By drawing the curtains around the unit the patient may be concealed from view and given complete privacy.

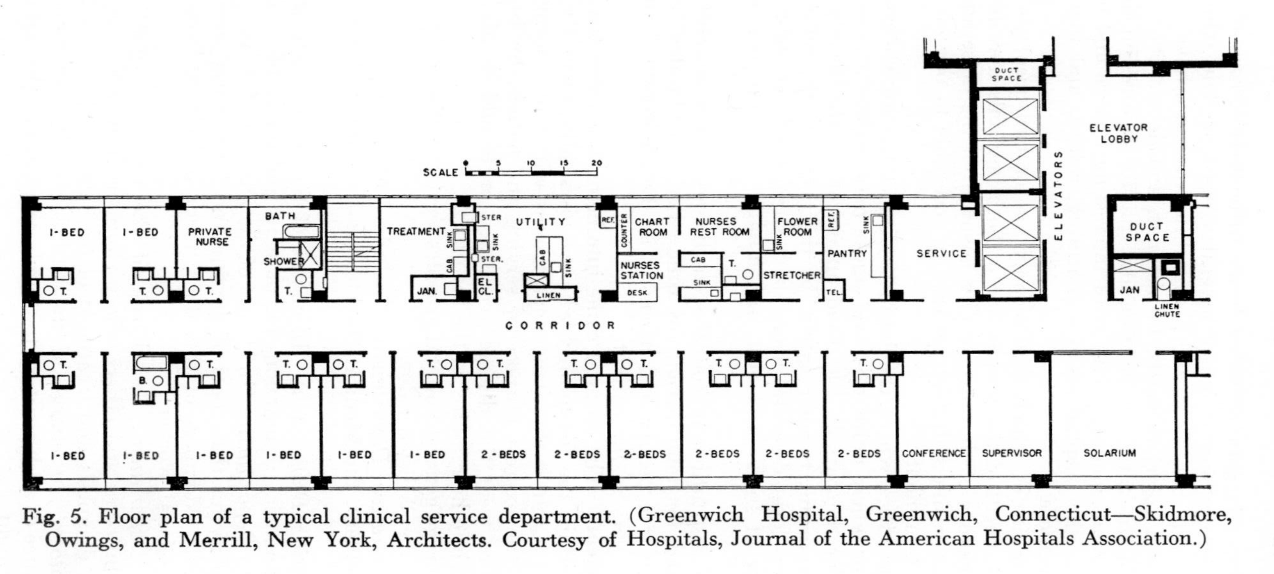

Fig. 5. Floor plan of a typical clinical service department. (Greenwich Hospital, Greenwich, Connecticut—Skidmore, Owings, and Merrill, New York, Architects. Courtesy of Hospitals, Journal of the American Hospitals Association.)

The hospital room of today bears little resemblance to the all-white, severely plain room of several years ago. The white walls, white curtains, bare floor, and plain white furniture, have given way to soft pastel colors in walls, furnishings, and decor. Cheerful floral drapes and slip covers, interesting and colorful pictures on the walls, and bedspreads made of cloth with interesting texture and attractive colors, give the hospital room a charming, restful, and more home-like atmosphere.

In communities which require only one or two hospitals to meet the health needs of the people, one or both hospitals may be located on the outskirts of the town or city, away from the noise and confusion of the business district yet readily accessible to persons needing care and treatment.

In large cities where the business district has grown around the hospital, or where noise, dirt, and smoke may become a source of discomfort for the patient, the disadvantage of an undesirable location can be overcome, to some extent, by the height of the building. Patient rooms located several floors above street level are comparatively quiet, free of smoke and dust, and usually well supplied with sunshine.

Mental institutions or convalescent homes, where patients may be hospitalized for long periods of time, should be located on ample grounds, where beauty and harmony in the environment may help insure recovery of the patient.

Departments. The hospital came into being to answer the needs of persons within the community who are physically, mentally, or spiritually ill. Each of the many departments within the hospital functions for the express purpose of serving the patient by helping to diagnose or treat the diseased condition or to add to his physical comfort while he remains in the institution.

The average general hospital provides services to the patient through the departments listed below:

Administrative Department. Includes the governing board, the Superintendent, the Medical Director, and administrative staff or assistants.

Accounting Department. In charge of the chief accountant; handles all financial transactions for patients and for employees.

Nursing Department. In charge of the Director of Nurses; assumes responsibility for the school of nursing and for nursing service given the patients. Members of this department include professional and non-professional workers.

X-Ray Department. In charge of the roentgenologist; includes x-ray technicians and others who perform services in the department to aid in diagnosis and treatment of patients.

Laboratory. In charge of the pathologist; its functions include performance of all laboratory tests and procedures needed for diagnosis and treatment.

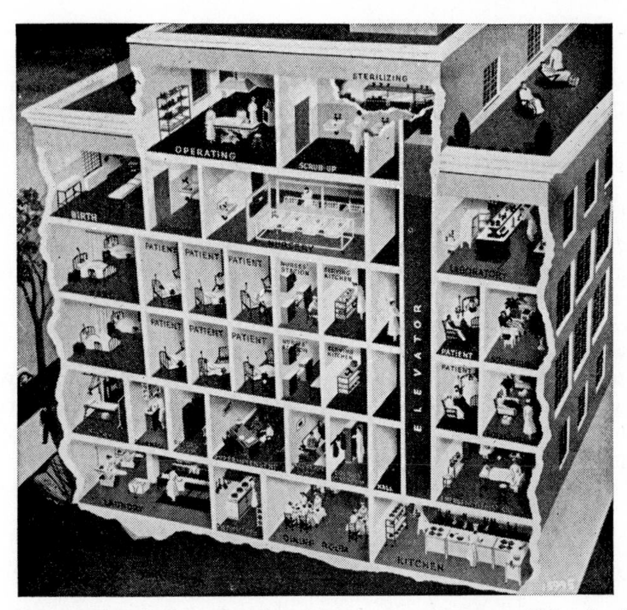

Fig. 6. Cross-sectional view showing various departments within the hospital. (Parke, Davis & Company, Detroit, Michigan.)

Dietary Department. Under supervision of the dietitian, who is responsible for buying, planning, preparing, and serving food and nourishment for the patients.

Housekeeping Department. In charge of the housekeeper who supervises the work of maids and janitors in keeping the hospital clean and neat.

Maintenance Department. Includes the carpenters, painters, electricians, and others who service the building and keep it and its furnishings in a state of good repair.

Laundry. In which all linen used in the hospital is washed and ironed. The sewing room is usually connected with this department, and torn linen is mended before being sent to the clinical departments for use.

Pharmacy. In charge of a registered pharmacist who supervises the filling of prescriptions and the supplying of medicine and of medicinal supplies to the clinical departments.

Stores Department. Where all supplies, including food, equipment, office supplies, etc. are received and dispensed to clinical departments as needed.

Out-Patient Department. Where patients are examined and treated without being admitted to the hospital.

Medical Records Department. Where all records pertaining to the patients are catalogued, filed, and made available for reference when needed.

Physiotherapy Department. This department gives treatments utilizing physical agents such as treatments by water bath, heat lamps, etc.

Occupational Therapy Department. Where various crafts or occupations are taught to the convalescent patient as a part of the program of rehabilitation.

Social Service Department. This department handles all cases requiring aid from agencies within the community which are organized to render such aid.

Central Supply Department. A centrally located department which furnishes needed equipment and supplies such as treatment trays, sterile solutions, and other articles to all clinical departments within the hospital. Oxygen equipment, orthopedic appliances, and rubber rings, hot water bottles, steam inhalators, etc. are also stored by Central Supply.

THE SCHOOL OF NURSING

Most schools of nursing are now owned and operated by general hospitals which provide the facilities for clinical practice.

After completing the basic course of study in nursing the student must meet standard requirements for nurses, set up by a Board of Nurse Examiners in each state, in order to become a professional or registered nurse.

For experience in special fields of nursing, such as communicable diseases, students are often sent on "affiliation" to hospitals which provide treatment and care only for that particular type of patient.

Administration. The educational director is in charge of the school of nursing and is directly responsible to the director of nurses. The number of instructors on the educational staff depends on the number of students in the school. The librarian for the school is also a member of the school faculty. Other members of the administrative or faculty group are the director of nurses, the counselor, the social director, the director of student health, and clinical instructors or supervisors.

Members of the medical staff of the hospital are not a part of the administrative body of the school, but are members of the faculty during the time they are lecturing to the student nurses. Lectures are usually given by doctors who are specialists in the particular subject.

General Requirements for Admission. Requirements for entrance to an accredited school of nursing may vary somewhat in different schools, although basically they will be much the same. Requirements as listed by most schools are:

The applicant must be a citizen of the United States or must have declared her intention of becoming a citizen.

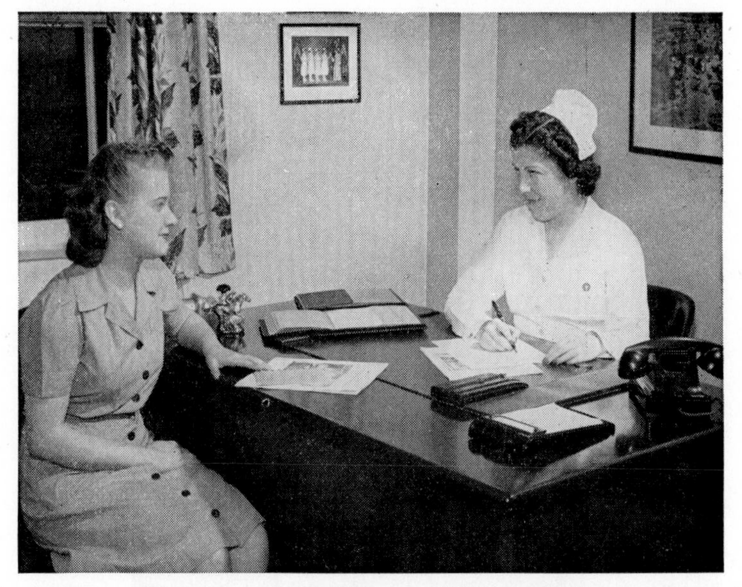

Fig. 7. A personal interview with the Director of Nurses. (Middletown Hospital School of Nursing, Middletown, Ohio.)

She must be between 17 and 30 years of age, and must be a graduate of an accredited high school, with a scholastic record which satisfies the requirements of the nursing school to which she applies.

She must be free of outside obligations during the entire course of study.

She must be in good health and able to pass a physical examination. Her hands must be free of eczema and other forms of dermatitis.

She must be able to furnish satisfactory references as to character, grooming, and sincerity of purpose, and must successfully conclude a personal interview with the director of nurses or the director of admissions.

Student Health Service. Although before acceptance the applicant to a school of nursing must submit satisfactory medical and dental records and be successfully immunized against smallpox and typhoid fever, during the first week she is enrolled she must pass a rigid physical examination conducted by members of the medical staff in charge of student health and by nursing personnel of the student health service.

Students are encouraged to report all minor illnesses to the student health department and are admitted to the infirmary for required bed rest or medical treatment.

The student health service is responsible for carrying out annual

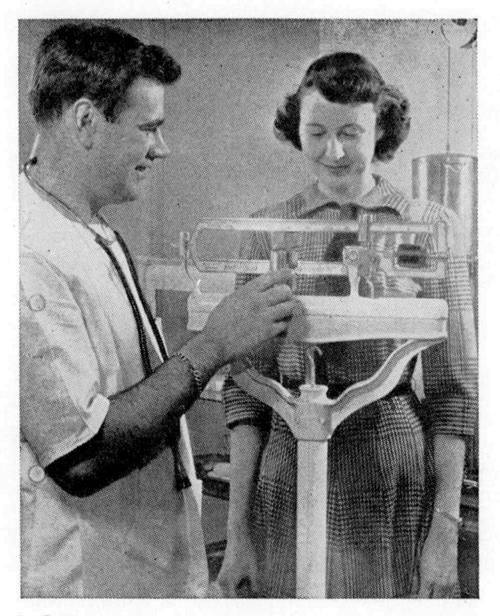

Fig. 8. The Student Health Service personnel are interested in the health of each student nurse. (Harper Hospital School of Nursing, Detroit, Michigan.)

physical examinations for all students and graduate nurses on the staff and for the immunization program required of all students going to other hospitals for classwork and clinical practice in special fields, such as communicable diseases.

Curriculum. The present tendency is for schools of nursing to become affiliated with colleges and universities, thus raising the academic requirements for admission. There is a definite trend, too, toward centralized programs of instruction, especially in the smaller schools.

The length of the basic nursing course is three years, and students are classified as to class membership as follows:

First six months	Preclinical student
Second six months	Freshman student
Second year	Junior student
Third year	Senior student

The first six months, or preclinical period of nursing, is considered a trial period for the student, during which she is given opportunity to decide definitely on continuing in the nursing program. This period also gives hospital authorities ample time to evaluate her achievement in theory and practice and to judge her qualifications for membership in the nursing profession.

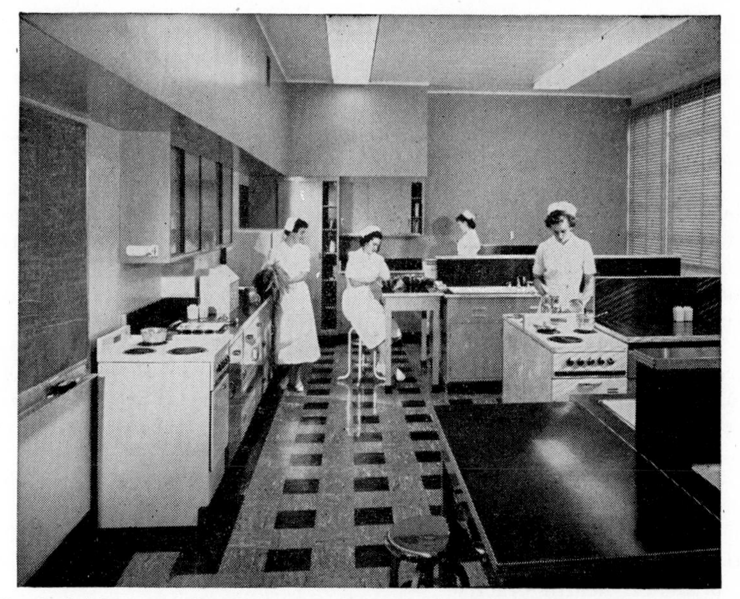

Fig. 9. A laboratory for the study of foods and nutrition. (St. Vincent's College of Nursing, Los Angeles, California.)

Although schools of nursing differ widely in patterns of basic nursing education, the fundamental principles found in various subjects contained in the curriculum presented show marked similarity in all schools. The main divisions of the basic nursing educational program are: (1) biological and physical sciences; (2) social sciences; (3) medical sciences; and (4) courses related to nursing care.

Biological and Physical Sciences. In the study of anatomy and physiology the nurse gains an understanding of the structure and function of the various parts of the human body. This knowledge enables her to safeguard her own health and that of others and to recognize the abnormalities which characterize disease.

Through knowledge gained in the study of chemistry the nurse reaches a better understanding of body processes such as digestion and the mechanical aspects of respiration, an understanding that is very necessary in the performance of procedures which make up the daily routine of nursing service.

In studying foods and nutrition the nurse learns why certain food elements are essential in the diet, and she is able to teach patients and their families, in an effectual manner, the importance of proper food habits in attaining and keeping good health.

Through such studies as microbiology and pathology the student nurse develops an understanding of how disease organisms are transferred and how such transference may be prevented. Without this knowledge she would be less able to protect herself, or to help her patients gain protection from communicable diseases.

Social Sciences. The subject matter contained in social sciences concerns the study of human behavior and includes all aspects of individual, family, and group relationships.

Through the study of psychology the student develops a better understanding of herself and of her patient. Making her own adjustments and modifying her own reactions will help her to a better understanding of the patient who is dependent on her for help in making the necessary adjustment to illness which can greatly facilitate his return to a normal state of health.

Tolerance and sympathy, although desirable attributes in any one, are essential to successful nursing. The study of psychology helps the student to understand motives underlying the patient's behavior and makes it easy for her to refrain from censuring a difficult patient or one with marked personality conflicts.

Sociology reveals many patterns of group behavior and forms the basis for recognition of cultural traits in patients and their families. Because she deals with people of all classes, races, and creeds, the nurse should learn to relate cultural behavior patterns and physical and mental health practices.

The nurse who would work well with other professional groups to achieve "worth-while social ends" must know and understand all the known agencies and available facilities in the community which will help to preserve and protect the individual or the family group.

A study of the history of nursing portrays the part played by the nurse in the past and should develop an appreciation of the attitudes and responsibilities which characterize nursing as a profession. By realization of the accomplishments of nursing in the past the student may be prompted to help promote needed reforms in the present and the future. Nursing history, by emphasizing the progress made in recent years, contributes to the preparation of the nurse by creating the desire for further progress through high standards of personal and professional conduct.

Medical Sciences. This group deals with the cause, signs and symptoms, prevention, treatment, and probable results of disease. The nurse is not expected to have a thorough knowledge of the science of medicine, but she should be able to recognize symptoms of disease and be familiar with accepted remedial measures or treatment.

After learning the general principles of medical science and general means of prevention and treatment, the student is ready to begin the study of specific conditions and to be instructed in the prevention, treatment, and nursing care of diseases such as tuberculosis and diabetes.

In medical sciences, too, the student learns of various community health agencies and comes to understand the importance of cooper-

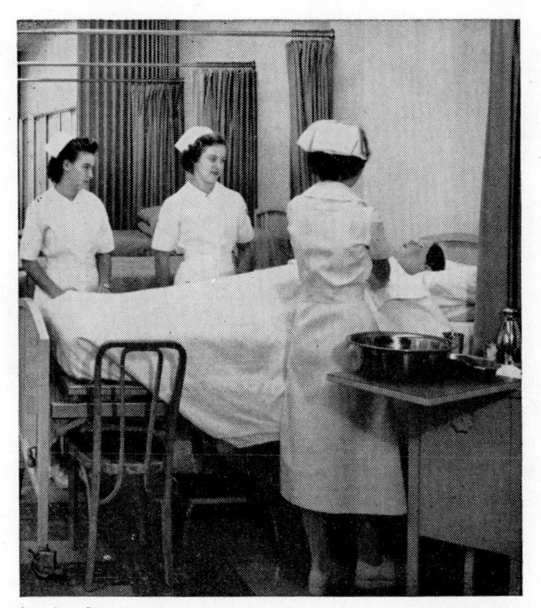

Fig. 10. Practice in the nursing arts classroom insures skillful clinical performance in the hospital. (St. Vincent's College of Nursing, Los Angeles, California.)

ating with other professional workers in behalf of the patient. Illness, to the observant nurse, may appear now as the *result* of social forces such as poverty, ignorance, malnutrition, and undesirable environment, and at the same time she is able to realize that illness can be the principal *cause* of social problems and individual maladjustment.

If the student understands that she is to play an important part in medical research she not only will be more interested in nursing but will be conscious of the need for accurate recording of observations and of the importance of giving proper assistance in improving methods of diagnosis and treatment. In many ways the nurse helps to build up the vast amount of data from which "medical discoveries" are made, and this aspect of her work should offer incentive for better cooperation with members of the medical profession.

Courses Related to Nursing Care. In the nursing arts courses the student learns to apply the knowledge of the sciences gained through studies mentioned above. She learns to recognize the nursing needs of the patient and to develop skill, through practice, in various procedures designed to answer those needs.

Usually the student is assigned to give routine daily care, such as baths and the serving of diets, to patients who are convalescent or only slightly ill. Working under the supervision of a competent graduate nurse she gradually is able to assume more responsibility and

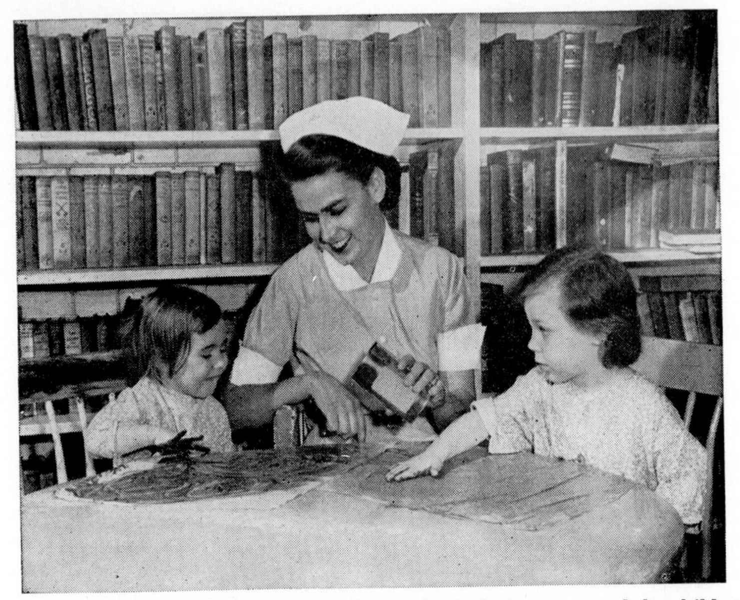

Fig. 11. The pediatric department can be fun for both the nurse and the children. (Johns Hopkins Hospital School of Nursing, Baltimore, Maryland.)

perform more complicated nursing procedures for the seriously ill patient or the patient with social problems of increasing complexity.

Through her work and study of medical-surgical patients, the nurse becomes experienced in caring for a large variety of injuries and functional disorders. In the special departments, such as the diet kitchen and operating room, she works under the direction of persons with advanced education and experience in these particular fields.

Continuing her progress in nursing arts courses the student spends several months in the obstetrical department, where she learns to care for the mother during labor and delivery and to give adequate postpartum nursing service. She is assigned to the nursery to learn to care for the newborn. In the obstetrical department the nurse finds ample opportunity to put into practice all she has learned in regard to a health teaching program. The young mother is not ill and is eager to learn health factors that will enable her to keep her baby in excellent physical condition.

In the pediatric department the nurse learns to care for well children as well as those who are ill. She must be able to distinguish normal from abnormal growth and development in children. She must be able to guide the parents in methods of health care for children and she must study and work with children until she is able to successfully interest, entertain, comfort, and teach them in a constructive and desirable manner.

Experience in psychiatric nursing enables the student to recognize and deal intelligently with behavior abnormalities in patients. Few illnesses are free from an accompanying abnormal mental behavior. Patients are all too often extremely depressed, irritable, critical, suspicious, apprehensive, or even hysterical, and the nurse must provide care that is adapted to the condition of the mind as well as to the physical condition.

In treatment of mental patients great emphasis is placed on occupational therapy and various forms of psychotherapy. The student who is really interested in helping the patient soon learns how to use effectively such therapeutic agents as games, handicraft, and other forms of recreational activities. Considerable attention is given to good hygiene and good health habits, too, since patients frequently recover with no other treatment than that of instituting healthful living conditions as a means of combating an injurious mental state.

To be adequately prepared for the duties of professional nursing, the nurse today must have a thorough knowledge of basic sciences related to her field. She must possess skilled technique in performing nursing duties, she must qualify as a teacher and be able to help in social work which serves to meet the health needs of individuals, families, and communities.

The Student's Orientation to Nursing. Even though today a large number of nursing schools have an orientation period of several days after enrollment, the adjustment to hospital environment and to nursing can still be an unpleasant ordeal for the girl who is beginning a new life in an atmosphere which is usually completely new to her.

The Big Sister. The practice of appointing *Big Sisters* among the Junior students in the school has been beneficial in helping the new student, or *Little Sister*, to more readily adjust to the nursing situation and to the nursing group.

If the beginning student has only a vague idea as to what will be required of her as a nurse, the Big Sister may smooth the path for her by explaining much that is new and, at times, rather frightening.

The Big Sister should discuss the regulations which govern student activity within the residence and student conduct within the hospital. She should explain that such regulations are a necessary part of every well organized school of nursing. The young student who accepts the regulations and understands the necessity for them will have already begun the process of making a satisfactory adjustment and will find it is not difficult to live harmoniously with other residents in the nurses' home.

Some factors which should be brought to the attention of the beginning student are:

The Class Schedule. The schedule of classes for the preclinical nursing student is usually more extensive than that of a high school

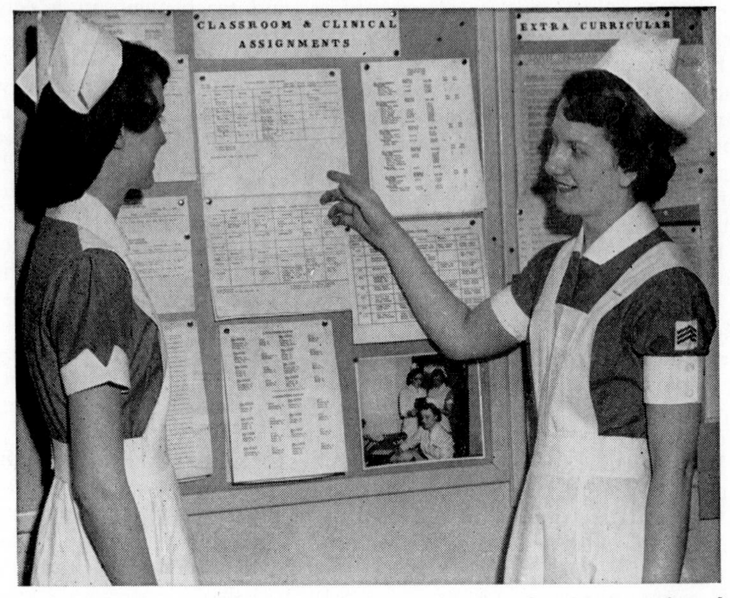

Fig. 12. The new student learns of classroom and clinical assignments from her Big Sister. (Miami Valley Hospital School of Nursing, Dayton, Ohio.)

student or of the freshman student in college. It is not uncommon for nursing students to carry six hours of classwork each day. Classes consist of the basic science courses, including anatomy, physiology, microbiology, and chemistry, as well as the courses related to actual patient care, as nursing arts and professional adjustments. The nursing arts course introduces the student to fundamental procedures she must learn to perform skilfully in giving nursing care to the patient.

In a school of nursing, the student is not permitted to be tardy or absent from class and lessons must always be prepared. Failing grades invariably lead to dismissal, for a careless or poorly informed nurse may make a mistake which can endanger the life of a patient. Students are closely supervised and are severely censured for indifference or carelessness. Their work is too closely related to the welfare of the patient to permit haphazard learning or only partial understanding of theoretical and practical instruction.

Daily Routine. The student in nursing, who is just beginning her course of study, will find most of her time for each day planned for her. She is "on schedule" from the time she wakens at 6 A.M. until she retires with "lights out" at approximately 11 P.M. She is expected to be up by 6 o'clock in the morning, to attend chapel services at 6:30, to eat breakfast at 6:40, and be ready to report for duty or for class at 7 o'clock. She must be punctual in reporting for class and for duty, or be held responsible for disrupting routine for her classmates and co-workers. She eats her meals at a scheduled time, observes quiet hours for study at certain scheduled times, and is assigned to duty at a designated time and place. To conform to residence regulations she may even find that the daily bath must be taken at a specified time. She will soon see that in order to live harmoniously with the other students the planned schedule for daily routine is necessary during the orientation program and for the entire time spent in the school.

Factors in Adjustment. The student of nursing will adjust more easily to her new environment if she takes into account various other factors which bear a direct relationship to her success or failure as a member of the nursing group.

Personal Appearance. Whether the nurse is endowed with beauty or outstanding good looks has little bearing on her appearance in uniform. The attractiveness of the nurse is a composite of many factors, and beauty of face or figure is of minor consideration. Good grooming, a pleasing manner, and a friendly disposition may readily compensate for any irregularity of features. Any young woman of average weight who wears the uniform of a nurse may answer all the requirements of good personal appearance by observing the following suggestions:

Make certain that white duty shoes are really white. Shoes should be shined at least once daily, shoelaces should be washed each evening, and the shoes should be kept in good condition. Run-over heels detract from appearance regardless of how clean and neat the shoes may be.

Always wear white duty hose that are clean, free from runs, and show no evidence of having been darned or mended even if such is the case. Seams should be straight and the hose should be held firmly in place by supporters of a girdle or garter belt. Even though uniforms are of a length which permits them to hang well below the knees and rolled stockings would not easily be detected, the use of circular garters is not advisable from the standpoint of health.

All underclothing should be spotlessly clean and in good state of repair. Slips are easily seen through the material of some uniforms and should be well fitting, not excessively decorated with lace or embroidery (a tailored slip is more in keeping with the tailored appearance of the uniform), and the length of the slip should correspond with the length of the uniform. Nothing detracts more from a nurse's appearance than a slip showing below the hem of the uniform.

A girdle or foundation garment should be worn if weight exceeds by even a few pounds the normal weight for a person of the same age and height. A brassiere which fits well and offers the needed support should be worn, especially if there is a tendency toward being what is adequately described as "buxom." Lingerie worn by the nurse should always be white, since colored materials, even of pastel shades, usu-

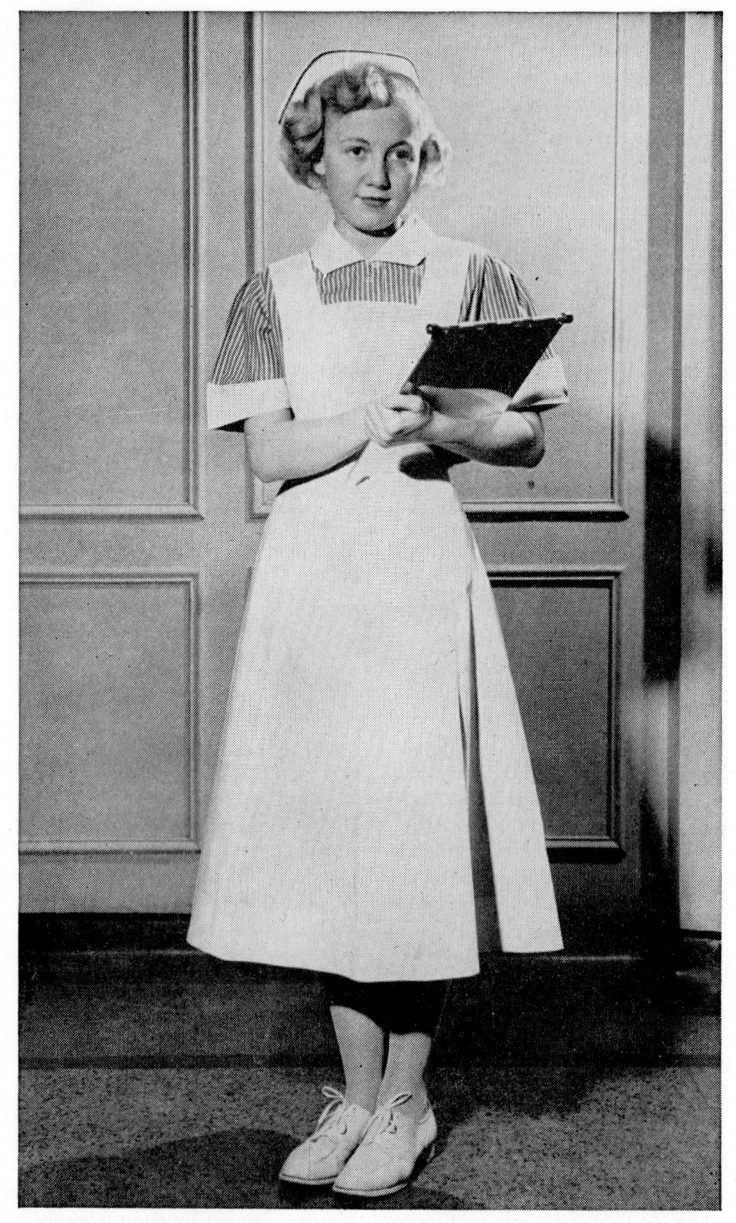

Fig. 13. Personal appearance is a determining factor in success in nursing. (Grant Hospital School of Nursing, Chicago, Illinois.)

ally show as darker areas under the uniform and give it a dingy or unclean appearance.

The uniform should be clean, well made, of perfect fit, and of the length currently considered correct. Torn uniforms should be mended provided they are in good condition except for the tear. If the mended areas are to be plainly visible, the uniform should be replaced with a new one. The cap should be clean, folded correctly, and worn in the manner prescribed by school regulations.

To make certain of an attractive appearance during working hours the nurse, whether student or graduate, should wear her hair in a neat arrangement which prevents it from falling below the collar of the uniform. Her skin should be clear and impressively clean. Only a conservative amount of make-up should be worn.

Jewelry, except for wedding ring and school pin, should not be worn with the uniform. Such practices as gum chewing, loud, boisterous talking, lounging in undignified positions, smoking just before reporting for duty, and gossiping about patients or hospital personnel should be assiduously avoided.

Teeth should be given proper care through systematic, daily brushing and by routine visits to the dentist at least twice each year. Hands should be carefully manicured; if nail polish is worn it should be modest in color and impeccable in condition. Chipped or carelessly applied nail polish will detract from the personal appearance of any young woman.

When in uniform nurses should not use perfume. Although pleasing at times to persons in good health, perfume may be quite distressing to a patient. People who are ill tend to be unduly sensitive to odors, and a heavy perfume may be just as obnoxious to them as the odor of an antiseptic or disinfectant. Use of a good deodorant and talcum powder or cologne will better meet the needs of the nurse who is desirous of pleasing the patients assigned to her care.

No discussion of the wearing of the uniform is complete without the admonition that all nurses should refrain from wearing the white "on duty" uniform on public streets or in public conveyances. The nurse who wears the uniform to the shopping district of her town or city, who appears in it at the bank or postoffice or on street cars and busses is careless indeed of the impression she may make on the numerous persons with whom she comes in contact.

The original purpose of wearing a white uniform in caring for the sick was to provide the cleanest possible dress, the one least likely to carry germs or to be contaminated. The patient, whose resistance is already lowered by the disease for which he is hospitalized, needs to be protected from all possible sources of further contamination by pathogenic microorganisms. The nurse who wears the "on duty" uniform to public places does a great injustice to each patient to whom she gives nursing care.

Factors such as conduct, behavior, and manners are discussed in

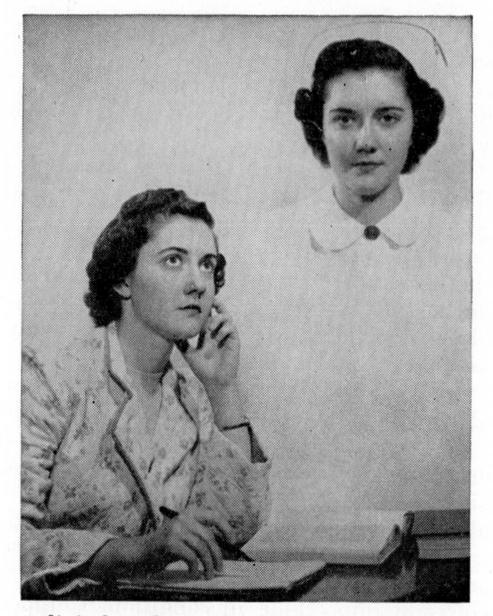

Fig. 14. The preclinical student nurse of today will be the graduate professional nurse of tomorrow. (Fresno General Hospital School of Nursing, Fresno, California.)

detail in a later chapter. The student, however, may be reminded here that she should remember to practice all the approved techniques of social usage to attain a happy and satisfactory social relationship with patients, students, and other hospital personnel.

Care of Property. In the nurses' residence the care of "common facilities" such as the kitchenette, bathroom, and lounges should be part of each student's responsibility to the other members of her group. She should not be extravagant or careless in the use of hospital supplies and equipment. She should be especially careful in handling property belonging to the patient (false teeth, spectacles and other personal articles broken or lost can be replaced only with difficulty and at great expense). She should respect the possessions of other students with whom she shares living quarters in the residence.

Recreation. With a heavy class schedule and long hours on duty the student in nursing has little time for recreation, yet she should plan so that she takes part in some recreational activity each day. By becoming interested in a hobby, a collection, or some other form of activity not associated with nursing she finds a means of renewing strength and enthusiasm for her nursing duties.

Religion. Nursing had its beginning in religious institutions and organizations. The student in nursing will be called on to minister to the needs of patients of many different religious beliefs and she will need to bear in mind that each of the various forms of religion contributed, to some extent, to the whole of religious knowledge. She should not attempt to impose her own religion upon a patient, but should encourage and inspire confidence in any faith the patient may profess to follow. Her own religious belief will help her to adjust to the new environment in which she finds herself.

By satisfactory adjustment to nursing and by successfully meeting the requirements in theory and practice for graduation from her chosen school, the preclinical student nurse of today becomes the graduate professional nurse of tomorrow.

Summary of Important Factors

Nursing is that service which helps an individual to regain or keep a normal state of body and mind, or helps him gain relief from physical pain, mental anxiety, and/or spiritual discomfort.

The professional nurse is one who has graduated from an accredited school of nursing, has met requirements for registration, and is permitted to work at nursing in the state in which the school is located and in other states in which reciprocity has been established.

The spirit of nursing has existed since the beginning of time.

Florence Nightingale was the founder of modern nursing.

The first schools of nursing in the United States were established in 1873.

The American Nurses' Association was formed in 1911.

Although the responsibilities and opportunities in nursing are constantly changing and expanding, the spirit of nursing remains the same.

Hospitals have developed to meet the health needs of the community in which they are located.

The chief functions of a hospital are to provide care for the sick and injured, prevent disease, promote health, provide for the education of doctors, nurses, and other personnel, and promote research in medicine and nursing.

Schools of nursing are usually owned and operated by general hospitals.

The curriculum in a school of nursing includes biological and physical sciences, social sciences, medical sciences, and courses related to nursing care of the patient.

The orientation program is designed to help the beginning student nurse to adjust to her new environment.

Effective study methods are necessary to the success of the nursing student.

Factors pertinent to satisfactory adjustment to nursing include appearance, conduct, manners, consideration for others, and establishment of good personal relationships.

Good grooming, a friendly manner, and pleasing disposition are necessary for an attractive personal appearance.

The uniform, shoes, hose, shoelaces, and cap should always be neat and clean.

A proper girdle and brassiere should be worn with the uniform.

The wedding band and school pin are the only pieces of jewelry that may be worn with the uniform.

Hands of the nurse should be carefully manicured. Chipped nail polish should not be worn.

Strong perfume, body odor, or the odor of cigarette smoke clinging to the uniform of the nurse may be very unpleasant for the patient.

The "on duty" uniform should not be worn in public places or on public conveyances.

Suggested Reference Reading

"The future of the registered nurse," Lucille Petry; Nursing World, January, 1952.

"Lipstick for that touch of color," Veronica L. Conley; Today's Health, February, 1952.

"Meeting the student's emotional needs," Dorothy Mereness; American Journal of Nursing, March, 1952.

"Nursing is nice work," J. P. Richardson; Modern Hospital, September, 1952.

"I was a nurse," F. Rich; Davis Nursing Survey, October, 1952.

"Acne needn't get you down," Jane P. Kirkpatrick; Today's Health, November, 1952.

"Why be fat?" Herbert Pollack; American Journal of Nursing, December, 1952.

CHAPTER 2

Effective Study Methods

TOPICAL OUTLINE

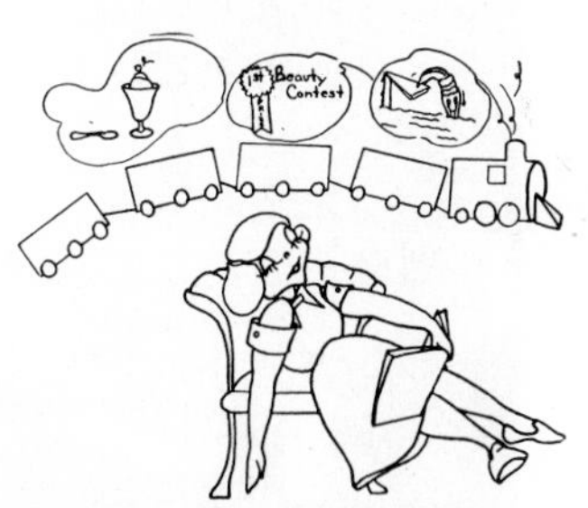

Many a train of thought is just a string of empties.

Good study habits may mean the difference between a student's being accepted as a member of the freshman class at the completion of the preclinical period or being asked to withdraw from the school. For that reason alone instruction in effective methods of study should be a basic part of the orientation of the student to the school of nursing.

WHY STUDY?

The student nurse, to develop good study habits and make use of suggested successful methods of study, will need to understand the important part study will play in the task she has undertaken. Without long periods of time spent in studying and without a knowledge of how to study effectively, she may be handicapped throughout the entire period of her stay in the school.

Good methods of study will help her to satisfactorily meet scholastic requirements, to take meaningful notes in lecture classes, to learn the complicated medical terminology which she must know, and to advance in her chosen work to the status of the graduate, registered nurse. Without making proper use of the basic requirements for study

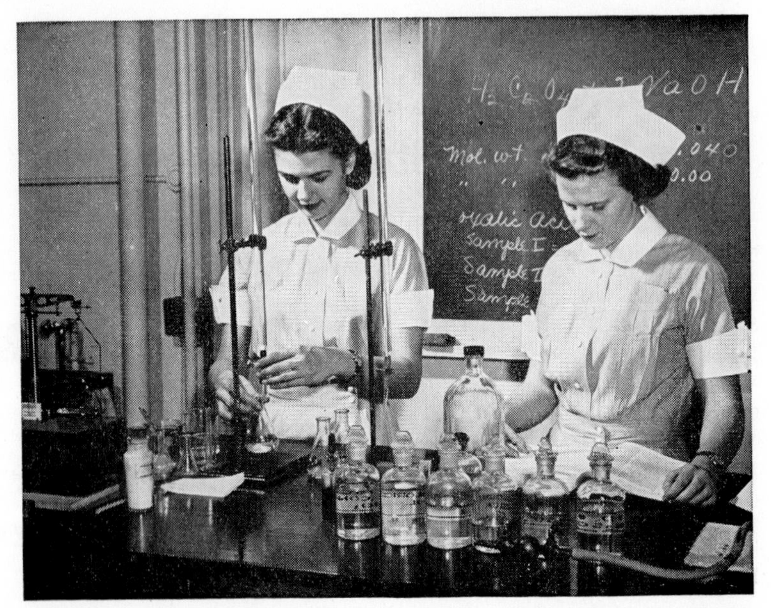

Fig. 15. The student must have the incentive and the will to study. (Johns Hopkins Hospital School of Nursing, Baltimore, Maryland.)

she will fail to understand the relationship between what she learns in the classroom and the work she will do in the hospital.

In a number of ways the administration of the school may help to promote good study habits among the students. Privacy in the nurses' residence where each student is provided her own room furnishes an important inducement to study. Adequate lighting, good ventilation, provision for quiet hours, and sufficient, up-to-date reference books in the library are some of the major considerations which are the responsibility of the school.

The student herself must have the incentive and the will to study. She must put forth the effort needed to develop the kind of study habits that will be of benefit to her. She must recognize that through study she may acquire the knowledge and skill necessary for her to achieve her aim of becoming a well qualified, registered nurse.

Appropriate answers to the question "Why Study?" include the following:

Most failures among preclinical students are due to ineffectual study methods and lack of application rather than to the student's inability to master the subject material of the nursing curriculum.

When lessons are well prepared the student will enjoy attending classes. If she goes to class without having studied the lesson the class hour will be one of uncomfortable awareness of lack of preparation and hope that the instructor will not give a quiz or call on her to recite.

To be a successful co-worker to the doctor, to understand and intelligently care for patients, and to benefit from her experiences in various departments in the hospital, the student will need to devote much of her time to study.

Another answer to "Why Study?" is for the student nurse to be able to pass state board examinations successfully and meet requirements for registration in the state in which she plans to work.

Well planned and meaningful study during the preclinical period will insure a good theoretical background for advanced courses in nursing. Successful mastery of the basic nursing program prepares the student for study in the field of her special interest and helps her benefit to the fullest extent by a postgraduate course or by advanced work in education.

Effective study methods and time spent in studying help the student achieve a high scholastic rating. The record made while the student is in school is used by future employers in judging the nurse's qualifications for a position that might be open to her.

It is advantageous to receive a certificate in nursing from a school with a recognized standing in medical and nursing fields. The high scholastic standard of any school of nursing can be maintained only through the combined efforts of students, faculty, and administrative personnel of the institution.

SPELLING

Although there seems to be little or no emphasis on spelling in the curriculum of the high schools, the student of nursing will find that she must know how to spell correctly not only words in general usage but technical terms as well.

For the student who knows that her spelling is limited the following suggestions may be helpful:

When a misspelled word is brought to your attention, look it up, learn to pronounce it correctly and to spell it.

When learning new words write them several times, being sure to spell them correctly.

Memorize spelling rules and use them when needed. One spelling rule that is helpful and can easily be remembered is: "*i* before *e* except after *c* (for example, conceit, deceive, ceiling), or when sounded like *a* as in neighbor and weigh."

Some words are spelled without logic and no rules seem to apply. Such words necessitate memory work. Facts to be memorized for correct spelling include: only one word ends in "-sede" (supersede); three words end in "-ceed" (exceed, proceed, succeed); others end in "-cede" (accede, recede, secede, etc.).

Faulty pronunciation may lead to misspelling. A few of the many words commonly misspelled because they are incorrectly pronounced are: athlete, arctic, government, interesting, laboratory, optimistic, perspiration, temperament.

Words that have a similar sound when pronounced yet differ in meaning may often be misspelled. Such words include: accent (to stress), ascent (climbing), affect (to influence), effect (to bring about), council (a group), counsel (advice), stationary (not movable), stationery (writing materials).

To improve spelling and to avoid embarrassing mistakes the student should have available for use a collegiate or standard dictionary which can be consulted whenever there is doubt about the spelling of a word.

One of the chief reasons for requiring a student nurse to spell correctly is the fact that she is responsible for notations on the patients' chart and all such notations should be meaningful, printed legibly and made up of words correctly spelled. The dictionaries in ward libraries will be helpful to the student who needs to check the spelling of certain words before recording on the charts.

To improve spelling of technical terms the student should practice spelling the word correctly as she learns the meaning of it and it is added to her increasing vocabulary of medical and nursing terms. A special effort should be made to memorize the correct spelling of words which are commonly misspelled.

Reading. One of the most important factors in determining success for a student is reading ability. Success in scholastic achievement may well determine the student's further educational development and influence the kind of life she will have.

Reading is important to school success, to job success, and to success in personal relationships. The more the student reads, the more information she will possess, and the more interesting she becomes as a person. She will also be better able to converse with patients of widely different backgrounds and interests. She will gain satisfaction through reading for recreation, and will discover the whole new world of varied and interesting experiences which awaits the person who learns to read well and to read for pleasure.

When reading ability has not been developed and the student reads slowly and with difficulty, there is no pleasure in it and she will tend to avoid reading the assigned lessons of the various nursing courses.

To evaluate her own reading ability, the student should know some of the faults in reading and should recognize them as they apply to herself. The most common faults in reading include:

(1) Word by word reading—the type of reading which is slow and laborious because the number of fixations made by the eye is excessive.

(2) Inadequate vocabulary—when much of the terminology in the textbook is unfamiliar to the student a great deal of time must be spent looking up words in the dictionary.

(3) Limited comprehension—lack of concentration, limited vocabu-

lary, and failure to recognize the important concept presented in the text all contribute to lack of understanding of material being read.

(4) Inability to read graphs or tables—the student who fails to understand the significance of graphs or tables and pays little or no attention to those included in the text contributes to her own deficiency in reading ability.

To read effectively it is necessary to read at a fairly rapid rate and with a high degree of comprehension. Reading rate should be adjusted according to the difficulty of the material being read. A simple article being read for pleasure may be read very rapidly, whereas an assigned lesson of technical material will probably require slower and more thorough reading.

The rate of reading depends on the number of fixations made by the eye as it travels across the page. The reader who reads word by word will read slowly because the eye fixates at each word and stops at very frequent intervals. The fast reader will read in phrases, with the eye making only a few stops as the sentence is being read.

Practice reading, if carried out in the correct manner, will increase reading rate and improve reading comprehension. The student should attempt to read rapidly while trying to remember or to get as much as possible from the material being read. Magazine articles, chosen so that they treat of progressively more difficult or complex subjects, provide excellent material for reading practice. The student who begins practice reading in an effort to improve reading ability should understand that only consistent practice will be of benefit. A schedule of time for such practice will need to be made and continued for several months if reading skill is to be developed and maintained.

Some faulty habits of reading which tend to slow reading rate and therefore should be avoided are: lip reading (making the same lip movements that would be made in reading aloud); whispering (pronouncing each word in a whisper while reading); and pointing with the finger (using the finger as a guide to point out each word as it is being read).

Correction of one or of all of such faulty habits will be necessary if rate of reading is to be increased.

Comprehension is defined as the power of understanding. Reading with comprehension is reading with definite understanding. Reading of lesson assignments must be reading with comprehension if the student is to benefit. The student who has learned to read correctly will be able to prepare lessons in a much shorter time than will the student who must read an assignment several times before beginning to understand the material being read.

To improve reading comprehension the following suggestions should be followed:

Improve vocabulary—Failure to recognize the meaning of a word may prevent understanding of an entire sentence or paragraph.

Recognize the basic concept (important point) in material being read—The person who reads with understanding soon is able to recognize the most important idea or thought of the material and learns to differentiate between it and that which is written as further explanation and merely to emphasize the main point.

Know when to scan and when to study—Material that is relatively unimportant can be read quite rapidly; that which must be learned will require more careful reading.

Read more—The slow or faulty reader is usually a person who reads very little; to improve reading habits more practice in reading will be necessary.

It has been estimated that 20 to 25 per cent of students attending colleges or universities are reading at or below seventh grade level. There are many causes of reading difficulties, some of the most common being:

Emotional problems—A student who is emotionally upset will find it impossible to read with comprehension since her mind is occupied with the problem or situation causing the emotional reaction.

Poor teaching—Students who were given inadequate instruction in methods of reading and who were permitted to "skip" words they could not pronounce or define usually fail to develop any appreciable skill in reading.

Inadequate teaching materials—Students who were deprived of suitable reading materials may have major reading difficulties.

Physical factors—Students who have impairment of vision or are handicapped by ill health are apt to show the effect of such physical abnormalities in their methods of reading and in other activities related to classroom work.

Lack of mental ability—Persons having a low I.Q. usually read with difficulty and with little comprehension.

Lack of interest—Persons who dislike reading will have little interest in reading well, and because they do not read well their dislike for reading tends to be increased.

If reading ability, in rate and comprehension, is to be improved, a systematic program must be designed to correct reading faults and be continued over a long period of time. Sporadic attempts at improved reading practices will be ineffectual, and any improvement thus gained will be only temporary.

A good or efficient reader displays the following characteristics: (1) a constant and consistent increase in vocabulary; (2) the habit of reading in phrases rather than in words; (3) the desire to read a wide variety of printed materials; (4) the ability to adjust the rate of reading to material being read; (5) a knowledge of how to use the library; (6) an enjoyment of reading.

Many reading tests which will determine the student's reading rate and comprehension are available. Most students in schools of nursing should read at the rate of approximately 300 to 350 words per minute. A reading rate below 275 words per minute indicates the need for im-

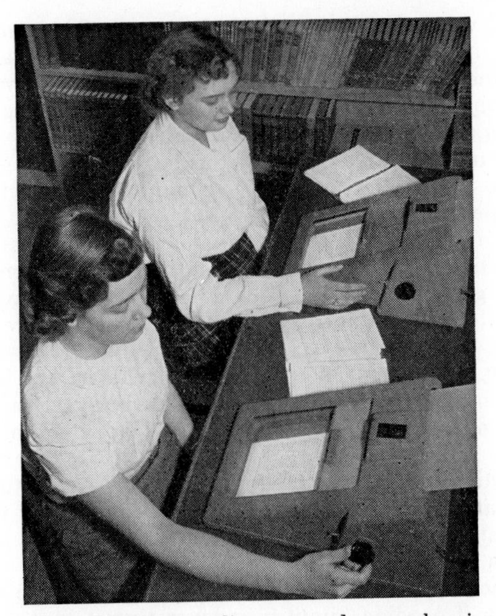

Fig. 16. Students can improve reading rate and comprehension through use of the reading accelerator. (Milwaukee Institute of Technology, Milwaukee, Wisconsin.)

proved reading ability. Practice reading, reading exercises, or the use of the reading accelerator may be helpful in enabling the student to read faster and better.

VOCABULARY

Reading skill depends to a great extent on vocabulary. So long as the reader encounters familiar words he is able to read rapidly and understand without difficulty what he is reading. When he is reading material that contains a large number of unfamiliar words he is forced to read slowly and to re-read whole sentences, and is somewhat confused as to the meaning of the material.

The student nurse will need two types of vocabulary: a general vocabulary—the words used in newspapers, books, and magazines dealing with items of general information, current events, or experiences of other persons, and a technical vocabulary, made up of medical and nursing terms and of technical terms in related fields, such as science and mathematics.

Vocabulary is very closely related to intelligence. The scores made on vocabulary tests show a high correlation with scores made on intelligence tests.

In nursing, vocabulary is especially important. The general vocabulary is made up of words that serve as keys for thoughts, and the more such words the nurse can command the better able she will be to express her thoughts. The technical vocabulary, pertaining to nursing, is essential to the student nurse for several reasons:

The nurse needs to understand medical and nursing terms in order to understand medical lectures and to comprehend subject material in the nursing textbooks.

The nurse needs to know the terminology of her profession in order to speak effectively and in a manner befitting her position.

Finally, a good vocabulary, general and technical, will help the nurse to build self confidence and to become a more interesting person.

To Improve Vocabulary. Both types of vocabulary can be developed or improved by systematic effort. The following suggestions, carried out as a part of improving methods of study, will help to improve vocabulary:

(1) In reading lesson assignments for all courses, the student should list words that are not familiar to her. She should then try to determine the meaning of the word by the way it is used, and then look up the word in a dictionary.*

(2) She should choose the definition which applies to the word as it is used and, if possible, simplify it by stating it in her own words. A simplified definition is much easier to remember than one which is highly complex or made up of unfamiliar terms.

(3) She should learn correct pronunciation and definition for terms commonly used in nursing. The student of nursing will find unfamiliar terms that she will need to learn appearing frequently in several different courses of study. The various courses of nursing have been integrated with related courses so that terminology for one may closely approximate that of another. If vocabulary work is part of the required study for each course it will help the student to observe the close relation that exists between courses.

(4) New words should be put into use after their meaning has been learned. By using them in conversation, in class discussion, and in written work for class new words soon become part of the student's total vocabulary. Through use, too, the words are learned so pronunciation is accurate when the word is spoken and spelling is accurate when the word is written.

The use of technical and medical terms indicates to members of the medical and nursing professions that the student now belongs to her own professional group. In illustration, one need only remind the reader that when the student begins work in the school of nursing she rapidly discards common phrases or terms which characterize the un-

* Simplified definitions of terms necessary to nursing have been compiled in "The American Nurses Dictionary" (A. L. Price, W. B. Saunders Co., 1949).

professional or lay person. She substitutes medical terms for common words or phrases which, up to the time of her entrance into the school, were accepted by her without question.

After being in the school only a short time she may return home to find that it sounds rather queer to hear a member of the family speak of Aunt Ruth having "cramps" or of Johnny being given a typhoid "shot," or say that baby Anne "threw up" her feeding. The student nurse has learned to speak of "dysmenorrhea" and "typhoid injections," and of "vomiting." She hears the technical terms used at school, finds them used in the textbooks, and has learned to substitute them for nontechnical terms which are still used by members of her family.

(5) To increase vocabulary the student should learn the many common prefixes and suffixes, in order to recognize new words in which they appear. Such prefixes and suffixes may be found listed in the dictionary, and familiarity with them will greatly facilitate improvement of vocabulary. Prefixes are placed before the word which they modify in meaning. Examples: *mono-*, meaning "one"—mononucleus, a cell having only one nucleus; *auto-*, meaning "self"—autobiography, a related account of one's own (self) life. Suffixes form the ending of the word whose meaning they influence. Examples: *-itis*, meaning "inflammation"—appendicitis, inflammation of the appendix; *-ectomy*, meaning "surgical removal"—appendectomy, surgical removal of the appendix, nephrectomy, surgical removal of a kidney, tonsillectomy, surgical removal of the tonsils.

(6) In learning the meaning of words that have been looked up because they were unfamiliar, the best method is the card system. The card system of learning vocabulary is really quite simple and much more effective than that of listing words with their definitions and studying from the list thus compiled.

Cards used should be small enough to fit easily into the pocket of the nurse's uniform. Carried in the pocket at all times, the cards will be available whenever needed. When the student has a few minutes of time, as while traveling to and from classes, while waiting in line at the cafeteria, while waiting for class to begin, while waiting to start a nursing procedure, to consult with the head nurse, to obtain the patient's record, or to receive an assignment, the cards may be studied and additional words added to a growing vocabulary.

The card should be printed in an easy-to-read form and should include the word, correctly spelled, marked for pronunciation and defined in terms that are understandable to the student.

When the word has been learned and put into use the card may be replaced by another which bears a different word. In this manner the technical vocabulary can be built up without definite time being taken from scheduled study time to achieve it.

When words are listed for study, each word bears an association relationship with the word above and below it and the student tends prognosis prŏg - nō′ sĭs

The probable outcome or result of a disease

Fig. 17. A card to be used in learning vocabulary.

to learn the word in relation to other words. When the card system is used each word is learned as a complete unit in itself and is not dependent on relationship with other words.

(7) To increase vocabulary the student may need to increase the amount of reading she does. By reading extensively and including a wide variety of reading material, vocabulary will be increased through familiarity with a greater number of words.

(8) By listening carefully to words used by others vocabulary may be increased. The student should pay particular attention to news commentators on radio and television, to doctors lecturing to classes of students, and to nurses and other hospital personnel who use technical terms in general conversation.

On hearing words that may be relatively new to her, the student may soon learn to incorporate them into her own vocabulary.

As a final suggestion for development of a sizable vocabulary the student may need to be reminded of the difference between a large vocabulary and a vocabulary of large words. The use of long or complicated and unfamiliar terms to replace a shorter one which is equally useful produces an effect of artificiality and egotism. To say that "Firemen hastened to the conflagration" is objectionable in ordinary conversation when "Firemen sped to the fire" will do. The use of long words *is* indicated, however, when the word will take the place of an entire phrase or sentence which might otherwise be needed. The statement "Man is a monogamist, as a rule" is preferable to the lengthy or wordy explanation "As a rule, man is of the belief that men should have only one wife—at least only one at one and the same time."

As vocabulary is developed, reading will become more rapid and the reader will gain a new respect for words, whether they are read, heard, or spoken.

CONCENTRATION

Students often ask, "How can I learn to concentrate?" They should be informed that concentrating on a subject of real interest is not difficult. The difficulty begins when they attempt to focus attention on an assigned lesson at a time when they would much prefer to visit with classmates, see a movie, or write a letter.

When study has no appeal the student may attempt to avoid or to postpone it by various time-wasting activities. She may sit at her desk, open the textbook and make sure that pencil and notebook are handy, and then decide to sharpen the pencil. She goes to the end of the corridor, where the pencil sharpener is located, and stops at the room next to her own to ask about the assignment (although she had written it in her notebook when it was given in class). She lingers there awhile and then returns to her own room.

At the desk once more she finds the page number of the assigned lesson, counts the total pages which must be read, looks through them to see how many photographs are included. Illustrations decrease the amount of printed material in the lesson. She hears another student at the telephone in the corridor, thinks of her own boy friend and wishes *he* would call *her*. She decides she would like a drink of water so goes to the drinking fountain. She then returns to her room, sits at the desk, and, with determined effort, begins to read. At the end of the first paragraph the thought occurs to her that she should have gone to the bathroom while in the corridor for a drink.

Upon returning from the bathroom she sits at the desk, adjusts the light, and begins to read. And though she remains at the desk and keeps her eyes focused on the printed page her mind wanders to other subjects. For such a student, the first half hour of time supposedly spent in study has been of no benefit from the standpoint of the amount of knowledge gained.

To develop proper study methods and to help focus attention on the lesson being studied, several courses of action may be considered by the student:

(1) She should develop the habit of sitting at her desk to study. Sitting upright at the desk will prevent the tendency toward relaxation prompted by sitting in an easy or comfortable chair. No attempt should be made to study while reclining on the bed. The bed is used primarily for sleeping and the habit has become firmly fixed. If the student settles herself comfortably in bed to study she will find that she has become so sleepy she can't remain awake in order to read the lesson. Sitting at the desk for each study hour will soon become a fixed habit for her and will promote the impulse to study.

As a rule students are able to study effectively in a library chiefly because it is a place designed for study, a place where others are studying, and a place to which they go with the express purpose of study in mind. By promoting a similar situation at her own desk the student nurse can learn to study there and form desirable study habits.

(2) Lighting for study should be adequate. The entire desk top should be illuminated and lights should be so arranged that there is no glare from the book or notebook being used in study.

(3) The room should be well ventilated. If the room is warm and the air stale because of lack of ventilation, the student will be lethargic and will have difficulty remaining awake.

(4) Only those materials needed for study should be on the desk where study takes place. Articles such as clocks, photographs, radios, and unanswered mail left on the desk may distract the attention of the student and interfere with study. There is no basis for the general belief that a student will be unable to study if a radio is turned on in the room. Some students study effectively while tuned to their favorite radio programs; others may find it necessary to keep the radio silent while they concentrate on the assigned lesson.

(5) The mind should be free of personal problems. If the student is unhappy, irritable, or worried, she may be unable to focus her attention on anything other than the problem which is disturbing her. If she is fearful of her ability to meet scholastic standards or is concerned about keeping physically fit, it may be impossible for her to study. If she is emotionally upset by some incident or happening at her home, or by a situation pertaining to her work in nursing, she may not be able to study effectively.

(6) Continuing suggestions for the improvement of study habits: When given several lesson assignments to prepare the student is more apt to work consistently and systematically if she studies to complete each assignment, as soon as possible after beginning work on it. If she works by the hour instead of by the job much time may be wasted before work on the assigned lesson is begun.

(7) In studying an assigned lesson, the student should anticipate questions that may be asked by the instructor during class or on an examination at some later date. In learning to anticipate questions she learns to recognize the important points in the lesson.

(8) The student should use good study techniques. Desirable study techniques are practices pertaining to study methods that help to produce good study habits and good results from study. Among them may be mentioned:

Making written assignments—when an assignment is made, if it is written by the student it will be available to her at the time she needs it and there will be no chance of an error being made in regard to what is required of her in preparing the lesson.

Taking good notes—notes that are brief yet meaningful will be of real benefit for review and for preparation for an examination.

Correcting all wrong answers on returned test papers. Such papers indicate areas of weakness which may require further study.

Preparing the assigned lesson soon after the assignment is made. When the subject, as discussed in class, is still fresh in the student's mind the assignment may be prepared with greater ease than after a lapse of several days. Early preparation of the assignment may prevent attendance at the class without any preparation. The student who postpones studying a lesson until the night before class may find unexpected circumstances interfering with her plan to study and leaving no time to prepare the lesson.

Studying to learn and to remember. Knowledge gained by the student through study will be used during the entire time she is active in nursing. All study should be done with the express purpose of adding to her store of useful knowledge. To study merely in order to pass the next examination is to create a very weak foundation on which to build a nursing career.

WRITING PAPERS

The writing of term papers, case studies, book reports, and study projects is part of the required work for the student of nursing.

As a member of a profession the nurse is expected to be able to write so that meaning is clearly conveyed through her choice of words. It has been said that "a good writer is one who is able to bring words together, as beads are strung, so that the effect is pleasing." All written papers should receive careful attention of the student since they furnish an opportunity to achieve good grades that will help to increase the grade average for a course that may be difficult for her.

The Term Paper. The simplest method of writing a term paper is that of preparing an outline, arranging it in proper sequence, then writing the paper. The outline should consist of the name of the subject, a list of topics to be discussed, subtopics, and notations. Such an outline can serve as the framework on which to build the composition.

The following illustrates the way in which an outline may be used effectively to write a paper on the chosen subject, "Food Requirements, Food Service, and Diets for the Hospital Patient."

The first step in writing the paper should be the preparation of a rough outline which will contain the various factors to be discussed. Such an outline might appear as:

define—food—nutrients
classify foodstuffs—carbohydrate, protein, fat, etc.
give requirements for normal nutrition (7 basic foods)—calories needed
allergies related to food
serving trays
feeding helpless patients
vitamins—minerals—salts—water
preparation of patient for mealtime
standard hospital diets
special diets
false teeth, care
rectal feedings

From such an original list a second list or outline should be prepared, with the items arranged in logical sequence for the paper. A few topics may be added, and some that appeared in the first list may be dropped. If necessary for clarification, several subtopics may be introduced. The second list might appear as follows:

Definitions:
  food
  foodstuff

diet
dietitian
allergy
nutrition
Introduction:
importance of diet in treatment of disease
nurse's responsibility in relation to diet
food is fuel for the body
understand food needs of normal (healthy) person to understand food needs for the ill
Classification of Foodstuff:
protein
carbohydrate
fat
Normal Nutrition:
food requirements—seven basic foods
fluid requirements—six to eight glasses water
vitamins—mineral salts
Diets:
standard hospital diets
special diets
Food Allergies:
Preparation of Patient for Mealtime:
Serving the Tray:
method of carrying tray
appearance of tray
Feeding the Helpless Patient:
never hurry, mention the food that is on the tray, pleasant conversation

While the student is writing the paper she may wish to add more subtopics or again make slight changes in the sequence of the topics. The paper should be written in an easy-to-read manner, and statements should be clear and meaningful. Care should be taken that the paper isn't merely a lot of words. Most instructors really read term papers.

Although other textbooks may be used in reference reading no attempt should be made to copy textbook material and incorporate it as part of the paper. The instructor is apt to recognize the fact that the paper has been copied.

Careful attention should be given to spelling, grammar, and punctuation in doing the paper. It is always a little startling to the instructor to come upon such statements as "the *vile* contained tincture of the drug," or "the *intervenious* was discontinued very soon after the *seditave* was given."

The final suggestion in regard to writing a term paper is that it be started immediately on assignment and completed several days before the date it is due. There is great satisfaction in completing such work soon after assignment and in knowing that it will be ready to submit to the instructor at the designated time.

THE BOOK REPORT

The method of writing a book report will depend on the kind of book read and the factors which the instructor has indicated should appear in the report. Most such reports include the name of book, name of the author, list of characters, synopsis of the plot, and the student's personal opinion or evaluation of the book as it is related to the course of study.

EXAMINATIONS

Examinations are of two major types, the subjective, or essay type, and the objective type. The subjective type examination requires that the student be able to recall and to reason in order to answer the questions correctly. The objective type requires ability to recognize or to guess.

To prepare for either type of examination the student should keep a complete file of good notes, preferably in outline form; frequently review material previously studied and discussed in the classroom; know the important factors or items for each lesson, and have an understanding of the different type questions which may be asked and the best method of answering them.

From previous examinations weaknesses in the course will have been pointed out and additional study time should have been given to correct those weaknesses.

The Subjective Type Examination. To better understand the suggestions that will be given to help answer the essay type question, several examples of such questions are given: (1) Give at least four good reasons for keeping the medicine cupboard locked. (2) Explain, and draw a diagram to illustrate, how to determine the site for an intramuscular injection. (3) What are the local signs and symptoms of inflammation? (4) Mention several important instructions that should be given visitors to patients in isolation.

In writing an examination of the type illustrated above the following suggestions are made to the student:

(1) Answer first the questions for which you are certain you know the correct answers. If you know the answers to several questions they may be answered rather rapidly and the remainder of the time then devoted to the effort required in answering questions which seem more difficult.

(2) Be sure you understand the meaning of the question before you attempt to answer it. Read it several times, if necessary, note if it has more than one part, and give complete answers to all the parts.

(3) Make the answer accurate, brief, and legible. Don't write several paragraphs of vague statements in an attempt to conceal the fact that you don't know the answer.

(4) Know what is meant by the terms *outline, name, describe,*

illustrate, explain, and *define.* Such terms are often used in essay type questions and the answers should carry out the specific instruction each term indicates.

(5) Don't give more information than is asked for in the statement of the question. If asked to *name* the various methods of performing physical examination for a patient, don't *name* and *explain* each of the five methods.

(6) If asked to *compare* two objects, make sure the answer tells how the objects are alike and also how they differ.

(7) Don't borrow an answer from the paper of the student nearest you. One of the chief benefits derived from examination is to learn where weakness exists and more study is needed. Borrowed answers will nullify the examination in this respect. Borrowing may lead to embarrassment, too, as in the case of the student who noted her neighbor had written, directly beneath the last question on the examination, "I don't know the answer," and who wrote on her own paper, "I don't know the answer either."

(8) Always review the completed paper before submitting it to the instructor. Make sure that all parts to all questions have been answered.

The Objective Type Examination. Objective tests are made up of several different kinds of questions. This particular type of examination can be answered with a minimum amount of writing by the student. Objective type questions are usually preferred by instructors and students since a greater number of questions can be answered in less time. Grading is objective and may be done more rapidly, and the responses indicate what the test is intended to measure, namely, knowledge of course content, rather than the ability to spell or to choose good words for expression of thoughts.

The following are examples of the questions asked on different objective type examinations:

True-False (indicate if the statement is true or false):

1. The subjective type question is the essay type question. ____________
2. About ninety per cent of body weight is water. ____________
3. Wilted flowers should be discarded regardless of the patient's wishes. ____________

Yes-No (answer the question "yes" or "no"):

1. Is a window deflector an aid to proper ventilation? ____________
2. Is inability to sleep termed "insomnia"? ____________
3. If the door to a hospital room is closed, may the nurse enter without knocking? ____________

Multiple Choice (underline the best answer):

1. Basic foods needed for health include milk, cheese, spinach.
2. Twenty-four drams of a drug would contain two ounces, three ounces, four ounces.
3. A drug which induces sleep is a hypnotic, emetic, cathartic.

Matching:

1. ( ) phobia	1. a drug used to relieve pain
2. ( ) hysteria	2. a drug used to induce sleep
3. ( ) narcotic	3. an abnormal fear
	4. lack of emotional control

Completion (supply the missing words or phrases):

1. Changing from a liquid or solid state into a vapor is termed ______________.
2. The three main types of fever are ______________, ______________, and ______________.
3. An ______________ is an agent that softens the skin.

Suggestions for writing objective type examinations include:

(1) Read directions carefully. Be sure there is understanding as to the way in which the answer is to be given.

(2) Know before beginning to write the test if omitted answers are marked as wrong answers. A penalty for omitting an answer may be greater than would be that of guessing.

(3) Answer first the questions which are not at all difficult, return later to those requiring more thought.

(4) Use relationship to determine the answer. Associate the question with a page from the textbook, a certain topic or an illustration.

(5) Remember that True-False questions containing the words, "all," "always," or "never" permit of no exceptions.

(6) If the question seems difficult, restate it in your own words. This may help to clarify the meaning.

(7) Review the completed examination paper before submitting it to the teacher. If an answer is changed, be certain it isn't being changed from a correct to an incorrect answer.

TAKING NOTES

The ability to take good notes may contribute largely to scholastic success for the student in nursing. The function of good notes is threefold: (1) to help in understanding subject material; (2) to help remember longer and more accurately that which is learned; (3) to furnish an outline for review before examination.

Efficient learning may be based on ability to take good notes, and the student who sincerely desires instruction in the correct method of taking notes should observe the following regulations:

(1) Know the topic or subject to be discussed. Read the lesson before attending the lecture so you will have some understanding of the subject.

(2) Make the notes brief and put them in outline form. All words such as *a*, *an*, *the*, *if*, and *but* should be omitted from notes, only essential words and phrases being used. Writing too much interferes with listening and thinking.

(3) Do not attempt to write exact words of the speaker. His thoughts and expressions should be put into simpler words and phrases.

(4) Organize notes effectively. Notes or statements should be arranged in proper sequence to show relationship to each other.

(5) Take notes in outline form. Notes that are very brief, arranged in outline form with main topics, subtopics, and explanations, furnish excellent study material.

(6) If, during the lecture, a statement or point is missed, leave a blank space on the page and continue taking notes as before. The omitted statement may be obtained later from the instructor or another student.

(7) Recognize important points in the lecture by the speaker's use of repetition, long pauses, and tone of voice to emphasize what he wishes the student to remember.

(8) Keep notes pertaining to one particular subject separated from notes of other subjects. Separate note books or separate sections of the same notebook should be provided for each course of study.

(9) The loose leaf notebook of standard letter size (8½ by 11 inches) is the most practical for use since it will accommodate usual mimeographed material. Additional pages may be added so it is possible to keep term papers and graded quiz or examination papers with the notes to be used for future study.

(10) Write the name of the course of study and the date at the top of each page of notes so they can be kept in correct arrangement within the notebook.

(11) Use abbreviations as much as possible so notes can be taken more rapidly.

Commonly used standard abbreviations (Table 1) will need to be memorized by the student and used extensively in recording on the patients' chart and in reading and understanding doctors' orders, laboratory reports, and data recorded by other hospital personnel. If the student learns the abbreviations early in her course of study she may put them to use in taking notes, thus increasing the speed with which good notes may be taken during lecture classes.

Example. The following example shows how brief notes may be made from subject material given by a lecturer or in a textbook. The subject under discussion is that of "Conversing with the Patient."

Discussion: Part of a nurse's duty to her patient is to converse easily and intelligently with him while performing such nursing procedures as giving a bed bath or while serving the tray. A few minutes each day spent in reviewing headlines in the daily newspaper or in reading from current magazines will enable the nurse to understand and respond to comments made by the patient in regard to current events.

Each student nurse should form the habit of reading for a short while each day from really good books and magazines. Just fifteen minutes a day devoted to this practice adds up to approximately seven hours of worth-while reading at the end of one month.

In a large city hospital recently the effect of such reading by one

Table 1. STANDARD ABBREVIATIONS AND SYMBOLS

ā̄a .... of each
abd .... abdomen
a.c. .... before meals
ad lib. .... as desired
A.M. .... morning
amt .... amount
aq .... water
ax .... axillary
b.i.d .... twice a day
B.M.R .... basal metabolic rate
B.P. .... blood pressure
C. .... centigrade
c̄ .... with
cc .... cubic centimeter
comp .... compound
C.S. .... central supply
dil .... dilute
dr .... dram
Dr .... doctor
E.E.N.T. .... eye, ear, nose & throat
E.K.G. .... electrocardiogram
elix .... elixir
ext .... extract
F .... Fahrenheit
fld .... fluid
fract. dos. .... divided doses
G.I. .... gastrointestinal
gm .... gram
gr .... grain
gtt .... drop
G.U. .... genitourinary
h .... hour
Hb .... hemoglobin
H.S. .... at bedtime
I.M. .... intramuscular
inf .... infusion
I.V. .... intravenous
kg .... kilogram
lab .... laboratory
lb .... pound
liq .... liquid
L.L.Q. .... left lower quadrant
m .... minim
mg .... milligram
min .... minute
no .... number
noct .... night
N.P.N. .... non-protein nitrogen
O .... pint
O.B. .... obstetrics
o.d. .... every day
O.D. .... right eye
o.h. .... every hour
Ol .... oil
O.P.D. .... out-patient department
os .... mouth
O.S. .... left eye
oz .... ounce
P .... pulse
p.c. .... after meals
per .... by
P.M. .... afternoon
p.r.n. .... whenever necessary
P.S.P. .... phenolsulfonphthalein
pulv .... powder
q.d. .... every day
q.h. .... every hour
q.2.h. .... every two hours
q.3.h. .... every three hours
q.4.h. .... every four hours
q.i.d. .... four times a day
q.s. .... sufficient quantity
R .... rectal, respiration
R.B.C. .... red blood cell
R.L.Q. .... right lower quadrant
℞ .... take
s̄ .... without
sat .... saturate
sig .... write
sol .... solution
solv .... dissolve
s.o.s. .... if necessary (one dose only)
sp. gr. .... specific gravity
spec .... specimen
sp .... spirit
s̄s̄ .... one half
S.S. .... soap solution
stat .... immediately
T .... temperature
tab .... tablet
T.B. .... tuberculosis
tbsp .... tablespoon
t.i.d. .... three times a day
tinct .... tincture
tn .... tension
T.P.R. .... temperature, pulse, and respiration
tsp .... teaspoon
U .... unit
ung .... ointment
V .... volume
V.O. .... verbal order
W.B.C. .... white blood cell
wt .... weight

of the student nurses was clearly demonstrated. A patient who failed to sleep well one night and seemed fully prepared to be disgruntled for the day because of that fact instead spent the day chuckling to himself and entertaining doctors, nurses, family, and visitors with the remark made by the student nurse to whom he had addressed the complaint about not sleeping. She had told him of reading the evening before about a man who "for three quarters of an hour lay awake all night"! The student had spent a few minutes reading the current issue of Reader's Digest and, remembering the clever witticism, had used it to good advantage for the patient.

The above in outline form (complete):

Nurse needs to be able to converse with patient
- better able to do this by reading newspapers and current magazines
- fifteen minutes each day adds up to seven hours per month—good reading
- A remembered bit of humor may do much to help patient's morale

The above in outline form (very brief):

Know how talk c̄ patient
- daily reading—newspaper, magazine, good book (few min. helps)
- remember bits humor—boosts patient morale

HOW TO USE THE SCHOOL LIBRARY

To use the school library effectively the student should be instructed in the correct use of the card catalog method of locating books on the shelves, the method of "signing out" a book and of being credited for it when she returns it to the library.

While being instructed in library procedure the student should be taught how to obtain needed information from such reference books as dictionaries, encyclopedias, almanacs, year books, and the "Readers' Guide."

Pamphlets. Much valuable subject material exists in pamphlet form and should be made available to students through the library facilities. Pamphlets may contain reprints of articles in magazines not on the library's subscription list. Other examples of pamphlet material are those from national, state, or local government agencies, or nursing, health, and welfare organizations. Pamphlets should not only be available in large numbers but should be classified, labeled, filed, and made readily available for use to faculty members or students.

Periodical Indexes. Printed indexes are available for completed volumes of magazines and should be included with the magazines as they are bound into one volume each year.

Bibliography cards prepared by the American Journal of Nursing provide a current index to the Journal and can be used until the printed index is available.

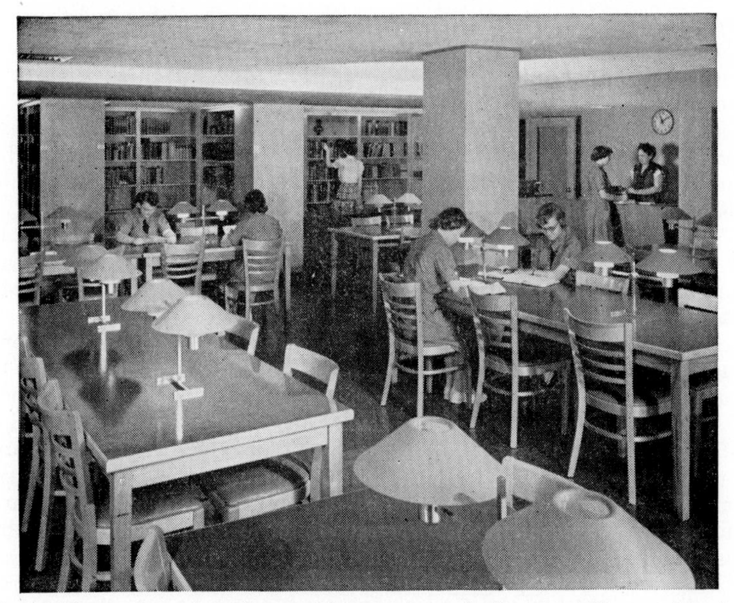

Fig. 18. The student of nursing spends many hours in the school library. (Presbyterian Hospital School of Nursing, Chicago, Illinois.)

Reference Service. The librarian may be asked a great many times each day for information which requires the use of reference material. She may also be required to procure from other libraries materials not available in the school library.

Use of the Library. All members of the library staff should be responsible for teaching students and faculty members how to use the library effectively.

New Books and Other Materials. The bulletin board and the library display shelf are logical places where the arrival of new books and other publications can be noted. The bulletin board for the school library may be a colorful and interesting means of publicizing recently acquired books and other materials.

The Ward Library. An up-to-date reference library located on each clinical department and made available to busy doctors and nurses is considered an essential tool of learning for most schools of nursing today. The ward library provides for quick and valuable information on such matters as the use of a new drug, the interpretation of laboratory reports, the treatment and nursing care of certain diseases, and the correct medical term for use in recording on the patient's chart.

Books Needed for the Ward Library. The general classification of the patient (surgical, medical, obstetrical, etc.), will determine the specific books that will be needed in the ward library. In an orthopedic department nursing care books pertaining to the diseases, abnormalities, and injuries to the skeletal system should be available. Basic texts required for all ward libraries include a medical or nursing dictionary, a standard English dictionary, a drug encyclopedia, a manual of charting, a pharmacology text, a nutrition text, and a text that treats of the clinical interpretation of laboratory tests. The nursing arts procedure book and a manual of laboratory tests should also be a part of each ward library.

The books should be catalogued and plainly marked with the name of the clinical department to which they belong. As an added precaution, the name of the hospital should be stamped across the side and ends of the book.

In this chapter on "Effective Study Methods" many suggestions have been made to the student. Few of the suggestions are easy to carry out, yet all of them will be helpful in correcting faulty methods of study. Any student who has poor study habits, or who studies ineffectively, will benefit by putting into practice these suggested means for improvement. The student who readily admits that her study habits are not good yet who continues to study in the haphazard manner she used before reading this chapter will benefit not at all by instructions given here.

The student who plays golf, or swims, or engages in some form of group activity for recreation must be given instruction in the particular activity, and then must practice before she acquires the necessary skill. The same requirements must be met if the student is to develop effective methods of study. After instructions have been given she will need to put into practice the suggestions which will help her overcome her study deficiencies.

Summary of Important Factors

Ineffectual study methods is the chief cause of failure of students in schools of nursing.

Reasons why the student should study are: (1) to make passing grades; (2) to enjoy classwork; (3) to benefit more from clinical experience; (4) to pass state board examinations; (5) to help maintain the school's good standing.

Use of spelling rules and of the dictionary will help the student to spell correctly.

Reading rate and comprehension bear a marked influence on scholastic success.

The most common reading faults are word-by-word reading, inadequate vocabulary, and limited comprehension.

Practice to improve reading must be consistent and extended over a long period of time to be really effective.

A reading rate below 275 words per minute indicates the need for improved reading ability.

Learning prefixes and suffixes helps to increase vocabulary.

The card system of study is the best means of learning vocabulary.

The student should sit at her desk to study.

Good lighting, adequate ventilation, quiet, and freedom from worry are needed for effective study.

Good study techniques include: (1) writing assignments; (2) taking good notes; (3) reviewing corrected examination papers; (4) preparing assignments early; (5) studying to gain information.

An outline of topics and subtopics is helpful in writing term papers.

Examinations may be subjective or objective in type.

In writing the subjective type examination the student needs to know the meaning of the terms *outline, define, explain, name, describe,* and *illustrate.*

Good notes are usually brief, well organized, and arranged in outline form.

Important reference books include dictionaries, encyclopedias, almanacs, year books, biographies, Readers' Guide, and bibliographies.

Knowing effective methods of study will not benefit the student who does not practice them.

Suggested Reference Reading

"Ward libraries," Edna Walker Colburn; American Journal of Nursing, March, 1951.

"Library services in a school of nursing," Helen W. Munson; American Journal of Nursing, April, 1951.

"How well do modern schools teach reading?" Paul Witty; Today's Health, November, 1952.

"Students can become more effective readers," Mary Jane Silence; American Journal of Nursing, March, 1953.

"The reading accelerator," Mary Jane Silence; American Journal of Nursing, March, 1953.

CHAPTER 3

Interpersonal Relationships in Nursing

TOPICAL OUTLINE

A chip on the shoulder always indicates there is wood higher up.

To give intelligent and effective nursing care to the patient the nurse, both student and graduate, must establish good relationships with members of allied professions or groups.

When on duty she becomes an important member of a team that must work in cooperation and harmony to bring to the patient all the knowledge and skill available for combating his particular disease or physical impairment.

She should make a special effort to get along well with those with whom she works and to accord them the respect and consideration that comes with understanding that each, in his own way, contributes to the total care and treatment being given the patient.

When a good working relationship exists between doctor, nurse, and other hospital personnel, the patient benefits. In a hospital where relationships are not good and each worker attempts to work independently of the others as much as possible, the patient suffers because planning for his total care is apt to be haphazard and inadequate.

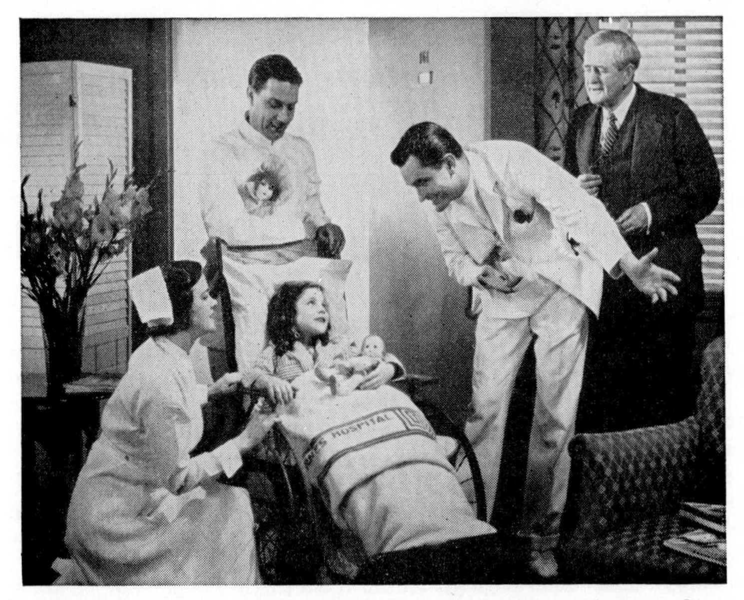

Fig. 19. The patient benefits by good relationships between doctor and nurse. (Parke, Davis & Company, Detroit, Michigan.)

When interpersonal and interdepartmental relationships are not good, treatments and nursing care procedures may be poorly timed, unskilfully administered, and rendered ineffective because of lack of cooperation of the personnel involved.

To establish good working relationships with members of the medical staff, members of other departments in the hospital, associates in the nursing department, and with the patient, the nurse must be cooperative and understanding. She should recognize the importance of working as a member of a team whose chief aim is to help the patient recover from illness or injury so he can return to a normal, active life.

THE NURSE AND THE DOCTOR

As changes take place in the science of medicine, in world events, in the standards evolved by nurse educators, and in social conditions affected by present economic and political trends, the relationship between nurse and doctor undergoes corresponding change and readjustment.

In the early period of nursing the nurse neither expected nor received recognition from the doctor, who considered her an undesirable member of society—a lowly creature, tolerated in the presence of so-called "decent" persons only because her services were so greatly needed.

With the advancement in nursing through organized nursing activities and through the efforts of nurse educators, the doctor gradually came to accept the nurse as a not too bright but very necessary servant to help him in the care of the sick.

For years the nurse was carefully instructed in the importance of blindly obeying every order and carrying out each prescribed treatment without thought of questioning either the wisdom or the integrity of the doctor.

Today, although the relationship continues to change and is dependent on localities, previous customs, and present conditions, the trend seems to be toward a more complete understanding of the two and a willingness to work together in the best interests of the patient.

Changes in hospital practice brought about by a greater demand for hospital care have effected changes in nursing service and in interpretation of what is meant by the phrase, "good nursing care."

Various members of the medical profession, depending on their specialty or field of work, think of different types of service and different procedures related to their specialty when asked for their conception of "good nursing care." The doctor chiefly concerned with treatment of medical patients would have the nurse be responsible for assisting with, or preforming in their entirety, a large number of complicated diagnostic procedures. He delegates to her the task of supervising or ordering collection of specimens and the proper timing of certain tests. Without giving any thought as to whether or not she has been thoroughly informed in such procedures, he makes her responsible for all preliminary preparations for cystoscopy, basal metabolism tests, electrocardiography, kidney function tests, and many other procedures that have little or no relation to "nursing care."

The medical specialist may expect the nurse to be familiar with the procedures of gastric analysis, diagnostic or therapeutic use of x-rays, and a host of other specialized forms of treatment.

The doctor who is chiefly interested in surgery may expect the nurse to be proficient in performing such procedures as intravenous injection, blood transfusion, and the administration of plasma or of recently discovered drugs; to recognize at once any symptom that might indicate surgical complications; to use, with efficiency and skill, all the complicated equipment needed to perform the operation, and to be thoroughly versed in oxygen therapy and in the use of Wangensteen suction or other apparatus used extensively in the care of the postoperative patient.

Many doctors are concerned with the amount of technical education required of the nurse today and are critical of the fact that she is being "over educated," yet they continue to relinquish duties to the nursing personnel that formerly were considered the definite responsibility of the physician. Continued delegation of such duties to

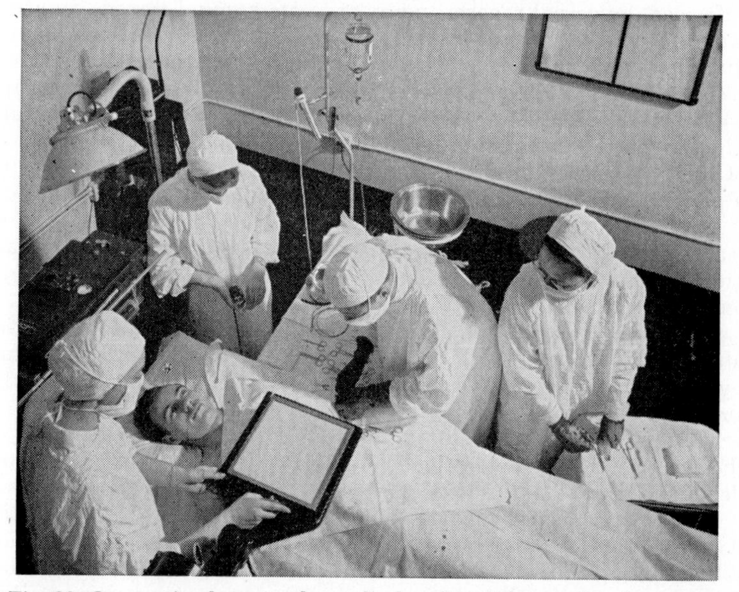

Fig. 20. Cooperation between the medical staff and the nursing department is essential since the work of one supplements that of the other. (Presbyterian Hospital, Chicago, Illinois.)

members of the nursing staff makes imperative the advanced educational training of nurses. As nursing duties expand to embrace former duties of the physician, it is vitally necessary that the nurse continue to be better educated if she is to be capable of accepting the responsibility for performing complicated and technical procedures.

Cooperation between the medical staff and the nursing department is of special importance since the work of one supplements that of the other.

Diagnosis of the patient's illness and orders for medication and treatment are primarily the function of the physician, yet the nurse is expected to know the correct dosage of medicines and to be familiar with methods of treatment that might be used. If a medicine is prescribed in such a way that the dosage is inaccurate and the nurse gives the medicine as ordered, despite the fact that she should know the dose is incorrect, the nurse as well as the doctor can be held responsible for the error. Although all nurses are expected to follow the doctor's order, no nurse is relieved of responsibility if she blindly follows orders to the detriment of the patient.

In working with the doctor the nurse is expected to observe and report symptoms of changes that may occur in the condition of the patient. She should know deviations from normal and keep the doctor informed, by verbal reports and by accurate hospital records, in every way that will be helpful in diagnosis and treatment. The most highly qualified nurse, however, is not capable of assuming the doctor's responsibilities and should never attempt to diagnose or to prescribe treatment. She may be well versed in the medical practices for certain diseases, but she is not qualified to assume the duties or responsibilities of the physician. When asked by friends or relatives to prescribe for a patient, she should recommend that a qualified doctor be consulted.

The relationship between doctor and nurse is usually that of teacher–pupil, since the doctor with whom she first becomes acquainted is likely to be a member of the medical staff who lectures on a subject contained in the curriculum of the nursing school.

The nurse, by being punctual in reporting to class, by paying strict attention to the medical lecture, by making a satisfactory grade, and by participating in class discussion, can show her appreciation for the time and effort expended by the doctor in teaching the class.

The attitude of the beginning student toward various members of the medical staff is determined largely by the attitude of older students and of graduate nurses.

In a school where medical and nursing ethics are observed the doctor is accorded the respect and loyalty which his position warrants. Through his social conduct, and his interest in and care of his patients, he merits the consideration and respect given him by the nurses.

The nurse, instructed not to accept verbal orders from a doctor, should be courteous and respectful in her refusal to do so, pointing out to the doctor who gave the order that her instructions apply to all doctors, and not merely to him as an individual member of the medical staff.

Familiarity between doctor and nurse is frowned on in most hospitals, not only because of social implications, but because it tends to destroy the dignified, co-worker relationship which is so necessary if both are to serve the best interests of the patient.

Nurses should be instructed not to consult members of the medical staff in regard to their personal health or adjustment problems. The health director in the school will arrange for medical consultation when needed.

Nurses should not attempt to impart information of a medical nature to patients or to persons outside the hospital. Such information should come directly from the doctor caring for the patient.

In all relationships the nurse must know what is expected of her by the other person involved. In order to derive the most from her association with the doctor she needs to know what he may rightfully expect of her as a nurse.

The important qualities which the doctor would expect of a nurse in addition to technical knowledge and practical application of that knowledge are loyalty, honesty, dependability, and a willingness to

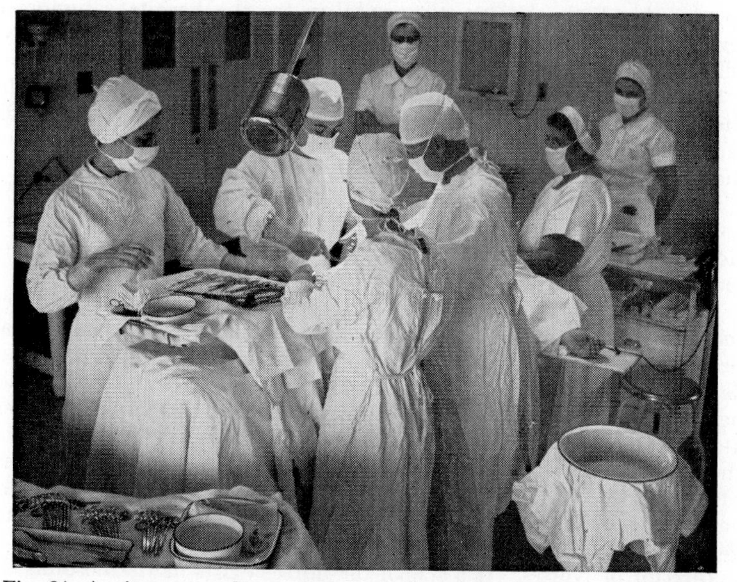

Fig. 21. An important department in the hospital where good interpersonal relationships are essential is the department of surgery. (Mercy Hospital School of Nursing, Hamilton, Ohio.)

carry out his planned course of treatment and care for the patient.

He expects the nurse to inspire the patient with confidence in him and in his ability as a doctor.

He expects her to understand the care and use of new and improved equipment and to be able to administer new medications intelligently.

Since the doctor and nurse have a common interest, in restoring sick people to health and in preventing healthy people from becoming sick, each needs the assistance and cooperation of the other if they are to work together to accomplish improved medical and nursing care.

ORGANIZATIONAL PLAN OF HOSPITAL PERSONNEL

With hospitals differing so widely in control and ownership and in the type of clinical services provided, it is not unusual to find many differences, too, in their organization or plan of management.

Made up of many different departments, which are staffed with trained and untrained workers, the hospital must be well organized and well managed if it is to function for the best interests of the patient.

Although each hospital has its own plan of organization and management, all follow a similar pattern made up largely as follows:

Board of Trustees. A governing board which may be elected or appointed, which assumes responsibility for the hospital's financial, legal, and moral obligations, and which appoints an administrative officer or superintendent to direct or supervise the entire institution.

Hospital Superintendent. Since the superintendent is appointed by the governing board he is directly responsible to its members for carrying out their directives and for coordinating the various departments of the hospital.

Medical Director. A registered physician who is responsible to the governing board. He is in charge of the medical staff, resident physicians, and interns, and serves as consultant to other departments on matters pertaining to medical practice.

Business Manager. As head of the business department the business manager is responsible to the superintendent and, with his approval, provides needed finances, facilities, and supplies to keep the various departments functioning properly. Under his direction the office personnel (clerks, stenographers, record librarian, switchboard operators), the purchasing agent, the dietitian, the pharmacist, the special therapy personnel, the maintenance personnel (engineers, painters, carpenters, mechanics, housekeepers, janitors, maids), and the laundry personnel perform their various duties and work harmoniously together to foster the safety and well-being of the patient.

Director of Nurses. If a school for nurses exists at the hospital the director of nurses is in charge of it as well as of nursing service. Under her direction the nursing department operates smoothly to give desirable nursing care to the patients. She is responsible to the superintendent of the hospital for maintaining adequate standards of nursing service and for conducting a school of nursing that is accredited by the State Nurses' Board. All nursing personnel and all nonprofessional workers in the department are under her jurisdiction.

THE NURSE AND HOSPITAL PERSONNEL

The interpersonal relationships existing between various members of the hospital staff may be said to revolve around the nurse, who is often the hub of such relationships. She is important in integrating the services of all departments within the hospital.

The personality of the nurse may be the determining factor in interpersonal relationships in nursing situations that arise each day. In every contact the nurse may have with other professional personnel and with nonprofessional workers there is a potential clash of beliefs, feelings, or behavior; there is also the potential of common understanding and mutual agreement.

The nurse who is able to understand her own behavior is apt to be more understanding of the behavior of others and, therefore, is in a better position to promote in others an attitude of respect and consideration.

The relationship between the student nurse and the graduate nurse

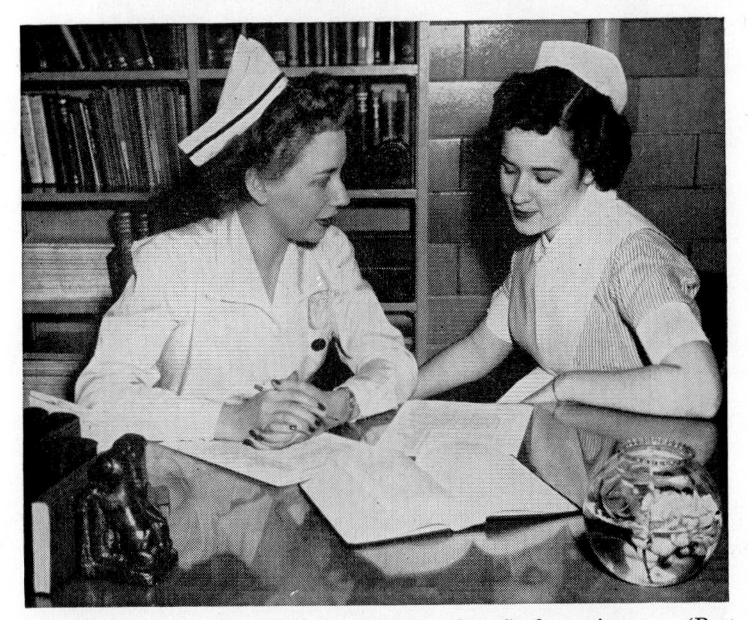

Fig. 22. Desirable student–faculty relationships benefit the patient too. (Protestant Deaconess Hospital School of Nursing, Evansville, Indiana.)

in a professional program will influence the behavior pattern of the student and largely determine the relationships that will exist, several years later, when she has become a graduate nurse and is in close association with students.

The nurse is only one member of a large group of persons whose work may affect the patient and be of importance in determining the final outcome of his illness. Nursing care given the patient is only part of the total plan set up for his benefit. The work of the doctor, dentist, dietitian, pathologist, social worker, psychologist, occupational therapist, physiotherapist, and clergyman is also very important and very necessary. The total plan may often be coordinated by the nurse, but only because she is in a strategic position to organize effectively the efforts of the others and because she is required to establish close relationship with the patient in the performance of her nursing duties.

All professional workers who are part of the hospital personnel should be interested in promoting the work of personnel in other departments so that the services of each will help to bring full benefit to the patient.

Good relationship between the personnel of different hospital departments must be maintained to satisfactorily serve the patients for whom the hospital exists. This is true whether the hospital is a small

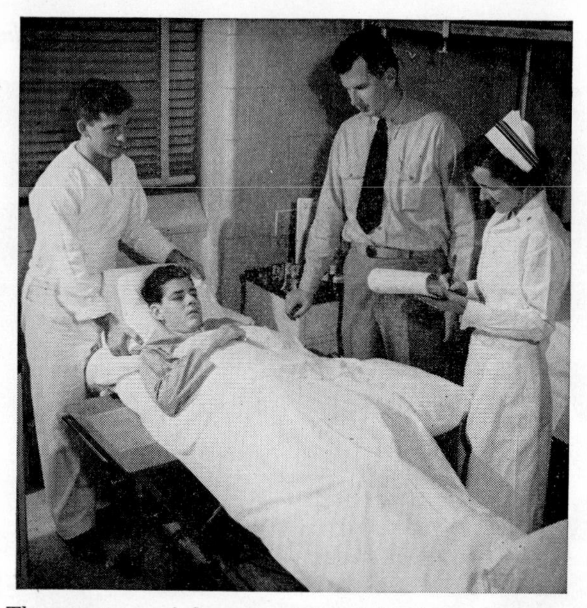

Fig. 23. The care-team of doctor, nurse, and hospital corpsman. (Bureau of Medicine and Surgery, Navy Department, Washington, D.C.)

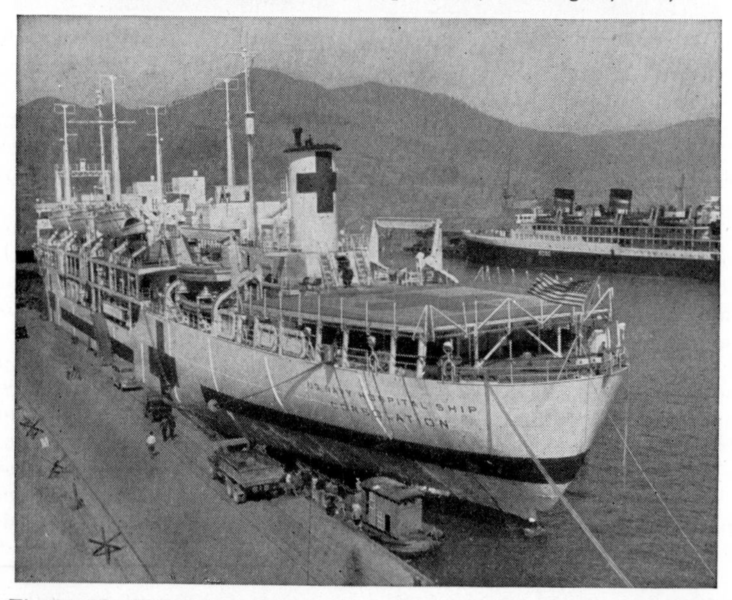

Fig. 24. The Navy's hospital ship, "Consolation," shown as she was tied up at Pusan, Korea, October, 1951. (Bureau of Medicine and Surgery, Navy Department, Washington, D.C.)

community hospital in a rural area, a large city hospital, or a hospital at sea, such as the Navy's hospital ship, "Consolation."

If the nurse is acquainted with the place and function of each department in the organization and how the work of the nursing department is coordinated with that of the others she is able to understand the importance of full cooperation in the work that is being done.

Interpersonal relationships for the nurse are important in her daily routine and in the development of an ability to get along well with others.

ORGANIZATIONAL PLAN OF NURSING DEPARTMENT PERSONNEL

Familiarity with the plan of organization of the nursing department personnel of the hospital will enable the nurse to understand her relationship and responsibilities to other members of the hospital staff.

The Director of Nurses is in charge of the school of nursing and of nursing service. She usually appoints a head of the school and a director of nursing service to share the responsibility of management.

The School of Nursing. The personnel of the school of nursing includes the following:

Educational Director. The nurse in charge of the school of nursing. Faculty personnel look to the educational director for organization and planning of class schedules, curriculum, and correlation of courses being taught.

Instructors. The specially trained, graduate, registered nurses who teach science or nursing arts and whose time is devoted largely to classroom work.

Clinical Instructors. Assistants to the instructors, who may help in formal teaching and help to supervise the work of students in the laboratory and in clinical practice.

Student Nurses. Nurses who are receiving education in theory and practice that will enable them to become graduate, registered nurses.

Counselor. A member of the faculty who may or may not be a graduate registered nurse and who has had special training in counseling and guidance. She may be required to teach a class in addition to the work being done in counseling.

Social Director. A faculty member qualified to help plan social activities for students and for faculty members.

The Nursing Service. The staff providing nursing service to patients in the hospital includes:

Director of Nursing Service. The director of nursing service is responsible to the director of nurses and acts as her assistant in directing the organization and administration of the nursing service as a whole. Her chief function is supervision of nursing care for all hospital patients.

Supervisor. A graduate, registered nurse in charge of a department or special clinical division of the hospital, supervising nursing

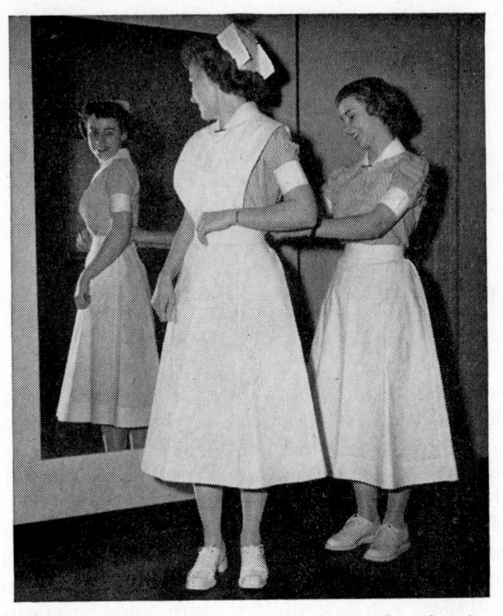

Fig. 25. The preclinical student nurse looks forward to the time when she also will wear the bib and cap. (Protestant Deaconess Hospital School of Nursing, Evansville, Indiana.)

care for patients in her department and organizing the activities of personnel assigned to duty there.

Clinical Supervisor. A graduate nurse who is primarily responsible for helping with supervision of student nurses in the department, and who works with the supervisor in assigning patients to students.

Head Nurse. A graduate nurse in charge of a single unit or department in the hospital. She is responsible for the organization and management of the unit, for nursing care given the patients there, and for helping in the clinical teaching program for students assigned to her unit.

General Duty Nurse. A graduate nurse who gives bedside nursing care and is senior member of the cooperative team of workers on the unit.

Private Duty Nurse. A graduate nurse who is employed by the patient and confines her nursing care to him exclusively. She is responsible to the head nurse for the kind of nursing care she gives the patient.

Student Nurses. Students enrolled in the school for the purpose of acquiring needed nursing skill by performing nursing service to patients in the hospital as part of the required clinical practice. The hospital serves as a laboratory for the student who learns to give nursing care to the patient by performing procedures which have been taught in the classroom.

Nonprofessional Workers. The Practical Nurse. A nonprofessional nurse who has had 9 to 12 months of instruction and clinical practice. Practical nurses are usually restricted to routine nursing procedures, as giving baths and serving trays. They assist graduate and student nurses in giving care to the patients.

The Nurse Aide. A worker who usually receives on-the-job training to help in giving nursing care and in bedmaking and care of linens, etc.

The Ward Clerk. A worker instructed in duties of a clerical nature, such as answering the telephone, delivering messages, filling out chart headings, etc., and who performs those duties as a part of the daily routine on the department.

The Orderly. A man assigned to the nursing department to assist in the nursing care of male patients. Most orderlies receive on-the-job training; their instructor is usually an experienced orderly or a clinical instructor.

The Maid. A worker who is responsible for housekeeping duties in the unit, such as sweeping, dusting, and cleaning service rooms.

Good relationships between various members of the professional and nonprofessional nursing service personnel are necessary if the unit or department is to function smoothly and the patient is to receive adequate nursing care.

Since the nursing department is one of the largest departments in the hospital organization, it is important that it be well staffed and well managed.

The student may readily see the importance of the role she is to play and the service she can render by establishing good relationship with other hospital personnel and by cooperating with them to provide better care for the hospital patient.

THE NURSE AND THE PATIENT

The relationship between nurse and patient is largely that of teacher–pupil regardless of the age, education, or experience of each person concerned. A patient admitted to the hospital enters a world that is apt to be totally unfamiliar to him, and throughout hospitalization he is dependent, to a great extent, on the nurse for guidance and instruction. She imparts information which will help him adjust to the daily routine of the new environment and to cooperate in accepting treatments necessary for his complete recovery of physical and mental health.

If the patient is to realize maximum benefit through his association with the nurse it is essential that he have confidence in her ability to perform nursing procedures and that he accept her guidance in matters pertaining to medicine and nursing which are beyond his understanding. To foster the patient's confidence in her ability and to be accepted as a competent guide or teacher the nurse must meet certain requirements which have become more or less standard since they are so necessary to the success of any member of her profession. Each nurse represents the whole profession to the patient she cares for, and her attitude toward nursing and toward the hospital is very apt to be reflected in the subsequent attitude of the patient toward other nurses and the institution.

Understanding the Patient. In her relationship with the patient the nurse is required to be keenly aware of the confusion and apprehension which he may experience mentally because of the physical condition which necessitates medical or surgical treatment.

The understanding nurse will recognize that restlessness, ill temper, and other symptoms of emotional strain are a part of the patient's reaction to the fears and anxieties brought about by physical pain or sudden illness. In addition to the anxiety he may have concerning the outcome of his disease, the patient may be vitally concerned as to the effect of his illness on the security or well-being of his family. Added to the mental strain of a sudden and drastic change from normal daily routine is the practically uncontrollable dread or fear of being alone in a strange and frightening environment. He reluctantly awaits the medical or surgical treatment which his physical condition may require. As a result of these emotional tensions the patient is likely to behave in a manner quite different from his normal behavior pattern. A person who is usually friendly and agreeable may become sullen, uncooperative, and hypercritical during his introduction to hospital routine.

If the nurse understands and is sympathetic toward the patient she can do a great deal to help him overcome the anxiety and emotional turmoil which so often accompanies illness. Her cheerful manner, her friendly concern for his welfare, and the ease with which she performs nursing procedures will all serve to reassure the patient. He will be greatly relieved and will feel more secure if she approaches him in a friendly manner, introduces herself, and by her initial remarks indicates that she is sincerely interested in helping him regain his health and resume normal activities. Her attitude should indicate that she sees nothing unusual in either his physical condition or his mental reaction to it.

The nurse can usually obtain full cooperation from the patient by assuring him that hospital personnel are available when needed and are thoroughly familiar with the therapeutic requirements of his particular illness.

By expressing confidence in the ability of his doctor, by explaining some of the procedures involved in his care, and by mentioning casually what is expected of him as a patient in the daily routine which will make up the greater part of his entire stay in the hospital, she offers the most help in making the adjustment from home to hospital surroundings.

A sympathetic and understanding attitude on the part of the nurse toward anxious relatives who may have accompanied the patient to the hospital will help alleviate the fear and depression of the patient, and will also serve to reassure the family as to the kind of care and attention the patient will receive. An explanation as to visiting hours and the necessary visiting regulations will benefit relatives and offer encouragement to them, since it invites planning for subsequent visits with the patient.

Good Manners. Good manners help to establish a desirable nurse–patient relationship. Meeting the patient for the first time, the nurse should introduce herself by mentioning only her *last* name. To give her first name to the patient is to encourage him to address her by it, which might be embarrassing to her if done in the presence of a member of the medical staff or of the nursing faculty.

If she calls him by his proper name, mentions the name of his attending physician, and indicates that she is pleased to do nursing duties for him she will have done much toward gaining his confidence and good will.

The tendency on the part of nurses to associate the room number, instead of the name, with the patients they care for is regrettable. The habit of referring to Mr. Brown as "108" or "234" should be discouraged. With practice a nurse can readily become proficient in remembering names.

To enter the room of a patient without knocking, to interrupt his conversation with the doctor or a visitor, to disregard the fact that he is listening to a radio or television program, to carelessly accept a gift or gesture of appreciation without showing gratitude, or to be thoughtless in regard to common courtesies and social customs, shows a definite lack of social grace and is even more unbecoming in a nurse than in persons of other walks of life.

Conversational Ability. In conversing with a patient the nurse should speak clearly and distinctly, refrain from the use of illiterate speech or poor grammar, and never use slang. To respond to a question from the patient with an unthinking "O.K.," or an equally disconcerting "Sure will," is indicative of a lack of education and of a questionable social background.

Nurses who use profane or obscene language, especially in the presence of a patient, show little regard for accepted standards of social conduct and are probably equally lacking in fundamental qualities which characterize the desirable members of their profession.

Self-training in the art of conversation is part of the developmental process of the student nurse. She should be able to converse intelligently on various subjects, yet refrain from a discussion of personal affairs, of other patients, or the hospital in which she is receiving her nursing education. She should be able, by close observation of the patient, to know when he wishes to talk and to recognize a reluctance on his part to talk or listen to conversation.

The nurse who chatters incessantly may be very trying to a patient and through this one social error can destroy the effectiveness of the nursing procedure she is doing, even though her technical skill in performing the procedure is highly satisfactory.

Conversely, the nurse who limits her conversation to a few well chosen remarks and then becomes an interested and sympathetic listener is well on the way to impressing a patient with her ability as a conversationalist.

Tone of Voice. The student nurse who wishes to do so can cultivate a good speaking voice. By reading aloud each day for ten minutes she can successfully overcome a lack of expression, add warmth to her voice while lowering its tone, and also correct such defects as poor enunciation and pronunciation. If possible, she should have a record made of her voice, study the faults that are apparent, and then take the necessary steps to correct them.

Conventional Behavior. Since nurses complain that some men patients tend to be unduly familiar, it is well to mention here that such attempts at familiarity are usually the result of the attitude of the nurse concerned. If she conducts herself in a dignified and professional manner few men will be other than courteous and gentlemanly. Conventions of society are respected by most men and they rarely transgress rules of conduct while in the hospital without having been encouraged to do so by a seeming lack of decorum in the actions and speech of the nurse.

The Very Young Patient. The nurse assigned to care for a child is expected to meet the psychological as well as physiological needs of her small charge. The average child who must be hospitalized is undergoing the experience of leaving a secure and familiar home environment for one that is altogether strange and frightening.

Doctors and nurses now realize that it is impossible completely to overcome physical disability unless psychological and social needs are also given consideration. The well qualified children's nurse, through the use of toys, books, and other recreational facilities, does a great deal to provide full opportunity for the very young patient to remain in close contact with articles familiar to him from his home environment.

The child of school age need not fall behind in classwork because illness interrupts his attendance at school. Instruction can be continued by the nurse, the social worker, or teachers hired to perform such duties.

The immediate environment of the child may be made bright and cheerful if the nurse is interested in providing for his greater contentment. The use by hospitals of bright colors on walls and floors, of gay draperies at the windows, and of paintings and murals depicting Mother Goose characters or scenes from circus life provides a

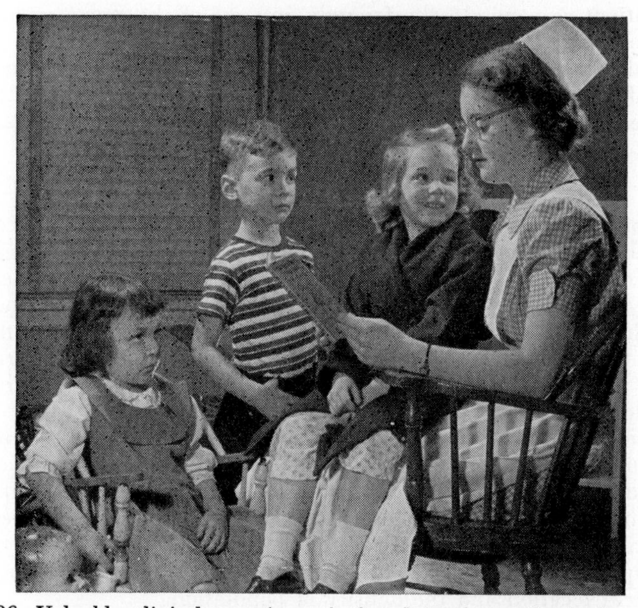

Fig. 26. Valuable clinical experience is found in the pediatric department. (Harper Hospital School of Nursing, Detroit, Michigan.)

source of constant enjoyment for child patients. Use of color books, special recordings, radio or television programs, and opportunity to talk with other children in the department play an important part in ultimate recovery.

The nurse becomes a substitute mother, friend, and teacher to the sick child, and she soon learns that the small patient who is entertained and amused, as well as treated for illness or injury, will cooperate more readily with hospital personnel directly concerned with his care.

Spiritual Needs of the Patient. A nurse is sometimes called on to provide for the religious or spiritual needs of her patient. She should bear in mind the statement of a hospital chaplain that "illness is basically a spiritual problem and health is a spiritual condition." Much of a spiritual nature is involved for each patient: in the apprehension and fear which cause some of them to delay seeking medical help, in the faith with which some finally accept need for medical or surgical treatment, in the mastery of physical pain and disability which some display, and in the way others meet death, the final crisis of illness. Spiritual needs of the patient are discussed in Chapter 37.

In the truly successful nurse–patient relationship the nurse inspires confidence, cooperates with others for the care of the patient, and performs nursing duties with skill and ease. Under such circumstances the patient responds to the friendly interest of the nurse and other hospital workers, accepts the treatment and medications offered him, and follows instructions not only for relief of present symptoms and cure of present illness, but for the prevention of future disability or disease.

THE NURSE AND THE COMMUNITY

In previous years the doctor and nurse were primarily concerned with the treatment and cure of disease and with measures to control its spread in the community. Today emphasis is placed on helping people of the nation to prevent disease and to maintain good health.

To help promote health the nurse should know the importance of preventing disease, of teaching health concepts, and of encouraging needy families to secure the benefits available through local health agencies.

"Community" Defined. To clarify the position of the nurse in the community it is necessary to define the term "community." Generally defined as "a group of people living within a certain geographical area and somewhat bound together through their common interests or activities," the term is similarly applied to the area occupied by such a group. A community may be rural or urban, depending on the geographical location and the density of population.

The rural community usually has less effective health organizations and a relatively smaller number of doctors and nurses, as well as a very small number of hospital beds available for care of the sick. The mortality rate in rural communities, however, is lower than that in urban areas.

The nurse who takes part in civic affairs derives satisfaction from performing important work in democracy. She enlarges her own horizon, broadens her interests, meets new and interesting people, and is not limited by her career as are other nurses who seem interested only in nursing.

Activities within the Community. The activities of family life, including the economic aspects of family or group living, are of special interest to the nurse concerned with public health, or the health of her community. She needs to know home backgrounds to better understand the effect of home life on the children. Her concern includes the amount and type of food served, the kind of furnishings in the home, the number of people living together as a family unit, and numerous other factors affecting the health and well-being of the entire group.

Besides understanding family life, the nurse should be familiar with the many aspects of community living directly related to the health record and the health problems of the community. She should have at least a basic knowledge of the industrial, professional, or agricultural activities which form the chief means of livelihood for the people. Her interest should extend to the housing facilities, and to problems resulting from lack of such facilities, crowded living conditions, and the ever increasing cost of establishing or maintaining a home. She should be interested in educational facilities for the training of adults as well as children. The local newspaper, the radio station, and the library should be considered as a means of making health education available to all within the local area.

The public health nurse should promote recreational activities within the community, helping in the effort to provide public playgrounds for children and entertainment of various forms for the adults. She may take part in religious activities and in activities concerned with transportation and communication. Above all, she should have a thorough knowledge of existing social service agencies which provide unemployment relief and care for the aged or poor, and promote health and general welfare of the public.

Social Services in the Community. Various social services in the community are supported financially by public funds, obtained by taxation, and by private funds which are contributed as gifts or obtained through community fund drives. The well known "Community Chest" fund helps to finance practically every known agency or institution serving the community.

Through "Family Services" aid is given to families in the form of food, clothing, rent, the finding of suitable shelters or homes, and, if possible, the securing of employment for the wage earner of the family. In offering aid of this kind to needy families an attempt is made to discover the cause of their apparent inability to provide the essentials of life and to prevent recurrence of a similar situation. Such organizations as the Y.M.C.A., Y.W.C.A., Boy Scouts, Girl Scouts, 4-H clubs, and others work with the youth of today to help make better citizens for tomorrow. Day nurseries, orphanages, child placement bureaus, institutions for the care of dependent or old people, and similar agencies are concerned with care of children and the aged.

Health Agencies in the Community. Through community health agencies the nurse is able to achieve her greatest service to the public. Much of her work is in the hospital, and the hospital is an integral part of the community health plan, not only serving to care for the sick but providing the means for education of doctors and nurses and playing an important role in preserving and promoting health.

The public health agencies, on the federal, state, county and city or local level, function to prevent disease and to promote general health. The most important of the federal health agencies include the United States Public Health Service, the Bureau of Home Economics, the Pure Food and Drug Agency, the Children's Bureau, and the Office of Indian Affairs.

In addition to agencies named above private agencies, such as the Visiting Nurse Association, are also concerned with health programs.

Through the V.N.A. care is furnished to the sick at a price which they can afford to pay or at no cost, if they are unable to pay. The three main types of service given are care of illness, care of maternity patients, and health teaching and supervision.

The City Department of Health, set up by law, usually provides for health education, compilation of vital statistics, control of communicable diseases, child welfare and maternity work, inspection of food and water supplies, control of the sale and use of drugs, laboratory service in relation to disease diagnosis and control, and public health nursing.

Nurses in public health service are on duty in schools and clinics, caring for maternity cases, helping to teach public health nursing to students in schools of nursing, and promoting health education to assist in prevention and control of such diseases as tuberculosis.

Progress Made in Community Health. The practice of "neighborly nursing" in some communities is helping to solve health problems in the particular area. In each community there are always mothers returning from the hospital with new babies, or those who are ill and have young children needing care. Married nurses in the community, working part time to care for the ill, help to solve some of the problems imposed by illness on neighbors and friends.

Nursing service is only a part of this community aid. Housekeepers, too, are on call and go where their services are needed. Volunteer workers do the marketing or see that the laundry is done, contributing their share of aid to the homemaker in need of such help.

By promoting good health for the community the people are assured a better community. Improved health care has resulted in an increase in life expectancy. Early in the 19th century the average length of life in United States was 40 years. Now life expectancy for men is 64 years and for women 68 years.

The advancement of education in regard to nutritional needs has been another accomplishment of community health programs. This country produces an abundance of food, and each year sees more progress in an effort to provide all its people with balanced, adequate diets. The relation of proper nutrition to good health is better understood, and more and more widely practiced.

Progress has also been made in medical science, leading to improved methods of diagnosis and treatment. The use of new and highly effective drugs has radically changed the accepted method of treating certain diseases. Educational programs have made people aware of the importance of early diagnosis and enabled them to recognize early symptoms of many different diseases.

Maternal and infant deaths have steadily decreased because of the effectiveness of improved prenatal care, premarital and antepartum tests for syphilis and its subsequent treatment, a greater knowledge in the field of obstetrics, and the use of drugs in controlling postpartum infections.

Communicable diseases have decreased due to effective immunization programs and to chemotherapy.

Current Health Problems. Despite the worth-while accomplishments in the field of public health there are still problems which merit the attention of public health agencies.

There is an increase in degenerative diseases such as heart disease, cancer, and diseases of the kidneys. The increase in these diseases is related to the increased span of life, even though the diseases may occur in the young as well as the aged. The incidence of chronic diseases, which create a large number of health problems, has greatly increased.

During recent years accidents have taken an increasing toll of human lives, until they now rate fourth place in the leading causes of death. The greater number of the deaths are the result of accidents in the home and on the highways, rather than of major disasters.

Although some communicable diseases have declined or become almost nonexistent, others continue to present major problems. At the present time no effective treatment or cure has been found for the common cold, which is one of the most annoying and most costly of all minor illnesses. Measles and whooping cough continue to be major hazards for young children. Tuberculosis has increased in rate since World War II, although the record for the past several years has shown a decrease in the number of patients affected.

The incidence of venereal disease shows a sharp increase, especially in the teen-age group. These diseases are among the most difficult to control and are high on the list of current health problems.

Mental illness occurs more frequently than all other diseases combined, and at the present time over 50 per cent of all hospital beds in the United States are occupied by mental patients. Although much has been done to provide treatment for the mentally ill, there is still a great and urgent need for more and better facilities and for doctors, nurses, and other personnel to provide the needed care.

To be of greatest service in the health program of the community, the nurse must recognize that she is an important factor in health education. She is expected to play a part in the prevention and control of disease, to assist in the care of the sick, and to teach health practices, not only by precept but by example. Nurses should be taught in their schools how to be good citizens as well as to become adept at nursing. Because of her technical knowledge and training, the nurse can be a decided asset in any civic organization. She usually knows better than other members of the organization the community problems related to health. Knowing that the health of the individual depends on his ability to gain for himself and his family the necessities of life, such as food, clothing, and shelter, the nurse must be interested in ways and means of helping the individual meet his responsibilities. To promote individual and public health she needs to continue to study the people, the conditions, and the health facil-

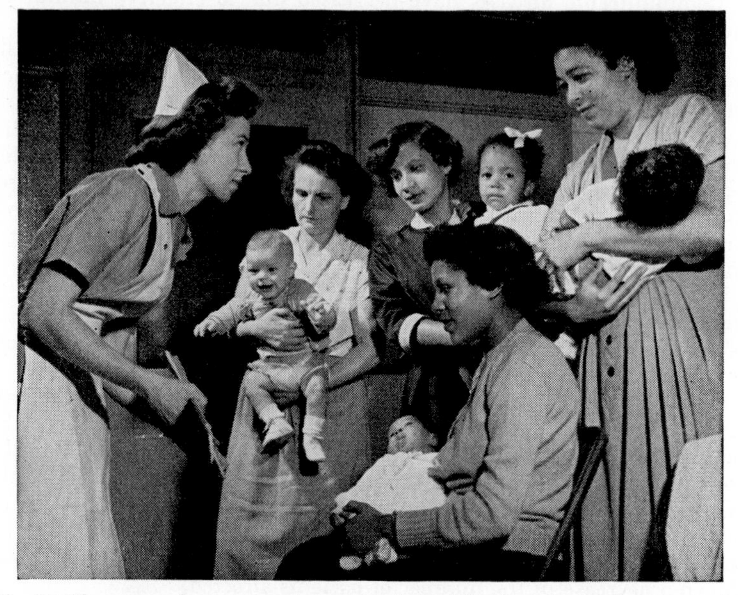

Fig. 27. The nurse plays an important part in health education in the community. (Washington University School of Nursing, St. Louis, Missouri.)

ities within the community in order to be instrumental in furthering the community health program.

Civil Defense. At a time when civil defense is of paramount importance, the professional nurse is expected to take an active part in the planning necessary to the program. The local communities are the core of the total civil defense effort, and the nurse plays a very important role in the defense program of her local community. Her work in the total program is discussed in Chapter 42, on "Radiation."

Summary of Important Factors

As the doctor delegates more medical procedures to the nurse she must be adequately prepared by education and practice to perform those procedures skillfully.

Relationship between doctor and nurse is usually that of teacher–pupil. Familiarity between doctor and nurse tends to destroy the dignity and co-worker relationship needed to serve the patient.

The nurse should not recommend one particular doctor to someone needing a doctor's services; she should name several, and let the patient make a choice.

The student nurse should not accept verbal orders from the doctor.

The nurse is responsible if she administers a prescribed drug in an amount that she should know would be harmful to the patient.

The nurse should never attempt to diagnose or prescribe treatment.

All personnel within the hospital have the common aim of rendering service to the patient. Each should cooperate with the others to achieve that aim.

The nurse should know the plan of organization for the hospital as a whole and for the nursing department so she will understand her relationship to others on the hospital staff.

The patient looks to the nurse for orientation to the hospital experience.

Personal appearance of the nurse is of major importance in establishing good nurse–patient relationship.

A nurse should (1) be able to recognize restlessness, fear, and irritability in the patient as abnormal reactions occasioned by illness; (2) be cheerful, considerate, reassuring; (3) express confidence in the ability of the patient's doctor; (4) establish good relationship with relatives of patients.

The nurse should be able to make introductions as necessary, giving her last name to the patient. She should knock before entering a patient's room, and refrain from interrupting a conversation between the patient and another person. In conversation she should refrain from the use of slang and poor grammar, be able to converse intelligently on current events, and never use profane or obscene language.

Planned care requires that the nurse cooperate with the doctor, dietitian, and others attending the patient, and that she explain procedures to the patient according to his ability to understand.

The child patient should be provided with toys, books, and other familiar articles to make him feel that the hospital surroundings are less strange. The nurse may also see that the child is entertained by radio, television, and association with the other children.

The nurse has a responsibility to her community: (1) to help prevent disease; (2) to teach health practices; (3) to refer families to local health agencies for help; (4) to help plan and execute a program for civil defense; (5) to make her knowledge and training available to the community for service in meeting health problems.

Factors To Teach the Patient

Confidence in the doctor should be fostered by the nurse's expression of her own belief in the doctor's ability.

The patient should be aware that all hospital workers are well qualified for the duties they perform and that his cooperation will insure greater benefit to himself.

Cooperation of the patient in taking medicines and accepting treatments will hasten recovery.

The best means of overcoming anxiety, fear, worry is the help that is available to the patient through social agencies and the clergy. Patients or their families should be referred to proper local agencies for needed assistance.

Members of the community should be taught: (1) how to protect themselves and families in an emergency; (2) how to care for the sick and injured at home; (3) how to serve best in time of disaster.

Suggested Reference Reading

"Nurses are citizens," Donald Faulkner; American Journal of Nursing, January, 1949.

"Neighborly nursing," Muriel Matson Kennedy; American Journal of Nursing, December, 1949.

"Does your voice defeat you?" Barbara Brice Lias; American Journal of Nursing, May, 1951.

"Status of the practical nurse," E. Turnbull; Hospital Management, February, 1952.

"It's true what they say about human relations," A. S. Kelsey; Modern Hospital, February, 1952.

"Personal relationships and nursing service," Lucy D. Germain; American Journal of Nursing, October, 1952.

"The patient's point of view," Patricia Jones; Canadian Nurse, October, 1952.

"What lights the lamp?" William S. Brines; Modern Hospital, November, 1952.

PART II

The Hospital Environment

CHAPTER 4

Hospital Housekeeping

TOPICAL OUTLINE

Care of Floors
Care of Furniture
Care of Linen
Care of Linen Closet
Care of Ward Kitchen
Care of Utility Room
Care of Flower Room
Care of Room After Dismissal of Patient
Control of Insects and Other Pests
Sanitary Facilities
General Cleanliness
    Cleaning of Equipment and Supplies

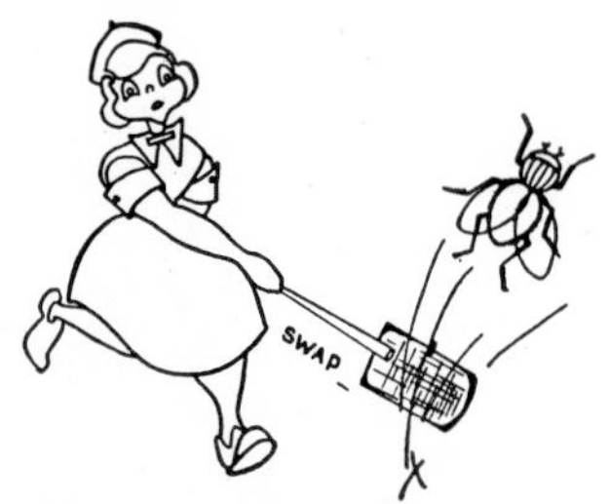

The hand is quicker than the eye, but somewhat slower than the fly!

Instruction given to students in schools of nursing would be incomplete without including information which would enable them to understand the basic principles of hospital housekeeping. Although the nurse is seldom called on to perform domestic services in the hospital she often must supervise or help instruct maids and other personnel whose duties include cleaning, dusting, and caring for hospital property. To be able to supervise such work she should know what is required, and she should be capable of performing the housekeeping tasks herself should the need arise.

The housekeeping department is under supervision of a housekeeper who is responsible for maintaining all departments and rooms in good condition and a state of cleanliness satisfactory to even the most fastidious patient. She is in charge of janitors and maids throughout the institution and is responsible to the business manager or hospital superintendent.

The housekeeper, while keeping the hospital clean, should also be responsible for making certain that hospital furnishings or equipment in need of repair is reported to the maintenance department. She should see that patient rooms and wards are comfortably and tastefully furnished, and all departments in the hospital are attractive and pleasant. By better understanding the functions of the housekeeping department, a nurse is better able to cooperate with that department while performing nursing duties.

Factors relating to housekeeping about which a nurse should be informed include the care of hospital furnishings and equipment, the care of various parts of the nursing departments throughout the hospital, the care of the patient's room or unit, and the control of insects or pests.

CARE OF FLOORS

The care of flooring within the hospital depends to a large extent on the material used in its construction and the way it is installed. Floors should be made of material that will resist wear and will not absorb odors; they must be attractive as well as durable, fire resistant, and easily maintained. The nurse's chief concern in floor care is for that in the patient's room or unit, care of his immediate environment becomes her responsibility. The cleaning and care of other floors is done by domestic workers under direct supervision of the hospital housekeeper.

Floors in private rooms or in ward units are usually of hardwood or linoleum.

Care of Linoleum Floors. Linoleum floors should be wet-mopped or scrubbed and, when thoroughly dry again, liquid floor wax should be applied and rubbed on until the floor is completely covered. Linoleum should be waxed and polished every 7 to 10 days, depending on the wear the floor receives. To protect linoleum, which is soft and easily dented, furniture shoes or glass cups can be placed under legs of the furniture. Waxed linoleum floors should be mopped carefully every day with a dust-proof mop.

Care of Wood Floors. Wood floors should be kept waxed and polished and mopped daily with a dustless mop to remove all lint or dust. They should be thoroughly cleaned, about every four months, with the electrical scrubbing machine, which makes use of a heavy brush and suction apparatus to scrub, rinse, and suction clean the floors in patient rooms and in hospital corridors.

CARE OF FURNITURE

Metal furniture may be adequately cared for by frequent washing with warm water and soap. Scouring powder may scratch the surface of the furniture and for that reason should not be used. In the daily cleaning of the room care should be exercised in moving the furniture so that it does not become marred or scratched. Metal furniture, as well as wood, should be handled carefully to prevent needless denting of its surfaces.

By use of modern furnishings in the clinical departments of the hospital beauty is combined with utility. Attractive, colorful furniture

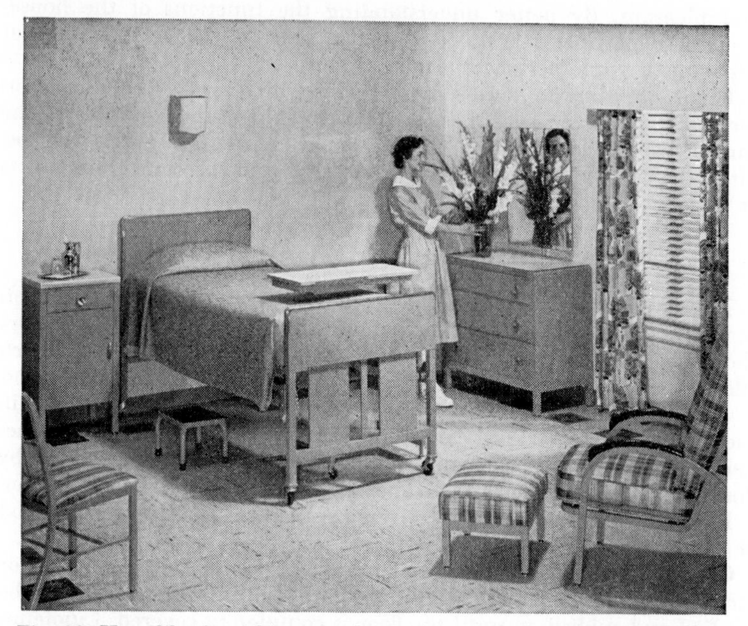

Fig. 28. Homelike furnishings for hospitals provide attractive rooms for the patients and simplify housekeeping tasks. (Simmons Company, Merchandise Mart, Chicago, Illinois.)

can be used with softly harmonizing colors in drapes and bedspreads to provide a cheerful, more suitable environment for patients. One very pleasing combination of color is achieved by use of natural wood furniture that is golden cream in color. Used with parchment shade walls, light brown inlaid linoleum, draperies of rainbow colors, and a bedspread of eggshell and brown chenille, the result is a beautiful and practical hospital room.

Most wood furniture used in hospitals has a water-proof finish and is made to withstand an excessive amount of wear. Each piece is simple in design and can be readily washed, cleaned, or disinfected, as necessary.

The following suggestions relate to the use and care of hospital furniture, whether it is of metal or wood:

1. In rooms where furniture is of a matching set, do not move the bed to another room when transferring a patient. The bed should remain with the set of furnishings for which it was made.

2. Do not force drawers or doors which are difficult to close—investigate to see if an article of equipment or linen has been crowded into the drawer or compartment thus preventing the drawer or door

from closing. To force closing in such an instance will damage the piece of furniture.

3. Report damage or breakage of furniture immediately so it can be repaired before it is damaged further.

4. Protect the dresser and bedside table by placing a suitable dish or container under each flower pot or vase brought into the patient's room.

5. When using the overbed table raise it high enough to clear the foot of the bed so it will not be damaged when moved.

6. When using the bed cranks—they should be pulled completely out when needed to elevate or lower the head or foot of the bed. If only partially in place the crank may hit the end of the bed, scratching or marring it as each rotation is made.

7. Use a tepid, mild soap solution to wash the furniture, and dry it carefully after it has been washed.

8. If anything is spilled on the furniture be sure that it is immediately mopped up. Report the incident to the housekeeper who may need to take additional precautions to prevent permanent damage to the finish.

9. Provide ash trays for the patient and his visitors who smoke so furniture need not be marred by careless handling of a lighted cigarette.

CARE OF LINEN

Another important phase of hospital housekeeping with which the nurse should be familiar is the distribution, use, and care of linen.

Linen is constantly being torn or worn out, necessitating mending or replacement. Linen articles that are only slightly damaged, yet cannot be satisfactorily mended, may be made over and used for other purposes. Linen too badly damaged or worn to be used as linen may still be utilized as cloths for cleaning and dusting.

Although the over-all distribution and care of linen is the responsibility of the housekeeper, each department supervisor should see that an adequate supply of linen is maintained for her department. Articles ordered by daily requisition should be in numbers large enough to meet the needs of the department yet should not seriously deplete the supply in the central linen room or greatly exceed that really needed on the department.

Removal of Stains. Although the removal of stains from linens or from bedspreads, drapes, and chair covers is the responsibility of the housekeeping department, the nurse may prevent the stain from becoming set by giving the matter immediate attention. If the article is taken at once to the housekeeper the stain may usually be removed without damage to the fabric.

Care of Linen Closet. A spacious linen closet is needed on each clinical department for storage of linen which will eventually be dispensed for use in that particular department. Shelves in the linen closet should be kept as clean as the linen that is daily placed on them.

All linen and other articles in the closet should be arranged on the shelves in an orderly manner. Before or while being placed on the shelves, the linen should be counted to make sure the proper amount has been received from the central linen room. All small articles such as T binders, wash cloths, and bedpan covers should be properly folded and placed on designated shelves or in cupboard drawers provided for them.

After the patients have had their morning care and baths, the linen closet should be put in order. During these procedures nurses tend to re-arrange linen or get it out of order by hastily removing items needed in bathing and caring for the patient.

The head nurse should assume charge of the linen closet and dispense all linen. Private duty nurses should be given the amount of linen required to care for their patients, but should not be permitted to hoard linen, thus needlessly depriving the rest of the department.

In the linen closet a circular pole (a broom handle of proper length) should be fastened so that it is parallel to the wall and about 8" from it. All rubber sheets not in use on the department should be hung over the pole. If they are folded to be put in storage, the rubber cracks and the sheet is rendered useless.

If the blanket warmer is located near the linen closet it may be checked and given daily care by the same person assigned to care for linen. Only a few blankets, which might be needed in an emergency, need to be kept in the blanket warmer at a given time.

The floor of the linen closet should be kept clean and free from lint.

CARE OF WARD KITCHEN

The kitchen or serving room on the various clinical departments is usually furnished and equipped the same, whether it is on a medical, surgical, obstetrical, or other special service department. It contains a stove, refrigerator, chest for cracked ice, a cupboard with plenty of shelf space for dishes and staple goods (as coffee, sugar, crackers, and bread), drawers for silverware, and a work table or counter. On the counter the toaster and percolater are kept so they will be ready for use at any time. Each kitchen contains a sink, a bulletin board, and the shaft with openings for dumb waiter service or a service elevator that opens into the room for transportation of the food truck.

All kitchen appliances, equipment, and supplies must be kept scrupulously clean. Usually a kitchen maid is assigned to work full time at keeping the kitchen neat and clean and helping with the preparation of food and nourishment for the patients.

Cupboard. If the cupboard is built of wood and painted with white enamel paint, it should be damp dusted daily and washed thoroughly at least once a week with hot soapy water.

Dishes and all other service utensils should be kept in designated places in the cupboard. If necessary, a diagram should be made so all personnel knows where each article belongs, and can replace articles so they are easily found when needed.

Stove. After a meal is served the stove should be cleaned. It can be rubbed with crushed newspaper and then with a cloth dampened with a thin oil.

If a gas stove is used all movable parts should be removed once a week and thoroughly cleaned with soap and water. The parts should then be allowed to dry before they are polished. All parts should then be replaced, tightly fitted, and the stove made ready for use again.

Sink. The kitchen sink should be kept clean at all times, being thoroughly washed and dried after each use. Greasy liquids should not be poured into the sink since grease will gradually accumulate in and clog the pipes. The small amount of grease present in ordinary dishwater will not affect the plumbing if the sink and pipes are flooded with hot water after the dishwater is emptied. A strong solution of bicarbonate of soda poured into the pipes before the hot water is turned on will help to cut the grease if there is an accumulation.

Scouring powder may be necessary to keep the sink white and clean. Metal fixtures should be kept clean and sparkling so the sink always presents an attractive appearance.

Refrigerator. The cleanliness of the interior of the refrigerator determines to a large extent the efficiency with which it does its work. To keep the refrigerator in good condition the following weekly care is recommended:

Remove all food from the refrigerator. Defrost the refrigerator, allowing plenty of time for all accumulated ice to melt and drain from the cooling unit. Remove all racks or movable inner parts from the refrigerator—wash all removable parts and the inside of the refrigerator with an ammonia solution. Rinse well with clear water, dry thoroughly, replace racks, then replace all food after making sure that food is put in clean containers, if necessary, and that food not likely to be used is discarded.

Each day the inside of the refrigerator should be given care and attention. Food not used the previous day should be discarded.

If medications are kept in the refrigerator they should be clearly labeled and the containers kept clean and in order.

Other Kitchen Equipment. The kitchen should be well equipped with such necessities as egg beater, sharp knives, fruit juicer, mixing bowls, and a generous supply of glass tumblers and drinking tubes.

Food served from a kitchen that is clean and neat will probably

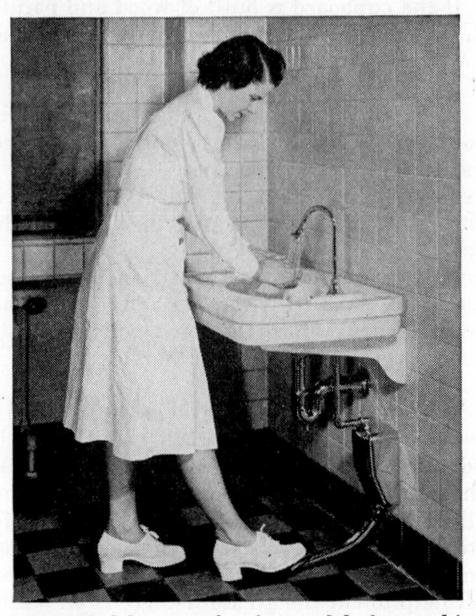

Fig. 29. Water, provided by use of a foot pedal, for washing hands in the utility room is an added convenience for the nurse. (Crane Company, Chicago, Illinois.)

look better and will surely be more palatable to the patient. The nurses and other personnel will enjoy serving trays if they come from a kitchen in which the kitchen maid obviously takes great pride.

CARE OF UTILITY ROOM

All personnel on duty in the various nursing departments should feel a responsibility for helping to keep the utility room clean. This room is often referred to as the "work room," since so many tasks are performed there. Each time equipment in the room is used it should be cleaned and made ready for use again. Tables or shelves on which stock solutions are kept should always be neat and clean. The sink should be kept as clean as the sink in the kitchen. If bedpans are emptied in an open hopper, a bedpan brush must be provided to be used in cleaning the hopper as well as the bedpan. Hot soapy water is the best agent for thoroughly cleaning the hopper and removing discolorations. If an open hopper is used a sterilizer should be provided so the bedpan may be sterilized after use.

New built-in bedpan cleaners and sterilizers provide for a cleaner and simpler bedpan technique. A foot pedal opens the sterilizer and the bedpan, with its contents, is placed in the space provided. The cover automatically closes, the bedpan empties itself and is washed with cold, then hot water, remaining in place the bedpan is then subjected to live steam and is sterilized. The steam automatically shuts off and the sterilizer can then be opened by means of the foot pedal.

If bedpans and urinals not in use in patient units are kept in the utility room they should be washed in soap and water at frequent intervals. Racks which hold the utensils should also be kept clean.

CARE OF FLOWER ROOM

After the cut flowers and plants have been suitably cared for each morning the flower room should be properly cleaned. An ideal arrangement is for the flower room to be located near the utility room so all dead flowers, paper boxes, and other refuse may be discarded into the incinerator. If the room is neat and clean the task of arranging or caring for flowers becomes much more pleasant.

In addition to a sink with running water, the flower room should contain a work table of proper height, a supply of flower baskets, vases, and bowls, sharp scissors, a knife and assorted needle holders and other articles needed in arranging flowers in their proper containers. The kind of container used and the way in which flowers are arranged will add to or detract from their appearance.

If possible, refrigeration should be provided in the flower room for those flowers which are not to be taken immediately to the patient. When cut flowers are discarded the vase or container in which they had been arranged should be cleaned and inverted so it will drain sufficiently to be ready for use again when needed.

CARE OF ROOM AFTER DISMISSAL OF PATIENT

After the patient has been dismissed from the hospital the room or unit he occupied should be cleaned and aired. The nurse is seldom required to clean the unit, but she may need to supervise the work as it is done by nurse aide or maid. Before beginning the actual cleaning procedure all windows should be opened wide to permit adequate ventilation of the room. Window shades or venetian blinds should be raised to the greatest height possible to permit sunshine to flood the room.

Enamelware, thermometers, and all other hospital equipment used by the patient should be taken to the utility room where it may be properly cleaned, sterilized or disinfected, and made ready for use again. The thermometer should be washed in soap solution, rinsed, and dried; the thermometer container should be washed, rinsed, and dried thoroughly. All enamelware, such as wash basin, urinal, and bedpan should be thoroughly washed; the bedpan and urinal should be sterilized. The bottle containing alcohol for back rubs should be washed outside and refilled with alcohol for use by the next patient. If the patient is charged for back rubbing alcohol, the partly used bottle should have been sent home with him and a new bottle be ordered for the next patient to be admitted to the room.

All old magazines, flowers, and other unwanted articles which the patient left behind should be discarded.

All used linen should be removed from the room, linen that was brought into the room, but not used for the patient, should be sent to the laundry along with the soiled linen. Even though the linen may not have been used it has been in contact with the patient or his immediate surroundings and would not be suitable for use for another patient.

Blankets and candlewick bedspreads, that need to be cleaned before being used again, should be labeled and turned in to the housekeeper. The mattress and pillows should be thoroughly brushed, using a whisk broom, they should then be placed in the room where air is circulating and they will receive direct sunshine for a while.

Any article of clothing or other personal belongings that have been left by the patient should be taken to the head nurse, who will give instructions as to how the article or property may be returned to its owner.

Window ledges and window sills should be washed. If necessary, woodwork in the room should be cleaned in the same manner. All light fixtures and lamps should be cleaned and polished. Furnishings in the room, including the inside of the dresser and the bedside table, as well as the springs and framework of the bed, should be washed with an antiseptic solution and immediately dried. The mirror on the dresser and the inside of the clothes closet should be cleaned. If any piece of furniture has been marred or damaged a report of repairs that are needed should be made to the nurse in charge. If slip covers on the chair or drapes at the window are soiled, the housekeeper should be notified. Clean slip covers and different drapes can be obtained to replace those being sent to the cleaner. All furniture which is not washed in cleaning the room should be dusted.

All throw rugs should be removed and cleaned with a vacuum cleaner. The nurse or housekeeper should see that the maid properly cleans the floor of the room, and if the radiator needs to be cleaned should instruct her in this procedure. A newspaper should be folded and sprinkled rather heavily with water then spread beneath the radiator. The radiator should then be cleaned with a long-handled radiator brush. After dust particles removed from the radiator have settled on the dampened newspaper it can be removed and placed in the incinerator. The radiator can then be dusted with the dry cloth used to dust furniture.

After the room has been thoroughly cleaned and ventilated, furniture should be placed in proper position, throw rugs should be returned to their place, and all enamelware and other needed equipment should be returned to the bedside table.

A complete towel set with wash cloth should be placed in the bedside table drawer. A bottle of alcohol to be used for back rubs and the clinical thermometer should be left in the room. A fresh cake of soap should be provided for the soap dish, which is kept in the bedside table drawer.

One of the dresser drawers should contain a woolen blanket to be used for extra cover at night. A bath blanket and a linen bag should also be left in one of the drawers of the dresser.

The bed should be made into a closed bed, with care taken not to tuck top covers in at the side so tightly that the bed will have to be remade when a new patient is admitted.

The signal light should be checked to see that it is functioning properly.

The window should be closed and the window shade should be drawn approximately 18 inches from the window sill.

The door of the room should be left slightly ajar and all lights should be turned off.

CONTROL OF INSECTS AND OTHER PESTS

The variety of insects which present a problem in the hospital depends to some extent on the geographic location of the hospital. In North America the most common hospital "pests" and the ones with which nurses are chiefly concerned include flies, mosquitoes, moths, bedbugs, cockroaches, centipedes, pediculi, fleas, mice, and rats (see Table 2 and Figure 30). Such pests are known to be responsible for the spread of communicable diseases by direct contact or indirectly through contamination of water or food supplies.

Most hospitals engage the services of an exterminating company to keep the institution relatively free of pests. Even with this method of control, nurses should understand the principles involved and cooperate in helping to eliminate or control hospital pests.

Flies. Flies are found wherever dirt and filth and unsanitary conditions exist, apparently thriving best in putrefying and fermenting organic matter.

Although the house fly is the most common species, several species are found wherever food is handled or dispensed. In hospitals, hotels, restaurants, bakeries, etc. may be seen the housefly, stable fly, food maggot fly, green bottle fly, and the blue bottle blowfly.

Flies are attracted to body excreta and other forms of filth. Contaminated by direct contact with dirt and filth, they carry microorganisms causing infection on their spiny, sticky feet and legs as well as on fine hairs protruding from their heads.

Scientific experiments have proved that the causative microorganisms of such diseases as typhoid fever, dysentery, and tuberculosis have been carried by flies. Intestinal infections which are often prevalent in babies are usually caused by contamination from flies.

To control flies public health agencies must be concerned with measures which provide for the destruction of breeding places, the enforcement of sanitary regulations in public eating places and other institutions and for effective campaigns against their growth and development.

In the hospital it is necessary for personnel of the various departments to wage continuous war on all housekeeping pests. Food should be kept in covered containers; garbage and other waste should be properly disposed of before it can be accessible to flies. Bedpans should be kept thoroughly clean. If necessary, fly paper, fly traps, fly swatters, and fly spray should be used to help eliminate the harmful insects.

D.D.T., used effectively during the war to control insects and pests

Table 2. COMMON HOSPITAL INSECTS

INSECT	WHERE FOUND	LIFE STAGES	LIFE CYCLE	AVERAGE REPRODUCTION RATE PER YEAR	EXTENT OF DAMAGE	IDENTIFYING FEATURES AND CHARACTERISTICS
Ant	On lawns. In buildings. In diet kitchens. Where food is found. In storerooms.	Egg Larva Pupa Adult	3 months. Thousands of eggs laid by the Queen.	2,000	Can do serious damage to rafters and beams in buildings. Destroys food.	Black in color, ¼ to ½ inch long. Home colonies contain as many as 2,000 to 3,000 workers.
Bedbug	In hotels, hospitals, and other institutions. In patient rooms and in lounge rooms used by employees.	Egg Nymph Adult	2 months. 50 eggs.	200	Attacks and bites humans—may cause serious infection.	Dark brown in color, ¼ inch long. Has piercing and sucking mouth parts. Casts its skin five times to complete growth.
Beetle	In flour mills and bakeries. In storerooms where flour, cereals, and grains are stored.	Egg Larva Pupa Adult	4 weeks. 400 eggs.	3,000	Ruins flour and other stored supplies; converts flour into a gray, useless mass.	Brown in color, ⅛ inch long. Worst of all pests in bakeries, flour mills, and rooms where grains are stored.

Booklouse	In flour mills and bakeries. In places where old books and papers accumulate.	Egg Nymph Adult	150 days. 60 eggs.	500	Presence is a source of annoyance.	Gray in color, wingless; 1/25 inch long. Lives on microscopic molds.
Centipede	In hospitals and other institutions. In damp basements, boiler rooms, and utility rooms.	Egg Adult (The egg hatches within the body of the adult.)	1–2 years. Eggs not laid; young are born alive.	10	Presence is a source of annoyance.	Gray in color, 1 inch long. Has 15 pairs of legs, last 2 pairs are longer than the others. Not a true insect. Feeds on insects.

Table 2. Common Hospital Insects (Continued)

INSECT	WHERE FOUND	LIFE STAGES	LIFE CYCLE	AVERAGE REPRODUCTION RATE PER YEAR	EXTENT OF DAMAGE	IDENTIFYING FEATURES AND CHARACTERISTICS
Cockroach	In industrial plants and institutions. In damp basements, wash rooms, kitchens, boiler rooms, elevator shafts, utility rooms.	Egg Nymph Adult	250–300 days. 30–40 eggs per egg case; 2–5 egg cases.	4,500	Destroys food stuffs, labels, and cartons. Leaves disagreeable odor. Carries filth.	Light brown color, 5/8 inches long. Has chewing mouth parts. Shuns light, runs crazily when exposed to sudden light. Casts skin six times to complete growth.
Cricket	In industrial plants and institutions. In damp basements and elevator shafts.	Egg Nymph Adult	18 months. 40–170 eggs.	10	Feeds on fabrics.	Black in color, 1 inch long. Jumps—similar to grasshopper. Produces chirruping sounds. Related to roaches; casts skin 9–11 times to complete growth.

Flea 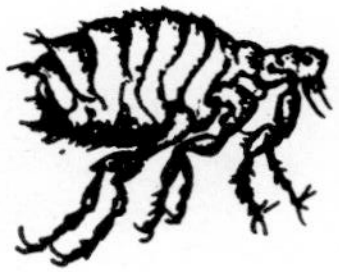	In institutions. Breeds in baseboards, cracks, crevices. On cats, dogs, and humans.	Egg Larva Pupa Adult	30–150 days. 300 eggs.	2,000	Attacks animals. Carries diseases. Attacks legs of human beings, may cause infections.	Reddish brown, wingless; body shiny and thin; 1/16 inch long. Legs suited to leaping. Found on cats and dogs and on plants and lawns where such animals are kept as pets.
Housefly 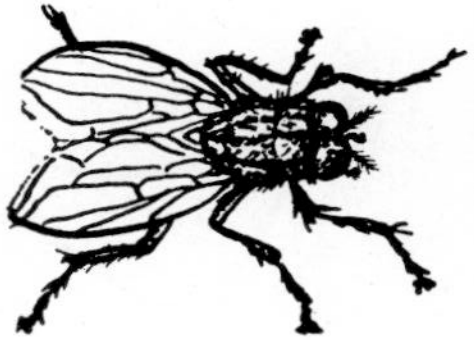	In homes and institutions. In kitchens, utility rooms, storerooms, and patient rooms. Where food is kept.	Egg Maggot Pupa Adult	8 days. 400–600 eggs.	50,000 10–12 generations in one summer.	Carries diseases such as diarrhea and typhoid fever.	Black in color, ⅜ inch long. Has two wings and a sucking tube.
Headlouse 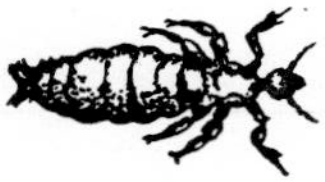	On human hair. Easily transferred from one patient to another.	Egg Nymph Adult	2–3 weeks. 50–200 eggs.	1,000	Causes severe itching—may be cause of infection from scratching.	Grayish—flat body, ½ inch long. Head narrow and pointed; body long and narrow. Eggs are sealed to human hair.

Table 2. COMMON HOSPITAL INSECTS (CONTINUED)

INSECT	WHERE FOUND	LIFE STAGES	LIFE CYCLE	AVERAGE REPRODUCTION RATE PER YEAR	EXTENT OF DAMAGE	IDENTIFYING FEATURES AND CHARACTERISTICS
Mosquito 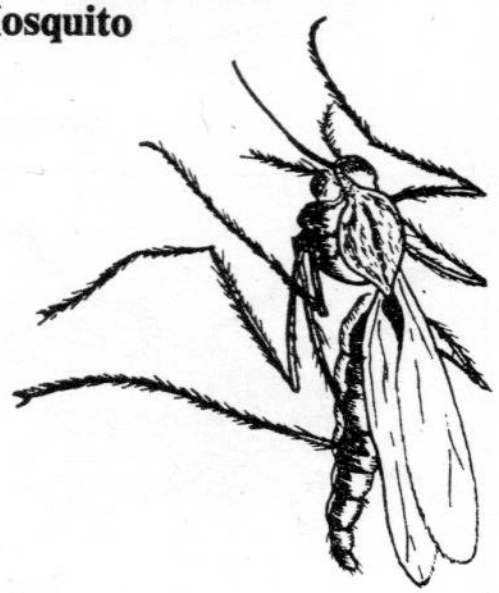	In homes and institutions. Breeds in swamps, sluggish streams, drain traps, tubs, and rain barrels.	Egg Larva Pupa Adult	30 days. 200 eggs.	10,000	Persistent hum is very annoying. Bites—may cause infection from scratching.	Transparent wings, 5/16 inch wingspread. Only the female mosquito can bite.
Moth 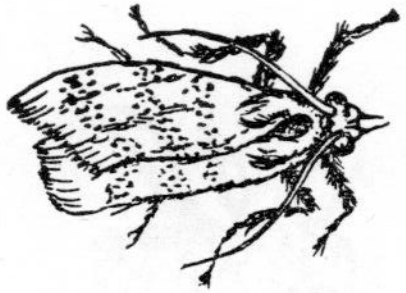	In homes and institutions. In carpets, drapes, upholstery, and clothing. In linen closets.	Egg Larva (see below) Pupa 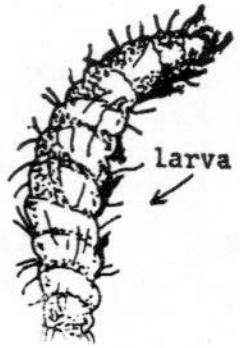 larva	6 months to 1 year. 200 eggs.	500	Only the larva can damage fabrics. Damages wool blankets and woolen garments.	Gray-brown in color; ½ inch wingspread. Spins webbing into cases.

Silverfish 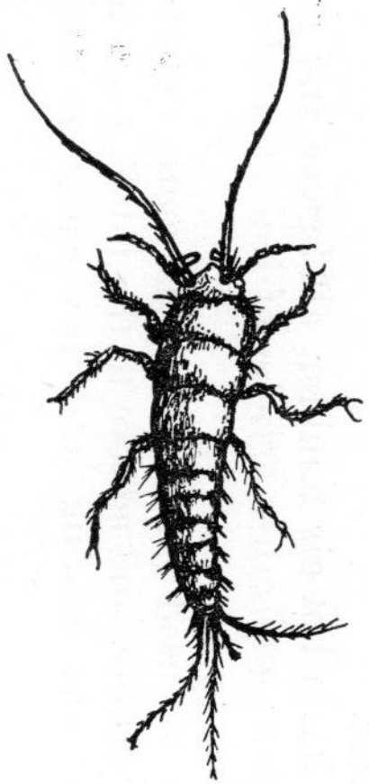	In institutions. Found near water pipes, in bathrooms, kitchens, utility rooms, and boiler-rooms.	Egg Nymph Adult	3 months to 3 years. 100 eggs.	100	Destroy labels and cartons.	Silver in color, ½ inch long. Covered with scales. Has chewing mouth-parts. Feeds on vegetable and animal matter.
Termite 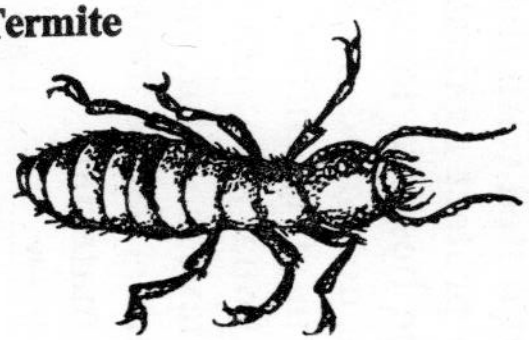	In wooden beams, institutions, foundations of buildings.	Egg Nymph Adult	6 months to 5 years. Thousands of eggs laid by the Queen	1,000	Destroys books, papers, and foundations of buildings.	White (workers), ⅜ inch long. Feeds in wood or other material containing cellulose.

in army quarters and on army clothing, is now used in attempts to disinfect and sanitize entire geographical areas. One midwest city recently, through the combined efforts of public health agencies and various fraternal and other public-minded organizations, put on a campaign which resulted in a systematic and effective eradication of flies, mosquitoes, roaches, etc., and led to improved sanitary conditions throughout the entire community.

As a means of protection against flies the miantenance department of the hospital should see that all screen doors and windows fit perfectly and are in perfect condition.

In the nursery and in the pediatrics department bits of food dropped on the floor should be immediately swept or mopped up so flies will not be attracted to the department.

If flies are to be sucessfully controlled, absolute cleanliness and order must be maintained and the destruction of flies must be an important part of all control plans.

Mosquitoes. Mosquitoes are known carriers of malaria, dengue, and yellow fever. The vigorous scratching of painful mosquito bites may cause an infection. They thrive in swamps, along river banks, and in fish ponds, fountains, cesspools, and gutters. They are most active at night and seem to attack some people more readily than others. All breeding places should be eliminated, screened, or, if possible, covered with a thin layer of oil which will destroy the larvae and pupae and in this way decrease the number of mosquitoes.

The hospital and nurses' home should be well screened and every effort made to protect patients and personnel from these obnoxious pests.

Moths. Moths usually tend to conceal themselves in darkened surroundings. They deposit their eggs in clothing, rugs, and upholstered furniture, where they later develop into worms which are capable of destroying the fabric.

Moths feed on wool, feathers, fur, and hair. They have been known to attack felt linings in a piano and to virtually destroy stuffed birds and animals.

In the hospital frequent inspection should be made of rugs and furnishings. Wool blankets and articles of clothing should be kept in mothproof bags. Mothballs should be used freely in chests and closets. Frequent dry cleaning of clothing and blankets will prevent their being infested with moths. Mattresses should be autoclaved at intervals also to protect against moths.

If the hospital laundry has a hot air tumbler, all larvae and moths will be destroyed on blankets and other articles of linen tumbled for approximately thirty minutes.

Cinchona alkaloids can be used satisfactorily as moth repellants. They have no odor, are invisible, and adhere to the fabric even when it is subjected to brushing and dusting, and they cause no damage to the material.

Tobacco, cayenne pepper, and sodium bicarbonate, contrary to popular belief, are of very little use in combating moths.

Bedbugs. Bedbugs are generally found in surroundings which are unclean and unsanitary. They live and breed in cracks and crevices of beds and walls, and because their bodies are very flat they can easily hide in the narrowest of crevices. They are active at night when they feed upon the blood of the human being they attack. They can subsist for long periods of time without food.

The bedbug has no wings, is dark reddish brown in color, and is smooth and hard in appearance. The young bedbug is light in color and very small. Bedbugs have a nauseating odor about them, and when they attack their victim they usually inflict a series of bites, raising a row or series of white elevations.

This particular species of hospital "pest" is usually brought to the hospital by patients, visitors, or employed personnel. To prevent infestation with bedbugs the hospital should be made as nearly insect-proof as possible. The use of metal beds and closely woven mattress covers deprives bedbugs of their breeding places and thus helps to eliminate them.

Patients who are restless and apprehensive and show characteristic symptoms of bitten areas should be transferred to a different bed so the suspected one may be thoroughly inspected. Bedbugs are difficult to find and even more difficult to destroy. Once their presence has been established the room may be fumigated and the mattress sterilized. The bed should be taken apart and painted with gasoline or kerosene. Hospital personnel in all departments should be very watchful to prevent these bugs from being brought into the hospital in clothing, luggage, or other personal belongings of patients and their visitors.

Cockroaches. Roaches are usually found around the woodwork and near plumbing fixtures where there is moisture and heat necessary for their growth and development. They may be brought to the hospital with fruits and vegetables from the wholesale storerooms. They eat paper and fabrics, as well as foodstuffs. Diet kitchens badly infested with roaches have a peculiar and characteristic odor. If a light is turned on suddenly at night large numbers of these hospital pests can be seen running crazily about in an attmpt to conceal themselves behind the nearest object.

Sodium fluoride is used extensively in an effort to exterminate roaches. Boiling water poured along the edge of ledges, plumbing fixtures, and on the wheels of food carts will also help to destroy them. Poisonous gas for fumigation is another method resorted to in control of these pests.

Centipedes. The centipede, or "thousand-legged" bug, is a long, slender insect with numerous pairs of tiny legs. It is thin in appearances and moves hastily and jerkily. Some persons are highly susceptible to the poisonous bite of the centipede and find it extremely painful.

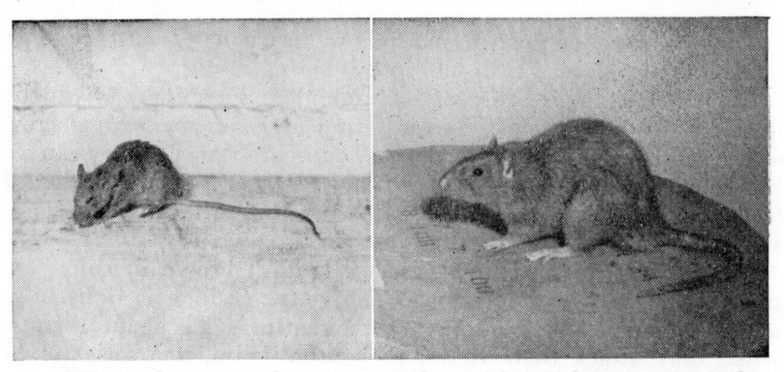

Fig. 30. Mice and rats are the most prevalent of hospital pests. (Agricultural Experiment Station, Purdue University, West Lafayette, Indiana.)

Control of this insect consists of destroying it wherever it is found. Storerooms and other places should be kept clean. Sodium fluoride dusted about in cupboards, closets, and storage space is effective in helping to control the centipede.

Pediculi. Pediculi, commonly called "lice," are parasitic, living on animals or plants. Their blood-sucking habit makes them dangerous to men because of local irritation to the skin and because of their capability of transmitting disease.

Epidemics of typhus fever in prisons, on shipboard, and in army camps are thought to be caused by the body louse that carries the disease from one person to another. Personal cleanliness is one method of control. Kerosene with liquid insecticides has been used effectively to combat lice.

In the hospital all newly admitted children should have their hair and scalp examined for lice, which are not uncommonly transmitted from one child to another through direct or indirect contact. A child with pediculosis, if not detected on admission to the hospital, may be the cause of infestation of an entire children's ward.

Fleas. Fleas are primarily a parasite on animals, although some species may prefer the human being for host. Fleas are thought to spread typhus fever and the plague which are not commonly encountered in America, so the chief menace to persons in this country is the irritating bite of the insect.

One means of preventing fleas is exclusion of animal pets from the house. Fleas may be destroyed by the use of insecticides in the form of a flea powder.

Mice and Rats. Of all pests, mice and rats seem to be the most universally prevalent. They feed on a great variety of foods, and in gaining access to ships by gangplanks and ropes have been known to carry disease from one continent to another.

These animals, in addition to carrying disease, have destroyed property by causing fires. Many youngsters have also been severely injured by rat bites.

In an effort to control these pests buildings are made as rat proof as possible and food is kept in containers which make it inaccessible to either mice or rats. Poison and traps are used effectively against them, and animal pets (cats and dogs) in homes are encouraged to destroy them.

Poisonous gases may be used in buildings badly infested with mice and rats, although extreme precaution is needed to prevent injury to personnel as a result of the hazardous procedure.

SANITARY FACILITIES

Water Supply. In the hospital of today, with public health authorities taking full responsibility for the purity of the water supply, there is little cause for concern in regard to this major sanitary factor. In event of sudden disaster as flood, hurricane, the outbreak of an epidemic, a communicable disease, or war-caused disaster, the persons of the area affected would be advised to boil all water used for drinking, bathing, and the preparation of food.

In rural communities where sanitary control is not so rigidly enforced, the water supply may become contaminated from a nearby toilet or from improper sewage disposal. When doubt exists as to the purity of water the nurse should always boil that to be used in the home or institution where she is employed.

Microorganisms which are found in polluted water are destroyed by heat, and water that has been boiled for a few minutes will be safe for drinking. Water that has been boiled has a peculiar, flat taste which is objectionable to most persons. The normal taste of the water can be restored by the simple process of pouring it from one container to another to reincorporate the air that was lost during boiling.

Waste Disposal. The disposal of wastes is another essential sanitary measure. Modern plumbing in homes and hospitals is highly efficient and has practically removed the danger of spreading communicable diseases through improper sewage disposal.

In order to keep waste disposal appliances in good working condition the nurse should make certain that plumbing fixtures are not misused. Careless disposal of objects such as broken tongue blades, bobby pins, soiled dressings, and fruit skins in toilets and hoppers will obstruct drainage pipes and interfere with the functioning of the entire plumbing system.

Discharges from nose and throat, facial tissue and sputum boxes, and all soiled dressings, including sanitary napkins, should be deposited in paper bags, then burned in the hospital incinerator.

Garbage Disposal. Disposal of garbage is a sanitary measure that should also be given consideration. Liquid garbage can be emptied into a sink, solid portions should be collected in metal covered pails. These pails should be emptied daily and should be thoroughly cleaned after each use.

The sanitation department of the community usually provides for the collection and disposal of garbage.

GENERAL CLEANLINESS

The atmosphere of the immediate surroundings of the patient depends to a great extent on the cleanliness and order of the room. If the room is clean and neat the growth of bacteria will be inhibited, and less dust will be set in motion by the activity of the patient and of hospital personnel.

The patient is more comfortable in a room that is clean and in order. His confidence in the nurse will be greatly increased if she helps to provide a desirable hospital environment which promotes greater peace of mind and a feeling of security.

Although the nurse herself is rarely called on to do the actual cleaning of the hospital room, she should be thoroughly versed in the correct method of cleaning and should feel a definite responsibility to see that the room is cleaned each day in a manner and at a time that is least disturbing to the patient. She should work harmoniously with the employees who do the actual cleaning and should be able, when necessary, to supervise the procedure, or to do the job herself if there is no one else available.

Cleaning of Equipment and Supplies. Articles made of aluminum, china, copper, enamelware, glass, porcelain, chromium, and monel metal should be washed in warm soapy water, then rinsed well and dried. Only mild abrasives should be used when scouring is necessary. To remove stains from aluminum use a metal polish; for copper use vinegar and salt, and for porcelain use iodine followed by the use of alcohol.

Articles made of rubber should be rinsed with cold water, washed in warm water with soap, rinsed well, and allowed to dry. Rubber goods should not be placed on warm radiators or in bright sunlight. Grease, oil, and acid will cause rubber to deteriorate. Rubber sheets and pillow cases should be hung across a rod to be stored, as folding creases and cracks the rubber.

Articles of furniture should be washed with warm water and soap and dried immediately with a soft cloth. Upholstered furniture should be cleaned periodically with a vacuum cleaner.

Summary of Important Factors

The nurse needs to know how to clean and care for hospital property in order to supervise the work of persons assigned to housekeeping tasks.

Care of floors is necessary to promote cleanliness and provide attractive surroundings.

Furniture should be kept clean and in good condition.

Torn linen should be sent to the sewing room for repair.

Personnel should be cautioned about being wasteful of linen.

Pillow cases should not be used as substitute linen bags.

All kitchen appliances and equipment should be cleaned at least once a week.

Greasy liquids should not be poured into the sink to cause clogging of the pipes.

All nurses should accept responsibility for keeping the utility room clean.

Thorough cleaning of the room after dismissal of a patient is needed to make it ready for another patient.

An exterminating company should be made responsible to keep the hospital free of insects and pests.

All personnel need to wage continuous war on flies, cockroaches, mice, etc.

Incoming patients should be examined for presence of pediculi.

Immediate waste and garbage disposal is essential for good sanitary practice.

Suggested Reference Reading

"Central linen room service," Anna Harmens; American Journal of Nursing, December, 1950.

"Color is more than beauty," Faber Birren; Modern Hospital, January, 1952.

"Odor problems," Hospitals, February, 1952.

"How to get rid of household insect pests," C. Lester Walker; Reader's Digest, April, 1952.

"Nursing looks to housekeeping for high standards of service," Dorothy M. Morgan; Modern Hospital, June, 1952.

"How to clean a hospital room," Hospital Management, September, 1952.

"Cleaning carnival," Sadie Mills Franklin; Hospitals, September, 1952.

CHAPTER 5

The Patient's Hospital Environment

TOPICAL OUTLINE

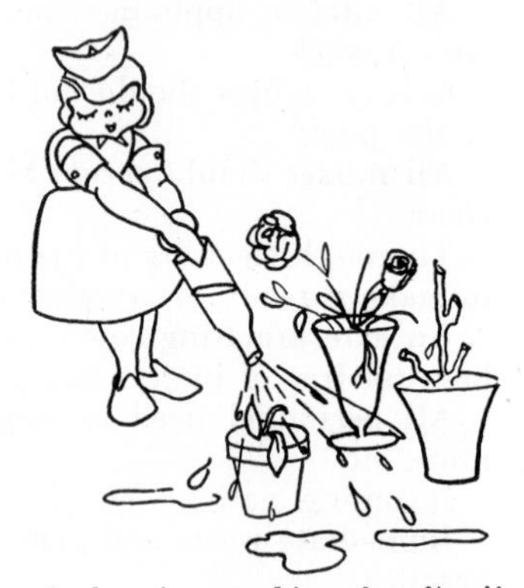

A plant is something that dies if you don't water it—and rots if you do.

ENVIRONMENTAL FACTORS RELATED TO HEALTH

The immediate surroundings of the patient have marked influence on his response to medical treatment. Cleanliness, which is one essential factor, has been discussed in detail in the preceding chapter, and safety, also of great importance, is the subject of the following chapter. The present discussion is concerned with other factors that must be given consideration in providing the patient with a healthful and pleasant environment during the time he remains in the hospital, including atmospheric conditions, lighting, prevention of noise, and esthetic factors.

Atmospheric Conditions. Factors related to atmospheric conditions which influence health are temperature, humidity, air movement, purity of air, and ventilation. The modern method of controlling atmospheric conditions is known as *air conditioning*, which involves circulating the air, washing it clean, and regulating its temperature and humidity.

Temperature. Because individuals differ in their reaction to atmospheric conditions there is no set indoor temperature which can be considered ideal for everyone. For each person the most suitable indoor temperature is that which is warm enough to prevent feeling chilly, yet is not warm enough to cause perspiration. Temperature ranging between 68 and 72° F. is usually best suited to most persons. At night when the person is covered with warm blankets the room temperature may be even lower than 64° F. Temperature above 80° F. is undesirable because excessive heat decreases the person's natural energy, causes perspiration, and results in an abnormal sensitivity to cold.

Humidity. As the humidity (the amount of moisture in the air) is increased, evaporation from the skin is retarded and the individual suffers more from extremes of temperature. Water is a better conductor of heat or cold than is air, and on extremely hot days when the humidity is high people are more uncomfortable than on days when the temperature is just as high but the humidity is less.

When a given quantity of air at a given temperature contains all the water vapor it can hold, the humidity is said to be 100 per cent. A humidity of 40–60 per cent is considered desirable by most persons.

In some disease conditions, such as asthma, a relative humidity that is quite low (10–20 per cent) is more comfortable for the patient.

Air Movement. Warm air weighs less than cold air, and for that reason tends to rise. Air movement, through currents of air of varying temperatures, has a refreshing effect. Air conditioning makes it possible to approximate the refreshing outdoor air within homes, hospitals, and public buildings. Electric fans may be used to secure air movement, but care should be taken to prevent chilling the patient with a too strong current of air from the fan.

The opening of windows and doors in a room will quite often provide for sufficient air movement to refresh the air within the room. If it is not possible to ventilate a room by having windows and doors open during cold weather, outdoor air may be admitted to an adjoining room, then permitted to enter the room where ventilation is needed.

Purity of Air. The usual impurities found in air are gases, dust particles, and microorganisms. Respiratory diseases may be spread by such impurities as lint from blankets and bed clothing. Microorganisms may be carried from one patient to another by the droplets sprayed into the air through sneezing and coughing. Ultraviolet rays and glycol vapor have been used to help control aerial contamination but have not been proved to be entirely effective.

Patients in wards need to be protected from droplet infection by the use of cubicles, isolation technique, freedom from dust, good ventilation, and ample space between the beds.

Ventilation. A room with windows on two sides may be cross ventilated by opening one window at the top, the other at the bottom. For the room with only one window, ventilation may be provided by opening the window at both the top and bottom so the air can circulate freely, the warm air rising and going out the top as cool air enters at the bottom.

Regardless of the method chosen to ventilate the room, care should be taken to avoid drafts. The use of wind deflectors is recommended. Screens placed between the window and the patient's bed may prevent a direct current of air from reaching the patient.

Lighting. Natural light, produced by rays from the sun, is extremely important in the care of the sick. Aside from the healing powers it possesses, light is necessary for warmth and cheer in a room and for stimulation of mental faculties.

According to some authorities on the subject, a room to be well lighted should have window space equal in area to about one fourth of the floor space provided.

Direct sunlight is effective in building up resistance to disease and has been of special therapeutic value in reducing susceptibility to such diseases as rickets and tuberculosis. It is thought by some to build up protection against colds and other infections.

In addition to its importance as an essential health factor sunlight provides illumination, and the amount of sunlight allowed to enter a room will control the degree of brightness and cheer which the room will have. Nurses realize the importance of cheerful surroundings and arrange blinds or shades to permit the entrance of sunlight. Bright light should not fall directly on the patient's face or shine into his eyes. Too much light or excessively bright light may cause discomfort to the patient and produce nervous irritability. Glare produced by sunlight can be most annoying and interferes with clear, accurate vision.

In some cases, as during serious illness or immediately after eye surgery, the amount of light permitted in the room should be greatly reduced. For many patients rest hours should be observed during the day, and at such times the room should be darkened while the patient rests or sleeps.

During the day, outdoor or natural lighting should be uniform throughout the room, furnishing enough illumination for distant corners and general background of the room. At night over-all lighting of the room may be supplemented by a light at the bedside. This light can be of greater intensity and confined to the area where it is needed for reading, sewing, or engaging in other forms of recreational or occupational therapy.

With such an arrangement of lighting the eyes of the patient need not make a constant adjustment between two different forms and strengths of light.

To be adequately lighted a room must have a certain amount of light which may be measured in terms of candle power. This standard unit of light intensity (termed a foot-candle) is the amount of illumination at a point on a surface one foot distant from the source of light of one international candle. Although the standard unit of light is termed "candle power" or "foot-candle," most persons are more familiar with the difference in light according to the number of watts with which the light bulb is labeled. For reading, sewing, or other so-called close work, a bulb of 60 to 100 watts is needed. For ordinary lighting, where a mellow light is needed, such as that for over-all lighting of a room, a smaller watt bulb may be used.

To prevent eye fatigue and to provide the correct amount and kind of light the nurse must understand the type of lamp and strength of bulb used and how best to adjust them to meet the needs of the patient.

In the hospital operating room lights with a complicated arrangement of reflectors are used so that no shadows are thrown on the field of operation by the movement of the surgeon's hands or by the instruments being used.

The use of soft, pastel colors in hospital interiors, to replace the plain white walls and ceilings of yesterday, have added to the eye comfort of patients. All-white walls, ceilings, curtains, and furniture reflected so much light that the entire room had a damaging effect produced by glare. Soft-toned maple wood in modern attractive furnishings, walls painted in peach, gray, blue, and other restful shades, and drapes that are bright and gay have made the hospital room cheerful and pleasant. With psychological as well as physical factors considered to be of great importance in medical treatment, attractive and pleasant surroundings play a major role in the well-being of the patient.

Prevention of Noise. Research has shown that noise in one's environment tends to produce physical fatigue and to cause various nervous or emotional disturbances. Loud noise may be actually harmful to a person forced to endure it for a prolonged period of time.

Noise is especially annoying to persons who are ill, and hospitals now make a concentrated effort to reduce the degree of noise to which a patient is subjected. Sound-absorbing materials are used in the ceilings of hallways, in serving kitchens, dining rooms, labor rooms, and nurseries. Rubber tires and rubber bumpers are used on dressing carts, stretchers, and wheelchairs; door silencers and other mechanical noise reducers are used. Noise made by elevators, electrical machinery, etc., has resulted in the location of patient rooms as far away from specialized departments and from elevators as the plan of the building will permit.

The greatest source of noise, and often the most disturbing, is the hospital personnel—loud talking, laughing, and heavy walking may greatly annoy the patient. Whispering and tiptoeing may be equally upsetting, since it tends to cause apprehension and uncertainty in the patient's mind.

The control of radios used in other patients' rooms may insure more quiet for the seriously ill patient. Many modern institutions are installing call systems or alarms that employ lights, instead of loud

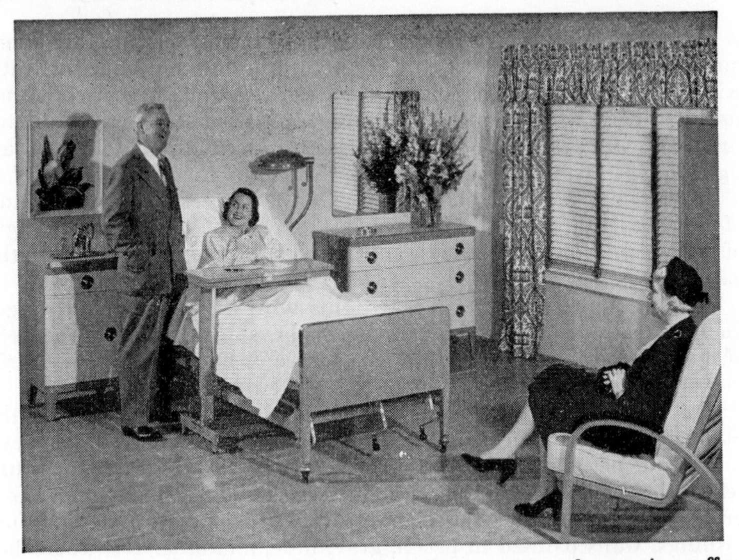

Fig. 31. A good arrangement of furniture helps to create a harmonious effect. (Simmons Company, Merchandise Mart, Chicago, Illinois.)

speakers, in an effort to reduce noise within the hospital. Nurses should move quietly about their work and speak in low, restrained tones, setting an example for other employees to follow. Although all employees should maintain an atmosphere of quiet in the hospital, the nurse is most responsible for the prevention of noise, because she is in direct contact with the patient and is concerned with nursing care.

Elimination of Unpleasant Odors. Since the reaction to odors varies so widely in individuals, the same odor varying from pleasant to obnoxious, hospitals have attempted to keep the immediate environment of the patient free from odors. Good ventilation and cleanliness are essential factors in controlling odors. Some motor-driven devices are available for use in patient units and have been received with some measure of satisfaction.

In a room where the air is stale there will be an inevitable odor of stuffiness until the room is properly ventilated.

Very objectionable odors are those of bad breath or body perspiration. Nurses who are interested in the comfort of their patients will not offend by being guilty of either when on duty.

Esthetic Factors. To answer psychological, as well as physical needs of the patient, the nurse must be aware of the important role played by the attractiveness of the patient's room. Although esthetic factors may not be accepted as being essential to good health, they are nevertheless of great value in establishing the desired psychological reaction and thus, at the same time, improving the physical condition of the patient. The arrangement of furniture in the room will help to produce a harmonious effect if it is orderly and pleasing to the patient. Color used to good advantage will help to make almost any room appear brighter and more interesting. Suitable pictures hung where they may be seen easily will result in pleasure to the patient. Color may be added by carefully selected drapes or bedspread, by very pretty gowns and bedjackets worn by women patients, and by plants or flowers sent by thoughtful friends and relatives.

Although a luxurious environment may be more pleasing to the patient, the nurse should recognize the difference between essential and non-essential health factors and should not be concerned if only modest necessities are provided for the daily care of the patient. A capable nurse knows that the patient receiving proper medical and nursing care usually recovers just as rapidly in an environment that is plain and simple as he would if surrounded by all the modern conveniences and the latest precept of interior decorating.

THE PATIENT UNIT

The patient unit has been defined as "the area, furnishings, and equipment necessary for the care of a single patient." The unit may vary in size; it may be a private suite (including living room, bedroom, and bath), a single room where furnishings, equipment, and supplies are used for the care and comfort of just one patient, or the immediate surroundings of a patient in a ward where several patients are placed in one large room. The very large ward of thirty to forty beds is seldom found in hospitals today, since most patients prefer the single room, the semiprivate (two-bed room), or the small ward of four to six beds.

Rooms for the care of a single patient are usually located on the outer sides of the hospital building where air, light, and ventilation are readily accessible. Workrooms, such as kitchens, utility rooms, and storage rooms are located on the inner side of hospital corridors.

Without interfering with facilities for carrying out nursing duties, hospital administrators have succeeded in making both private rooms and wards cheerful, colorful, and attractive. Many patients who dreaded the experience of leaving familiar surroundings of home for a necessary period of hospitalization are pleasantly surprised to find that their hospital room is no less attractive than the room they occupy at home.

The patient who remains in his own home should have a room near the bathroom and one that is far enough removed from the center of the family's activities to be quiet and restful. As much as the plan of the house will permit, the patient's room should be located away from street noises or from other disturbing outside influences.

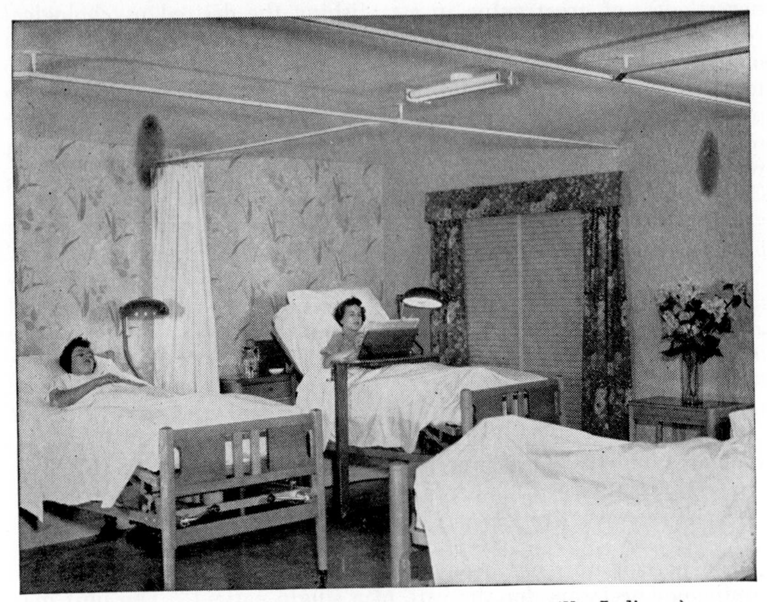

Fig. 32. The four-bed ward. (Hill-Rom Co., Batesville, Indiana.)

For the patient at home, if possible, a twin size bed should be used in giving nursing care. The bed should be elevated to proper height on blocks of wood, or two mattresses may be used to raise the bed level to approximately the desired height. Improvised back rests may be provided by a canvas-covered wooden frame, by an inverted straight chair, or by a suitcase on which pillows are supported. In many urban areas hospital beds may be rented, and their use will greatly facilitate caring for a patient in the home.

In the ward, the same as in a private room, the area immediately surrounding the patient (including the furnishings and the equipment needed for his care), is termed the "patient unit." Each ward unit contains the essential articles that are available to patients in private rooms. The ward patient who desires or whose condition demands privacy may be screened from view of other patients by curtains which hang from a rod fastened to the ceiling, and when the curtains are pulled to their full extent the entire unit is enclosed. If hanging curtains are not available, portable screens may be used to separate one patient unit from another in the semiprivate room or wards.

Furnishings Needed for the Unit. The pieces of furniture which have come to be standard equipment for a patient's room or unit include the hospital bed, bedside table, tray table, and straight chair. A comfortable chair, screen, dresser, lamp, and footstool are provided

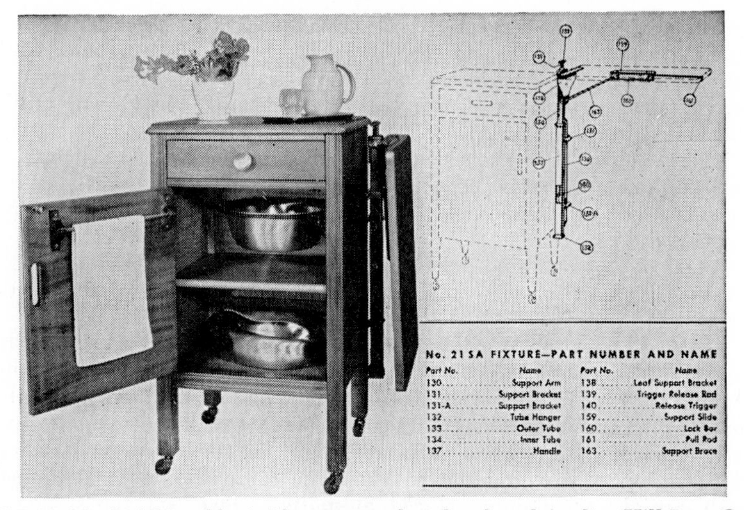

No. 21 SA FIXTURE—PART NUMBER AND NAME

Part No.	Name	Part No.	Name
130	Support Arm	138	Leaf Support Bracket
131	Support Bracket	139	Trigger Release Rod
131-A	Support Bracket	140	Release Trigger
132	Tube Hanger	159	Support Slide
133	Outer Tube	160	Lock Bar
134	Inner Tube	161	Pull Rod
137	Handle	163	Support Brace

Fig. 33. The bedside table (with parts numbered and explained). (Hill-Rom Co., Inc., Batesville Indiana.)

for all private rooms and for many units in a semiprivate room or ward. Drapes, bedspreads, and pictures for the walls make the room more attractive. Hanging screens usually separate ward units and may be closed to provide privacy. Most hospital furniture is made of metal or of sturdy wood and is provided with casters so it may be moved about easily.

The Bed. The hospital bed that is commonly used is the Gatch bed, which is described in detail in Chapter 7.

Bedside Table. A variety of tables are available, any one of which may be satisfactory if it answers the need for a working table top at the side of the bed and for storage space for equipment used in giving care to the patient. All cosmetic necessities, including toothbrush and toothpaste, are to be kept in the drawer of the bedside table. The lower part of the table should be used to keep bedpan, urinal, wash basin, and other equipment out of sight when not in use.

Tray Table. Tray tables vary in design even more widely than bedside tables and range from the simple tray supported on legs which may be folded back on the table itself when not in use, to the highly efficient over-bed table which is an extensive framework placed on casters so it may readily be moved. In the home, an ironing board or a leaf from the dining room table supported on two piles of books, one on either side of the patient, may serve as an overbed table. Whatever the design of tray table used, its chief purpose is that of holding the tray on which meals are served to the patient.

Straight Chair. The straight chair is another essential part of the working equipment for care of the patient. It is used for clean and soiled linen during the time the patient is being given a bath. It is used as additional space for treatment trays as nursing care requires. During visiting hours the straight chair is often the only chair available for visitors in wards.

Wastebasket. A wastebasket helps to keep the room neat and in order and should be so placed in the room that facial tissues, candy wrappers, scraps of paper, etc., can be dropped into it when discarded by the patient.

Footstool. As each hospital bed is much higher from the floor than an ordinary bed, it is essential that the patient unit be provided with a footstool.

Lamp. The lamp in the patient unit should match other furnishings in the room in design and color. The most desirable lamp is one which offers indirect as well as direct lighting, giving plenty of light for reading or for treatments and also capable of adjustment to give soft, indirect illumination to permit light in the room for nursing care without disturbing the patient. The lamp should be equipped with a night light dome placed at mattress level for the standard hospital bed.

Screen. Screens are used to separate one patient unit from another in a ward. Whatever the design or type of screen used, its chief purpose is to provide privacy for the patient.

Dresser. Each private room has a dresser included with standard furnishings, but the ward of two or more beds may have one dresser provided for the use of several patients. Blankets and other necessary supplies for care of the patient are kept in the dresser drawers.

Linen Requirements in the Patient Unit. In working daily with standard pieces of hospital linen, especially linen used in making the hospital bed, the nurse soon learns to recognize and handle all such material with ease and efficiency. In addition to the articles necessary for making the bed, discussed fully in Chapter 7, the linen needed to supply each patient unit includes:

Bath Blanket. The bath blanket is a light weight, cotton blanket, somewhat narrower in width and about the same length as the blanket used for warmth.

The bath blanket is used to cover the patient during the bed bath and serves as a drape for the bath and for other nursing procedures or treatments. The bath blanket should be used to protect the patient from drafts when he is transferred from one department to another by wheelchair or cart. For the patient who is permitted to sit up for short periods of time, the bath blanket should be used as a light covering for the lower extremities.

Face Towel. The face towel, about 18 by 36 inches in size, is made of cotton and linen and is used to dry the face after it has been bathed. Face towels are also frequently used as hand towels for the bath procedure and for afternoon care.

Wash Cloth and Bath Towel. These articles, used as their name implies, are made of terry cloth. The wash cloth is about 12 inches square. The bath towel usually measures 22 by 44 inches.

Other Equipment Needed in the Patient Unit. Patient unit equipment has become standardized to include the various articles kept at the bedside and used each day for giving routine nursing care to the patient. Such articles include:

Wash Basin. The wash basin is a rounded basin of enamel or stainless steel which holds the water used for bathing the patient.

Emesis Basin. A kidney-shaped basin of enamel or steel, used daily in care of the mouth and used as a container to receive vomitus. It may also be used as a small waste container during surgical procedures.

Mouthwash Cup. A cup or container for the solution used in cleansing the mouth and teeth.

Soap Dish. The standard soap dish with a shelf or drain which prevents the cake of soap from becoming water soaked.

Bedpan. The bedpan is a special container used to receive waste products of urine and feces from the patient who must remain in bed. The high front and shallow back permits proper placement for use with minimum effort on the part of the nurse and the least amount of discomfort to the patient.

Urinal. The urinal is a vase-like container designed to receive urine from the male patient who is unable to be out of bed. One side of the urinal is slightly flattened to prevent spilling of its contents. The entire urinal is about 10 inches long; a large side handle permits easy handling by patient or nurse.

Although care of the patient unit may be considered primarily as one of the duties of the housekeeping department, it is a very important factor in the care of the patient and as such must be accepted as a responsibility of the nursing staff.

A clean, neat, and pleasant environment for the patient is necessary if he is to receive real benefit from medical treatment and nursing care. If the nurse is sincerely interested in the welfare of the patient she will assume responsibility for care of the unit to the extent that, if it becomes necessary, she will clean and care for the unit each day when routine nursing care is being given the patient.

Daily Care of the Patient Unit. Although the nurse is rarely responsible for the cleaning of the patient unit, she must know exactly what should be done in order to properly supervise the maid or aide who is assigned to the cleaning task. During the time the patient remains in the hospital, the room or unit must be properly cared for each day, but does not necessarily have to undergo a thorough cleaning.

Daily care of the patient unit should include the following:

Faded or withered flowers should be removed from the room. Water should be changed on all cut flowers which are to be returned to the room.

All extra blankets used during the night should be folded and put away unless the patient needs an extra blanket while the room is being aired.

Throw rugs should be removed from the room. They should be cleaned on an outside porch or in the cleaning room (to avoid additional dust in the air rugs should be cleaned by a vacuum cleaner).

The room should be aired by opening windows and doors (in winter and on cold days the patient should be kept warm with additional blankets while the room is being aired).

All old newspapers, magazines, fruit, and refuse should be discarded.

The wastebasket should be emptied.

All furniture in the room should be dusted, including window sills. A non-scratching, lint-free cloth should be used. It should be remembered that dusting is to remove the dust, not merely to displace it and scatter it throughout the room to settle again on the furniture. Be very careful in dusting not to bump against the bed as all surgical patients and many receiving medical treatment are highly sensitive to such sudden slight shocks.

All articles from the top of the bedside table should be put away if they belong in the drawer or lower compartment. Articles left on the table should be neat and orderly.

The mirror of the dresser should be cleaned with a damp cloth and dried immediately by rubbing with a dry cloth.

A dustless mop should be used to remove all dust and dirt from the floor.

Cleaned rugs should be replaced. Rugs should not be thrown or flipped into position, but should be placed evenly and quietly where they belong.

Each piece of furniture should be correctly placed in relation to the bed and other furnishing.

All lights which are not in use and are not needed by the patient should be turned out.

Window shades or venetian blinds should be adjusted as desired by the patient. If there is more than one window in the room, blinds should be adjusted to the same height.

The door should be completely or partially closed, as the patient desires.

While cleaning the room a non-professional worker should not attempt to talk with a patient who is acutely ill, sleeping, or unaware of what goes on about him. The patient's wishes in regard to flowers, lights, shades, or the closing of the door will be known to the nurse responsible for his care, and she will attend to all such matters as they relate to the cleaning procedure.

Even if the patient is convalescent and quite able to talk, the maid or other person doing the cleaning should not attempt to carry on a conversation. Under no circumstances should a maid discuss one patient with another or give out information concerning the hospital. Any nurse who observes an untrained worker conversing freely with patients as she cleans the rooms should notify the head nurse, especially if the conversations are chiefly concerned with matters pertaining to the hospital.

After dismissal of a patient the unit must be thoroughly cleaned and made ready for occupancy by another, as directed in the detailed

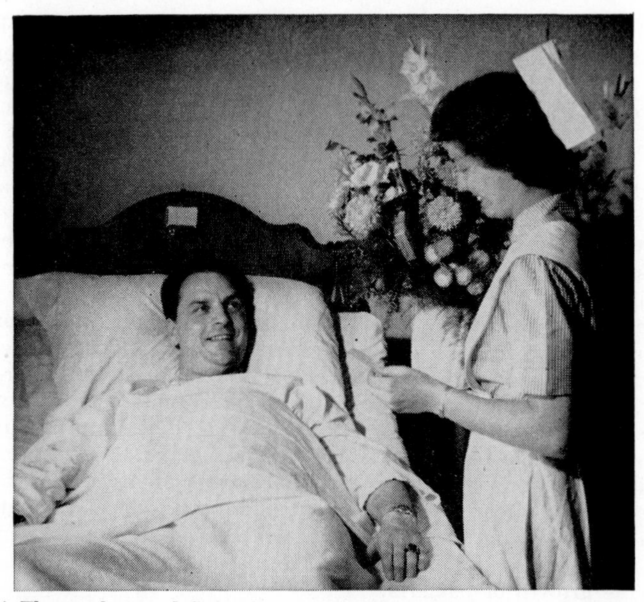

Fig. 34. Flowers have a definite therapeutic value. (Presbyterian Hospital School of Nursing, Pittsburgh, Pennsylvania.)

instructions for cleaning the unit or room given in Chapter 4, "Hospital Housekeeping."

CARE AND ARRANGEMENT OF FLOWERS

The nurse will soon realize that flowers have a definite therapeutic value, especially for the patient who may not often have visitors or who may be fearful and distressed because of his illness. A gift of flowers usually brings hope and cheer, linking the patient with the world of home and work and the familiar surroundings he has been forced to leave. Flowers help to satisfy the mental and spiritual needs which, in some instances, may be of greater importance than the patient's physical requirements.

That flowers have a very special meaning to their recipient is evidenced by the fact that many patients will cling to a single flower or a bouquet of flowers, long after their original beauty and freshness has been lost. The observing nurse learns early in clinical practice that it is unwise to discard even a much wilted bouquet of flowers, without first asking permission from the patient.

Hospitals now provide flower rooms where delivery of flowers is made and care may be given them. Hothouse flowers do not adjust quickly to changes of temperature. If they have been in a delivery truck for several hours in very cold weather, they should be left for some time in their wrappings in the flower room. Flowers that are received in a wilted condition should be placed immediately in cold water.

All flowers delivered to the flower room should be given proper care and should be tagged for proper identification until they can be delivered to the patient to whom they are addressed.

Care of Cut Flowers. Whether flowers are removed from the patient's room each night or left in the room, they should be taken each morning to the flower room for proper care for the day.

The flowers should be removed from the vase and placed on the sink where they can be spread over a large, flat surface. The vase should be washed with soap and water and refilled with clear, cold water. The end of the stems should be held under running water, while they are cut with a very sharp knife. A long slanting cut will prevent the stems from resting flat on the bottom of the vase, thus insuring free access of water into the stems. Stems should be cut under running water so air cannot enter the stem to block the entrance of water. Leaves on the stem below water level should be removed, since they tend to decompose and become unsightly, as well as promote the growth of bacteria.

When flowers are first cut, they will benefit by being placed in deep containers so the blossoms float on the surface of the water for a few hours. Flowers that show definite signs of wilting may sometimes be revived by having their stems placed in hot water. The heat tends to draw air from the cells, thus promoting better circulation of water in the stems. Cut flowers should be placed in fresh cold water at least once each day. The stems should be submerged in water to at least half their length. Cut flowers should be kept away from strong drafts and should not be placed in direct sunlight or near a hot radiator or other source of heat.

Care of Potted Plants. Potted plants should be placed in containers which provide for drainage. The flower pot should always be placed on a dish or other receptacle so that furniture or window ledge will not be damaged by moisture from the pot or from the plant.

Plants should be given water each day. The frequency of watering depends on the temperature of the room, the amount of light they receive, and the dryness of the soil in which they are growing. Water should not be poured over the leaves and stems of the plant, but should be directed over the soil at the rim of the pot or container. During the winter when plants may not get as much light as they require, they may benefit greatly by being placed beneath an ordinary electric light for several hours each day. House plants may do well if submerged at least once each week in a sink or in a bucket of water, so that water flows just over the top of the pot.

Flowers in the Hospital Room. A profusion of flowers in a hospital room gives the room a cluttered, crowded appearance which is not desirable. Most patients who are deluged with flowers readily accept a suggestion from the nurse that one or several bouquets be sent to nearby wards or to rooms where patients who have no flowers of their own may enjoy them.

Knowing where to place flowers in the room is just as important as knowing how to arrange them. The dresser top is the place usually chosen to display flowers which are tall or are arranged so that a lot of space is needed for them.

A small bouquet or even a single flower placed so that its beauty is reflected in the mirror may do a great deal to provide cheer and hopefulness for the patient. Small bouquets may be placed on the window sill, to one side of the overbed table, or on the bedside table, although other articles are kept on the tables. The flower arrangement placed where other articles must also be used must be small enough not to be in the way of patient or nurse.

Numerous flower arrangements which are sent to patients in the hospital are made up by the florist and delivered ready to be presented to the recipient; however, many flowers are boxed and delivered and the arranging is left to the nurse or attendant. If an effort is made to arrange the flowers attractively, the pleasure they bring the patient will be greatly increased.

Patients who have a profusion of flowers and plants will usually leave most of them at the hospital when they are dismissed. Nurses should distribute them to other patients and in this way provide the cheer and hopefulness which flowers can bring to those who might otherwise be deprived of such valuable therapeutic aid.

Summary of Important Factors

Temperature of the patient's room should be 68° to 72° F. during the day and somewhat lower at night.

Humidity of 40 to 60 per cent is considered desirable for patients.

Ventilation may be obtained by opening a window slightly at top and bottom.

Direct sunlight is beneficial to the patient; glare should be avoided.

Lamps with 60 to 100 watt bulbs should be available for reading or sewing.

The nurse should protect the patient from unnecessary disturbance by noise.

Odors should be removed from hospital rooms—by mechanical or electrical devices if necessary.

Esthetic factors as color in the hospital room help in providing psychological benefits to the patient.

The patient unit includes area, furniture, and equipment needed for the care of a single patient.

The housekeeping department is usually responsible for cleaning the unit, with the exception of the bed and bedside table. (These are the responsibility of the nurse.)

The patient will be more comfortable if the room is neat and clean, unnecessary lights turned out, and window shades or blinds drawn to uniform height.

Furniture needed for the unit includes a bed, bedside table, straight chair, tray table, lamp, wastebasket, footstool, and screen, the latter to afford the privacy needed for certain procedures or treatments.

Equipment needed for the unit includes a wash basin, emesis basin, soap dish, urinal, bedpan, mouthwash cup, and signal bell.

Linen needed for the unit includes bedspread, wool blanket, bath blanket, face towel, sheets, drawsheets, rubber sheet, wash cloth, pillow cases and covers, and bath towel.

Flowers have a definite therapeutic value for the patient.

The flower stem should be held under water and cut slantwise with a sharp knife.

Leaves on the stem below the water level should be removed.

Potted plants should be watered each day.

A profusion of flowers in the hospital room makes it seem cluttered and crowded.

Knowing where to place flowers in a room is just as important as knowing how to arrange them.

Factors To Teach the Patient

That discarding old newspapers, magazines, withered flowers, and waste is essential to keep the room clean and neat.

That cooperation is needed in keeping food in covered containers to prevent flies, roaches, mice, and other hospital pests.

That cooperation with the hospital personnel in maintaining correct temperature, humidity, ventilation, and lighting for the unit is necessary.

That direct sunlight in the room can be beneficial.

That radio and television volume should be controlled so as not to disturb other patients.

If a mechanical or electrical device is needed to control odors in the hospital room the patient should be told why the device is being used.

That the rubber sheet is needed to protect the mattress; when the mattress doesn't need protection the rubber sheet can be removed.

That it is important to help keep the unit clean, especially if it is part of a ward.

That furniture and articles of equipment within the unit should be used properly.

That regulations or practices which provide for privacy of other patients in a ward must be observed.

That sharing flowers with other patients is one of the best means of enjoying them.

Situation Type Problems

1. A student nurse assigned to care for the patient in a private room found the room practically overflowing with flowers and was forced to put two bouquets of cut flowers on the floor in order to have working space on the bedside table for giving the bath. While bathing the patient a ward aide brought in two more vases filled with flowers. None of the flowers were in condition to warrant discarding them. What would you have done?

2. A patient in a private room of a hospital complained to the doctor that she was displeased with the room because the window needed to be washed. The window washers had just completed washing the outside windows a few days before, but a series of rainstorms had left the windows badly spotted on the outside. The inside of the window was clean. The doctor asked a student nurse to see that the window was washed. What would you have done?

3. A student nurse assigned to the care of patients in a four bed ward found the large room greatly in need of attention from the housekeeping department maid. The mirror needed to be dusted, the wastebasket was overflowing, there was a large spot on the floor near the bed where some glucose solution had been spilled. The maid insisted that she had already cleaned the room and said emptying the wastebasket was the duty of another employee. The head nurse asked the student to report the matter to the head of the housekeeping department. The housekeeping department head was ill and would not be on duty that day. What would you have done?

Suggested Reference Reading

"Color is more than beauty," Faber Birren; Modern Hospital, January, 1952.
"The lighting of hospitals," Howard Haynes; Hospital Management, May, 1952.
"Paintings for patients," S. E. Walker; Hospitals, October, 1952.
"Flower rooms on every floor for therapeutic purposes," Hospitals, October, 1952.
"Hospital flowers," Jan Struther; What's New, December, 1952.

CHAPTER 6

Safety Measures

TOPICAL OUTLINE

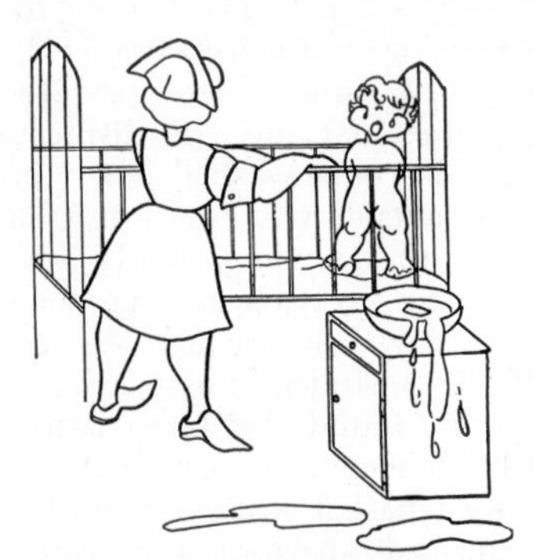

Children usually have no fear of water—unless soap has been added.

Safety measures related to nursing are primarily concerned with prevention of the many unfortunate occurrences or mishaps that may befall an individual patient, as falling from a bed or wheelchair, being burned by a hot water bottle, or receiving a wrong medication. In a larger sense, "accidents to patients" may refer to a disastrous fire or explosion in a hospital or other institution with resultant loss of life, or serious injury, to many patients and to hospital personnel.

From the standpoint of the hospital, safety measures must provide protection for the worker or employee as well as for the patient.

If large-scale disasters and individual accidents are to be prevented for patients and workers, each worker must be aware of the potential dangers of his job and be instructed in the use of all safety devices available in the institution. Each worker should be carefully selected for the job he will perform, there should be adequate supervision of all workers, and all persons in the institution should cooperate in observing safety regulations.

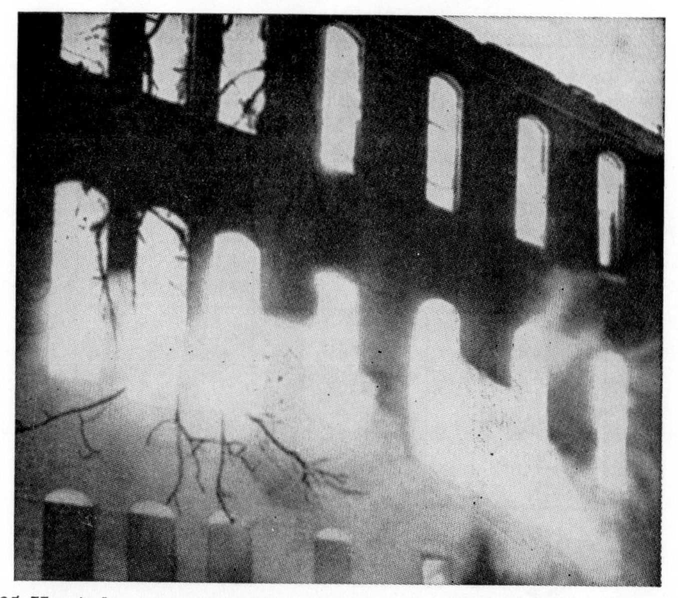

Fig. 35. Hospital construction of fire-resistant materials does not guarantee safety from fire. (Grinnell Company, Inc., Providence, Rhode Island.)

FIRE IN THE HOSPITAL

In the United States, according to national fire protection records, there are some three institutional fires each day. Fires occur each year in a number of hospitals and other institutions where patients are housed. Hospital management must accept the grave responsibility of fire prevention in an effort to protect patients and personnel within the institution.

Most hospitals are now constructed of fire resistant material, but that alone does not guarantee safety from fire. The building should be designed to prevent the spread of fire from its point of origin, and stairs and elevator shafts should be protected so that fire in the basement or lower floor will not spread to upper stories.

Each department in the hospital should have at least two safe exits as a means of escape from fire. In areas where patients are housed the exits should be wide enough to accommodate hospital beds.

Boiler rooms, kitchens, laundries, and paint shops, which have more than ordinary fire hazards, should be in separate buildings or separated from other areas by fire resistant walls and ceiling. Fire doors should be at all openings to such rooms, and automatic sprinkler protection should be provided.

The hospital should be amply protected by hose systems and chem-

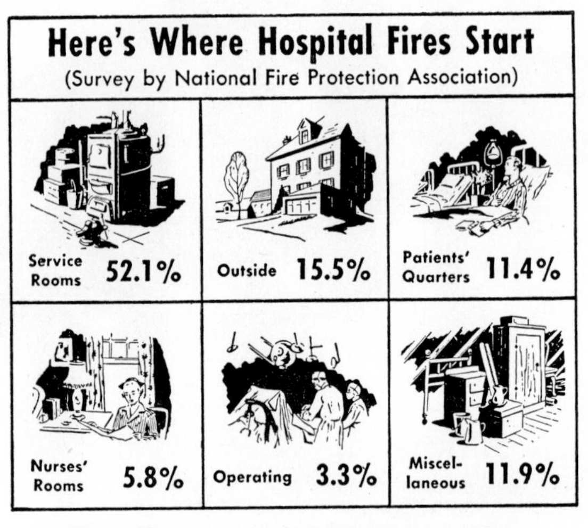

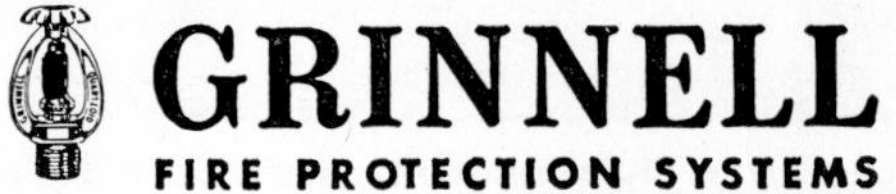

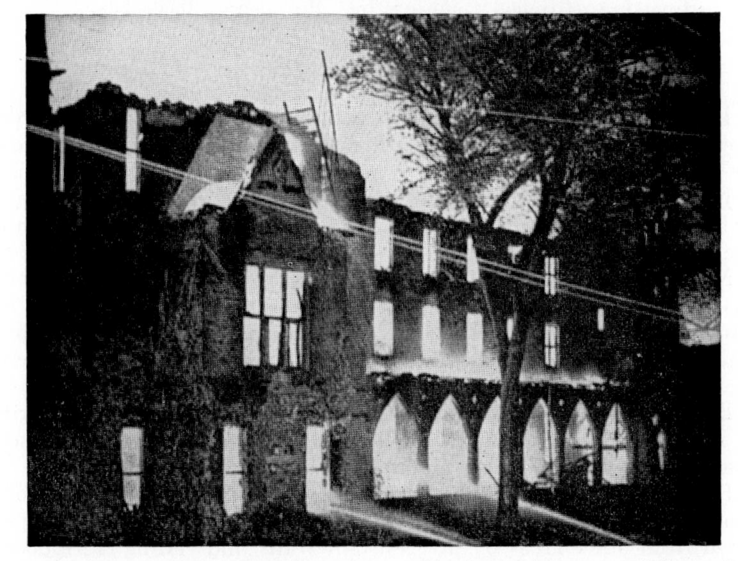

Fig. 36. More than half the hospital fires start in the service rooms of the institution. (Grinnell Company, Inc., Providence, Rhode Island.)

ical fire extinguishers. Automatic fire detection and alarm systems are essential. Such systems provide prompt notification should fire occur in storerooms, attics, or other unoccupied areas.

The most effective means of preventing hospital fires involves education of personnel in all possible causes of fire, and their cooperation in eliminating such causes and preventing fires.

Causes of Hospital Fires. *Careless smoking* or handling of cigarettes is one of the most frequent causes of hospital fires. Sand-filled receptacles for cigarette butts should be placed at elevator entrances and in corridors. Smoking stands and ash trays should be provided in all rooms where smoking is permitted. Wastebaskets of metal should be used throughout the hospital and smoking by patients should be carefully supervised. "No Smoking" signs should be prominently displayed in rooms or areas where smoking is dangerous, and all employees should be warned of the danger. Smoking where oxygen is stored, or in use, and where inflammable anesthetic gases are used or stored should be strictly forbidden.

Patients who smoke in bed may set fire to the mattress and cause a serious hospital fire. The nurse should either remove cigarettes and matches from within reach of the patient who is incompetent and irresponsible, or remain with him to see that careless handling of the cigarette does not start a fire.

Defective electrical equipment is another common cause of fires within hospitals. *Short circuits from misuse of equipment and defective electrical wiring* may also cause hospital fires. Since much of the equipment used for patients is handled by the nurse, she should be alert to the danger of improper or careless use of such equipment. Frayed cords, loose plugs, and worn connections should be noted and articles sent at once to the maintenance department for needed repair.

Spontaneous combustion may cause a hospital fire. Although the responsibility is primarily that of the housekeeping department, the nurse should help eliminate the hazards of this third largest cause of hospital fires. Materials subject to spontaneous combustion include rubbish, oily rags, sawdust, and agricultural products. Storage areas should be properly ventilated, oily materials should be kept in metal containers, rubbish should be disposed of before it collects in large amounts, and all spilled greases or inflammable liquids should be immediately removed. The nurse should remove all dirt, lint, or oil which may be present on electric motors of equipment used in treating patients.

Oxygen and other agents used in inhalation therapy may be the frequent cause of hospital fires.

Prevention of Hospital Fires. The first line of defense against hospital fires is a properly informed and trained personnel. Each hospital employee should know how to sound an alarm, how to operate the available fire extinguishers, and the proper procedure to follow when a fire occurs. Every new employee and each new class of student

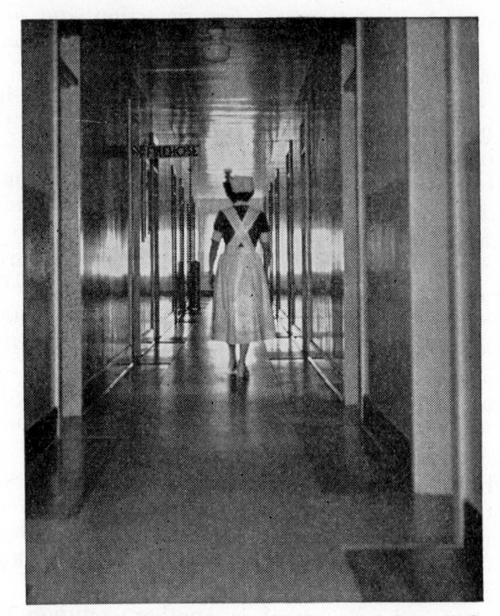

Fig. 37. Two main lines of defense against hospital fires: informed personnel and adequate fire protection equipment. (San Diego County General Hospital School of Nursing, San Diego, California.)

nurses and interns should be given fire-fighting instruction and taught to use fire-fighting equipment. The nurse should also know how to avoid or control panic among patients and employees. Panic at such a time may be more dangerous and cause more harm than the flames or smoke of the fire.

Each member of the hospital staff should know the location of fire-fighting equipment in the hospital, should know how to use it effectively, and should be familiar with written safety instructions on the best means of controlling fire in their own particular department of the hospital.

Fire drills should be repeated for everyone at regular intervals. Only by an understanding of the importance of fire prevention and correct fighting of fire on the part of everyone can the probability of fire be lessened.

Basic Rules if a Fire Occurs. Each hospital should have its own carefully worked out plan of action in case of fire. Although such plans will differ in detail, they will be basically the same.

The briefly outlined plan of action below is used in many institutions, and will be of great value to a nurse who may be forced to take charge of a dangerous situation should fire break out in her department.

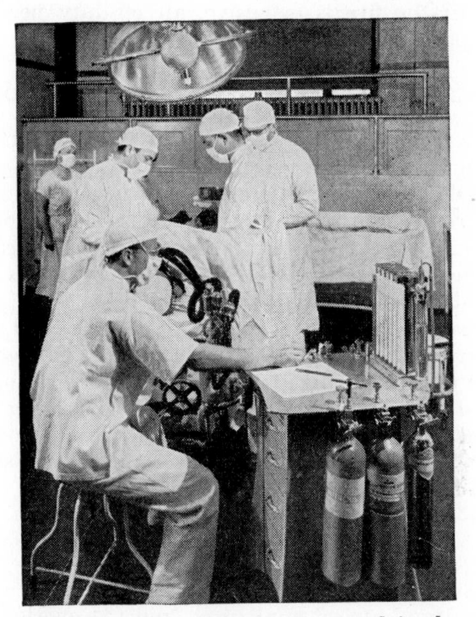

Fig. 38. Danger from fire and explosion is increased in the operating room. (Boston City Hospital, Boston, Massachusetts.)

1. Notify the switchboard to call the fire department and administrative officers, give exact location of the fire to the switchboard operator.
2. Assign one person to remain at the telephone to relay instructions.
3. Be calm—reassure patients and workers.
4. Have workers and ambulatory patients close all doors and windows.
5. Turn off all oxygen equipment and all electrical appliances.
6. See that all possible exits are clear.
7. Place wet blankets under closed doors if needed to keep patient rooms free of smoke.
8. Remove all patients in close proximity to the fire: (a) those nearest danger to be removed first; (b) ambulatory patients to help remove those in wheelchairs if hospital personnel is limited; (c) helpless patients to be removed on mattresses or on stretchers; (d) removal of patients should be accomplished in an orderly fashion, and all patients should be accounted for by the nurse in charge.
9. All nurses and other hospital personnel who are off duty at the time a fire occurs should be prepared to report at once to the department to which they are routinely assigned. If personnel on duty need

assistance or if the fire is extensive, all off-duty personnel will be notified to report for duty.

FIRES AND EXPLOSIONS IN OPERATING ROOMS

The danger from fire and explosions in the operating rooms is increased through daily use of electrical machines and equipment and because of the use of anesthetizing gases.

Static electricity is a hazard in the operating room, and because of that fact nurses who work in the surgery department may be restricted in the wearing of nylon uniforms. Uniforms of nylon are known generators of static sparks.

Suction pressure machines, cautery apparatus, and various x-ray and diathermy machines may also be a source of danger.

In an effort to decrease the incidence of fires and explosions hospitals have installed conductive flooring in their operating rooms. They have provided for better grounding of electrical currents and have prohibited the wearing of woolens, silks, and rubber-soled shoes by workers in the department.

FIRE IN THE NURSES' RESIDENCE

The three chief causes of fires in nurses' residences are : (1) smoking in bed, (2) faulty electrical appliances, and (3) overloaded electrical outlets. Correction of these faults would markedly decrease the number of fires which occur in nurses' residences each year.

Should fire occur in the nurses' residence the same basic rules as outlined for fire in the hospital should be followed. The switchboard operator or person in charge of the residence should be notified so the fire department may be called. Each nurse should be responsible for sounding the alarm on her corridor and should make certain that her nearest neighbors are awake and alerted to the danger. Nurses should vacate the building quickly and in an orderly manner. All residents should be warned not to return to the building or attempt a return to their room even though it may seem to them that the immediate danger is not great enough to prohibit them from trying to salvage a valuable belonging.

When the fire has been extinguished and residents are permitted to return to the building they should remain alert for evidence of recurrence of the fire.

ACCIDENTS TO ADULT PATIENTS

Accidents may be caused by carelessness on the part of hospital personnel, by thoughtlessness of the patient himself, or by faulty equipment.

The hospital administrator depends on the nursing staff to safeguard the patient. To do this effectively she must be aware of the kinds

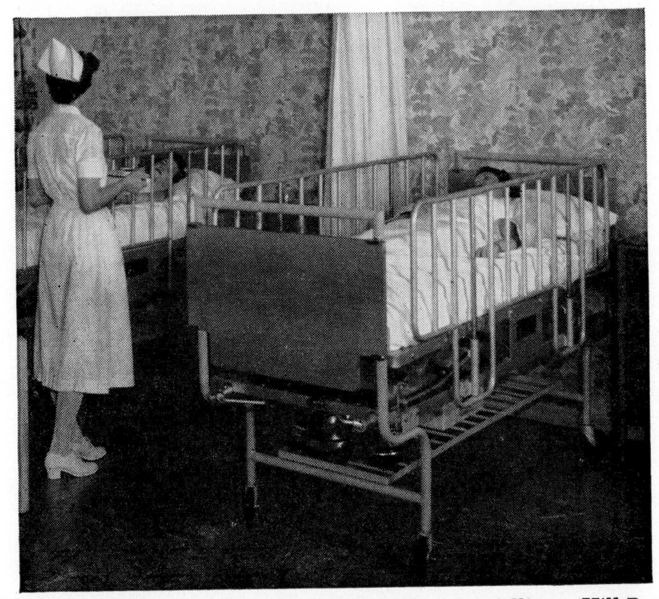

Fig. 39. Side rails on the bed protect the patient from falling. (Hill-Rom Co., Inc., Batesville, Indiana.)

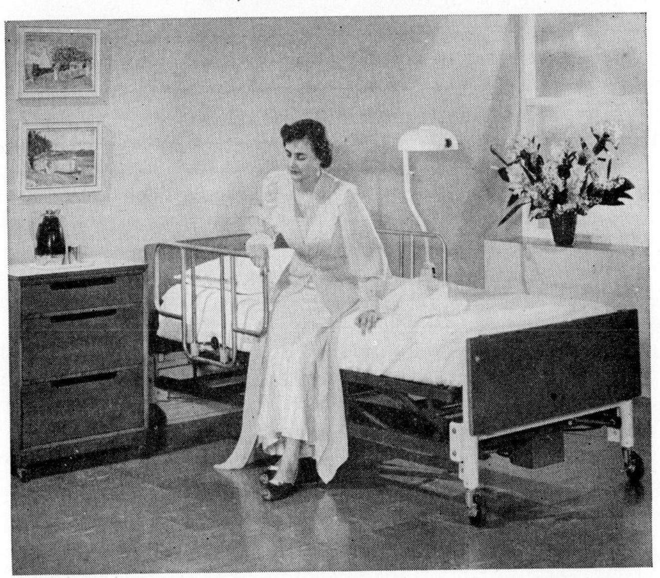

Fig. 40. The Hilow bed with permanently attached Safety Sides is a modern, effective means of preventing serious injury from bed falls. (Hill-Rom Co., Inc., Batesville, Indiana.)

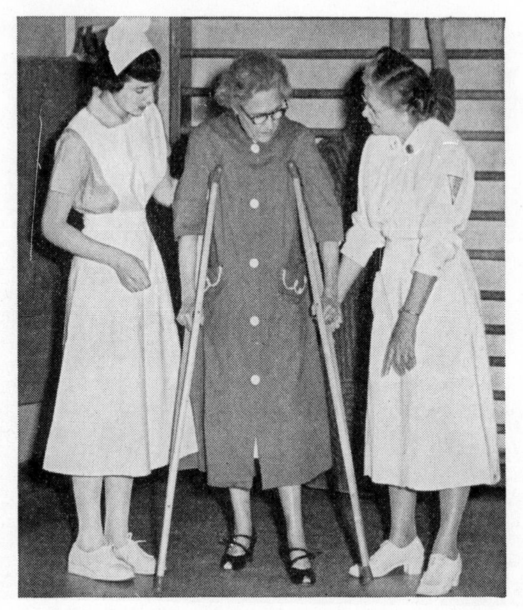

Fig. 41. Danger of falling is increased for patients who are on crutches. (Kansas City General Hospital School of Nursing, Kansas City, Missouri.)

of accidents that occur in hospitals and of various means of preventing them.

Falls. Falling from bed has been, for many years, a common and much dreaded form of hospital accident. Long side rails often cause more serious injury by tempting the patient to climb over them.

The modern Hilow bed, with Safety Sides attached, is recognized as a safe bed for hospital patients. The bed should be kept always in the "low" position except when medical or nursing care is being given the patient. The safety sides do not *restrain* the patient, but give him something to grasp when getting out of bed. Serious injury is also prevented by lessening the distance should the patient fall.

Patients may fall on floors that are highly polished or on small rugs that do not have a non-skid backing. Spilled liquids on floors are responsible for falls by patients. All such liquids should be cleaned from the floor immediately after being spilled.

Workers who mop large areas of a floor at one time may cause a patient to fall. Corridors should be mopped so that only one half the corridor (lengthwise) is wet at one time, and patients may walk on the part that remains dry.

Elevator operators should make sure that the floor of the elevator is in perfect alignment with the corridor floor when the elevator

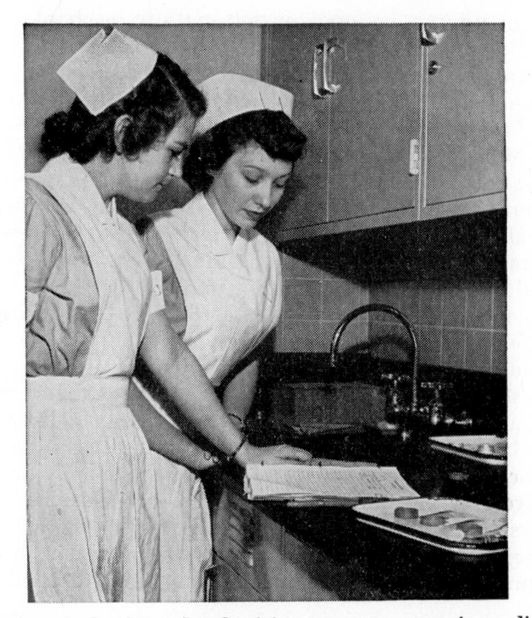

Fig. 42. A written order from the physician prevents errors in medication. (Alabama Baptist Hospital School of Nursing, Birmingham, Alabama.)

makes its stops, or persons stepping from the elevator should be warned to "step up" or "step down."

Amputees may fall and injure themselves if they are inadequately instructed or insufficiently trained in the use of crutches.

Patients should be assisted in and out of wheelchairs or be instructed on getting in and out without causing the chair to tip over. Anti-tip devices are now available for wheelchairs and should be put into use in all hospitals.

Falls from windows are usually the result of willful action on the part of the patient and can be prevented by installation of devices that will prevent opening the window more than a few inches.

Burns. Burns from hot water bottles are another common accident to the hospital patient. Through carelessness or negligence on the part of the nurse, many patients receive such burns. Hot water used in hot water bottles should always be tested, with a bath thermometer, to make sure that it never exceeds 125° F. in temperature. The nurse should keep in mind when preparing a hot water bottle that patients who are very old, very young, or very ill are more susceptible to burns. The skin in the very young and in the very old patient is thin and less resistant to heat. The very ill patient is usually unable to react normally and is therefore less protected.

Electric Shock. Water is a conductor of electricity, so electrical equipment should not be used or left within reach of patients in bathrooms. Patients should be warned of the danger in handling electrical appliances with wet hands. Electric heating pads and blankets should not be allowed to become damp or wet and should be watched carefully when in use by patients.

Errors in Medication. Another very real hazard for the hospital patient is that of errors in medication made by nurse, pharmacist, or doctor. Poisoning by chemicals or drugs should be guarded against by keeping all such medications under lock and key, in special cupboards separate from the medicine cabinet that is in general use. Nurses should be carefully instructed and supervised in the giving of medicines to limit the chance of error through lack of information or knowledge.

As a further protection against errors in medication no treatment or medicine should be given without a written and signed order from the physician. If the prescribed drug or dosage of a drug seems to differ from the usual kind and amount given, the nurse should question the order to eliminate the possibility of a mistake by the doctor.

Other sources of possible accidental injury to patients are broken thermometers or drinking tubes, needles that break off when a hypodermic is being given, and the careless use of razors, safety pins, sharp instruments, or other potentially dangerous articles.

ACCIDENTS TO CHILDREN

Accidents to children in the hospital are usually caused by negligence or carelessness of an adult. Nurses assigned to the care of children should know that large numbers of children under 15 die in accidents each year, the number of accidental deaths exceeding that of death caused by known childhood diseases. Such deaths result from suffocation, burns and scalds, falls, ingestion of poisons, and drowning.

Cause. Children may be hospitalized because of an accident, and are subject to accidents that may occur during hospitalization. A nurse in the pediatric department should be responsible for the safety of the young patient, but may inadvertently become the cause of accidental injury for him. Because of lack of awareness of danger, distractions and interruptions caused by other patients, an especially heavy assignment of work, and personality factors or weaknesses, such as habitual carelessness, the nurse may cause harm to the child.

Prevention. To prevent falling by hospitalized youngsters tall children should not be placed in very small cribs, the sides of which are too low and permit the youngster to fall over them. The nurse should never leave an infant or very young child in a crib with the sides down or on a sink or table where falling is possible.

When lifting or holding an infant the nurse should support its head and back in proper manner.

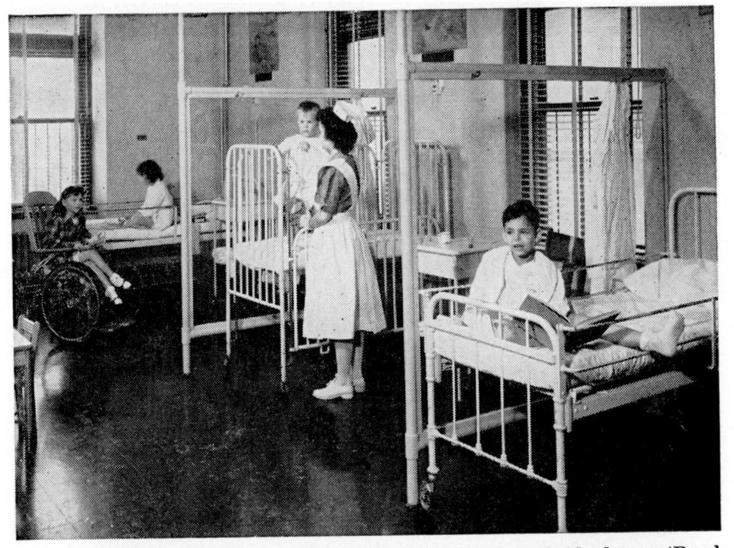

Fig. 43. A child should not be left alone in a crib with the cribside down. (Presbyterian Hospital School of Nursing, Chicago, Illinois.)

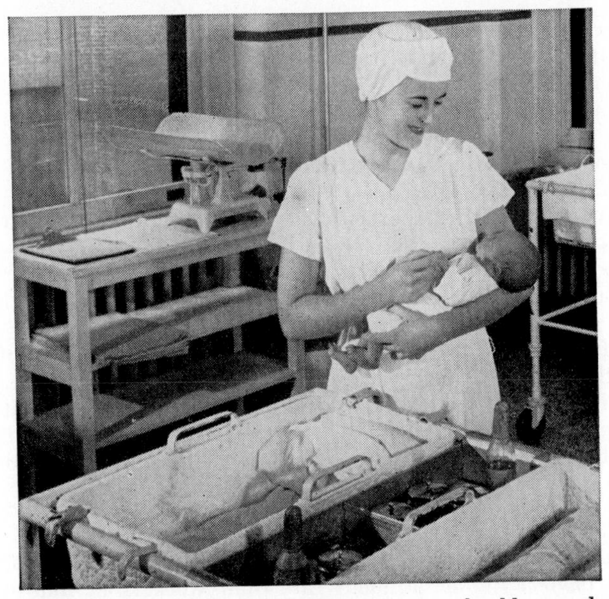

Fig. 44. When lifting or holding an infant the nurse should properly support its head and back. (Johns Hopkins Hospital School of Nursing, Baltimore, Maryland.)

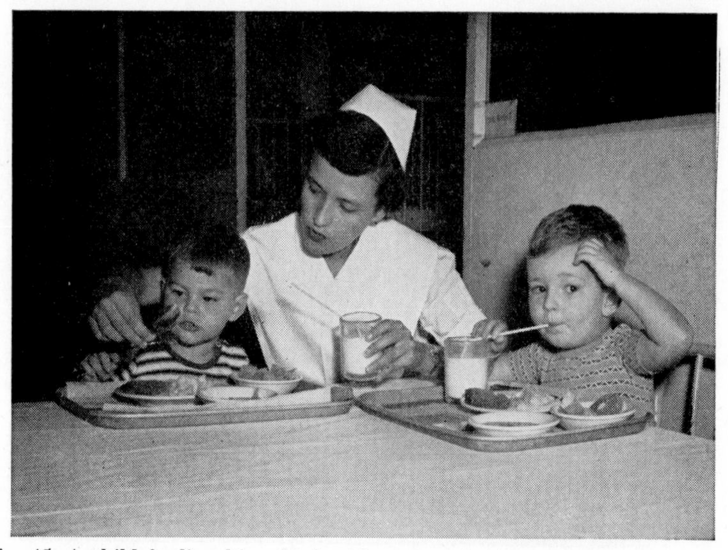

Fig. 45. A child feeding himself should not be left alone. (Indiana University Medical Center School of Nursing, Indianapolis, Indiana.)

Other rules to be followed in protecting the child patient from accidental injury include:

Never leave dangerous objects (safety pins, matches, cleaning fluid, breakable objects) within reach of a youngster. Don't permit a child to place small objects in his mouth.

Never force feedings on a child or leave him alone if he is feeding himself.

Always test, with a thermometer, the temperature of water to be used in a hot water bottle.

Have assistance when giving a hypodermic injection to a resisting child, and never leave him alone when rectal temperature is being taken.

Carefully select toys, remove unnecessary pillows from the crib when the child is sleeping, carefully inspect the nipple on the bottle before feedings, and see the child frequently during the night and at rest periods during the day so that close supervision can eliminate some of the hazards that are present for all hospitalized children.

ACCIDENTS TO NURSES

Statistics from the National Safety Council show that hospital employees have a higher accident rate than workers in industry, and for that reason the nurse needs to cooperate with other personnel to prevent accidents to staff members as well as to patients.

The chief hazards for employees in hospitals include those related to the use of oxygen and ether, lifting of patients or of heavy objects, breaking glass ampules, handling sharp surgical instruments, and autoclaving supplies with subsequent danger of being seriously burned by live steam.

Falls on stairways or near elevators, injury from swinging doors, and exposure to patients not known to have communicable disease are hazards that continually confront the nurse.

To prevent this high rate of accidents to nurses and other personnel, hospitals should put into effect well planned and well executed safety programs. The basic responsibilities of such a program would be to make the entire hospital staff "safety conscious" through instruction by department heads in the fundamental rules of accident prevention, to inspect each department periodically for hazards, and to correct all potential causes of accidents.

The most common accidental injuries to nurses each year are: strain from lifting patients, cuts from sharp instruments or broken glass, and bites or blows received from children and from uncooperative or irresponsible adult patients. Eye injuries are not uncommon among nurses; the eyes may be injured by a foreign body, by spilled solution, or by contact with contaminated hands. Collisions, falls, and electrical shock also cause injury to nurses.

For her own protection the nurse must be constantly aware of the danger of accidental injury and take precautions to prevent such accidents. She should be particularly careful when passing through swinging doors, walking up and down stairs, or stepping off elevators, and she should never touch an electrical connection when her hands are wet.

In learning safety measures for her own protection the nurse becomes better acquainted with methods of safeguarding the patients from accidental injury and becomes better able to cooperate with the administration in preventing accidents within the hospital.

ACCIDENT CONTROL

Accidents to patients can be controlled if the nurse and other hospital personnel are alert to causative factors of accidental injury. Most accidents suffered by patients are caused by unsafe equipment or conditions, or by unsafe acts of the nurse. If she is conscientious and careful in the administration of drugs and in the handling of potentially dangerous equipment, and remains alert to possible danger to the patient, she may help to substantially reduce the number of accidents that occur each year.

Safety measures which should be effective in helping to control accidents to patients include:

Periodic fire drills, routine check of fire-fighting equipment, and enforcement of "No Smoking" rules. All paints, oils, and other in-

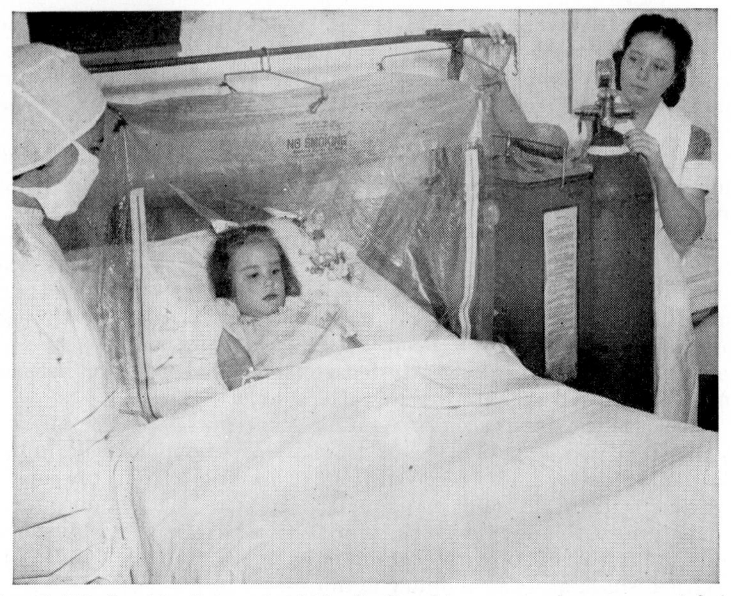

Fig. 46. "No Smoking" signs should be displayed in a room where oxygen is being used. (Mississippi Baptist Hospital School of Nursing, Jackson, Mississippi.)

flammable materials kept in proper containers in safe location, and repair of defective equipment when needed. Electric fans fastened securely in place.

Well lighted stairs with hand rails, treads in state of good repair, and kept free of all hazards such as mops, pails, boxes, etc.

Caution in handling of glass articles, sharp instruments, etc., and observance of proper methods of lifting and moving patients.

Use of side rails on beds, and wheel chairs equipped with anti-tip devices.

All hospital personnel should be encouraged to use care in performance of duties, being constantly aware of dangers to themselves and to patients. The nurse can well afford to be more safety conscious, and should welcome educational programs instituted by the hospital to help protect herself as well as the patient from accidental injury.

REPORT OF ACCIDENTAL INJURY

Any accident to a patient or to a hospital employee should be immediately reported to the nurse in charge. Forms used to report such accidents are usually made up to suit the needs of each particular hospital. Information required for complete reporting of an accident includes:

Date of accident — Exact time of accident — Name of patient — Diagnosis — Age — Sex — Marital status — Religion — Room or bed number — Department — Injury sustained — Condition of patient before accident — Names of witnesses — Doctor who examined patient — Time patient was examined — Complete report of what occurred — Report of examination findings — Treatment given.

Reports of accidents are usually required in duplicate so individual copies may be sent to designated administrative offices within the hospital. A report should be made regardless of whether the accident involves a patient, a member of the hospital staff, or another person who may be on hospital property when an injury is incurred. Even very minor accidents should be reported, since it is not unusual for injuries which apparently are of no consequence to be the cause of impaired functioning of a part at some later date.

In reporting accidents the nurse should make her statements brief and meaningful, giving only the essential facts needed to explain what occurred, but not placing blame for the accident on any one person. She should not include in the report comments which reflect her own personal opinion in regard to any factor or phase of the accident.

ACCIDENTS IN THE HOME OR COMMUNITY

Because accidents are high on the list of leading causes of death, and the nurse shares the responsibility for teaching accident prevention, it is essential that she be informed as to accidents that commonly occur in the home or in the community.

The nurse on active duty in a hospital and the nurse no longer concerned with active nursing but an interested and active member of her community are each in a strategic position to play an important part in accident prevention.

Safety Measures for Infants. Infants up to the age of 12 to 18 months need to be protected from accidental injury by close observation and careful attention to their needs and activities.

The infant should be watched closely when placed on a table, scales, or bathinette, and should never be left alone where there is danger of falling. Crib sides should always be up and fastened securely into position when the baby is in his crib. When the baby begins to walk, gates should be placed at the head and foot of stairs to prevent attempts at climbing and to safeguard him from falling.

Extra pillows and blankets should be removed from the crib when the baby is sleeping. Small objects such as toys, safety pins, whistles, etc., should be kept out of the baby's reach. The baby of crawling

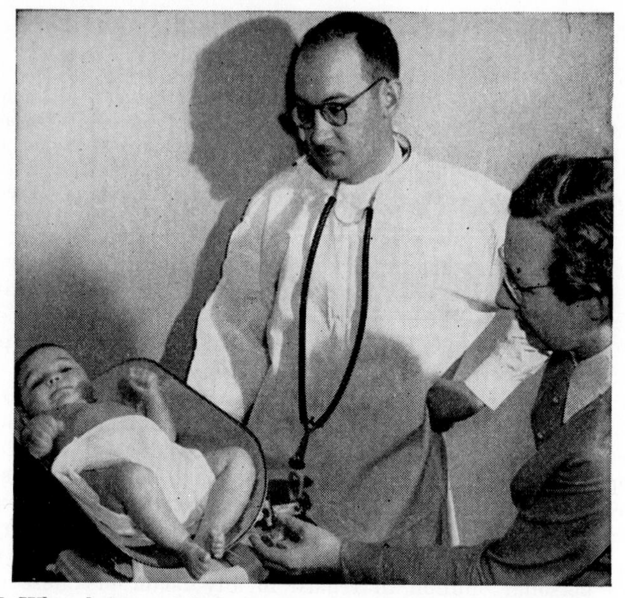

Fig. 47. When being weighed, the baby should be well balanced on the scales and should not be left alone. (Presbyterian Hospital, Chicago, Illinois.)

age investigates all such objects by placing them in his mouth, a practice which can result in strangulation.

The baby should never be left alone while in the bath, and young toddlers should be supervised at play if they are near small bodies of water, as a lily pond or swimming pool.

All electrical outlets within reach of the baby should have guards placed over them.

Containers of hot foods or liquids should be pushed back from the table or stove edge. The handles on such containers should always be turned inward. Matches and other dangerous articles should be kept out of the child's reach. The high chair should always be placed so it is a safe distance from the stove.

All medicines or drugs should be locked away from curious youngsters and medicines should be given only as prescribed by a doctor. Insecticides and disinfectants should be kept out of the child's reach.

Safety Measures for the Preschool Child. Doors leading to potential danger (basement stairs, etc.) should be kept locked and windows should have guards. Dangerous toys should not be given him. The stairs should have a strong hand rail and be kept free of toys, mops, brooms, etc. Non-skid rugs should be placed on waxed floors. Children should be cautioned not to cross the street and to remain near home while at play.

Safety Measures for the School Child. Careful instructions should be given the child in regard to crossing streets, he should be told to cross at intersections only, cross with the green light, learn traffic signals, and obey traffic regulations, stop at the curb and look both ways before crossing. Children should use the safest route between home and school, and never play in the street.

When riding a bicycle he should always have lights on after dark. He should go down feet first on slides. He should stay away from excavations, railroad yards, and empty houses unless he is accompanied by an adult.

A child should learn to swim, but should never jump or dive into cold water, and should never jokingly call for help. He should look for rocks before diving, and float when rest is needed.

Safety Measures for the Adult. Measures which should be adopted to assure safety for adults in the home include the following:

A screen in front of fireplaces, and non-skid backing on all scatter rugs. A firm kitchen step stool for climbing.

Wastebaskets made of metal.

Heavy pot holders to remove hot dishes from the oven.

Sharp knives kept in a wall rack instead of a cabinet drawer. Poisonous drugs plainly labeled and locked in a cupboard.

Rooms adequately ventilated.

Old razor blades discarded into a proper disposal unit.

A hand hold on the bathtub, and a rubber mat in the bottom of the tub to prevent falling.

Protection from electrical shock is achieved when each light cord pull chain is provided with an insulating link, and all worn electric cords are replaced. Radios, fans, and other electrical appliances are kept out of the bathroom, and electrical appliances are not touched with wet hands.

Halls and stairways should always be well lighted and carpets repaired.

Garden tools put away after use, and the clothesline placed high enough to avoid catching anyone who might walk beneath it. The burning of leaves and rubbish should be closely supervised, and the basement and attic should be kept clean.

The garage door should always be open before the car motor is started, thus preventing an accumulation of carbon monoxide gas. When backing the car from the garage the driver should be sure no children are in the driveway.

Safety Measures for the Aged. In addition to the general safety measures for adults the elderly person who doesn't see or hear well and is not able to move swiftly should be further safeguarded. For such persons curbs, street crossings, high steps on busses and differences in floor levels are sources of danger. Low, portable pieces of furniture, as footstools or floor fans, may be the cause of falls, since old people often fail to notice them.

Water should be run into the tub just before the bath is to be given. Serious accidents have resulted when hot water is left running and the older person becomes confused. He may not be able to turn off the water or get out of the tub in time to prevent being scalded.

Doors should be locked at night to prevent the elderly person from wandering out of the house. Safeguards are needed on gas appliances —old people have been known to turn on the gas and then forget to light it. The hazards for aged persons in the home are increased as the sense of sight and hearing is gradually lost and the person's physical condition approaches senility.

Summary of Important Factors

Prevention of accidents to patients is a major responsibility of the nurse; protection of herself and of other hospital personnel is also part of her duty.

Fire-resistant material used in hospital construction does not make the building fire proof. Education and training of personnel is the most effective means of preventing hospital fires.

Careless smoking of cigarettes is the most frequent cause of hospital fires. "No Smoking" signs should be prominently displayed in areas where smoking is hazardous, and the regulation should be strictly enforced.

Periodic checking of electrical equipment and repair when needed is an important part of fire prevention activity.

Water is a conductor of electricity. Electrical appliances should not be touched with wet hands. Heating pads or blankets should not be used if they become damp.

Rubbish and oily rags should not be allowed to accumulate because of the danger of spontaneous combustion.

Fire is a potential danger where oxygen equipment is in use and protective measures are necessary.

Each hospital employee should know how to sound an alarm and how to operate available fire extinguishers.

The nurse must remain calm. She will need to control panic in others at the time a fire occurs.

Basic rules if fire occurs: Sound alarm—notify switchboard; assign person to remain at telephone; close windows and doors; disconnect all oxygen equipment and electrical appliances; remove patients in close proximity to the fire.

If fire occurs in the nurses' residence each nurse should see that her neighbors are alerted.

After leaving because of fire no one should return to the building until the danger is over and permission to return has been given.

The nurse must be constantly aware of hazards to help prevent accidents to patients. Common accidents to patients include: falling; burns; errors in medication; fire from smoking in bed; cuts from broken glass and careless use of sharp instruments.

Children suffer such accidents as suffocation, falls, poisoning, drowning, burns, and scalds.

The nurse, by being aware of potential danger, may prevent accidental injury to herself and others. All measures of accident control should be studied and practiced by the nurse.

When making a report of an accident all necessary information should be given.

The nurse should know the chief causes of accidents in the home and should instruct the patient in various means of preventing such accidents.

Factors To Teach the Patient

That smoking a cigarette in bed is a dangerous procedure and deserves his utmost attention and care.

That one should not smoke in an area where smoking is extremely dangerous and "No Smoking" signs are prominently displayed. That because oxygen aids combustion, smoking should not be permitted in areas where oxygen is being used.

That water is a conductor of electricity—electrical appliances should not be touched with wet hands. Heating pads or electric blankets that are damp should not be used.

That panic at the time of a fire may be more dangerous than the fire.

If fire occurs patients should cooperate with the nurse in charge of the department, remain calm, and (if ambulatory) help with wheelchair patients; if restricted to bed, await help from hospital personnel.

That falling may be prevented by use of such protective measures as side rails on the bed; non-skid backing on rugs; avoidance of walking on waxed floors; hand rail on stairs; watching alignment of elevator and floor; extreme care when smoking in bed; proper instruction or assistance in getting in and out of wheelchair and in walking with crutches.

That a hot water bottle should not be hotter than the prescribed 125° F.

Measures for prevention of accidents in the home include: all poisonous drugs should be kept in a locked cupboard; dangerous articles should be kept out of reach of small children; window guards, stair hand rails, non-skid rugs, bath mats of rubber are all needed to prevent falls; a protective screen should be kept in front of the fireplace; wastebaskets should be made of metal; worn electric cords should be replaced, appliances disconnected after use, and care taken not to overload electric circuits; chairs should not be used as a substitute for a kitchen step stool; an electrical appliance should never be touched with wet hands; persons should not get into bath tub with hot water running; extra precautions are needed for old people who do not see or hear well, cannot move quickly, and become easily confused.

Situation Type Problems

A student nurse on duty in the nursery was asked to place a hot water bottle at the foot of a baby basinette which had been prepared

for a newborn baby. She was told to be certain that the temperature of the water used did not exceed 115° F. The basinette was empty at the time the order for the hot water bottle was given.

The student had learned that hot water bottles for anesthetic beds need not be placed in a cover and that the temperature of the water used in filling them was not important since they were removed from the bed before the patient was returned from the operating room. She filled a hot water bottle and, without taking the temperature of the water or covering the bottle, tucked it in the space beween the mattress edge and the foot of the basinette.

The nurse who brought the baby to the basinette a few minutes later failed to notice the hot water bottle. The baby was placed, still wrapped in blankets, into the basinette and the nurse returned to her duties in the delivery room. The nurse in charge of the nursery observed that the new baby was breathing normally and crying lustily, so she went on with her task of feeding another infant.

The baby in the basinette continued to cry, so when the student nurse returned from lunch she was asked to give her immediate attention to that baby.

The student carried the baby to the work counter at the sink and removed the folds of blanket. She noticed that the baby's feet were unusually red and the baby screamed as though in pain when she took hold of them. Investigation disclosed that large blisters had formed on both heels of the infant, where the feet had been lying against the too hot hot-water bottle. What would you have done?

Suggested Reference Reading

"Accident prevention in pediatric nursing," Gaylord W. Graves; American Journal of Nursing, January, 1949.
"Fires in hospitals and nurses' homes," Dorothy Pellenz; American Journal of Nursing, January, 1949.
"Our firetrap hospitals," Miriam Zeller Gross; Reader's Digest, October, 1951.
"A hospital emergency and receiving department," Lelia G. Parrish and Ruth Wallis; American Journal of Nursing, December, 1951.
"Fire safety is everybody's business," Modern Hospital, May, 1952.
"Safe sun baths for your child," Adeline Bullock; Parents, June, 1952.
"Teach them cycling safety," Thomas Powell; Today's Health, September, 1952.
"Toys for toddlers," Anne Leonard; American Journal of Nursing, December, 1952.
"Errors in giving medication," Anne K. Byrne; American Journal of Nursing, July, 1953.

CHAPTER 7

Bed Making

TOPICAL OUTLINE

THE BED
LINEN NEEDED TO MAKE THE BED
MAKING THE BED
- The Mitered Corner
- The Box Corner
- The Closed Bed
- The Open Bed
- The Bed for the "Up" Patient
- The Occupied Bed
- The Anesthetic Bed

THE BED CRADLE
CARE OF BED LINEN

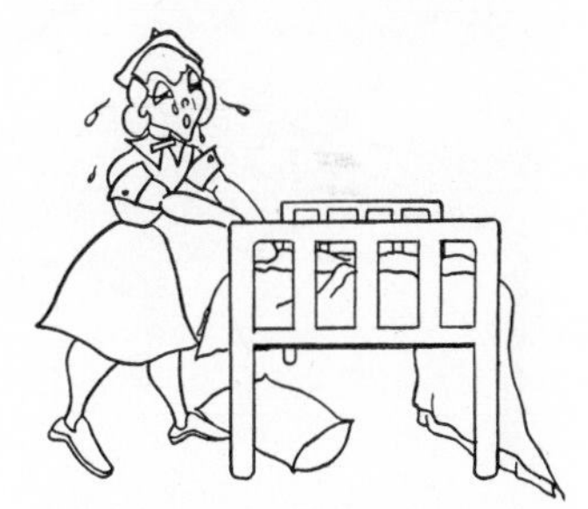

Life is made up of smiles, sobs, and sniffles—with the sniffles predominating.

Making a bed properly is one of the first procedures taught to the student of nursing. The skill developed by the nurse in performing this particular procedure determines, to a great extent, the comfort of the bed patient. It is a factor in the immediate surroundings of the patient, since the way in which the bed is made and the manner in which bed linen is arranged will influence the attractiveness of the room or unit which he occupies.

If the student nurse has learned to use her hands effectively in making beds, washing dishes, and helping with household tasks at home she should have little difficulty in learning to handle the various articles of bed linen and should soon be able to make a hospital bed in the proper manner. The girl who has had very little practice in handling bed linen may find the procedure somewhat difficult but, with practice, will soon be able to make a bed that will pass inspection from even the most demanding instructor.

Relatives of a very ill patient will readily admit that the nurse is better able to secure comfort for the patient than they seem to be, even though their ministrations are an expression of love and tenderness. The nurse has been carefully instructed in the best method of freshening pillows, tightening sheets, and arranging covers so that she performs the procedure skillfully, requiring no exertion on the part of the patient.

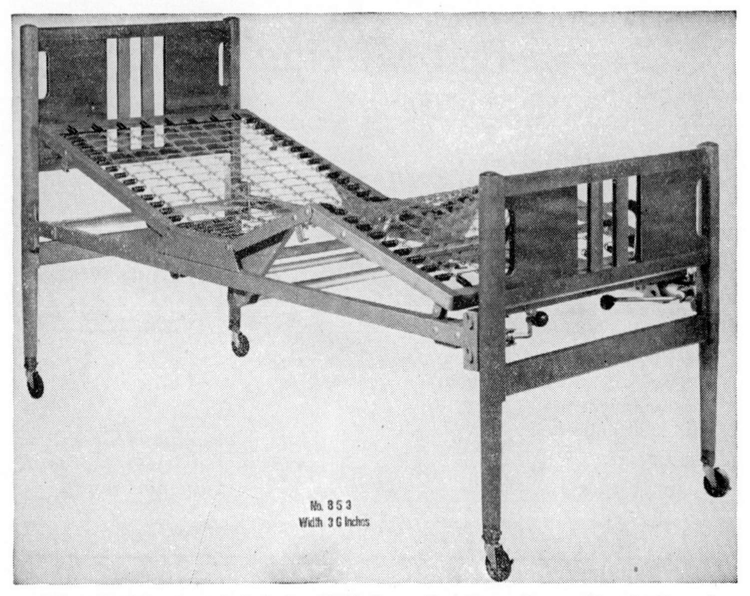

Fig. 48. The hospital bed. (Hill-Rom Co., Inc., Batesville, Indiana.)

THE BED

The hospital bed most widely used is the Gatch bed, with springs of woven wire which are durable, comfortable, and easy to clean. The metal frame to which the springs are fastened is divided into three sections, which may be raised or lowered, by means of hand cranks at the foot of the bed, to change the patient's position. The adjustable parts of the bed provide complete support while making the patient comfortable and insure correct position of the body for various treatments or nursing procedures.

The standard hospital bed is 6½ feet long, 3 feet wide, and 27 inches from the floor. The bed will accommodate the average patient and is high enough from the floor to be convenient for the nurse as she performs routine nursing duties. The height of the hospital bed prevents undue strain and fatigue for the physician, nurse, and other hospital personnel who help in the care of the patient.

For most patients innerspring mattresses are more comfortable than any other kind, and large numbers of hospitals use mattresses of that type. When innerspring mattresses are not available, mattresses of horsehair are usually preferred. Whatever the type, the mattress should be smooth and firm to give needed support to the body.

For patients who must remain in bed for long periods of time and for very thin patients a sponge rubber or an air mattress may be preferable. Such mattresses are better suited to prevent pressure on any one area and thus protect the patient from the development of pressure sores.

Each bed should have two pillows, one filled with horsehair which is cool in summer and best suited for the needs of the patient with an elevated temperature. The other pillow should be filled with feathers, which make it soft and comfortable. In addition to the two large pillows, several small pillows should be available to give support to various parts of the body and to help in making the patient comfortable. Pillows are used primarily to support head and shoulders of the patient but may also be used for support to other parts of the body when the patient is turned from one position to another. Two large pillows (standard size—20 by 28 inches and weighing 2½–3 pounds) and one or more small pillows should be provided for each patient. Pillows are usually made of stout cotton ticking, with washable covers to protect the pillow from dust and lint.

Some patients are allergic to many different types of pillow fillers, and for them the kapok-filled pillow is usually satisfactory. The allergic patient may use a feather pillow if it is securely covered with a plastic type cover fastened with a zipper. Such covers should always be used on pillows for patients with head injuries or with operations about the face or head, or when the pillow is apt to be soiled from discharge or from dressings.

LINEN NEEDED TO MAKE THE BED

Before beginning to make the bed the nurse should bring all linen that will be needed into the room and place it on the chair beside the bed. If arranged on the chair in a reverse order to that in which it will be placed on the bed, there will be no necessity to handle the entire supply while searching for each piece as it is needed. The following articles of linen will be in proper order for making the bed if placed on the chair in the order listed: Pillow cases—pillow covers — spread — blanket — sheet — draw sheet — rubber sheet — sheet (— mattress pad — mattress cover).

The *mattress cover* is made of heavy cotton and is used to protect the mattress from dust or soil. It may be changed frequently so that it is clean when used for more than one patient.

The *mattress* pad is a full length quilted pad which covers the top of the mattress and protects it from dust and soil.

Bed *sheets* need to be of sufficient length and width to permit them to be tucked well under the mattress at the head and sides of the bed, or, in the case of the top sheet, to be tucked under the mattress at the foot of the bed and to be folded back over the blanket and spread, to protect them from coming in contact with the patient. Sheets for hospital use are approximately 72 inches wide and 108 inches long, and are made of cotton. The usual practice, in making up the patient's bed, is to place the top sheet, which has been in use for one day, on the mattress as the lower or foundation sheet, and to provide a clean sheet for the top sheet.

Skin irritations may occasionally be caused by sheets which are not thoroughly rinsed in the laundry so careful washing and rinsing is needed to remove all harsh soap or chemicals.

The *rubber sheet*, made of rubber sheeting, is used to protect the mattress. Heavy ticking sewed on each end of the rubber sheet reduces the amount of rubber used in the sheet (and so reduces expense) and also provides a better substance or material for tucking under the mattress to hold the rubber sheet securely in place. The rubber sheet, made of heavy rubber which does not allow for evaporation of perspiration in a warm atmosphere, may cause discomfort to the patient. If the rubber sheet is hot and uncomfortable, the patient may request that it be removed from the bed. (Some hospitals require that the patient sign a record form which states that he accepts responsibility for having the rubber sheet removed and will pay for any damage that might result to the mattress.) To prevent discomfort from the rubber sheet, it may be placed directly on the mattress, then covered with the foundation sheet and draw sheet. A quilted pad covering the rubber sheet will also reduce discomfort for the patient.

The rubber sheet should be wide enough to cover approximately two-thirds the length of the mattress.

Substitutes for rubber sheets that may be used in the home include oilcloth and plastic, or other waterproof materials. If none of these materials is available, several thicknesses of newspaper will afford some protection for the mattress.

The *draw sheet*, a specially made sheet for hospital use, consists of two layers of material, stitched together. Used to cover the rubber sheet when placed on the bed, it is wide enough to extend about three inches beyond it at either edge, and is long enough to tuck securely under the mattress at each side.

The draw sheet may be changed often, if necessary, with only a minimum amount of disturbance to the patient. For incontinent patients or those with profuse perspiration or an excessive amount of drainage, the draw sheet may be changed at frequent intervals to keep the bed clean and dry.

The *blanket* used in making a hospital bed should be warm and light in weight. It should be long enough to be tucked under the mattress at the foot of the bed and still extend upward far enough to cover the patient's shoulders. Blankets are usually about 75 per cent wool and 25 per cent cotton. The latter prevents excess shrinkage. Although kept on the bed during the time the patient remains in the hospital, the blanket does not come in direct contact with the patient, so it may require cleaning only at infrequent intervals.

The *spread* is used to make the bed more attractive in appearance

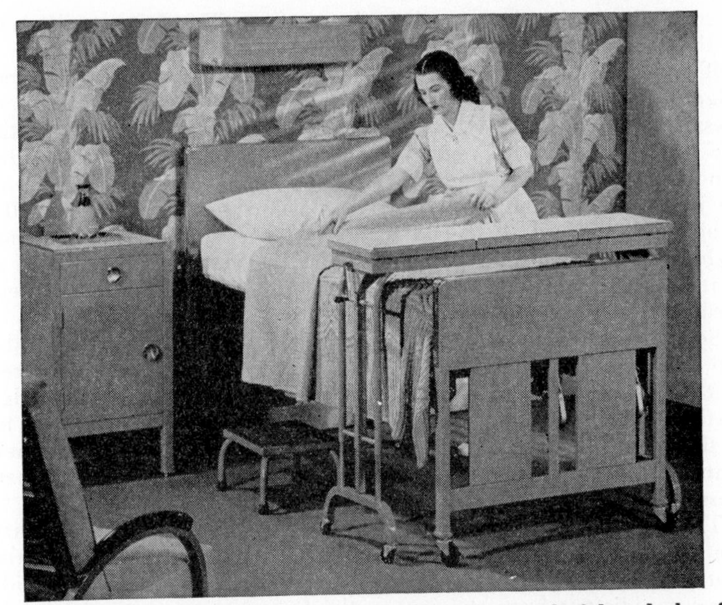

Fig. 49. Pastel spreads help make the hospital room colorful and cheerful. (Simmons Company, Merchandise Mart, Chicago, Illinois.)

and to protect the other linen. It should be light in weight, washable, and large enough to be tucked in well at the foot and to completely cover the entire top surface of the bed. Spreads of various pastel shades help to make the hospital room or ward colorful and more cheerful.

Pillow cases, usually of muslin, are made so they are a few inches wider and several inches longer than the pillow. Pillow cases are changed at least once each day or more often if necessary.

MAKING THE BED

The first step in bed making is moving the mattress toward the head of the bed and to the side as needed so that it rests evenly on the bed springs.

The mattress pad should be placed so that it covers the entire length and width of the mattress. The lower or "foundation" sheet should be placed so that the smaller of the two hems is even with the foot edge of the mattress. Kept in the correct position, it should be stretched smoothly into place and tucked securely under the head end of the mattress. If the sheet is not fastened securely at the top and sides it tends to wrinkle toward the foot of the bed, as the patient tends to slide downward on the mattress. This is especially true if the backrest of the bed is elevated during the day.

The rubber sheet should be placed across the bed so that the upper edge of it is approximately 15 inches from the top edge of the mattress. (The distance may be measured by placing the elbow at the top edge of the mattress and extending the arm and hand. The distance from elbow to fingertips is approximately 15 inches.) About 30 inches of the mattress will extend below the lower edge of the rubber sheet. The draw sheet is placed over the rubber sheet, stretched tightly across the bed, and tucked under the mattress at each side so that the foundation of the bed is very tight and smooth and held securely in place.

So that the top sheet will be right side up when folded across the top covers, it is placed on the bed wrong side up. It should be placed so that the larger hem is at the top and is brought to the top edge of the mattress. Placed on the bed in this way the top sheet will be of the right length to fold down over the top edge of the spread and blanket. The top sheet should be long enough to tuck under the mattress at the foot of the bed.

The blanket should be placed so it is centered on the mattress with the top edge of the blanket about a foot from the top edge of the mattress. If the blanket is not centered on the bed, with the side edges equidistant from the center, the top covers may tend to slide off the side of the bed where the blanket is longer.

The spread should be placed on the bed with the top edge of the spread even with the top edge of the mattress and the bottom edge tucked under the foot of the mattress. All top covers are allowed to hang free over the sides of the mattress.

Pillow covers and pillow cases should be placed on the pillows. The end of the cover should be snap fastened or tied in place and the open end of the pillow cover should be inserted into the pillow case so it will then be at the closed end of the case.

Pillows should be placed on the bed so that the open end of the pillow case is away from the door or entrance to the patient unit.

The sheets and spread used in bedmaking are fastened into proper position by having corners mitered. The blanket is held in position by box corners made at each corner at the foot of the mattress.

The Mitered Corner. In making the hospital bed the distinguishing feature of the mitered corner must be given attention. By mitering is meant the formation of a smooth-fitting corner by folding the sheet or spread in such a way that a 45 degree angle is made with one or both of them and the corner of the mattress sharply outlined.

As the sheets are placed on the bed the corners are mitered and the sheet then tucked under the mattress to be held firmly in place. The spread is mitered at the corners at the foot of the bed. Since the spread is used to enhance the appearance of the bed the mitered cor-

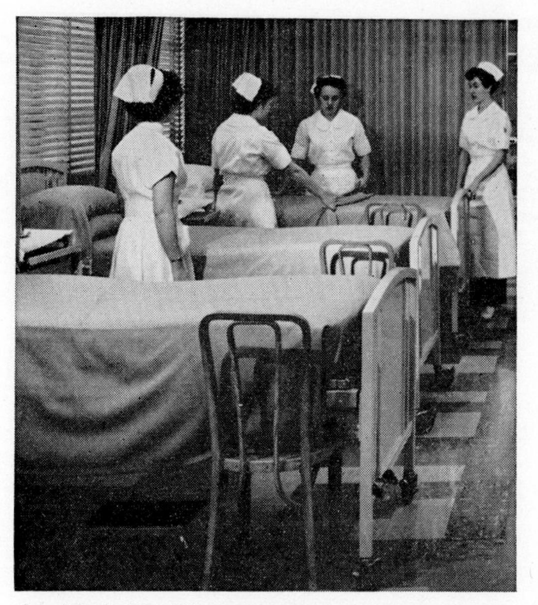

Fig. 50. The closed bed. (St. Vincent's College of Nursing, Los Angeles, California.)

ners are not tucked under the mattress at the sides. After the mitered corner has been made the sides of the spread are allowed to hang free.

The Box Corner. Box corners serve the same purpose as the mitered corner, to cover the corner smoothly and anchor the cover into place. Box corners are used for the blanket at the foot of the bed. The blanket is of heavier material than sheet or spread and use of the box corner is indicated. The fold in the blanket is adjusted so that it is even with and parallel to the edge of the mattress which forms the corner. The 45 degree angle of the mitered corner would leave a ridge of blanket which could not be concealed by the spread. By making the box corner the blanket fits smoothly around the mattress corner and can be held in place by being tucked under the edge of the mattress. The spread can be placed over the blanket and will be smooth and neat at the corner when the mitered corner is made.

The Closed Bed. The term "closed bed" is used to designate the hospital bed which remains empty until the admission of another patient. It is termed "closed bed" because the top covers are so arranged that all linen beneath the spread is fully protected from dust and dirt.

In the closed bed the top 10 or 12 inches of the upper sheet is folded down over the top edge of the blanket and smoothed into posi-

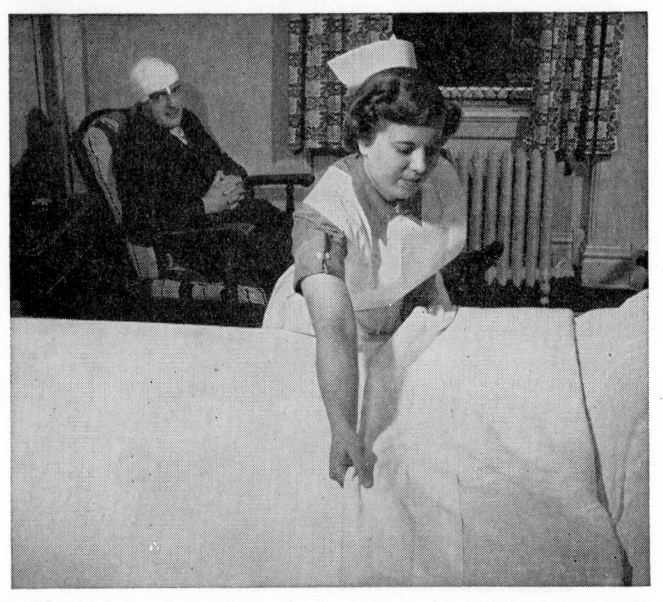

Fig. 51. The bed for the patient who is up and about. (Presbyterian Hospital School of Nursing, Chicago, Illinois.)

tion across the mattress. The spread is then placed so that its top edge is even with the top edge of the mattress and it completely covers the entire top surface of the mattress. The hospital bed should be made up as a "closed bed" during the time it remains unoccupied.

The Open Bed. The term "open bed" is used to designate the hospital bed when it is occupied, or about to be occupied, by a patient.

In the open bed the upper sheet is placed so that the wide hem rests along the top edge of the mattress. The blanket is then put in place. The spread is placed over the blanket and the top 10 or 12 inches of spread is folded under the top edge of the blanket. After the spread has been folded into position the top edge of the sheet is folded down across the folded edge of the spread, making an envelope cover for spread and blanket. The "open bed" is used for all occupied beds in the hospital.

The Bed for an "Up" Patient. The bed for a patient who is allowed to be up should be neat in appearance and made so that it can easily be converted to an "open bed" for the patient when he must return to it for rest or sleep.

For this type bed the top covers are arranged as described above for the open bed. As soon as the open bed has been completed the top covers—spread, blanket, and sheet—are grasped in both hands and folded with their top edge to the foot of the bed. The top edge is then brought toward the head of the bed, until it is directly above the center fold originally made.

Placing the Pillows. For each of the three types of beds described above the pillows are placed in position after the top covers have been arranged. The first pillow is placed, open end of pillow case farthest from the door, against the head of the bed and centered so that the ends are equally distant from the sides of the mattress, the pillow should be flat on the mattress and smoothed into position. The second pillow is placed directly on top of the first one, in exactly the same position.

The Occupied Bed. The nurse should be thoroughly familiar with the procedure of making an empty bed before she attempts to make a bed occupied by a patient.

Since the spread may be used more than one day, depending on its appearance when the bed is made, it should be carefully folded each time it is removed from the bed.

If the patient has been using more than one pillow, all extra ones should be removed from the bed. One pillow is left beneath the head of the patient, if he wishes, since sudden removal of all pillows tends to give the impression that the head of the bed is lower than the foot. The sensation of almost standing on one's head is an unpleasant one and most patients object when all pillows are removed for bedmaking.

As top covers are taken from the bed the patient will need to be covered with a bath blanket to prevent exposure. Before any attempt is made to remove the foundation or bed linen from beneath the patient, it will need to be loosened from under the mattress at the head and along both sides of the bed.

To work effectively in making the occupied bed, the patient must be turned or moved to one side of the mattress and made comfortable and secure in that position so there will be no danger of his falling out of bed. The nurse may then go to the opposite side of the bed and begin to remove soiled linen which is to be replaced with clean.

The soiled draw sheet should be rolled smoothly, its entire width, across the bed and pushed against or slightly under the patient.

The rubber sheet should be fanfolded and pushed against and slightly under the folded draw sheet, then the foundation sheet should be rolled and pushed against and slightly beneath the rubber sheet. Care must be taken so that all folds or rolls of linen are even and extend smoothly across the mattress. The excess length of the foundation sheet which had been tucked under the head of the mattress should be rolled or folded and pushed aside at the top edge of the mattress.

When pushing the rolled draw sheet, rubber sheet, and foundation sheet against the patient the nurse should place one hand on the patient's hip or side, which is not resting on the bed, as a steadying measure so he will not feel that he is being pushed out of bed.

The clean lower sheet should then be placed on the bed lengthwise so that it covers at least half the width of the mattress. The part of the clean sheet that will cover the side of the mattress on which the patient is lying is pushed in a loose roll against the center line folds already made by the linen being removed from the bed. The excess length of the sheet is tucked beneath the top of the mattress, the upper corner is mitered, and the sheet is then tucked under the mattress at the side of the bed for its entire length.

The rubber sheet may then be pulled toward the nurse from the center roll and stretched smoothly across the clean foundation sheet which has just been placed in position.

The clean draw sheet is put in place with the side not tucked under the mattress fanfolded against the draw sheet that is to be removed from the bed.

The patient may then be turned so that he is resting on the half of the bed which has just been made fresh with clean linen. The soiled linen is removed from the opposite side of the bed and placed in the linen bag.

The clean linen should then be brought into place on the side previously occupied by the patient, corners mitered, and edges tucked under the mattress to complete the foundation of the bed.

So the foundation of the occupied bed will be made taut and firm the sheets should be pulled tightly across the mattress after the patient has been turned to the clean side of the bed. If done properly the tightening of the sheets across the bed will move the patient slightly toward the side on which he was formerly resting. This tightens the sheet on the side of the bed which was made first, and the weight of the patient holds the sheets firmly in place while the nurse then tightens and secures them on the side of the bed being made.

To place the top covers in position and get them centered correctly on the bed, the patient should be turned on his back and moved to the center of the bed. Top covers will be straight and even if the nurse places them on the bed so the center crease in sheet and spread and center fold of the blanket follow the center line of the mattress when it is lined up with the center of head and foot boards of the bed. In placing top covers on the bed enough room should be allowed for the patient's feet. If necessary a pleat may be placed in the top sheet and blanket. The patient should be instructed to keep his feet upright as the bed is being made. Loosening the top covers slightly at the foot of the mattress will also help to provide sufficient room for the patient's feet.

Clean pillow cases should be placed on the pillows each day even though other articles of linen on the bed are not changed as often. The pillows should be placed beneath the patient's head and shoulders with the lower pillow extending below the shoulder line a few inches and the top pillow placed about 6 inches nearer the head of the bed than the lower. The open end of both cases should be turned away from the entrance to the patient's room.

In making an occupied bed the nurse should work quietly and efficiently, and avoid jarring the bed or walking around it more than is absolutely necessary. Care must be taken in turning the patient to see that the bath blanket remains in the position needed for proper draping.

Soiled linen should be placed in the laundry bag immediately when taken from the bed, under no circumstances should it be left on a chair or allowed to fall to the floor. Clean linen should be handled in all bed making procedures so that it never touches the floor.

The Anesthetic Bed. The anesthetic or ether bed is one which is made ready to receive a patient who has had a general anesthetic. Although making of the anesthetic bed is a part of the procedure of caring for an operative patient it is a task often assigned to the preclinical student and for that reason is included as a part of this chapter.

The anesthetic bed is made so that the operative patient may be placed in it very quickly without undue exposure. For this type of bed, linen must be given additional protection, provision must be made so the bed will be warm, and precautions may be needed to protect the patient from injury to himself while he remains unconscious or while consciousness is being re-established.

Extra blankets will be needed to keep the patient warm. Additional rubber sheets should be placed on the bed, at the upper part of the mattress, to protect the foundation sheet from perspiration and vomitus.

The top covers of the anesthetic bed should be placed so the head and foot, as well as both sides, are folded upward to clear all but the top of the mattress and thus may easily be turned back to admit the patient. When the patient has been placed in the bed the top covers may then be arranged as for the occupied bed.

If hot water bottles are placed in the anesthetic bed they should not be covered with hot water bottle covers; they should be removed before the patient is placed in the bed.

Articles needed for the anesthetic bed, in addition to those used in making an empty bed, include: one rubber sheet to cover the head of the mattress not already covered by the regulation rubber sheet; one draw sheet to cover the additional rubber sheet; two bath blankets placed over the foundation linen of the bed to provide additional warmth to the patient; gauze bandage to tie or fasten into position the pillow which protects the patient's head from the head board of the bed.

Articles needed to equip the bedside table for care of the anesthetic

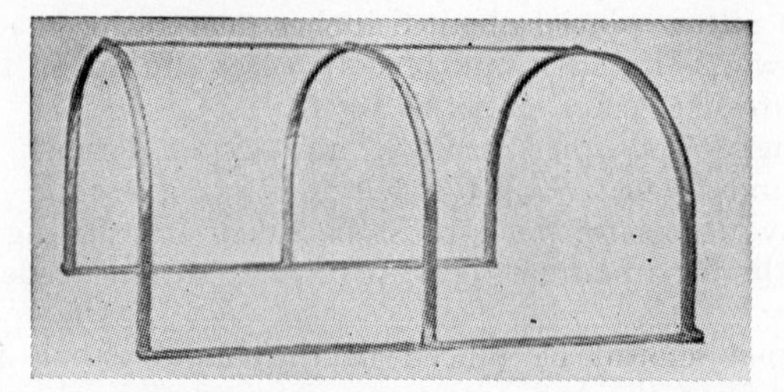

Fig. 52. A bed cradle. (Hospital Equipment Corporation, New York, New York.)

patient include: 2 emesis basins; 2 face towels; mouth wipes; paper bag; pad and pencil; tongue blades; safety pins; sphygmomanometer; stethoscope.

THE BED CRADLE

The bed cradle is made of wire, iron, or wood in the shape of three or more half hoops resting on flat runners and held in position by crossbars. It is used to support top covers, thus preventing them from touching or resting on the patient's body, or on a part that may be injured and in need of protection.

The size of the cradle depends on the part to be protected. Cradles used to protect an injured leg or foot are comparatively small, whereas those used to protect the whole body are large enough to cover the lower two thirds of the bed.

Making the bed when a cradle is in use is comparatively simple. For the smaller cradle the top covers may be placed on the bed as before and draped across the cradle. Corners may be mitered and top covers arranged in much the same manner as for the empty bed. When the large cradle is used additional sheets may be needed to cover the cradle adequately and still serve as covering for the patient.

The top covers should be placed on the bed so their upper edge, folded as for an open bed, extends upward to cover the patient's chest. Additional sheets and blankets are then placed to extend over the cradle and to allow their being tucked in at the foot of the bed. The bed will be neater in appearance if the spread is placed over the cradle and brought to the foot and tucked under the mattress there. A clean sheet folded across the upper part of the bed will make the usual envelope fold for top covers and still extend down to meet the spread, thus giving a finished appearance to the bed. Made in this way the covers may be moved aside to permit care of the patient without removing the entire top covering of the bed.

THE FRACTURE BED

The fracture bed is used to provide a firm support for the fractured limb and to prevent top covers from causing discomfort to the patient or interfering with traction or other therapeutic apparatus.

The fracture board placed under the mattress should be wide enough to rest on the frame of the bed and should be so placed that it will be held securely in the desired position. The foundation of the bed is made as for the open bed.

Fracture beds, made with the mattress in sections which can be moved to facilitate care of the patient, are made with the linen arranged to accommodate the various movable parts of the bed and may still present an appearance similar to that of the standard hospital bed.

In changing linen on a fracture bed, if the patient cannot be turned from side to side, soiled linen may be removed from the head to the foot of the bed and clean linen put into place in the same manner. The patient is supported while the linen is moved into place beneath him. Fracture beds with overhead frames facilitate changing of bed linen since the patient may use the hand trapeze to help lift and support himself while the bed is being made.

CARE OF BED LINEN

As the nurse is taught the fundamentals of bed making she will need to receive instruction from the head nurse in the care and handling of linen and of articles used in bed making. If necessary, regulations regarding the use of linen may be formulated, including the following:

1. Return torn or damaged articles of linen to the sewing room for repair or replacement.
2. Use stained linen for patients being treated with ointments or lotions which contain drugs that will cause staining.
3. Protect the woolen blankets by properly folding sheet and spread over edge of blanket in making the bed. Blankets should be cleaned at intervals. Stored blankets should be protected from moths and dust during the time they are in storage.
4. Refrain from fastening the signal cord to sheets with a safety pin.
5. Refuse to use linen for purposes other than that for which it was originally intended.
6. Do not be wasteful of linen, and discourage private duty nurses to hoard linen in their patient's room.
7. Remove the sleeve of the gown from the arm of a patient before a cast is applied. It will not then be necessary to cut the sleeve in order to remove the gown later.
8. Refuse to allow patients leaving the hospital to wear or take with them articles of linen belonging to the hospital.
9. Discourage the use of pillow cases as a substitute linen bag when baths are given. Seams will burst if the pillow case is filled with soiled linen from the bed. Linen bags made of heavy, long-wearing material should be provided for all departments within the hospital.

Care of Equipment after Use

All soiled linen removed from the bed should be placed in the linen hamper for removal to the laundry.

Blankets containing wool should be cleaned rather than sent to the laundry.

Rubber sheets, when not in use, should be hung from a pole or rolled around a pole to be put away. Folding will cause the rubber to crack and break. Care should be exercised in giving treatments in which oil is used so that oil is not spilled on the rubber sheet. Oil tends to soften the rubber, causing it to disintegrate.

Mattresses and pillows may be cleaned with soap and water and a stiff brush and should be placed outside for sun and air after the dismissal of a patient.

In some institutions mattresses are autoclaved at intervals to insure cleanliness.

Summary of Important Factors

The bed is the most important part of the patient's environment.

The way the bed is made is important to the comfort of the patient, the appearance of the bed and unit, and the facility with which care is given.

All linen should be brought to the unit before bed making begins.

The empty hospital bed should be made as a closed bed.

For a patient able to be up, the bed should be made as illustrated.

The occupied bed should not be bumped or jarred when being made.

Bed linen should never be allowed to come in contact with the floor.

The mattress needs additional protection when an anesthetic bed is being made.

Torn linen should not be used in making the bed.

Old or stained linen should be used for patients receiving treatments with drugs that will stain bed linen.

Rubber sheets should not be folded when taken out of use temporarily, as folding will crack or break the rubber.

Care should be taken that oil does not come in contact with rubber sheeting, as oil causes rubber to deteriorate.

Factors To Teach the Patient

The method of turning so the bed can be made without undue exertion on the part of the patient.

If a drug that will stain linen must be used in treatment, old and stained linen will need to be provided, even though it may not make a good appearance on the bed.

By lying still, in the center of the bed with feet held at right angles to the leg, the patient can assist the nurse in placing top covers correctly on an occupied bed.

Improvised equipment, such as oil cloth, may be used in the home to protect the mattress if a rubber sheet is not available.

The bed for the patient who remains at home may be elevated on wooden blocks or raised to correct height for nursing care by adding a second mattress.

Scientific Principles

Anatomy and Physiology. Muscle tone is diminished when the patient must remain in bed.

The body exerts uneven points of pressure against different areas of the mattress.

The buttocks may become the site for a pressure sore because of pressure and a depleted blood supply.

Chemistry. Woolen fibers from the blanket may cause irritation to the skin of the patient.

Strong soaps and bleaches used in the laundry may cause skin irritation to the patient if the bed linen is not thoroughly rinsed.

Microbiology. Bed linen becomes contaminated if allowed to touch the floor.

If linen is folded away from the nurse microorganisms are not so likely to be transferred to her uniform.

Bed linen should be changed frequently to insure cleanliness.

Frequent washing of her hands will protect the nurse from microorganisms contacted through handling bed linen for various patients.

Physics. When lying horizontally the position of the body should approximate, as nearly as possible, the standing position; the foot at a right angle to the leg, arms and legs in correct alignment, with chest up and head erect. A small support under the knees to keep them slightly flexed will reduce strain.

The patient in a horizontal position can be turned from side to side without being lifted.

Excessive heat loss during the bed making procedure can be prevented by keeping the patient well covered.

Psychology. Explanation of how he may cooperate in the procedure will help the patient adjust to the unfamiliar practice of having a bed made while he remains in it.

Privacy can be provided by means of screens.

The skill and efficiency of the nurse in doing the procedure will reduce exertion required of the patient.

If the procedure brings comfort and relaxation to the patient, his attitude toward it will be beneficial.

Sociology. Conversing with the patient as the bed is being made enables the nurse to learn about the patient and to take advantage of opportunities for teaching.

The nurse should know how to listen as well as talk.

The nurse should know that subjects of conversation of interest to the patient include his condition, his family, his work, his recreation or interests, and happenings that are of national interest. To satisfy such demands the nurse should keep informed by reading newspapers and magazines, by observing others, by hearing radio and watching television, and through other conversations.

Situation Type Problems

1. A preclinical student nurse was assigned to the task of making an occupied bed. The patient wished to talk while she was doing the procedure. He asked her several questions regarding the political campaign which was in the last week before election. He questioned her as to her reaction to a recent rioting of prisoners in a prison not far from the hospital, and attempted to get her opinion as to which college football team she thought would most likely win the Big Ten championship. The student nurse was unable to discuss any of the events mentioned as she had not been interested in any of them. The student was somewhat embarrassed, so explained to the patient that her class schedule was so heavy she had no time to read the newspaper. The patient stated that he would prefer to have the bed making a little less perfect if it would give the nurse a little time to become somewhat informed on what was going on in the world. What would you have done?

2. A preclinical student was assigned the task of making an anesthetic bed for a patient soon to be returned from the operating room. The bed was only half made when a senior student came in and started helping her with the procedure. The senior told the younger student to prepare the hot water bottles for the bed while she finished making it. The bed was carelessly made and did not look neat when completed. The clinical instructor criticized the preclinical student because of the appearance of the bed. When the student explained that the bed had been made by a senior student the instructor criticized the preclinical student for not having done the task assigned to her. What would you have done?

Suggested Reference Reading

"Posture and modern bedding," Catherine M. Thomas; Trained Nurse and Hospital Review, August, 1946.

PART III

Basic Procedures for Preclinical Study

CHAPTER 8

Local Applications of Heat and Cold

TOPICAL OUTLINE

Regulation of Body Temperature
Local Application of Heat
- Uses
- Effects
- Reflex Action
- Contraindications
- Methods of Application

Local Application of Cold
- Uses
- Effects
- Reflex Action
- Contraindications
- Methods of Application

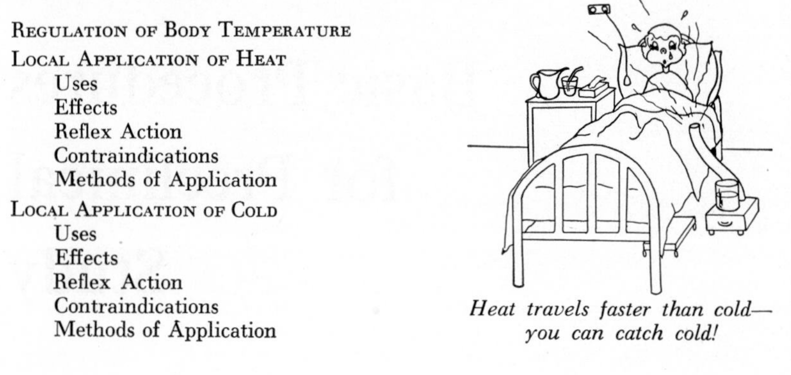

Heat travels faster than cold—you can catch cold!

The use of physical agents (sunlight, water, heat, cold, and massage) in the treatment of disease and for relief of pain has been a part of medical practice for centuries. Hot springs known and used for therapeutic purposes by early Greek and Roman physicians are still in use today.

REGULATION OF BODY TEMPERATURE

In order to function normally the body is equipped with a temperature-regulating mechanism which strives to maintain a balance between heat production and heat loss so that body temperature remains fairly constant at or near 98.6° F. Heat generated within the body by chemical action is effectively balanced by heat loss from the body by several different means. This constant level of body temperature may be maintained by man and other so-called warm-blooded animals, regardless of the temperature of their environment.

In Chapter 16, on Food Requirements and Food Service, the way in which food intake yields heat and energy for muscular activity and for various body processes is discussed. In order to maintain body temperature at normal level, heat loss must be increased in direct proportion to the amount of heat gained. Heat may be transferred (gained or lost by the body) by one of three principal methods: (1) conduction—contact with a heated object such as a hot water bottle to gain heat, or with a cold object to effect heat loss; (2) convection—transfer of heat from another source, as that gained from a heat lamp, or heat transfer from deeper organs of the body to the skin or superficial tissues; (3) conversion—transfer of heat by means of electrical currents of high frequency, such as that of diathermy or short wave.

Other means by which heat is lost from the body include: (1) evaporation from the skin through perspiration; (2) expiration (liberation of CO_2) from the lungs; (3) warming of inspired air; (4) elimination of urine and feces.

Since the greater heat loss from the body is through the skin (by radiation and evaporation), several factors pertaining to anatomy and functioning of the skin are reviewed here.

Nerve endings in the skin (receptors that keep the individual aware of environmental conditions) pick up sensations of heat or pressure and, according to the kind and degree of stimulus, register pain.

Numerous sweat glands in the skin excrete perspiration which, through evaporation, effects heat loss from the body.

Capillaries in the skin, by vasodilation and vasoconstriction, influence circulation of the skin surface and help regulate body temperature. When the capillaries are dilated the amount of blood in the skin is greatly increased, and heat is lost from deeper organs and from the body surface through radiation. If the capillaries are constricted less blood is held in the skin and less heat is lost to the environment.

A temperature-regulating center in the midbrain acts to keep body temperature "normal" when sensory nerve endings in the skin relay needs for temperature adjustment. The temperature-regulating center of the brain functions to control body temperature in much the same way that a thermostat regulates temperature in the modern home according to needs as indicated by change in room temperature.

LOCAL APPLICATION OF HEAT

Heat supplied to the body is usually accomplished by local application of heat to the skin.

Uses. Warming a part of the body surface by local application of heat may be important in providing comfort for the patient. The most common method of applying heat for comfort is application of a hot water bottle or heating pad to cold feet to help promote rest and relaxation. The nurse may apply heat locally without a written order from the physician.

Heat is also applied locally to relieve pain, inflammation, and congestion, to increase metabolism, and to hasten the process of suppuration in any given area.

The effect produced by local application of heat is only part of the therapeutic benefit to be derived from heat. In various forms heat is also used to produce a general or systemic reaction. The more extensive application of heat, as hot packs or baths, is discussed in Chapter 10. Applications of heat by special methods and for treatment of specific disease conditions such as those requiring medicated stupes and hot sterile compresses will be treated in Chapter 25, on Compresses, Fomentations, and Stupes.

The use of local application of heat and the method of application depends on the condition being treated, the area of the body affected, the severity of the disease, and the preference of the attending physician. To carry out the prescribed treatment intelligently and effectively, the nurse will need to know the purpose for which heat is applied and the proper method to use. She should also understand the reaction that takes place when heat is applied locally.

Effects. The effects produced when heat is applied to the skin may be quite varied. Even though heat may be applied by means of placing a hot water bottle to the affected area, the resulting reaction may involve not only the skin surface but far distant parts or internal organs.

The physiological action of heat depends on such factors as the method of application, the condition of the patient, whether moist or dry heat is used, the intensity of heat produced, the temperature of the application, whether it remains in place for a limited or prolonged time, and the area of body surface covered by the application.

When heat is applied locally to a definite area of body surface heat is given off from the application. The temperature-control mechanism of the body attempting to keep the temperature of that area of skin surface the same as that of the rest of the body sets in motion local phenomena related to heat loss. The capillaries of the affected area become dilated, more blood comes to the skin surface, and the area becomes reddened. This local reaction to the application of heat is termed hyperemia. The increased flow of blood to the area means increased metabolism, with resultant improved nutrition which hastens repair of the diseased or injured tissue. With more blood in the vessels of the skin there is less blood in the tissues under the skin. In this manner blood may be drawn from an inflamed or congested area. Pain may be relieved by the lessened pressure on sensitive nerve endings. Moderate heat relaxes muscle tissue and in doing so relieves cramps and fatigue.

With application of heat skin secretions are increased and the affected body surface becomes moist as well as reddened. If the application is prolonged tissues of the skin are softened and its resistance is lowered.

The effect of heat on the body results from its action on the nervous system (heat-regulating mechanism) and the circulatory system (vasodilation and vasoconstriction). Since so many factors influence the effect of application of heat the nurse should be guided specifically by orders of the physician so that desired results of the use of heat will be obtained.

Reflex Action. In addition to the effect of heat at the site of application there are reactions of internal organs and of parts of the body some distance from the involved local area. The distant part or the internal organ reacts because nerve cells in those parts have been stimulated by impulses traveling from a skin area to the brain or spinal cord. Sensory and motor nerves which innervate the skin also supply the distant part of the body.

The effects produced in the reflex areas are like those produced in the local area, although it has not been clearly established whether reflex action depends on reflex stimulation entirely or whether part of the benefit derived may be due to the fact that drawing blood to the surface of the body reduces the blood supply in more distant parts.

The areas of the body affected by local application of heat and cold are as follows:

Surface or Skin area	*Reflex area affected*
head, face, hands, feet	brain
back of neck	mucous membrane of nose
chest	lungs
area above heart	heart
lower right front chest	liver
lower left front chest	spleen
upper abdomen	stomach
lower abdomen	intestines
lower abdomen and groin	pelvic organs
lumbar region of back	kidneys
lumbar and sacral region of back	pelvic organs

Contraindications. Heat should not be applied locally when the process of suppuration or abscess formation should be retarded or averted. In appendicitis, in which there is danger of abscess formation, heat should not be used in an attempt to relieve abdominal pain. Infections of the teeth or of the ear should not be treated by local application of heat.

Methods of Application. Factors to be considered in choosing the method by which heat is to be applied locally include: the condition of the skin (if highly sensitive to temperature of the hot application), the duration of the treatment, and the results desired. If there are abrasions or open wounds heat may need to be applied with sterile supplies and equipment. The age of the patient should be taken into consideration, as well as his general physical condition. Patients most sensitive to heat and therefore most in danger of being burned by application of heat are the very old, the very young, and the very ill.

Other factors involved in the choice of method that should be used are: the area to be covered, the weight of the application, facilities that are available, and the preference of the physician.

Different methods used in applying heat locally include:

Hot Water Bottle. Before the hot water bottle is filled it should be carefully checked for leaks. The temperature of the water (bath thermometer to be used in checking temperature) should not exceed 125° F. If the hot water bottle is to rest on a body part, as to cover a dressing on arm or leg, it should be filled to approximately half its full capacity. If it is to be placed at the feet of a patient, it may be three-fourths full. Air should be removed from the bottle by compressing the sides or by placing it flat on a table or work counter to insert the cap in the mouth or opening.

A hot water bottle should always be placed in its flannel cover before being taken to a patient. When being used for an unconscious patient, a patient in shock, or an infant the hot water bottle should be placed outside the blanket covering the patient. Severe burns have been caused by careless use of the hot water bottle. In continuous treatment the hot water bottle should be refilled about every two hours.

It is not unusual for patients to complain that the hot water bottle is not warm enough. Hospitals and other institutions have enforced regulations regarding the maximum temperature of the water to be used because of the frequency of hot water bottle burns. Student nurses should remember there is very great danger of burning a patient unless they carefully adhere to regulations in regard to temperature of the water to be used in a hot water bottle.

Electric Cradle. The electric cradle is used to provide continuous dry heat from ordinary electric bulbs. Used especially for treatment of circulatory disturbances of the lower extremities, the cradles are equipped with several bulbs, 25 watt strength, which are enclosed in wire cages to prevent burns to the patient and accidental fire from contact with paper, linen, or blankets. The number of lights used in the cradle is determined by the needs of the patient.

Electric Heating Pad. Many patients prefer a heating pad to other means of applying heat locally. The patient should be warned of the danger in using the pad and only those pads which have automatic control should be used in the hospital. Electric heating pads should not be used to keep wet dressings hot since there is danger whenever electricity is in contact with moisture or water. The nurse should examine the cord and the plug on the heating pad to determine if the pad is safe for use before connecting it to the electric outlet in the patient's room.

Chemical Heating Pad. This type of heating pad is used for the

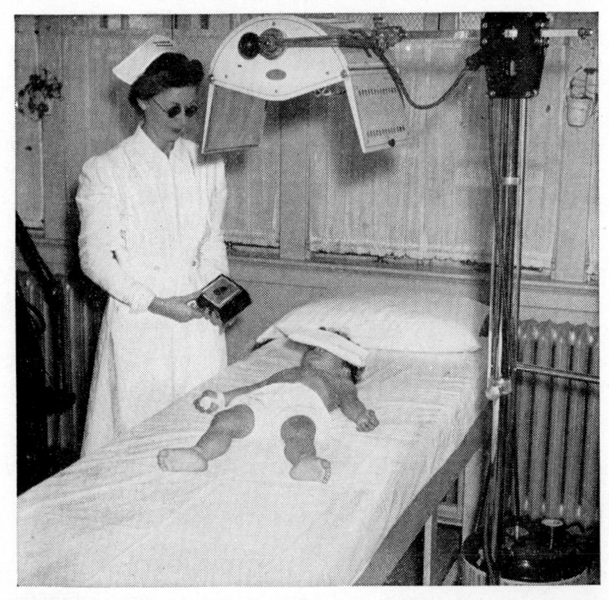

Fig. 53. Ultraviolet rays are obtained from sunlight or produced artificially by lamps and burners. (Presbyterian Hospital, Chicago, Illinois.)

same purpose as the hot water bottle. The pad is somewhat heavier than a hot water bottle, and for that reason is not desirable for use with compresses or dressings. Heat is produced by addition of a small amount of water to the chemical contents of the pad. It may remain quite hot for as long as 8 to 10 hours, depending on the amount and kind of chemicals used.

Heat Lamps. Carbon arc lamps used to provide ultraviolet radiation are another means of applying heat. Ultraviolet rays are obtained from sunlight or may be artificially produced by lamps and burners. Moderate radiation reddens the skin and stimulates growth of tissue cells. Intense radiation will destroy tissue and produce undesirable changes in the blood.

Infrared lamps heat the skin surface but do not penetrate to tissues beneath the skin. Hyperemia is produced by use of the lamps and there is danger of burning the patient if exposure to the infrared rays is prolonged. Too intense radiation will cause blister formation. To be effective the skin must be exposed and be free of ointment or other medicinal applications. Infrared lamps are portable and may be brought to the patient's bedside for treatment of such conditions as sinus infection, asthma, sprains, perineal lacerations, and impaired circulation in an extremity.

LOCAL APPLICATION OF COLD

Uses. Cold applications, like those of heat, may be used effectively in the treatment of certain disease conditions and, like heat, if improperly used, may be harmful to the patient.

When cold is applied for short periods of time only, it may be used to check hemorrhage, to slow the action of the heart, to reduce body temperature, to check inflammation, and to prevent discoloration and swelling of a bruised or injured part. If it seems wise to avoid or to delay suppurative processes, such as abscess formation, cold applications will help check the action and growth of bacteria. Cold is effective in relieving pain caused by pressure when used to reduce congestion and circulation in the affected part.

The nurse must understand the action of cold and the danger involved in its use if she is to effectively protect the patient from its harmful effects.

Effects. The effect produced by cold applications depends on such factors as: the method used in making the application, the length of time the cold application remains in place, the area or surface involved, the condition of the skin, and the general condition of the patient.

The primary effect of cold is contraction of blood vessels in the skin by stimulation of nerve endings there that are connected with the vasomotor center in the brain. Cold also causes the involuntary muscles of the skin to contract, exerting pressure on skin capillaries. Thus the amount of blood in the skin is greatly decreased and the involved area has the appearance of marked pallor.

Cold acts as a depressant to vital body functions to slow heart action and decrease pulse rate. By contracting blood vessels cold acts to increase blood pressure. Cold checks the activity of all living cells and in that manner will check the growth of bacteria. In the treatment of inflammation cold checks the inflammatory process and symptoms of pain, swelling, heat, and loss of function. Intense cold is capable of affecting sensory nerves so they are numbed and lose their ability to transmit sensations of taste or pain.

The secondary action of cold is that of dilation of blood vessels, increased cell activity, and increased sensitivity of nerve endings. Prolonged applications of cold will destroy all sensation in the affected part. By interfering with normal functioning of nerve cells cold will cause the vasomotor center to fail in its function and circulation will be retarded. Veins in the skin become relaxed and congested and give to the skin the characteristic blue or purplish appearance. Such disturbance of circulatory processes will interfere with the supply of food and oxygen to body cells and if continued will cause death of the affected tissues.

Prolonged cold, by lessening the activity of body cells and by lowering the temperature of the body, may cause death. The nurse should be well versed in the harmful effects that may result from cold applications and should recognize at once the first symptoms (blue, purplish, mottled appearance of the skin, with stiffness and numbness of the part) of undesirable effects of prolonged cold applications.

The effect of heat and the secondary action of cold are essentially the same, and either may be used in treatment of certain conditions.

Summarized, the effect produced by heat and cold applications would be as follows:

First Effect of Cold Applications	*Second Effect of Cold Applications and of Applications of Heat*
decreased circulation and suppurative process	increased circulation
decreased congestion	decreased congestion and swelling
	increased perspiration
increased nerve sensitivity	decreased nerve sensitivity
decreased action of bacteria	increased action of bacteria
strengthened muscular functioning	relaxation of muscular spasm
	relief of pain
	sedative action
	stimulate body processes
reduced temperature of affected part	increased temperature of affected part

Reflex Action. The effect produced on an internal organ by reflex action of the application of cold is the same as that at the area of application. When making cold applications to relieve symptoms related to the condition of an internal organ, the skin at the site of application should be carefully watched. If it becomes blue and mottled in appearance and numbness is present the application should be immediately discontinued since surface tissues may be damaged and the beneficial reflex effect will not ensue.

When making applications of cold to the body a hot water bottle should be placed at the patient's feet to prevent an undue sensation of chilliness.

Contraindications. Local applications of cold would be contraindicated if the patient shows symptoms of impaired circulation in the skin. Such applications would cause further impairment and aggravate an already undesirable condition. If the area to be treated has been injured so that tissues are damaged, or broken, cold should not be applied. Cold should not be used on a part where nutrition has been questionable. Poor nutrition would usually exist in an extremity or part in which circulation is impaired. In anemic conditions cold is contraindicated.

As local applications of cold affect circulation of the area being treated, the use of cold should be avoided if the effect on the tissues is such that impairment of circulation may cause discomfort or pain to the patient.

In some gastric disturbances cold may have a detrimental effect on digestion. Cold inhibits the secretion of gastric juice by causing contraction of tissues in the stomach and for that reason the drinking of ice water at mealtime or after oral administration of medicine should be discouraged.

Patients who are extremely sensitive to cold or who have been ill for a long time may react unfavorably to cold applications, so that the desired reaction is not obtained or harmful results ensue. Infants or very young children and the aged or senile patient may be easily shocked by low temperatures. Such patients do not respond satisfactorily to applications of cold and may not receive beneficial effects from the treatment. An extremely nervous patient or the known neurasthenic may not react favorably to applications of cold.

Methods of Application. Applications of cold should always be started gradually and increased in intensity as the patient is able to tolerate the treatment. The nurse should explain the procedure to the patient and tell him the expected or desired results, since a more favorable effect will be noted if the patient understands why the cold application is being used.

Methods of applying cold locally include the following:

Ice Cap. This container for particles of ice is commonly applied to the head for relief of headache or for treatment of fever, delirium, or skull fracture. It is placed over the right lower quadrant of the abdomen for treatment of acute appendicitis. For an acute cardiac condition it may be placed on the chest just over the heart.

The ice cap should be tested for leakage before use by filling it about half full of water, screwing the stopper into position, and inverting the cap. If leaks are present the water will spurt or drop from the site where the leak exists.

In filling the ice cap pieces of ice about the size of a walnut should be used and the cap should be filled to one half or two thirds of its total capacity, depending on the area where it is to be applied. When filled to less than its total capacity the ice cap will readily conform in shape and fit snugly against the part being treated. Pieces of ice with sharp edges should be held under running water to round or remove such edges. Sharp or jagged pieces of ice may puncture the rubber of the ice cap.

After the ice cap has been filled to the desired capacity all excess air should be removed by lightly twisting and compressing the sides of the cap just below the opening. The outer surface should be thoroughly dry before the cap is placed in its cover, which is made of flannel, heavy stockinette, or absorbent toweling.

If the patient is in a sitting position or the cap is applied to an area where it may tend to become displaced, a harness made of gauze bandage may be quickly made to hold the cap in proper position. Use of the breast binder to hold an ice cap in position to the cardiac region is not uncommon.

Ice caps usually will need to be refilled 30 to 60 minutes after application. Before the ice cap is reapplied, the area to which application is being made should be carefully inspected for signs of undesirable effect of the cold treatment.

Ice Collar. The ice collar is another method of applying cold locally, its shape permitting its use around the neck. The ice collar is used to relieve pain following tonsillectomy and for other conditions affecting the throat.

Other applications of cold, such as cold baths, sponges, or compresses, are discussed in Chapter 10 and Chapter 25.

In applying cold, whether for surface or deeper penetration, the patient must be closely observed for symptoms of shock or sudden chilling and for symptoms of stasis, the blue-purplish mottled appearance of the skin. To prevent such undesirable effects of prolonged treatment cold should be applied for only one or two hours, then removed for the same length of time to permit re-establishment of normal circulation before cold is applied again.

Care of Equipment after Use

Hot Water Bottle. The cap should be removed and the bottle emptied. The exterior should be dried, and the bottle should be inflated with air to prevent the sides from adhering to each other. With the bottle inflated the cap may be screwed loosely into place. The bottle should be hung in a cool dry place until needed for use again.

Electric Cradle. Light bulbs should be removed and stored in a safe place to prevent breakage. The cradle should be washed thoroughly with a strong antiseptic solution and stored until needed again.

Heating Pads. Chemical heating pads should be stored so that they are protected from dust and dirt. Electric heating pads should be examined closely to make sure the electrical parts, including cord, are in good condition. The pad should be placed in a box to be stored.

Heat Lamps. All heat lamps should be disconnected after use and returned to their proper storage place. If the lamp needs to be cleaned it should be washed with an antiseptic solution and dried immediately.

Ice Caps and Collars. The ice cap or ice collar should be emptied, washed, dried, and inflated with air, and the stopper put into place to prevent the sides from collapsing and adhering to each other. Such articles should then be put into storage until needed again.

Summary of Important Factors

Body temperature is maintained through action of a temperature-regulating mechanism in the brain.

Local applications of heat are used for comfort, for relief of pain and inflammation, and to hasten suppuration.

Factors that influence action of heat applications are: method used, age and condition of the patient, intensity of heat produced, duration of application, and the area covered.

Reflex action of heat is the same as that produced at the surface area.

In appendicitis or infection of teeth or of an ear, use of heat is contraindicated.

Heat is applied locally by hot water bottle, electric pad, chemical heating pad, heat lamps, and infrared lamps.

Cold applications are used to check hemorrhage, slow heart action, reduce body temperature, relieve pain, and check inflammation, discoloration, and swelling.

Secondary action of cold is the same as the action of heat.

Prolonged application of cold may be very harmful to the patient, causing shock, chilliness, and blue mottled appearance of the skin, indicating that circulation is impaired and tissue damage is imminent.

Local application of cold is contraindicated when surface tissue is broken, when circulation is impaired, and in some gastric disturbances.

The very old, the very young, and the very ill may be easily burned by heat applications and receive undesirable effects from applications of cold.

Cold is applied locally by ice cap or ice collar.

Cold applications continued for a long time should be alternated with periods when the application is removed to permit re-establishment of normal circulation in the part.

Factors To Teach the Patient

That because of danger of burns from a hot water bottle the maximum temperature of water permitted is 120–125° F.

That prolonged application of cold is dangerous, signs of undesirable effects being cold, blue-purplish mottled skin, and numbness of the part being treated.

That burns from heat applications and harmful effects from cold are more apt to occur in the very old, the very young, and the very ill.

That hot water bottles, ice caps, and ice collars should always be covered before being applied to the body.

That secondary effect of cold is the same as that produced by local application of heat.

That cold applications continued for a long time should be alternated with periods when the application is removed to permit reestablishment of normal circulation in the part.

That heat is contraindicated when symptoms of appendicitis are present or when abscess formation is to be inhibited.

Scientific Principles

Anatomy and Physiology. Practically all parts of the body, through blood vessels and nerves, will react to application of heat or cold to the skin. There are so many capillaries in the skin that, when distended, they can hold the major portion of the blood in the body. Moderate heat applied to the skin will provide general warmth to the body. Moderate heat also increases perspiration.

Heat dilates blood vessels in the skin to aid healing processes and to promote suppuration.

Heat relaxes the muscles and relieves fatigue.

The local effect of heat is the same for all the different methods of application.

Cold contracts involuntary muscle and blood vessels in the skin by action of the nervous system.

Internal organs are affected by application of heat or cold to the skin.

A prolonged application of extreme heat or cold will cause destruction of body tissue.

Chemistry. Heat, increasing the speed of a chemical reaction, speeds up body metabolism.

Sodium salts are used in chemical heating bottles. The formation of crystals causes the bottle to become warm and to hold the warmth for a long time.

Microbiology. Covers used for hot water bottles, ice caps, and ice collars should be sent to the laundry after each use.

Hot water bottles, ice caps, and ice collars are kept free of bacteria by soap and water washing and careful drying.

Sterile technique must be used, as well as sterile supplies, in applying heat or cold to wounds with a break in continuity of tissue.

If sterile technique is to be used for cold applications the container of sterile solution may be set into a bowl of chipped ice.

Cold inhibits the formation and absorption of poisons from bacteria.

Pharmacology. Irritant drugs used with heat applications intensify the action of the application. Turpentine and mustard are the substances commonly used for their irritant effect.

Physics. Heat is one of the most valuable of all physical forces.

Heat is transferred by conduction, convection, and radiation.

Pressure should not be exerted on a hot application, as the danger of causing a burn is increased by reduction of the air layers in the application.

Electrical appliances are insulated with rubber, which is a poor conductor of electricity. Water is a good conductor of electricity, and the nurse should not handle electrical equipment if her hands are wet.

Ice bags become wet on the outside because the greater coldness of the bag condenses moisture from the air.

Psychology. Patients may fear that heat or cold applications will produce pain. The nurse should explain the procedure and prepare the patient for differences in the temperature of the application. Cooperation on the part of the patient is necessary for successful treatment by heat or cold applications.

Applications of heat or cold should be closely supervised so the patient will not be harmed by the treatment.

Sociology. The patient at home may be dependent on the visiting nurse for hot or cold applications.

Burns caused by carelessness or negligence are common causes of legal suits against the hospital.

Situation Type Problems

1. The student nurse filled a hot water bottle one-half full (water temperature 125° F.) and placed it at the feet of the patient who had complained that his feet were cold. The patient stated that the hot water bottle was not hot enough and asked the nurse to fill it again, using water that was really *hot*. What would you have done?

2. A patient suspected of being diabetic entered the hospital for diagnostic tests. He complained that his feet were cold and asked the nurse aide who admitted him if he might have a hot water bottle. The nurse aide explained to him that heat and cold applications had the same effect, that she was unable to find a hot water bottle so had filled an ice cap to place to his feet. In placing the ice cap she noticed a large reddened area on the big toe and asked the patient if his toe was sore. The patient stated that the toe had seemed somewhat more sensitive than usual, but was not exactly "sore." A few minutes later the patient informed the student nurse who had come in to check his blood pressure that "The ice cap which the nurse aide had placed to his feet still felt cold instead of warm," and asked if he should continue to use it. What would you have done?

3. In the pediatric department a baby girl of six months cried almost continually for the first two hours she was in the hospital. The head nurse suggested that a hot water bottle be placed at the baby's feet since they felt cold to touch.

The nurse who filled the hot water bottle did not take time to take the temperature of the water, but did test it by pouring some across her inner wrist. Because there was only one hot water bottle cover in the linen closet she decided to use the hot water bottle without a cover for the baby. She knew the baby would not complain about the appearance of the hot water bottle and that her other and much older patient for whom a hot water bottle was needed would object to having a hot water bottle without a cover. What would you have done?

Suggested Reference Reading

"Deep freeze unit for ice bags," Fred G. Carter; American Journal of Nursing, March, 1948.

"Keeping hot packs hot," from study made at University of Minnesota; American Journal of Nursing, July, 1952.

CHAPTER 9

Cleansing Baths—Personal Hygiene—Routine Care

TOPICAL OUTLINE

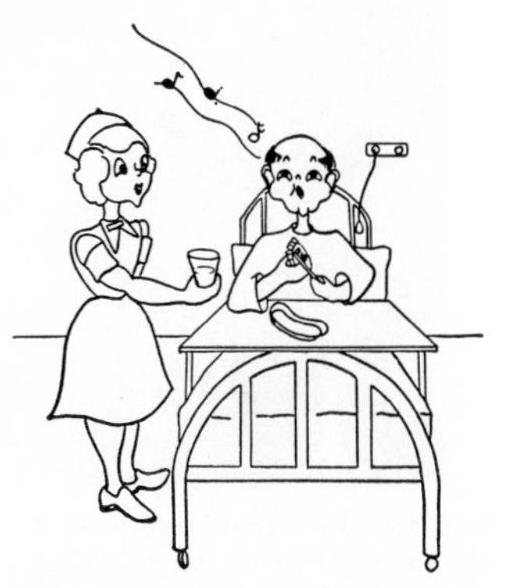

Seems there's one advantage to being old—you can whistle while you brush your teeth.

Hygiene, the science of health, is a basic factor in the nurse's responsibility for teaching good health practices as well as providing nursing care for patients.

Personal hygiene for the patient is a continuous process of learning about and observing desirable health practices. Some patients come to the hospital with good health practices already well established and need only continue those practices as much as is permitted by their physical condition. Other patients will need instruction in matters of hygiene and for them the nurse becomes a health teacher. In giving daily care to the patient she has an opportunity to demonstrate all the essential procedures for personal cleanliness and to set an example by observing good health practices herself.

Cleanliness is essential to the comfort and welfare of the patient and is the basis for many nursing procedures performed in giving

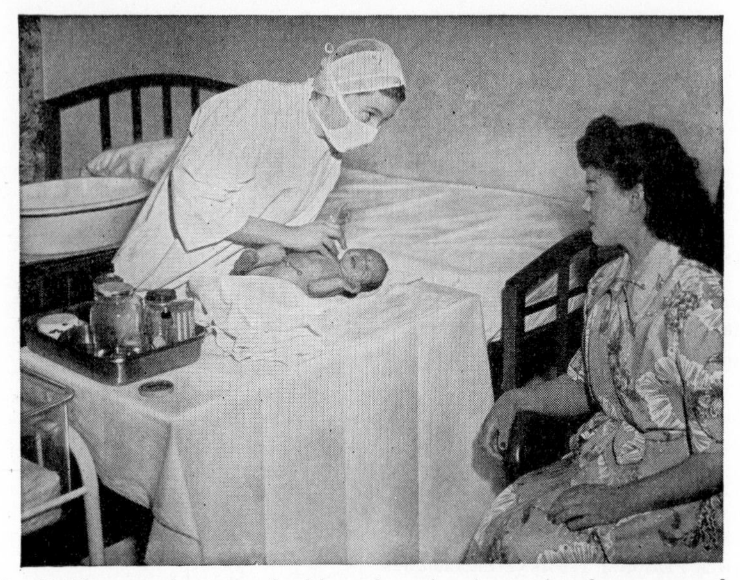

Fig. 54. The nurse becomes a health teacher when instructing the young mother on how to bathe the baby. (Mercy Hospital School of Nursing, Denver, Colorado.)

daily care. It is especially important that the patient's body be kept clean and his skin in good condition.

The condition of the skin furnishes an accurate index to the health of the individual. During illness, when part of the body is not functioning normally, the skin will show the effects of such abnormality. No amount of creams or lotions applied externally and no one ingredient in the ever growing list of cosmetics can successfully camouflage the real character of a skin lacking in the qualities that are produced by good health.

For the well person, proper care of the skin is one of the major factors in maintaining good health. For the person who is ill skin care becomes even more important. If the skin is not kept as clean as possible, it will not be able to function normally. To give adequate skin care to patients the nurse needs to understand the various functions of the skin.

FUNCTIONS OF THE SKIN

The skin forms a surface covering and protects the body by forming an effective barrier against the action of microorganisms. Any break in the skin surface may become a portal of entry for bacteria.

In the skin is located endings of sensory nerve fibers which transmit the stimuli causing sensations of pressure, temperature, and pain.

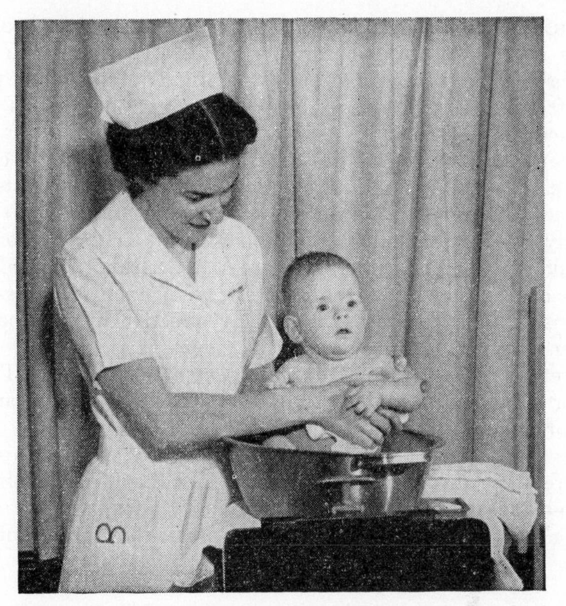

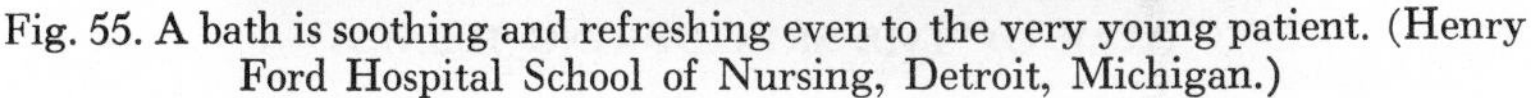

Fig. 55. A bath is soothing and refreshing even to the very young patient. (Henry Ford Hospital School of Nursing, Detroit, Michigan.)

The skin is also an important organ of excretion, since it helps to eliminate waste products from the body by means of perspiration.

The skin is a heat-regulating organ, helping to keep the temperature of the body at 98° F. even when climate and other environmental conditions change and the body must adjust to the changed conditions.

The skin secretes an oily substance which keeps it smooth and supple. If baths are given frequently, this natural oil may need to be replaced by the use of creams or lotions to prevent chafing or cracking of the skin. An exceedingly dry skin is subject to abrasions, scratches, and other breaks in its surface through which microorganisms may enter.

Although it has never been satisfactorily established that daily or frequent bathing is absolutely essential for health, it is known that adequate cleansing of the skin promotes a feeling of comfort and well-being.

A bath is soothing and refreshing to the patient, aids the skin to function normally as a heat-regulating organ, and facilitates the elimination of the increased amount of body wastes occasioned by illness.

Cleansing the skin is of major importance in personal hygiene for both patient and nurse. The nurse, by means of a daily bath and careful use of deodorants, can maintain the attractive, healthful appearance which is needed for her to look her best in uniform. Cleansing her hands by frequent washing is a means of protecting herself from excessive contamination by microorganisms found in abundance in hospitals.

The patient, deprived of the exercise which stimulates circulation and increases perspiration and elimination of waste products from the skin, needs the aid to elimination which a cleansing bath can give. The daily bath and change of linen add much to his comfort and feeling of well-being, which promotes a desirable mental attitude. The use of a deodorant to control offensive odor is necessary since the cleansing bath may not be entirely effective in eliminating odor from the body. There are numerous sweat glands under the arms, and secretion from this area does not evaporate quickly. The underarm odor that results may be eliminated only by use of an antiperspirant or deodorant.

Nurses should particularly include the use of a deodorant in their daily care since nursing procedures require that they reach across or bend over the patient, and close proximity increases the danger of offending if they are careless in this particular matter of personal hygiene.

CARE OF THE SKIN DURING ILLNESS

A cleansing bath not only removes perspiration and waste products from the skin but serves also to stimulate circulation so that the condition of the skin is improved and pressure areas are less apt to develop. The daily bath helps to quiet the nerves of a restless patient and adds immeasurably to the comfort of those confined to bed with limited movement or activity.

A mild, pure soap and plenty of warm water should be used for bathing a patient. The skin of the face is essentially the same as that covering the rest of the body and is not harmed by use of soap.

Some patients, such as those who are incontinent, unconscious, or suffering from a debilitating disease, will require special and frequent care of the skin. In such cases thorough cleansing with soap and water may need to be repeated several times each day, and the use of oils, creams, or lotions may be indicated.

Some systemic diseases cause changes in the skin which can be treated successfully only by treatment of the disease. Patients with specific skin diseases require special treatment and care as indicated by a qualified dermatologist.

Various types of baths have become a part of the routine daily care for the hospitalized patient. The type of bath given the patient will depend on his age and physical condition. Patients who are able to be out of bed may be permitted tub or shower baths. Critically ill

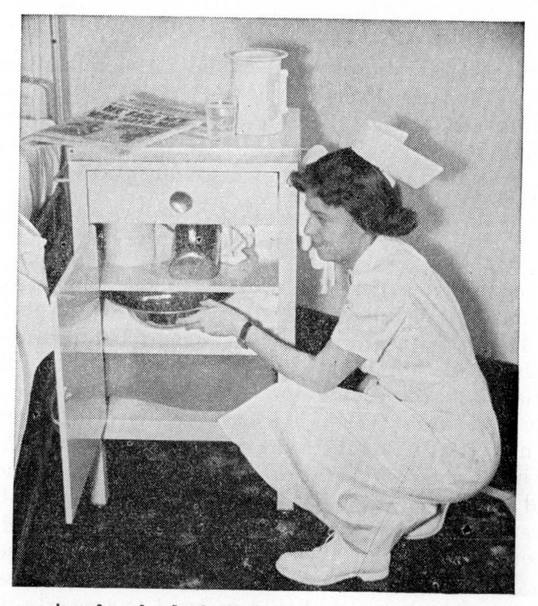

Fig. 56. Preparation for the bath includes preliminary assembling of needed supplies and equipment. (Presbyterian Hospital, Chicago, Illinois.)

patients usually receive a complete bed bath each day. Some bed patients may be given a partial sponge bath each day or on alternating days.

PREPARATION FOR THE CLEANSING BATH

The room in which the bath is to be given should be comfortably warm (70°–75° F.). Windows and door should be closed so the patient is protected from drafts, and provision should be made for privacy during the procedure. All supplies and equipment that will be needed for the bath should be assembled before the actual bath procedure is started.

The bath may be given before breakfast or postponed until an hour after breakfast. Stimulation of the skin in bathing increases circulation at the surface of the body and in doing so withdraws some blood from internal organs. To prevent interference with digestive processes the bath shouldn't be given for about half an hour after the patient has eaten breakfast. Before the bath procedure is begun the patient should be offered bedpan or urinal so there will be no need to interrupt the bath to attend to elimination needs.

PURPOSE OF THE CLEANSING BATH

The cleansing bath, whether bed or tub, or complete or partial, is given for the following purposes: (1) to cleanse the skin and thus increase elimination through that organ; (2) to stimulate circulation through slightly active or entirely passive exercise; (3) to refresh the patient by relieving fatigue and discomfort.

ROUTINE BATHS

For the acutely ill patient the daily bath should be given so that only a minimum amount of exertion is required. Even when bed linens are being changed the patient should be turned only once and then should be assisted by the nurse so that little effort is expended. The basin containing the bath water should be filled approximately two-thirds full of warm water (temperature 120° F.). The nurse may test the temperature of the bath water by immersing her elbow in it; she can readily tell if the water is too hot. A soap dish should be provided so that soap need never be left floating in the bath water, a practice which is careless, expensive, and wasteful.

Throughout the procedure the unit should be properly screened so that privacy is accorded the patient. To avoid embarrassment the bath blanket and bath towel should be used to properly drape each part of the body as it is being bathed.

THE BED BATH

The bed bath is given in the order usually practiced by a person in bathing himself. The face and neck should be washed first. Soap used in bathing must be thoroughly rinsed from the skin to prevent itching or dryness that could result if the soap remained in contact with the skin for a prolonged period of time. Although dermatologists agree that soap is no more harmful to the face than to the skin on any other part of the body, the patient should be consulted as to his wishes before soap is applied to the face. In giving the bath the nurse should fold the washcloth about her hand to prevent wet, dangling ends of the cloth from coming in contact with the patient. After the face and neck have been washed the bath procedure should be continued, to include arms, hands, chest, abdomen, legs, feet, and back in that order.

"Finishing the bath," the term applied to washing the genital area, is done by the patient if he is able. If he is unable to complete this final part of the bath procedure for himself the nurse should do it for him, making sure that the entire area is gently but thoroughly washed, rinsed, and dried. If she is tactful and dignified in manner, she need feel no embarrassment at giving this nursing care to the patient who is too ill to adequately care for himself. Bath water

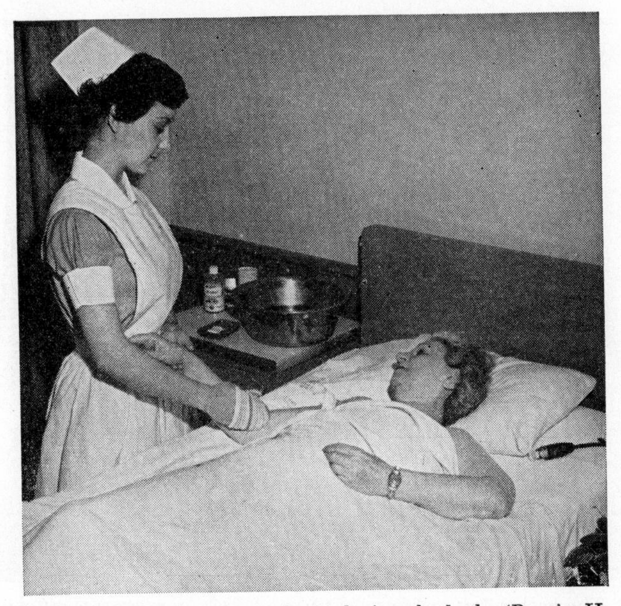

Fig. 57. The bath blanket becomes a drape during the bath. (Baptist Hospital of Alabama School of Nursing, Birmingham, Alabama.)

should be changed after the feet have been washed so that clean, warm water is available for washing the back and for "finishing the bath."

Throughout the bath firm, gentle strokes should be used in washing as well as in drying the part. Conversation between patient and nurse should be restricted mostly to information needed by the patient as to the cooperation expected of him so the bath will have a refreshing and restful effect. The patient who is able to converse and wishes to do so during the procedure should be permitted to make the conversation as limited or as lengthy as he desires. The nurse should not chatter incessantly nor remain absolutely silent. If she limits her remarks to a few well chosen words which indicate that she is attentive to what the patient is saying she will have demonstrated her ability to satisfy conversational requirements.

The Alcohol Back Rub. As soon as the patient has been given a bath he should be turned to his side and properly draped for the alcohol back rub. For the older patient, or one seriously ill, the back rub should be gentle and soothing, with little pressure being exerted by the nurse's hands as the back is stroked or rubbed. For the younger or convalescent patient vigorous stroking and firm pressure exerted against the back will be stimulating and beneficial. Vigorous stroking should be used at the beginning of the back rub since it increases

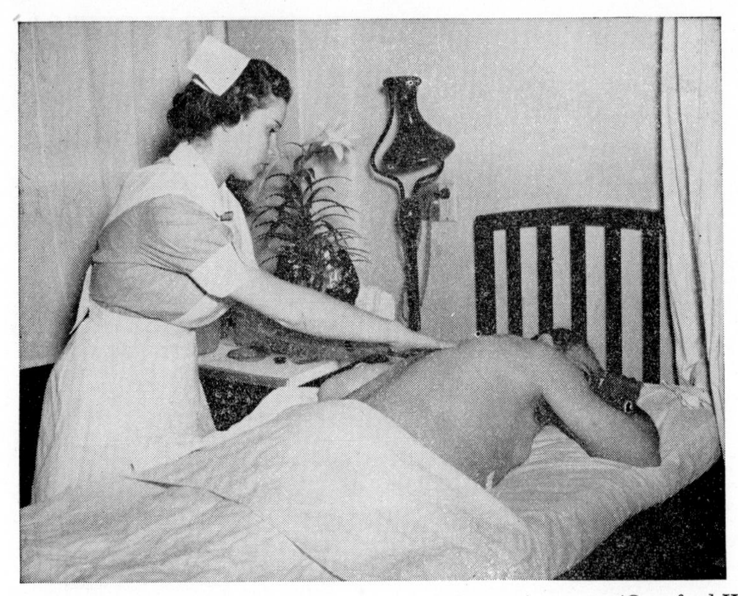

Fig. 58. The back rub is an important part of daily nursing care. (Crawford W. Long Hospital School of Nursing, Atlanta, Georgia.)

peripheral circulation and stimulates normal skin functioning. The rub should be completed with light, soothing strokes to make the patient more comfortable and more relaxed.

The solution usually used is 50–75 per cent alcohol. Its astringent, cooling effect on the skin is beneficial as a prophylactic measure in the prevention of pressure areas.

The patient may be startled by the sudden application of alcohol to the back because it feels cool. To avoid causing the unpleasant sensation of chilliness the bottle of alcohol should be placed in the bath water and left there during the bath so its contents will be warm when applied to the body. Special lotions and creams with an oil base are now available for use in giving back rubs. They help to keep the skin of the back soft and pliable and may be preferred by many patients.

For the back rub procedure the nurse should stand with her feet about 18 inches apart and should lean forward slightly in order to reach the patient's shoulders with arms extended. With fingers separated and fingers and palms of the hand resting firmly against the surface of the back, she should begin rubbing with long, smooth effleurage movements. The nurse should move her body back and forth in making the long, stroking movements, rather than bending the elbows as the downward stroke is made. Special kneading movements may be included as part of the back rub, with particular attention to bony prominences and to the pressure area at the end of the spinal column.

The cooling effect of the alcohol, combined with the long stroking movements of the nurse's hands, make the back rub a pleasant and refreshing sequel to the bath.

The back rub procedure should be completed by covering the back with a light film of talcum or bath powder and by making long, stroking movements of effleurage. The powder helps to keep the skin dry and prevents irritation or friction where skin surfaces are in contact with each other. The use of a suitable deodorant should be included as part of the bath procedure so that offensive body odor may be eliminated.

When the bath and back rub have been completed, clean linen should be put on the bed and a clean gown put on the patient. The bath soothes and relaxes the patient and, if he is encouraged to do so, he will rest and perhaps sleep for a few hours after the procedure.

When assigned to perform the bath procedure for a patient the nurse should accept the responsibility of also caring for the patient unit or room so that it is neat and orderly. Window shades should be raised or lowered to a uniform height. Electric lights not in use should be turned off. The room should be correctly ventilated. Magazines or books should be placed within easy reach of the patient and arranged in an orderly fashion.

If the patient wears spectacles the lenses should be examined and cleaned if not entirely free of dirt or smudges. If spectacles are placed on the bedside table or in a drawer, they should always be placed so that they rest on the frames rather than on the lenses. Lenses in contact with table or drawer surface may become scratched or broken.

If not cared for by ward attendants, flowers should be given proper care by the nurse. If there is a radio or television set in the unit or ward it should be placed so the patient can reach it for frequent selection of stations or channels and for adjustment of volume. Patients who have such mediums of entertainment should be taught to keep them operating on low volume so other patients will not be needlessly disturbed.

THE TUB BATH

For the patient whose condition allows him to be out of bed the doctor may permit a tub bath. The bathroom should be quite warm (78–80° F.) and the bath should be no more than 10 minutes in duration. Water should be drawn into the tub and all needed supplies placed close at hand before the patient is brought to the bathroom. Bathrobe and slippers should be worn by the patient to the bathroom and kept in readiness for use after the bath.

In most hospitals bathrooms designed for patient use do not have a lock on the door. If there is a lock the patient should be instructed not to lock the door. If he is able to bathe himself he may be left alone in the bathroom, but during the time he is in the tub the nurse should be close by. If the bathroom adjoins the patient's room the nurse should make the bed and put the room in order while the patient is bathing.

Characteristic splashings from the bathroom will indicate that the patient is in satisfactory condition during the bath. An absence of such sounds should lead the nurse to ask "Are you all right?" and to investigate at once if there is no audible response.

If a female patient is too weak or nervous to be left alone during the bath she may be assisted by the nurse, who takes an active part in the procedure. If a patient becomes faint or dizzy, water should be drained from the tub and her head lowered. The nurse should not attempt to lift from the tub a patient suddenly overcome with faintness. Such a patient will be extremely heavy and the surface of her body will be wet from the bath. Under such conditions it would be impossible for the nurse to support her or to prevent her from falling.

If a male patient needs assistance in taking a tub bath the orderly is instructed to remain with him and to help with the procedure. For the patient at home, whether male or female, the nurse will assist with the tub bath. Those who are mentally ill or in a very weakened condition should not be permitted to be alone while they remain in the tub.

All patients should be warned that there is danger of being burned or scalded if hot water is added to the bath while they are in the tub. They should be instructed never to touch electric wires or fixtures or attempt to turn on an electric light while they are standing or sitting in a tub of water. Many persons have been electrocuted by just such thoughtless actions.

To prevent accidental falling in the bath, a corrugated rubber mat should be placed on the floor of the tub. As soon as the patient leaves the tub he should be quickly dried by brisk rubbing with heavy turkish towels and should be dressed in clean pajamas and robe or in a clean gown to be returned to bed for further rest and relaxation.

THE PARTIAL BATH

As the name implies, "partial bath" is the procedure as performed for the convalescent patient or the patient not in need of a complete bed bath. For a partial bath the face and hands of the patient are bathed. The underarm area and back, including the buttocks, should be bathed and the alcohol back rub given. The patient should be asked to finish the bath or the nurse or orderly should perform that part of the procedure for him.

Partial baths should be given on alternate days if the practice has been adopted to save time for nurses. Using this method, the patient will then receive a complete bath on alternate days. If clean linen is available in sufficient quantities the bed should be changed after a partial bath in the same manner as after a complete bed bath.

THE SELF-ADMINISTERED BATH

If a patient is confined to bed but is able to give himself a bath, he should be encouraged to do so. The nurse should prepare the patient for the bath the same as if the bath was to be administered by her. All needed supplies and equipment should be brought to the bedside. Top covers should be removed and replaced with a bath blanket. After all needed equipment and supplies have been provided for the bath, a basin of warm water should be brought to the bedside at the time the bath is to be started.

When the patient has completed the procedure of bathing himself the nurse should bathe his back and buttocks and give an alcohol back rub. The linens on the bed should be changed according to the supply available, the condition of the patient, and the appearance of the used sheets and spread.

OTHER PERSONAL HYGIENE PROCEDURES

In addition to the daily bath, other procedures related to personal hygiene are necessary to the daily care of the patient.

Shaving the Male Patient. The interruption of daily routine to which the patient has long been accustomed is one of the factors of hospitalization which is apt to be annoying and may be the immediate cause of development of an undesirable mental attitude. Most men, when well and carrying on activities of normal living, start the day by removing the growth of beard which has appeared on their face during the previous 24 hours. The practice of shaving is a fixed habit, and any departure from it may cause physical and mental discomfort.

A barber is usually available to the hospital patient and will come to the room or unit to shave him. Hospital orderlies or attendants are often called on to shave the male patient, but in some instances shaving has become the responsibility of the nurse.

If the patient is able to shave himself, the nurse will need to see that he has the necessary equipment and supplies, as a basin of hot water, shaving soap, brush, towel, paper tissues, razor, mirror, and after-shave lotion. A good light will be needed, and a wastebasket should be placed nearby. If brushless shaving cream is used, the brush will not be needed. If an electric razor is used, an extension cord must be provided if no suitable electrical outlet is located near the bed.

In many hospitals the patient will not be permitted to keep a razor (other than electric) at his bedside. In such event, the nurse

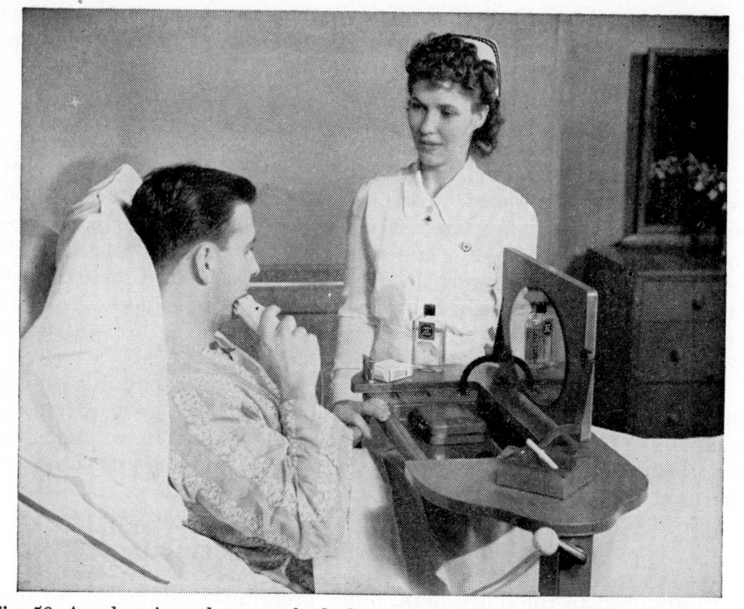

Fig. 59. An electric outlet near the bed or an extension cord will be needed if the patient uses an electric razor. (Hill-Rom Co., Inc., Batesville, Indiana.)

must have permission from the physician to give the patient the razor to be used for shaving. She is then obligated to remain with the patient while he is shaving.

If the nurse is responsible for shaving the patient she should not be hesitant about doing so even though she may have had little or no previous experience in handling a razor. The following suggestions may be of help if she is not experienced in shaving patients.

Before beginning the procedure see that the patient is in a comfortable position and draped so that his clothing and the bed linen will be protected. The face should be generously covered with lather from shaving soap or cream. This lather emulsifies the oil surrounding the hairs of the beard and allows them to be softened by the soap and water. The razor should be drawn smoothly over the face with firm, even strokes. The beard tends to grow in a certain direction, and a smooth shave is obtained by drawing the razor across the beard in the direction of growth. Paper tissues should be used frequently to keep the razor free of lather and particles of hair which have been removed by one or two previous strokes across the face.

When the shave has been completed the face should be gently moistened, for removal of excess shaving lather, and patted dry with

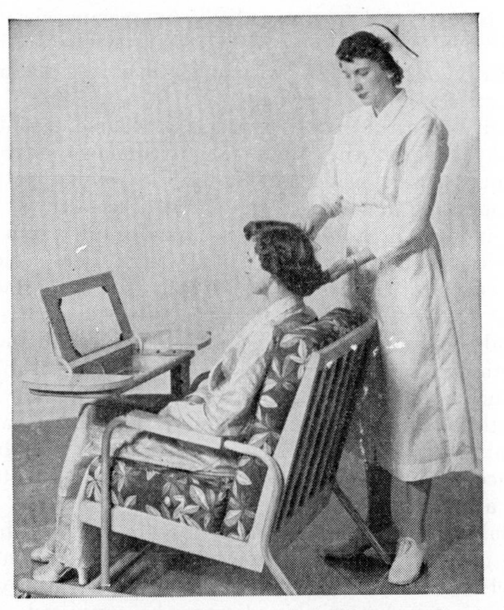

Fig. 60. Proper care of the hair promotes a desirable mental attitude. (Hill-Rom Co., Inc., Batesville, Indiana.)

a soft towel. After-shave lotion should then be applied to the palms of the nurse's hands and, through contact, to the patient's face.

Care of the Hair. Proper care of the hair is part of routine nursing care given each patient and is another means of maintaining a desirable mental state when poor physical condition tends to cause depression and discouragement. The hair should be thoroughly combed and brushed at least once each day. The best time for caring for the hair seems to be in the morning after the bath has been given. Although condition of the hair is determined largely by the patient's physical condition, its appearance is due largely to the care and attention given it by members of the nursing staff.

More time and attention must be given to the care of hair for the female patient than is required for the male. Women wear their hair longer than do men, and in some instances their hair may be more difficult to comb. If tangles are present they may be more easily combed out if the hair is moistened slightly with 95 per cent alcohol. If the tangles cannot be combed out, portions of the hair may need to be cut. The consent of the patient or of a responsible relative must be obtained before the nurse or other hospital employee is permitted to cut hair.

Brushing the hair once or twice a day helps to keep it clean and lustrous and is beneficial to the scalp by increasing circulation. The brush should have moderately hard bristles, and the brushing should be done in firm, even strokes, which begin at the scalp and move outward toward the end of the hair.

The style in which the hair is worn is, of course, a matter of individual choice, although the nurse may frequently be consulted or asked to suggest a hair arrangement for the woman patient who is desirous of appearing at her best, in spite of ill health.

If the hair is long, it should be parted and braided into two braids, at either side of the head, just back of the ears. Two braids are indicated so the weight of the hair is divided and neither braid will seem heavy to the patient. The braids should be securely fastened with a rubber band, hair ribbon, or piece of 1-inch gauze bandage.

While combing the hair, it is necessary to protect the bed from loose hairs and dandruff by placing a face towel under the patient's head during the procedure. If there is more than the usual or normal amount of dandruff in the hair and on the scalp it may be necessary to apply an accepted solution of dandruff remover, loosen the dandruff by massage, and then comb it from the scalp and hair. Dandruff is merely the flaking or peeling of bits of dried skin from the scalp and should cause no alarm, unless it appears in excessive quantity and is unusually persistent. For any abnormality of the scalp or hair, it is essential that a specialist in skin diseases be consulted.

Now that it is common practice for patients to remain only a few days in the hospital, the problem of shampooing the hair is an infrequent one. However, for the patient who is hospitalized for a long period of time, regular shampoos may be indicated. For the majority of patients who require shampoo, the procedure should be given every 7 to 10 days.

Care of the Nails. As part of the daily routine to promote personal hygiene for the patient, care of the nails must be given consideration. Well kept fingernails not only enhance the general appearance of the patient but are an added protection against infection which may result from scratching the body surface with dirty fingernails or from eating food that has been handled by hands with nails that are not clean.

Dirt and microorganisms lodged beneath fingernails may be a constant source of danger to a patient. The patient who has been confined in a hospital for several days and still displays unsightly, unkept hands and nails shows that the nursing care he receives leaves much to be desired.

It may be impossible, during the admission bath, to thoroughly cleanse hands and nails of a patient whose hands are badly soiled, such as a worker on a farm or a garage mechanic, but subsequent baths and attention to fingernails should result in a state of cleanliness acceptable to even the most fastidious of persons.

At regular intervals fingernails should be trimmed or filed so they are of a desirable length. If nails are trimmed with scissors, they should be cut to form a rounded end that protrudes only slightly beyond the end of the finger. An emory board should be used to smooth the nail edge and remove any possible irregularities or roughness which may have resulted from the cutting. In caring for fingernails it may be necessary to push back the cuticle with an orangewood stick; a pointed or sharp instrument should not be used since there is danger of cutting or tearing the skin at the base of the nail. Frequent washing of the hands with mild soap and warm water helps to keep nails clean and facilitates the prevention of hangnails. Pushing cuticle back each time the hands are washed and use of a lotion or cream at night will improve the condition of the nails.

The care of toenails becomes important if the patient remains more than a few days in the hospital. If toenails are allowed to grow too long they may cause discomfort when the patient walks about in bedroom slippers. Even when the patient remains in bed, toenails that aren't carefully cut at intervals may tend to turn under or to become deeply imbedded in the soft tissue of the toe at the side of the nail. This condition, if allowed to go uncorrected, may result in a break in the skin and subsequent infection. Toenails should be cut straight across to prevent the tendency for growing inward, and they should not be cut shorter than the tips of the toes. If toenails are cut too short the end of the toe is left unprotected.

Toenails and fingernails show a tendency to become hard and brittle with advancing years. Older patients whose nails need special attention may require the services of a chiropodist, who is specially trained and has special instruments for giving proper care to elderly patients whose nails cannot be cared for as a part of the nursing service.

Care of the Mouth. Probably no other phase of personal hygiene affords more opportunity for the nurse to effectively assume responsibilities of a teacher than the care of the mouth and teeth.

Great emphasis is now placed on the importance of "brushing the teeth twice a day and seeing the dentist twice a year." Dental products are widely advertised, and the general public is constantly reminded of the importance of good oral hygiene in maintaining health. Despite these attempts to educate the public, patients continue to come to the hospital with unclean and decaying teeth, halitosis, mouth infections, or other conditions caused by an excessive number of bacteria in the mouth.

Predisposing causes of tooth decay and of unhealthy gums and mouth tissues include poor general physical condition, faulty nutrition, and lack of daily care and attention to keeping the mouth clean.

The mouth is the portal of entry for numerous pathogenic microorganisms and soon becomes, through lack of proper care and cleanliness, an incubator for the growth and development of bacteria. The mouth is warm, moist, and contains deposits of carbohydrate and

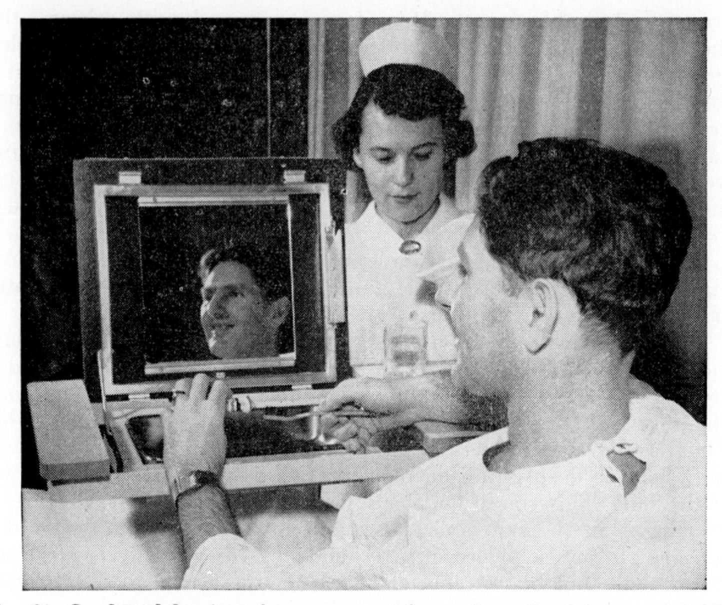

Fig. 61. Good oral hygiene is a necessary factor in maintaining good health. (Presbyterian Hospital, Chicago, Illinois.)

other food stuffs which become a perfect medium for bacterial growth unless proper hygienic measures are taken to insure adequate cleanliness.

A healthy condition of teeth and gums depends, to some extent, on proper nutrition. The doctor, dietitian, and nurse should work together to provide the patient with a diet that supplies adequate amounts of calcium, vitamins, and other elements needed for the maintenance of sound teeth. Foods that require chewing, thus furnishing the exercise and activity needed for teeth and gums to keep them in good condition, should be contained in the diet. Although the nurse has little to do with planning the diet or the selection and cooking of food, she is responsible for serving the tray or feeding the patient, and should encourage the patient to eat the food provided for his particular dietary needs.

In giving proper mouth care to the patient the nurse should be familiar with basic requirements for a satisfactory dentifrice and toothbrush. The toothbrush should have bristles that are moderately stiff and uneven in length from front to back, unless the dentist has prescribed a special type of brush. The dentifrice, which may be a liquid, paste, or powder, may be chosen for the flavoring agent used and the effectiveness with which it cleanses and polishes the teeth. A strong salt solution (made from ordinary table salt) may be used as a substitute for a commercial dentifrice if the patient has come to the hospital without adequate supplies for proper care of the mouth and teeth.

If the patient is able to brush his own teeth, he should be permitted to do so. If instructions are needed for carrying out the procedure, the nurse should demonstrate the proper method of holding the toothbrush, explaining how to do the circular and up-and-down movement so the teeth are brushed downward or upward away from the gumline. When the teeth have been thoroughly brushed the mouth should be rinsed well. Water used for this purpose should be lukewarm, since very cold or very hot water can be injurious to the gums and may cause discomfort to the patient.

For the patient who is allowed to sit up in bed, the nurse need do little more than provide the equipment and supplies which are needed for mouth care.

For the patient who must remain in a horizontal position, more assistance will be needed from the nurse. The patient should be turned to his side with a face towel properly placed to protect the bed and his clothing. An emesis basin should be placed in position just beneath the lower jaw. The use of dentifrice for cleansing and of clear water for rinsing the mouth is governed by the patient's needs and the thoroughness with which the nurse carries out the procedure. If the patient is unable to brush his own teeth, the nurse should be prepared to do it for him, being careful not to injure the gums by too vigorous brushing.

The use of a mouthwash, for patients who are given restricted diets or no food at all, and to cleanse the mouth at intervals during the day when brushing the teeth is not indicated, is an effective means of keeping the mouth clean and wholesome.

Oral hygiene procedures should be carried out as part of the routine daily care for each patient. Close observation of the condition of the patient's mouth will enable the nurse to detect early symptoms of infection. Such symptoms may include excessive dryness, foul breath, deposits on teeth and gums, and complaints of pain or of soreness in the mouth, which may be noted particularly when the patient is eating.

Teeth should be brushed before breakfast each morning and after each meal during the day. To provide the best service, the patient should have two tooth brushes and both should be cared for so they are clean at all times. After use they should be thoroughly rinsed with cold water and kept well apart while drying. At least once a week they should be washed with soap and water and immersed for a time in an antiseptic solution. New brushes should be obtained frequently.

Care of Artificial Dentures. If the patient is wearing artificial dentures, it is necessary for the nurse to care for them and see that they are not misplaced or broken.

When not in the patient's mouth, the dentures should be immersed in a mild antiseptic solution. A suitable container should be used, labeled clearly and kept in the bedside table drawer, where there is little danger of the dentures being broken or lost, and where the patient may have access to them at any time.

The same equipment used for cleaning natural teeth will be needed for cleaning dentures. A paper towel, folded several times, should be placed in the sink and, while dentures are being brushed and rinsed under running water, they should be held close to the towel as a safety precaution. If a partial plate or bridgework is being cleaned, all clips or braces should be thoroughly freed of deposits of food or other substances. Careless handling of such pieces may cause the edges to become roughened and cause damage to the teeth to which they are anchored in the mouth.

Secretions from the mouth make dentures slippery and difficult to handle. If the patient is able to do so, he should remove the dentures and hand them to the nurse. An emesis basin padded with gauze squares or paper toweling should be held in readiness to receive the plates. The labeled container for the dentures should be washed and filled with fresh solution at the same time the dentures are cleaned. After the dentures have been cleaned they should be placed in the container to be returned to the patient.

All nurses should be aware that artificial dentures are extremely fragile, very expensive, and difficult to replace when lost. Extreme caution should be exercised in their handling and care.

ROUTINE DAILY CARE FOR THE PATIENT

Daily care for the hospitalized patient consists primarily of different combinations of basic nursing procedures. Modifications of these procedures are required in meeting the needs of the individual patient. Although the number of possible combinations of basic procedures is practically unlimited, certain ones are generally used in giving care to the average patient throughout each 24-hour period and have come to be accepted as "routine."

Early A.M. Care. Care given the patient in the early morning, just prior to serving breakfast, includes washing face and hands, offering bedpan or urinal, oral hygiene (brushing teeth, care of dentures, use of mouthwash), combing hair, and placing patient, if allowed to sit up, in comfortable position in bed as part of the preparation for receiving the breakfast tray.

Routine A.M. Care. The routine nursing care, which is accorded all patients each morning after breakfast and takes up much of the nurse's time each day, includes giving bedpan or urinal; oral hygiene (which includes brushing of teeth); bed or tub bath; alcohol back rub; care of hair and nails; change of bed linens; change of patient's gown or pajamas; making the patient comfortable and doing necessary tasks to put the room in order.

P.M. Care. P.M., or evening care, routinely given to patients each

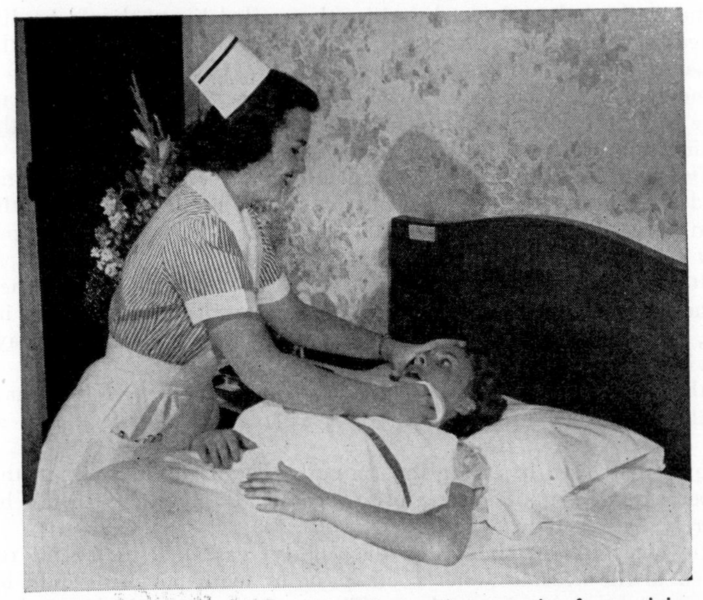

Fig. 62. Early morning care is an essential part of preparation for receiving the breakfast tray. (Delaware Hospital School of Nursing, Wilmington, Delaware.)

evening soon after the evening meal, includes giving the bedpan or urinal; oral hygiene, with the patient being assisted in brushing his teeth or with dentures being cleaned by the nurse; washing the patient's back and rubbing it with alcohol or a suitable skin lotion; tightening the foundation linen of the bed and brushing it free of crumbs. Linen that has become soiled during the day should be replaced. The room should be put in order and fresh drinking water placed at the bedside.

Care at H.S. Care given in the early evening, after the patient has received H.S. medications, includes offering the bedpan or urinal, and adjusting the bed so the patient is in a horizontal position and made comfortable for the night. An extra blanket should be folded across the foot of the bed so it will be ready for use if needed during the night, the room should be adequately ventilated, all lights should be turned out (except for the night light), and the signal bell should be placed within easy reach. The entire hospital corridor should be kept quiet so the patients' sleep will not be disturbed.

Care of Equipment after Use

After the Bed Bath. The wash basin should be thoroughly cleansed and dried and returned to the bedside table. Soap should be placed on the tray in the soap dish and put away until needed again.

The wash cloth and towels, with other soiled linen, should be discarded into the linen chute. Clean towels should be placed on the proper rod or shelf in the bedside table.

The top of the bottle of alcohol should be securely fastened in place; the bottle, with powder can or box, should be left in the bedside table.

After the Tub Bath. The tub should be cleaned with scouring powder. Used towels and wash cloths should be discarded into the linen chute. Soap and talcum or body powder belonging to the patient should be returned to his bedside table.

After Shaving. The wash basin should be cleaned and returned to the bedside table. The razor should be cleaned and replaced in its case, the shaving brush should be rinsed thoroughly and put away. Shaving cream or soap should be put away until needed again.

Other Equipment. The comb and brush used in caring for the hair should be washed in soap and water at intervals and kept free of hair combings at all times.

Equipment used in caring for the nails should be put away in the proper case or container after use. Tops on all containers should be securely tightened.

The emesis basin should be thoroughly washed, rinsed, and returned to the bedside table. Tooth paste or tooth powder should be kept in tightly closed containers. The toothbrush should be washed and rinsed thoroughly after each use.

Dentures should be kept clean and, when not in the patient's mouth, should be kept in a clearly labeled container.

Summary of Important Factors

The skin protects the body from microorganisms and serves as an excretory organ to help eliminate waste products through perspiration.

Cleanliness is essential for the nurse as well as for the patient.

Baths should be given in a room that is comfortably warm and free from drafts.

The term "finish the bath" needs to be explained to the patient.

The alcohol back rub should be a part of any bath given to make the patient more comfortable.

The patient should not be permitted to lock the door of the bathroom when taking a tub bath.

A nurse should not attempt to lift a patient who has fainted while in the bathtub; she should open the drain and let the water out of the tub.

Additional hot water should not be added to the bath while the patient is in the tub.

A person standing in a tub of water should never touch an electrical appliance—there is danger of being electrocuted.

The patient should be adequately and correctly draped for the bath procedure.

The hair should be brushed and combed at least once each day.

Fingernails should be kept clean and should be filed at frequent intervals.

Toenails should be cut straight across to prevent them from growing inward.

Oral hygiene is an important part of daily care for the patient.

Dentures should be carefully cared for and kept in a clearly labeled container so they will not be lost or broken.

Factors To Teach the Patient

Good habits of personal hygiene and their importance in maintaining good health.

The functions of the skin and necessity for keeping it clean, especially during illness.

The meaning of the term "finish the bath."

Frequent washing of hands will help to prevent disease; washing of hands should always be a part of preparation for eating.

Adaptations of the "bed bath" procedure to meet the needs of the patient being cared for in the home, including ways in which the patient may cooperate to make his care easier for the untrained person who will perform the nursing duties in the home.

That dangers involved in taking tub baths include: a locked bathroom door may delay needed assistance; a person may be electrocuted by touching electrical apparatus while standing in a tub of water; a person may become chilled if temperature of the bathroom or of the water is allowed to become too low; that a person may be burned or scalded if hot water is added while he is in the tub; risk of falling while in the tub.

Desirable effects of using alcohol and powder in giving skin care. Action of soap when used in bathing, and why water alone will not effectively cleanse the skin. Proper methods of care for hair, nails, and teeth.

That indiscriminate use of hair dyes may be harmful.

The importance of proper diet to oral hygiene.

The importance of care of nails, because nails can be a breeding place for microorganisms.

Social agencies that are available for help if the patient is worried about finances, employment, personal relationships, or future plans.

Scientific Principles

Anatomy and Physiology. The skin is made up of two layers, the epidermis (outer layer) and the corium or derma (true skin). The epidermis is made up of four layers, the outer one is being constantly shed and replaced from the layers beneath. The derma is a layer of connective tissue which contains glands, blood vessels, nerves, and the hair roots.

Glands of the skin include: sebaceous, which secrete oil or sebum, and the sweat glands, which secrete perspiration.

Appendages of the skin are hair and nails.

The skin plays a major role in regulating body temperature.

The skin is a protective covering guarding the underlying tissues against injury and invasion by microorganisms.

Nerves in the skin make it a sense organ conveying stimuli producing sensations of heat, cold, pain, and pressure.

Waste products from glands, dust, and bacteria need to be removed each day by a cleansing bath.

Hair is found on all parts of the body except palms of the hands and soles of the feet.

Color of the hair is due to pigment in the intercellular spaces of the cortex.

Stimulation of circulation by brushing is desirable for healthy hair.

Excessive secretion of sebaceous glands causes oily hair.

The mouth is lined with mucous membrane.

Teeth are the most important structures in the mouth, from the standpoint of hygiene.

Normal tooth development is helped by chewing hard fibrous foods.

Chemistry. Hard water is not suitable for bathing since it does not easily form a lather with soap.

Rubbing alcohol combines with proteins of the skin; the resultant hardening then makes the skin more resistant to pressure.

Excess alkalinity of soap may remove protecting oils from the skin.

The skin has an acid reaction which destroys some forms of bacteria. Powder may be used to keep the skin dry and to provide some astringent and antiseptic effect.

The chemical basis of nails is keratin.

The enamel of the teeth is made up of about 97 per cent mineral matter.

Tartar consists of mineral matter and food debris.

Gold and silver are used in dental repair because the secretions of the mouth do not affect them.

Microbiology. Bacteria found normally on the skin can enter the body only if there is a broken or open place on the skin. A mechanical or chemical injury permits such bacteria to invade the body; the injury may be very slight, as a tiny cut, or it may be extensive, with a large area of skin involved.

Bathing is necessary to remove dirt, oil, and the outermost cells which are constantly being shed from the skin.

Soap, necessary for bathing, acts by lowering surface tension of the water. When soap is used it must be thoroughly removed by rinsing, to prevent irritation to the skin.

Hand lotion or hand cream should be used generously, especially during winter months, to keep the skin smooth and free of chapping or of breaks.

Antiseptic treatment of the skin after a small injury may prevent infection.

Hands are readily contaminated with microorganisms and the nurse may spread disease by failing to wash her hands between patients.

Careful and frequent washing of hands safeguards the nurse and prevents the spread of disease from one patient to another.

Biting fingernails introduces dirt and bacteria into the mouth.

Ingrown toenails may be caused by tight shoes or hose.

An unclean scalp is incapable of functioning normally.

Oral cleanliness helps to prevent dental caries. The mouth has all the requirements—warmth, moisture, food, and protection—for the growth of bacteria. Teeth most liable to decay are the molars. Dentures should be well cleaned after each meal. Poor oral care may lead to gingivitis, pyorrhea, and sordes.

Pharmacology. Alcohol and witch hazel are astringents and tend to harden or strengthen the skin.

Cocoa butter is used to soften callused areas on the skin.

Mild antiseptics are needed as precautionary measures in slight injuries to the skin.

Cornstarch, which is smooth and without grit, makes an excellent dusting powder for the skin.

Sodium bicarbonate may be used successfully as a tooth powder.

Sodium chloride is abrasive for a tooth powder but, in solution, makes a good mouth wash.

Glycerin and lemon juice aids in softening dry lips.

Superfluous hair will be less noticeable if bleached with hydrogen peroxide.

Physics. Water is an excellent conductor of heat, so water for baths should be warmer than body temperature to prevent the patient from being chilled.

Water and alcohol evaporate from the skin; evaporation is a cooling process.

Friction is reduced by moisture, a lubricant, or a powder, and for that reason alcohol, a lubricant, or a powder is used for the back rub to lessen friction between the nurse's hands and the skin of the patient's back.

Pressure against blood vessels in the skin reduces the amount of blood that flows through them; if the pressure is continued for a long time, a pressure area may develop, with damage to the involved tissues.

In giving a bed bath the nurse can maintain balance easily and prevent fatigue or strain by standing with her feet about 18 inches apart on the floor. Also, by moving the patient to the side of the bed so she need not reach across the bed, fatigue is prevented.

A body put into water displaces an equal volume of water. When giving a foot bath or tub bath that fact should be given consideration.

If a denture is placed in cold water, friction will be prevented and it will slide easily into place.

Psychology. Privacy should be insured the patient for bath procedures.

Resentment by the patient of close supervision for a tub bath may be overcome by the nurse's explanation in regard to need for safety measures. A bath often bolsters the morale of a woman patient, especially if it becomes the starting point for such small attentions as a new hair style, or for use of cosmetics, cologne, and a becoming gown and bed-jacket. Little attentions, such as combing hair, placing of a ribbon in the hair, a manicure, and the use of perfumed soap, give the patient encouragement and help morale.

Care of the nails may be an interesting diversion for the patient. Hair or scalp ailments may create feelings of inferiority.

An unshaven face may embarrass and annoy the male patient. If he is unable to shave himself, a barber should be called, or the nurse should shave him.

When bathing the patient the nurse has ample opportunity to listen to complaints or to the talk which may serve to relieve mental strain for the patient. Conversation during the bath procedure should be governed by the patient's condition and desires.

Performing the bath procedure with skill and with a manner that indicates confidence in her own ability, the nurse inspires the patient's confidence and gives him a needed feeling of security. In caring for the patient, the nurse's hands should be smooth, warm, and gentle. The nurse should be agreeable, skillful, and herself hygienically clean, when giving care to the patient.

Sociology. If the patient must remain in bed after being sent home from the hospital, the Visiting Nurse Association will provide nursing service so that the bath procedure can be continued. If a member of the patient's family is responsible for the care of the patient she can be taught to give the bed bath and to perform other nursing duties in a competent manner.

In teaching the patient hygienic measures that promote good health, the nurse should inform him of social agencies in the community that will be helpful to him. Such agencies include The Family Service Bureau, The American Red Cross, Salvation Army, Tuberculosis Institute and the Y.M.C.A. and Y.W.C.A.

Situation Type Problems

1. An instructor in a nursing school explained in detail to a class of beginning students that there was little real basis for the belief some women have that soap cannot be used in washing the face. The instructor convinced the students that the skin of the face reacts to soap

and other mildly antiseptic solutions exactly the same as the skin of the rest of the body.

Next morning one of the students was informed by a patient, for whom she was preparing to give a bath, that soap was not to be used in washing the face.

The student told the patient that soap was no more harmful to the face than to the feet and proceeded to use a generous amount of it in bathing the patient. Although the patient submitted to having her face washed with soap she continued to express her apprehension as to the effect. Next day the patient's face showed the appearance of an undiagnosed "rash" and she blamed the nurse, saying that the soap used in giving the bath the previous morning was responsible. What would you have done?

2. On three different occasions a head nurse had reprimanded a student for wearing an engagement ring while on duty in the hospital. The head nurse had explained that the engagement ring should not be worn with the uniform, that it was a means of harboring and transmitting disease organisms since settings cannot be thoroughly cleaned by merely washing the hands, and that there was danger of scratching a patient with the ring while performing nursing procedures. The student was told that if she persisted in wearing the ring the matter would have to be referred to the Nursing Office.

Three days after receiving the warning the student was wearing the ring while bathing a patient. The patient turned unexpectedly as she was preparing to help him to turn, and she jerked her hand away in an attempt to keep it out of the patient's way. In so doing, she made a deep scratch on the patient's buttock with the ring. The patient was indignant and reported the incident to the head nurse, suggesting to her that it might be well for the school to have a regulation prohibiting students from wearing jewelry that could cause injury to a patient. As the head nurse, what would you have done?

Suggested Reference Reading

"Soap and cleanliness," A. Smith; American Journal of Nursing, April, 1935.
"Body odor," Joseph Jordan Eller; Trained Nurse and Hospital Review, August and September, 1945.
"Some skins need the doctor," Bernice Peck; Mademoiselle, January, 1952.
"Building better teeth," M. O. Lerrigo; Today's Health, March, 1952.
"Are you up to date on dental health?" W. Philip Phair; American Journal of Nursing, February, 1953.

CHAPTER 10

Therapeutic Baths—Special Care

TOPICAL OUTLINE

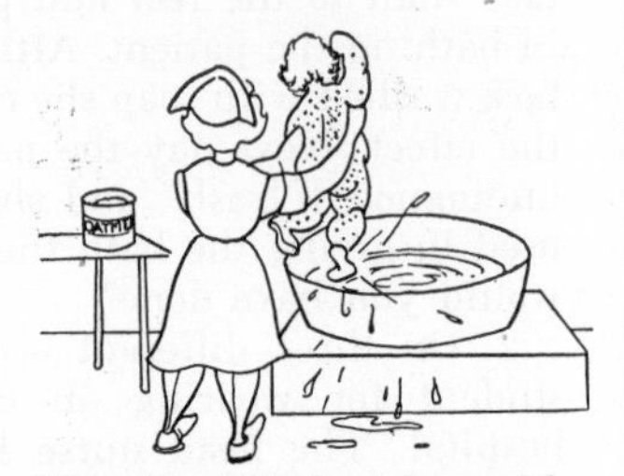

Why be difficult, when with a little more effort you can be impossible?

THERAPEUTIC BATHS

Baths have long been used for their physical effects, and a therapeutic bath is one given to produce a certain desired physical reaction. Patients should be under close observation of the nurse during the entire procedure and for a time later to make sure there are no resultant ill effects.

In general, warm or hot baths are soothing to the nerves, help to relax tired and aching muscles, and relieve pain, fatigue, and discomfort.

Cold baths tend to cool the body and to stimulate reaction.

Medicated baths are given for a specific effect, as to allay skin irritation or to serve as a sedative for the patient.

IMMERSION BATHS

Baths in which a part or the entire body (except for the head) is immersed in water, are termed immersion baths. They are further classified according to the length of time the bath is continued, the area or part of the body being treated, and the desired results to be obtained.

The most commonly used immersion baths at the present time in-

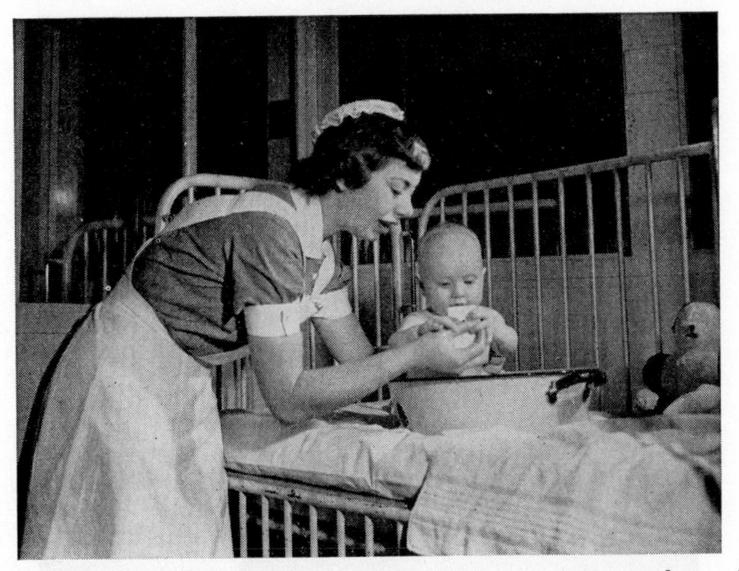

Fig. 63. An immersion bath for the baby requires constant attendance of the nurse. (Massachusetts General Hospital School of Nursing, Boston, Massachusetts.)

clude the continuous bath, relaxing bath, hot water bath, hot foot bath, Sitz bath, and arm soak.

The Continuous Bath. The continuous bath is used in the treatment of emotionally disturbed patients for its relaxing and sedative effect. The patient is placed in the tub on a special canvas or similar support so that the entire body, except the head, is under water. The room should be warm and quiet. The temperature of the water should be about the same as normal skin temperature (94–96° F.). On hot summer days the water temperature may be as low as 90° F. If the patient feels chilly, water temperature may be increased to as much as 100° F. The water should be maintained at an even temperature and should be checked about every half hour with a bath thermometer during the time the patient is in the tub.

The patient's face should be washed and dried several times during the procedure and he should be protected from drafts while being removed from the tub at the end of the treatment.

Patients in a state of excitement, or other mental aberration, should be closely observed while in the tub, since there is danger of drowning resulting from accident or suicidal intent.

The Relaxing Bath. This type of immersion bath is used in treatment of insomnia. The patient is made comfortable in a horizontal position in the tub, with only the head above water. The bathroom

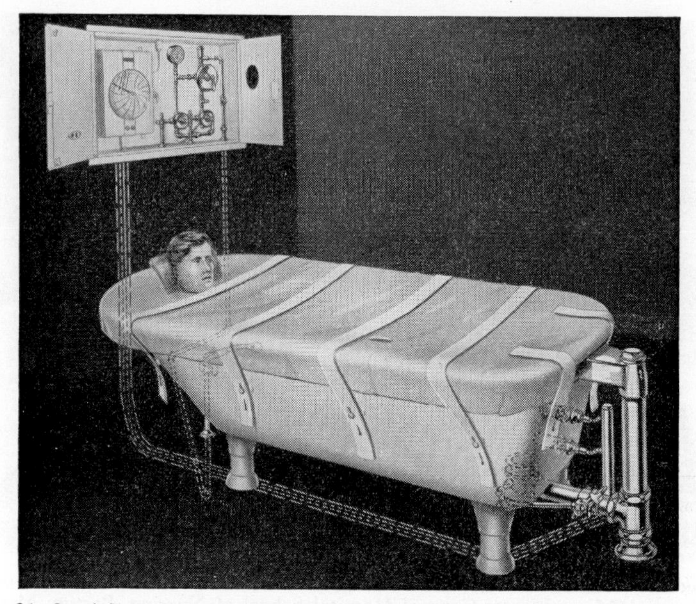

Fig. 64. Semi-diagrammatic representation of the apparatus used for the continuous flow bath. (Crane Company, Chicago, Illinois.)

should be warm and quiet. The bath water temperature should be about 95° F. The patient should be encouraged to lie in a state of quiet relaxation, to close his eyes, and to refrain from conversation.

The bath may be continued for as long as an hour if no undesirable effects are noted. After that time the patient should be patted dry with a turkish towel, placed in a warm, dry bed, and made ready for a nap or for sleep at night.

The Hot Water Bath. The hot water bath is used as a means of overcoming muscular soreness and strain. The temperature of the water should be about 100° F. The patient may remain in the tub for about 10 minutes. On being removed from the bath he should be dried quickly and placed at once into a warm bed; to avoid drafts. This bath may be used as treatment for sprains (ankle or wrist) by immersing only the affected part. The part being treated should be bathed for 10 to 15 minutes, or until the skin has become reddened.

The Hot Foot Bath. The hot foot bath relieves congestion in deeper organs or in a distant part of the body (the head). Temperature of the water used for the hot foot bath is about 100° F. when the bath is started and should be increased, by adding additional hot water, until it reaches 110 to 115° F., as tolerated by the patient.

The tub with the patient's feet immersed should be wrapped snugly in blankets so that the water will retain its heat. The treatment should be continued for 20 to 30 minutes, depending on the physician's orders. After the bath the patient's feet should be dried, and he should be kept for an hour or so in a warm, dry bed.

The Sitz Bath. The term "Sitz bath" refers to prolonged immersion of buttocks, thighs, and lower trunk in water ranging in temperature from 100 to 120° F.

The purpose of the treatment is to relieve congestion and inflammation of pelvic organs (as in dysmenorrhea), to relieve pain following cystoscopy, to induce urination, and to relieve discomfort caused by hemorrhoids.

The bath should be given in a warm bathroom. The patient sits in the tub of water and hot water is added to raise the temperature as the patient is able to tolerate it up to 120° F. When adding the hot water the nurse should hold her hand between the patient's body and the stream of water, to prevent any possibility of a burn. To prevent chilling of the upper part of the body a warm bath blanket should be draped around the patient and fastened securely at the neck. Ice compresses should be applied to the patient's forehead, or an ice collar placed about his neck to prevent headache.

Many hospitals have specially constructed tubs for Sitz baths so that the patient's feet may be placed in a foot bath of 110° F. The patient may be permitted to drink cold water during the treatment.

After 20 minutes the patient should be helped from the bath, dried, and assisted into clean dry linens. Dressings removed for the bath should be discarded and new dressings applied after the treatment. The patient should be returned to bed and kept warm so that chilling will be prevented.

The Arm Soak. The arm soak is used to make local application of moist heat, to relieve inflammation, and to facilitate removal of necrosed tissue. Temperature of water used for the bath ranges from 105 to 120° F.

A special portable tub or soak basin, of proper size to allow the entire arm to be submerged, is used for the treatment. The curved edge of the basin fits well up under the axilla and should be padded so the patient will be comfortable during the procedure. After the arm has been lowered into the water the cover of the basin should be put in place and a warm bath blanket draped over the shoulder and over the covered basin so heat of the water may be maintained for a longer period. In giving an arm soak the nurse should be certain that the basin is placed so the patient may keep the affected arm in the correct position in the bath without straining shoulder muscles or becoming unduly fatigued.

The treatment may be continued 40 to 60 minutes, depending on the physician's orders and the effect on the patient. The affected arm should then be gently dried with a turkish towel and wrapped in a bath blanket for half an hour.

If there is an open wound on the affected arm, sterile solution must be used. The equipment must be sterile, and the procedure should be carried out with sterile technique. Dry, sterile dressings should be applied after the soaking period has ended.

THE WHIRLPOOL BATH

Used extensively in physiotherapy, the whirlpool bath is effective in treatment of various conditions affecting the extremities.

The tub used for the bath is so constructed that whirling water is introduced into it and an overflow drain is provided so the desired water level may be maintained. Air pressure causes the water to enter the tub with a whirling motion; temperature of the water may range from 110 to 115° F.

The heat of the water relaxes the muscles and stimulates circulation in the part. The gentle massage-like movement of the water is soothing to the patient and relieves tension and discomfort. The whirlpool bath is used in conjunction with other forms of physiotherapy, such as massage and passive exercise.

SPONGE BATHS

Sponge baths are given for reducing body temperature, aiding elimination, and relieving restlessness or nervousness. They comprise one of the most commonly used forms of treatment for reducing body temperature when it is 102° F. or more. It is not unusual for body temperature of the patient to show a marked decrease (two degrees or more) in a relatively short time after a sponge bath has been given. For all sponge baths a washcloth may be used to apply the solution.

The Cold Sponge Bath. Cold sponge baths are given only on order of the physician and usually when the patient's temperature is 104° F. or higher. Before beginning the treatment the room should be made comfortably warm and the mattress should be protected with a rubber sheet. The bedpan should be offered the patient; an ice cap should be placed on his head, and a hot water bottle at his feet. A bath towel should be used to apply friction just before sponging. The temperature of water used for a cold sponge should be approximately 60 to 70° F.

A basin of ice cubes should be at hand so the water used for the sponging can be kept at the desired low temperature.

The patient should be draped as for a bed bath. The entire body surface should be sponged, including the face. As each part is sponged it may be loosely covered with the bath blanket. No attempt is made to dry the area after sponging. In sponging the abdomen friction should be omitted. After the front of the body has been sponged the patient should be turned to permit sponging the back and back of the legs.

The treatment requires approximately 15 to 20 minutes. As soon as it is completed the ice cap and hot water bottle should be removed and the patient should be made comfortable in a clean, dry bed. Thirty minutes after the procedure is completed the patient's temperature, pulse, and respiration should be taken and recorded.

The Tepid Sponge Bath. The tepid sponge bath is given for the same purpose as the cold sponge bath and is performed in the same manner. The only difference is in the temperature of the water, which for the tepid sponge should be approximately 90° F.

The Alcohol Sponge. Alcohol 70 per cent, with an equal amount of water, at a temperature of 90 to 100° F., is the solution used for the alcohol sponge. The cooling of the body is accomplished by evaporation. Since alcohol is drying to the skin, sponging of the face may be omitted in an alcohol sponge bath.

MEDICATED BATHS

A large variety of medicated baths are used primarily for the relief of skin disorders or for a soothing or sedative effect on the nervous system.

Such baths may be given as sponge baths, although usually they are given in the bathtub filled one-half to two-thirds its total capacity. The body of the patient should be immersed in the solution for 15 to 30 minutes, depending on the physician's orders. Temperature of the water may range from a cool 75° F. to a comfortably warm 96° F. After the patient has been in the bath for the specified length of time, he should be wrapped in a warm, dry sheet and returned to his bed. Some of the commonly used medicated baths and the methods of preparation are given here.

Sodium Bicarbonate Bath. Used in 5 per cent solution in various skin diseases for its soothing effect or to relieve itching. Sodium bicarbonate should be dissolved first in a small amount of hot water and added to the bath water.

Bran Bath. Used to soften and soothe an irritated skin. Two pounds of bran should be tied in a loose, muslin bag and placed in a deep basin. Boiling water should then be poured over it and permitted to stand 10 to 15 minutes. Moisture should be pressed from bran and all the fluid added to the bath water.

Mustard Bath. Given as a stimulant and to relieve muscle spasms and convulsions. For an adult, 1 tablespoon mustard is added to 1 gallon of water. For a child, one-half this amount is used. The powdered mustard should be dissolved in a small amount of tepid water and added to the bath water.

Saline Bath. A 2 per cent solution of sodium chloride, used as an artificial sea water bath, for its stimulating effect on nerves of the skin. The sodium chloride is dissolved in hot water and added to the bath water.

Starch Bath. Used for its emollient effect on the skin and to relieve irritation. One pound of corn starch should be mixed with cold water, and boiling water added to make a thin solution. The solution is then boiled 1 or 2 minutes and added to the bath water.

Oatmeal Bath. A soothing bath used in the treatment of skin diseases. Three cups of oatmeal and two quarts of water should be boiled together to make a porridge, which is then poured into a cheese cloth bag and one cup of baking soda added. With the mouth of the bag tied securely, the bag should be twirled around in the water, freeing the desired mucilaginous material into the bath water and leaving the residue in the bag.

Sulfur Bath. Used in treatment of acne and in skin diseases caused by parasitic organisms, as scabies. One-half to two ounces of sulfur (sulfurated potash) should be dissolved in a small amount of hot water and then added to the half tub of water drawn for the bath. The patient should remain in the bath for approximately 20 minutes. Friction should not be used in drying the patient after the bath.

Sulfur is harmful to all metals so equipment used (including the bathtub) should be thoroughly cleansed as soon as the treatment has been completed.

Special Care

When routine care is inadequate for maintaining proper functioning of certain parts of the body it becomes necessary to give added attention and care to the patient. Special care is given to the part affected, while the rest of the body is maintained with routine daily care. Such special care may involve the skin, to prevent skin disorders and to prevent or treat decubiti; the hair, if the patient remains in the hospital for a long period of time or needs treatment for pediculosis; or the mouth, in patients whose body temperature is greatly elevated or who have infections involving the mouth.

SPECIAL CARE OF THE SKIN

Decubitus Defined. Pressure areas are those areas of the body which are subject to greater pressure because bony prominences of the skeletal framework come very near the surface. There is little subcutaneous tissue in these areas, and the skin serves as the only protection to the projecting part. Such sites are most subject to the development of a pressure sore, or decubitus ulcer, because of impairment of circulation and the subsequent lack of nutrition to the part.

Areas of the body where decubiti are most apt to occur include the buttocks, hips, elbows, heels, ankles, toes, shoulder blades, back of the head, and the ears. Continuous pressure on these very susceptible areas will produce a reddening of the skin. If pressure is not relieved the skin breaks down and surrounding tissues are rapidly involved. A fully developed decubitus ulcer or pressure sore may result.

Causes of Decubiti. The immediate cause of a decubitus ulcer is

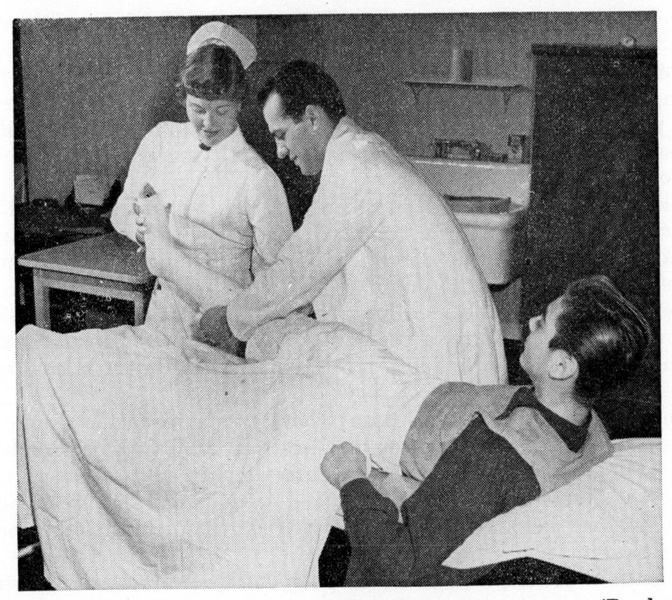

Fig. 65. A plaster cast may cause development of a pressure area. (Presbyterian Hospital, Chicago, Illinois.)

pressure or friction on the involved area. Other contributing factors are lowered vitality, incontinence, impaired circulation, obesity, anemia, emaciation, old age, paralysis, lack of cleanliness, and failure of the nurse to keep the bed dry and smoothly made. Any condition in which there is impairment of circulation to a part may be a predisposing factor in the development of a pressure sore.

Prevention of Decubiti. It is much easier to prevent the formation of a pressure sore than to treat effectively one that is fully developed. Daily good nursing care plays a most important part in the prevention of pressure sores. The primary aim of the nurse is to eliminate, so far as possible, all predisposing and immediate causes of pressure or of friction, to any part of the body.

To effectively prevent the development of a pressure sore the patient should be turned frequently, the bed should be kept dry and free of wrinkles or crumbs, and pressure areas should be massaged frequently with alcohol, which helps to stimulate and toughen the skin. All available devices, such as rubber and cotton rings, should be used to prevent pressure to certain areas. Talcum or body powder should be used liberally to absorb moisture from the skin. The nurse should also be diligent in making certain that the position of the patient is changed at frequent intervals.

The application of a cast to any part of the body may cause additional and excessive pressure so that a pressure sore soon develops. The nurse should examine the part in the cast frequently and should report at once to the doctor any change in color of the affected limb. Complaints by the patient of pain or discomfort or of numbness of the part in the cast should receive the immediate attention of the nurse, and measures should be taken to relieve pressure causing the discomfort.

The patient should be kept clean and dry. Several baths each day may be indicated during very warm weather. If the patient is incontinent back and buttocks should be washed frequently with soap and water and massaged thoroughly. The buttocks may be further protected by use of a rubber cushion. The use of infrared light rays may be helpful in preventing a pressure sore. Tincture of benzoin applied to the affected region to add a protective covering to the skin is sometimes helpful.

For an obese patient the area where two skin surfaces may rub together is a potential area of pressure sore development. Pendulous breasts or abdomen should be carefully tended, and measures taken to prevent pressure of one skin surface on another. The use of an air mattress may help to equalize pressure caused by the weight of the obese patient.

A patient predisposed to development of pressure sores is usually given a diet high in protein. By increasing intake of protein substances needed in the building of body tissue, resistance to pressure sore development is achieved.

For the patient with a very sensitive skin the chemicals used in the laundering of hospital linen may cause irritation to areas which come in contact with the linen. Care given to such areas should be the same as that used in preventing development of pressure sores from other pressure or friction.

Treatment of Decubiti. Treatment of pressure sores consists primarily of increased effort to prevent development of additional pressure areas. Effort is also made to prevent enlargement of the pressure sore as well as to promote its healing. The use of ultraviolet or infrared rays is indicated. Various drugs, such as penicillin or sulfonamides, may be used locally and systemically to control infection. Antiseptics such as chlorine and gentian violet are sometimes used. In all cases the ulcer should be exposed frequently to the air by turning the patient to a prone position and removing all dressings from the wound. Zinc oxide and other ointments may be used to prevent moistness of the affected area, especially if the patient is incontinent.

Some cases have been treated effectively by sealing the pressure sore with a pliofilm dressing and liquid adhesive, the exudate from the ulcer acting as its own foreign protein to stimulate growth of new tissue. Pressure sores which do not respond readily to medical treatment may be treated surgically, with cutting away of all necrosed tissue, cleaning the area of debris, and suturing, or grafting skin to the affected area.

While assisting in the treatment of a pressure sore the nurse should devote special effort to preventing the development of pressure sores in other areas. No matter how much time and effort is necessary for their prevention, it is only a small portion of that required to insure successful treatment of an open pressure sore.

Other means of preventing and treating pressure sores should be brought to the attention of all nurses. Although the results have been varied, each of the following methods is worth trying when healing has not been effected by known medical measures.

Sawdust therapy has been used effectively when other treatment has failed. The procedure is simple. Finely sifted sawdust is poured into the center of a muslin covered rubber ring. The patient is placed on the ring so that the ulcerated area is in the center of the sawdust, which may be as much as 1½ to 2 inches thick. The pressure area should be kept thoroughly clean, and the sawdust changed several times during the day. If the treatment is effective, improvement will be noted in a few days.

Sheepskin treatment is another method of promoting healing of pressure sores which have not responded to other corrective measures. The sheepskin, woolly side up, is placed under the patient so that the open wound comes into direct contact with the wool. The sheepskin should be large enough to avoid causing pressure on bordering areas. It may be cleaned simply by washing in warm, soapy water. It should be rinsed well and allowed to dry at room temperature. Do not place on a heated radiator or in an oven, as heat will dry and stiffen the sheepskin. The resiliency of the wool reduces pressure against the affected area. The wool absorbs moisture, and the patient is often much more comfortable than with other, more well known forms of treatment.

SPECIAL CARE OF THE HAIR

Special care of the hair may be required for patients who are hospitalized for a prolonged period of time, for those infected with head lice, and for those with hair that shows evidence of neglect.

In sickness, even more than in health, the general practice of a weekly shampoo should be followed. The condition of the hair is largely determined by the patient's physical condition; however, the appearance of the hair is due in large measure to the care and attention it receives. Patients who have been in poor physical condition for a long period of time may still have hair that is clean and attractively styled—hair that responds to frequent brushing, combing, and washing, and adds greatly to the personal appearance of its owner.

The nurse who dutifully gives a bath to the patient and conscientiously changes bed linens each day yet allows several weeks to go by without giving care to the hair fails to take advantage of an excellent means of fostering optimism and boosting morale for the patient.

Dandruff is thought by some to be a disease condition caused by an unnamed fungus. Others believe dandruff to be the visible and entirely normal shedding of flakes or particles of skin from the scalp. Whatever its origin, dandruff is conceded to be unsightly and a possible factor in contributing to undesirable skin eruptions of face, neck, and shoulders. The only successful treatment of the condition is frequent brushing and combing of the hair and thorough shampooing of it each week or every two weeks.

If the patient is extremely weak or in a serious condition he should avoid any form of exertion, and the shampoo or special care of the hair may need to be postponed.

When it is necessary to wash the patient's hair, several methods may be considered. The one which is less tiring for the patient and is given with ease by the nurse is that of transferring the patient to a stretcher and taking her to the bathroom, where all the necessary equipment has been assembled and the shampoo may be readily given.

Bed Shampoo. Although in most hospitals a written order from the doctor is required for a bed shampoo, few doctors will fail to respond to the request for such an order since they are aware of the mental benefit of the procedure to the patient. The written order was necessary when patients were likely to develop upper respiratory infections at the slightest provocation and when pneumonia was a very serious complication which all too often, before the discovery of antibiotic drugs, could not be treated effectively.

There is now little or no danger to the patient who is given a bed shampoo. The treatment may be done in the patient's room, which should be comfortably warm and free of drafts. With modern supplies and equipment, and careful preparation, the shampoo can be given in a few minutes, and in a very short time the patient's hair can be thoroughly dried, combed, and arranged in the usual manner.

Several factors should be given consideration by the nurse who is to do the procedure.

The bed should be adequately protected with rubber sheets and the patient should wear a make-up cape to protect her gown or clothing.

The room should be of correct temperature. To avoid the possible exposure of the patient to the unpleasantness of the common cold, the room in which the shampoo is to be given should be comfortably warm; temperature of approximately 76 to 78° F. is desirable. During the procedure the windows and door to the room should be closed so there is no danger of the patient being in a draft.

Two nurses should work together to perform the procedure. The bed shampoo can be done by only one nurse, but with two working together to give the shampoo less time is required and the patient is less likely to become tired and consequently less apt to develop a cold or to react unfavorably. Running water and a hose is seldom available in the patient's room; the second nurse is needed to help in handling the large quantity of water that should be used if the shampoo is to give adequate and satisfactory results.

The patient should be placed in a comfortable position before the procedure is started. Although the position of the patient may depend to some extent on her physical condition, it may be governed too by the kind of equipment used and the plumbing facilities available.

The patient lies on her back across the bed in a position so that her head is near the upper side edge of the mattress. Care should be taken to furnish adequate support for the head so there is no strain on the patient's neck. The head should be tilted backward so that water will run freely away from the face and ears, but no undue pressure should be put on the head. The patient should at no time during the procedure experience strain or discomfort in neck or upper back.

If the patient is required to remain in a sitting position, as in some forms of dyspnea, use of the backrest and proper placing of equipment will facilitate the giving of a bed shampoo.

The hair should be thoroughly brushed before the shampoo is given. A smooth-surface towel should be used to protect the bed from loose hair and dandruff as the brushing is done. A brush with stiff, strong bristles should be used, and the hair should be brushed briskly with firm, even strokes for several minutes. The scalp as well as the hair should be brushed, the stroke being made with the brush beginning each time at the scalp and descending toward the ends of the hair. Brushing not only removes dandruff, loose hair and dirt from the head, but assists in increasing circulation in the scalp.

All equipment should be assembled before the procedure is started. If running water is not available in the unit, several large pitchers of water will be needed. Other articles needed include a Kelly pad or an improvised trough made from a rolled blanket and rubber sheet to serve as a drain board, soap or liquid shampoo, several gallons of warm water, and a large pail or tub in which to collect the water used in rinsing the hair.

Liquid soap is preferable since it is more easily removed in the rinsing. To be effective, the liquid soap should be rubbed until a definite lather is produced. If the hair is oily, more soap will be needed. After the initial lather has been rinsed completely away a second application of soap and subsequent brisk rubbing is necessary to produce a lather for the second time. Hair with soap applied only once will be difficult to rinse and will be dull and unattractive in appearance because much of the soap film will remain on the hair. After the soap has been applied the second time and the hair has been rinsed free of all remaining traces of oil, dirt, and perspiration, the hair should be rinsed with water to which a small amount of vinegar or lemon juice has been added, and then finally with clear water. The final rinsing should leave the hair clean and shining.

The hair may be dried by several different methods, the most commonly used being that of rubbing with a heavy turkish towel. An electric hair dryer, a heat-giving lamp, or an electric pad are also effective means of drying the hair. When the electric pad is to be used it should be placed inside a clean pillow case and the hair spread across it to dry.

The bed shampoo is not a difficult procedure to perform and is one of the most rewarding of nursing duties since it benefits the patient in a mental and spiritual as well as a physical way.

Treatment of Pediculosis. The term pediculosis is defined as "the state of being infested with lice." Lice, or pediculi, are small wingless, blood-sucking insects which are parasitic on warm-blooded animals. The species *Pediculus humanus,* the only one which is parasitic on man, exists in two varieties, *Pediculus capitis,* found on the hair and scalp, and *Pediculus corporis,* found on the body and in clothing that has been worn by an affected person.

The body louse is capable of transmitting disease. The lice multiply rapidly and are easily transferred from one person to another. Infestation is usually associated with poor environment and lack of personal cleanliness, as when large groups of people are forced to live in close association and in an environment that may be totally lacking in cleanliness and sanitation. Under such conditions DDT, a powder which destroys the lice and which can be dusted or sprayed on large groups of people, has been used effectively. Clothing may be deloused by being subjected to extreme degrees of heat, as in autoclaving.

Body lice are rarely discovered on a patient, but it is not unusual to find a patient with head lice and displaying all the signs and symptoms characteristic of the condition. Even persons who are scrupulously clean may become affected, since the lice are readily transmitted from one person to another.

The patient with head lice may complain of severe itching of the scalp and will resort to almost continuous scratching of the head. An observant nurse will examine the hair and scalp of any patient displaying such symptoms and will find lice in large numbers if the condition has existed more than a few days. Nits or eggs of the louse are deposited on the hair and are sealed fast to the hair shaft. In severe cases the hair may appear to be heavily sprinkled with dandruff.

The destruction of nits may be extremely difficult; since those not destroyed will produce more lice, two or three treatments are often necessary to rectify the condition entirely.

Several years ago the standard treatment for head lice was application of a solution of equal parts tincture of larkspur and kerosene,

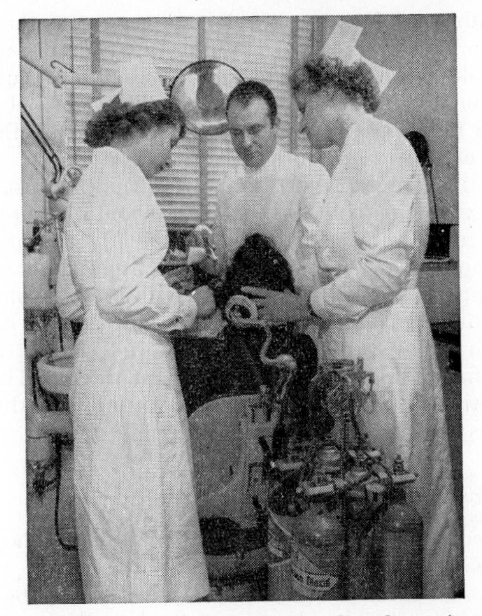

Fig. 66. Special care of the mouth may require that the patient be treated by a dental surgeon. (Chicago School of Dental Nursing, Chicago, Illinois.)

followed by a shampoo 8–12 hours later. Today preparations are available which act much more quickly and will destroy the nits as well as the lice.

After any treatment for pediculosis the hair should be combed with a fine-tooth comb and then thoroughly washed, rinsed, and dried.

If the skin is abraded from scratching extreme care must be taken in using any strong chemical preparation since it has an irritating action on the skin and will be doubly irritating where abrasions are present.

SPECIAL CARE OF THE MOUTH

The patient who has a very high fever or is seriously ill may require special care to mouth and teeth. Quite often such patients are unable to brush their own teeth so it becomes necessary for the nurse to perform the procedure. Special care is essential if the patient's mouth is to remain clean and in good condition. Care to the mouth should be given about every two hours during the day and at intervals during the night when the patient is awake and is being given other treatment or nursing care.

For the patient on a liquid diet the use of a mild antiseptic mouth wash at frequent intervals will suffice to keep the mouth clean. For the patient with a tendency to develop sordes, or for the unconscious patient, additional care is needed. Cotton applicators saturated with a solution made by dissolving a small amount of equal parts of sodium bicarbonate and sodium chloride in a glass of tepid water should be used frequently to remove accumulated secretions and prevent offensive odor of the breath.

To keep the lips, tongue, and inside of the mouth moist and smooth, a mixture of glycerine and lemon juice should be used. A small amount of the mixture may be applied to the affected areas by means of a cotton applicator. The same mixture applied to fever blisters which may appear around the mouth will prevent undue dryness and the formation of unsightly crusts when the blisters heal.

If the mouth is infected the frequent use of sodium perborate or potassium permanganate mouth wash may be ordered. These preparations are effective disinfectants capable of inhibiting the growth of microorganisms within the mouth.

Care of Equipment after Use

The tub used in giving immersion baths should be thoroughly cleaned after each use.

When medicated baths are given all supplies should be replenished and containers securely closed and returned to their proper storage place. Sulfur is harmful to metal so equipment used, including bathtub, should be cleaned immediately after a sulfur bath.

Special trays used in the treatment of decubiti should be returned to Central Supply to be cleaned and made ready for use again.

Sawdust used in treatment of decubiti should be burned.

Sheepskin used in treatment of decubiti should be washed in warm soapy water, rinsed well, and allowed to dry at room temperature.

Equipment used for a bed shampoo should be cleaned and returned to its proper storage place.

Combs used in removing lice and nits from the hair should be cleaned and sterilized before being used again.

Supplies used for special care of the mouth must be replaced. Utensils on the tray should be cleaned and sterilized. Tongue depressors and applicators should be discarded and burned.

Summary of Important Factors

Warm baths soothe nerves and help relax fatigued muscles.

Cold baths tend to stimulate reaction.

Immersion baths are frequently given to induce relaxation.

A Sitz bath is given to relieve pain and congestion in pelvic organs.

During arm soak procedure the patient should be made comfortable.

Solutions used for soaks must be sterile if there is an open wound on the affected limb.

For all bath procedures the patient should be adequately and correctly draped.

Temperature, pulse, and respiration should be taken and recorded half an hour after a sponge bath is given for reduction of body temperature.

Friction should not be used in drying the patient after a medicated bath.

Special care of skin is needed to prevent decubiti for many chronically ill patients.

Pressure or friction is the immediate cause of pressure sores. Predisposing causes of pressure areas are: lowered vitality, incontinence, impaired circulation, anemia, obesity, old age, paralysis, emaciation, and application of a cast.

Treatment consists of keeping the area dry and encouraging normal circulation.

Daily brushing of hair and a weekly shampoo will help to overcome dandruff.

The clothing of the patient and the bed linens must be protected when a bed shampoo is given.

Liquid soap is more easily removed from the hair in bed shampoo.

Treatment of pediculosis may require tactful handling of the patient because of the stigma attached to the condition.

Special care of the mouth is needed for patients with prolonged high fever.

Factors To Teach the Patient

When taking immersion baths for soothing or relaxing effect to refrain from conversation and to close their eyes and relax.

To avoid drafts during and immediately after warm baths are taken.

After a hot foot bath, to remain in bed for an hour or so.

Never to turn on hot water from the shower or a faucet when in a tub bath.

To avoid exertion of movement while receiving a sponge bath.

To refrain from scratching when medicated baths are given to relieve itching in skin diseases.

To help overcome predisposition to pressure sores by eating a proper diet.

Observe rules of good oral hygiene as a necessary part of treatment when body temperature is elevated.

Scientific Principles

Anatomy and Physiology. Oil secreted from the glands of the skin prevents dryness and helps to keep the hair in good condition. The skin protects underlying tissues from trauma and invasion by germs.

Special care to the skin is necessary to prevent pressure sores and to overcome the effects of impaired circulation to parts close to the body surface.

Immersion baths have a soothing relaxing effect because of numerous nerve endings in the skin.

Over bony prominences, as at the elbows, ankles, and knees, the skin is subject to irritation and the development of pressure areas.

Chemistry. Perspiration is a clear fluid, slightly acid in reaction. Its principal inorganic ingredient is sodium chloride, and its principal organic constituent is urea.

Rubbing alcohol tends to coagulate or harden protein of the skin, thus toughening the skin and making it resistant to pressure sores.

Microbiology. Bacteria require moisture for growth and reproduction; special care to the skin therefore includes keeping it dry.

Infection may be caused by scratching the irritated scalp when head lice are present.

Lack of care to the mouth may result in foci of infection for disease in other parts of the body.

Sordes is an accumulation of food particles and mucus on teeth, gums, and lips, when the mouth isn't kept clean.

Fever may cause the lips to become dry and cracked and a portal of entry for microorganisms if they aren't kept well lubricated with an oil such as mineral oil.

Pharmacology. Alcohol evaporates quickly so is cooling. It is used for this effect in sponge baths to reduce body temperature.

A vinegar rinse following the shampoo after treatment for pediculosis loosens the nits from the hair by dissolving the adhesive substance that attaches the nits to the hair shaft.

Salt solution is an effective and inexpensive dentifrice and mouthwash. A mixture of glycerine and lemon juice aids in keeping the inside of mouth and lips moist and smooth.

Physics. A limb or the entire body placed in an immersion bath displaces an equal volume of water.

Pressure against an affected area is reduced by use of sheepskin because the wool is resilient.

Constant pressure causes impairment of circulation.

Friction from rubbing produces heat at the skin surface, causing blood vessels to dilate and more blood to be brought to the affected area.

Heat produced by the activated water in the whirlpool bath relaxes the muscles and stimulates circulation.

Pressure from a cast may be the immediate cause of a pressure sore.

Psychology. Expected benefits of therapeutic baths should be explained so cooperation of the patient will be gained.

Care of the nails, especially if polish is worn, helps to create a sense of good grooming which is beneficial to the patient.

Special care is required to keep nails in good condition if hands or feet are being treated by immersion baths.

The very ill male patient should be shaved regularly to keep up morale and create a desirable mental attitude.

The patient may be very much embarrassed if head lice are found and treatment is started. Privacy during treatment should be provided.

Sociology. Baths given to relax and quiet the patient require that conversation between patient and nurse be kept at a minimum.

Excited or depressed patients need to be under constant observation during immersion bath treatments to avoid intentional or accidental drowning.

Situation Type Problem

1. In the Nursing Arts classroom an assistant instructor told a group of preclinical students that when a patient developed a pressure sore it was an indication that that patient had not received adequate nursing care. The instructor stated that all pressure sores could be prevented by good nursing care.

A short time later, on duty in one of the clinical departments, the student was assigned the duty of giving P.M. care to a patient who had been hospitalized for several months. The patient was receiving special care for a rather large pressure sore of the buttocks. The preclinical student watched a graduate nurse give the prescribed care for the pressure area and at the first opportunity she asked the graduate nurse why the patient had been neglected so that a pressure sore developed. The graduate nurse explained that the patient had been confined to bed for several months, and that emaciation, anemia, and other predisposing factors had made preventive measures ineffective at the time the pressure area developed.

The student remarked that "all pressure sores could be prevented by good nursing care."

The graduate nurse looked at her coolly for a moment, then said "I guess you're right—I'll suggest to the head nurse that you be assigned to give nursing care to the patient admitted yesterday. She's quite old, quite thin and partially paralyzed. Most of the time she is incontinent. A pressure area is already developing. I hope you won't mind if I watch you give good nursing care to her so I can learn how to prevent pressure sores for such a patient." What would you have done?

Suggested Reference Reading

"Effects of flying as related to teeth," Bulletin U. S. Army Medical Department, Washington, D.C., September, 1946.

"Decubitus ulcers," Anastasia M. Zahler; American Journal of Nursing, June, 1949.

"Sawdust bed therapy: Study at Teachers College, Columbia University," American Journal of Nursing, October, 1949.

"Is it ringworm," Samuel Ayres, Jr.; American Journal of Nursing, December, 1949.

"Dental caries can be prevented," Joseph F. Volker; American Journal of Nursing, February, 1950.

"A study of the care of decubiti," Helen C. Delabarre; American Journal of Nursing, February, 1950.

"Nursing care of patients having dermatologic conditions," Marguerite Wilkinson Bozian; American Journal of Nursing, July, 1952.

"Dermatitis in industry," Helen M. Wallace and Margaret A. Losty; American Journal of Nursing, January, 1953.

CHAPTER 11

Comfort Measures

TOPICAL OUTLINE

Causes of Discomfort
Providing for Physical Comfort
Moving, Turning, Lifting the Patient
Mechanical Comfort Devices
Posture and Position
Positions for Comfort or Care
Various Activities of the Patient
Restriction of Movement for the Patient
Providing for Mental Comfort

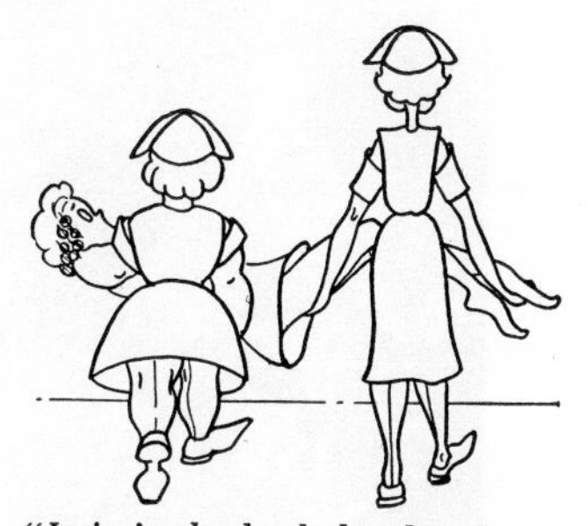

"It isn't the load that breaks us down—it's the way we carry it!"

Although the term "comfort" as related to nursing is used almost exclusively to denote physical well-being of the patient, members of the medical and nursing professions now recognize that mental and spiritual factors are also of extreme importance.

It is virtually impossible for a patient to be comfortable unless both mind and body are at ease. Nursing measures designed to promote physical comfort may be rendered ineffective if the patient is mentally distressed or in need of spiritual aid.

For the sake of simplicity and to give coherence to subject material, these important aspects of comfort will be treated separately. The student is to understand that in caring for the patient it will be necessary for her to employ the utmost skill in both phases of nursing care so that mind as well as body will benefit.

Comfort has been defined as "a feeling of physical and mental well-being; freedom from worry, fear, or pain." Factors that influence comfort concern rest and relaxation, attitude of mind, state of soul, relationship with others, and physical condition. To obtain comfort the patient must have physical rest, peace of mind, and spiritual ease.

Discomfort is defined as "want of comfort or ease; pain; annoyance." Discomfort as well as comfort is derived from both physical and mental sources.

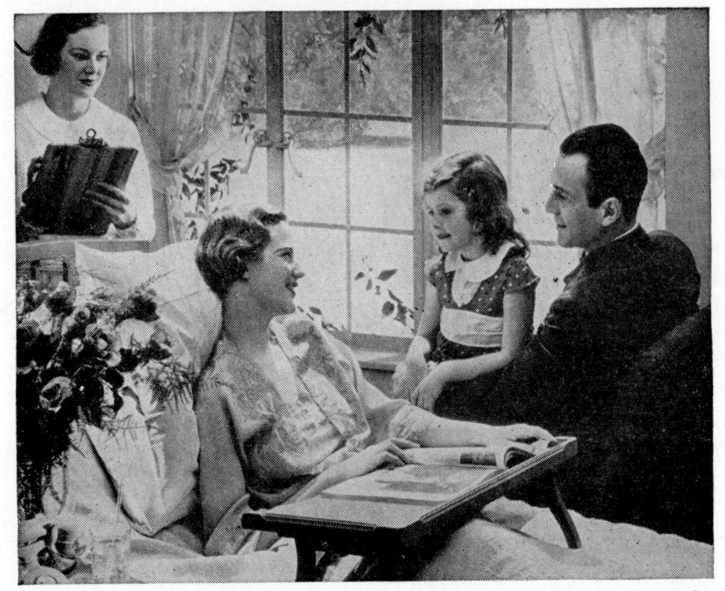

Fig. 67. The patient obtains comfort through physical rest, peace of mind, and spiritual ease. (Parke, Davis & Co., Detroit, Michigan.)

CAUSES OF DISCOMFORT

Causes of *Physical* Discomfort. Besides pain and restricted movement, often brought about by illness, a variety of causes may produce physical discomfort. The bed may be soiled, wet, or untidy, with sheets badly wrinkled; light from lamps or from a nearby window may be too bright and glaring; pillows may be improperly arranged; the body or part of the body, as an arm or leg, may not be properly supported; there may be delayed or inadequate attention to personal needs, such as cleanliness, elimination, and nourishment.

Physical discomfort may be caused by corrective devices which are necessary to treatment, as plaster casts, splints, and other orthopedic appliances.

Pressure areas on the skin may become a source of marked discomfort for the patient who is forced to remain in bed for a prolonged period of time.

Causes of *Mental* Discomfort. The mental discomfort of a patient may vary from slight annoyance to actual mental anguish. The degree of discomfort depends on whether it is caused by a problem that may be readily solved or one for which the patient can find no solution.

Fear and anxiety in regard to the illness, concern for the family, and, in the case of the father and wage earner, worry about the job he has been forced to leave may be major factors in causing the patient to be mentally disturbed.

Interruption of habits formed by daily routine at home may cause discomfort to a patient. If one has become accustomed to caring for teeth, hair, nails, and body needs in a particular manner, one may be annoyed at being unable to continue in that same manner.

A very neat and orderly person may be distressed by a disorderly room, by neglected flowers or plants, or by evidence of carelessness in hospital housekeeping.

Noise from nearby elevators, service rooms, kitchens, or telephones may be disturbing. Loud talking in the corridor or whispered conversations within the room may cause distress.

A patient who is quite modest in regard to her person may be made acutely uncomfortable by a nurse who has little understanding of such modesty. Failure to provide privacy for such a patient or to use concealing drapes in carrying out procedures of a very personal nature will lead to embarrassment and discomfort.

PROVIDING FOR PHYSICAL COMFORT

Before the student nurse is given instruction as to the proper method of moving or lifting a patient, she needs to learn basic procedures which are included in nursing care given to provide physical comfort for the patient.

Whenever a patient is to be moved or lifted it is usually wise to first place him in the dorsal recumbent position, lying flat on his back with arms at side and legs extended, and to have the mattress flat on the bed with backrest and knee rest lowered to horizontal position.

All movements made in handling the patient or the mattress and pillows, as well as bed linens, should be made gently and gradually. If the movements are made correctly there need be no jerking, painful motion felt by the patient.

When a second person is needed to help the nurse, another nurse, an orderly, or a nurse aide may be asked to assist in moving or lifting the patient. A member of the patient's family, if properly instructed by the nurse, may provide the additional help that is needed.

To Move Mattress up on the Bed. When the patient is unable to help, the nurse will need a second person to help move the mattress up on the bed.

Before movement is attempted, the backrest should be lowered so the weight of mattress and patient is evenly distributed over the entire length of the bed springs.

Two persons, standing at opposite sides of the bed, should grasp the mattress at the lower center on each side and, working together, move the mattress over the springs until it is well up on the bed. This should be done as linens are being changed. If the mattress is moved upward *before* the clean foundation sheet is put into place, the tightly made foundation of the bed will not be disturbed as it is certain to be if the mattress is moved later.

If the patient is able to assist in this procedure, the nurse may be able to move the mattress without asking help from another person. If the patient is to assist in moving the mattress toward the head of the bed, he should be instructed to grasp the rails or top (if the bed is very low) of the head board. He should then be told to flex his knees and to pull upward toward the head of the bed. At the same time, the nurse, standing at the side of the bed, should push the mattress toward the head of the bed.

The mattress will move without difficulty when the procedure is done in unison by patient and nurse, but it may be necessary for the nurse to walk around the bed and push the mattress into proper position, since it tends to move not only upward but to the opposite side.

To Prevent Patient from Slipping Down in Bed. The natural tendency is for the patient to slip downward in bed, especially if the backrest is elevated at intervals; it then becomes necessary to take measures to help him maintain a correct position in bed.

A well padded block, placed at the patient's feet and resting firmly against the foot of the bed, will prevent the patient from slipping downward. The use of a knee support, whether by means of the Gatch bed, a knee roll, or a pillow, will also help in preventing the patient from slipping down in bed.

To Turn Pillow at Patient's Back. Turning the pillow, on which the patient has rested for an hour or so, is a simple means of giving comfort. The procedure can be done quickly and smoothly and will usually leave the patient feeling refreshed. The nurse should stand at the side of the bed, passing one arm under the patient's head with hand beneath and around the patient's shoulder. The other hand is then placed for support against the patient's other shoulder where it touches the bed. The patient should then be instructed to flex the arm nearest the nurse and to rest the hand of that arm on the nurse's shoulder.

Standing with feet about a foot apart and firmly planted on the floor, the nurse may gradually raise the patient into a sitting position. Using one hand to help support the patient in this position the nurse should, with the other, remove the pillow from the bed.

If the patient is unable to sit alone in bed he may gradually be lowered to a reclining position, the pillow shaken and patted into a freshened state and placed beside the patient. The patient may then be raised again as before, so the pillow can be put back in proper position.

Pillows for Patient in Sitting Position. When the patient is allowed to have the backrest elevated two pillows are needed to make the position comfortable. One pillow is placed at the patient's back, the

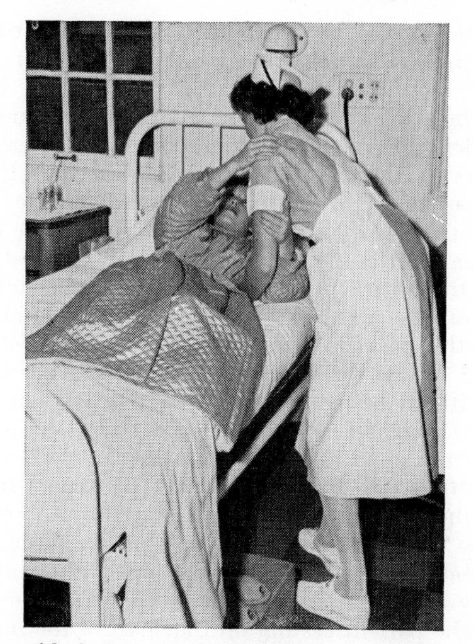

Fig. 68. To get out of bed, the patient must first be brought to a sitting position. (Good Samaritan Hospital School of Nursing, Phoenix, Arizona.)

other extending upward about 6 inches beyond the first. If necessary a small pillow may be used to give support to the patient's head.

Pillows for Patient Who Must Sit Upright. At least six standard size and two small pillows are required to create a comfortable and relaxing position for the patient who must sit upright. Four larger pillows should be arranged back of the patient, each overlapping the one beneath by about two-thirds its width, in an ascending manner. The small pillows will be needed to support the head. The remaining large pillows should be placed, one beneath each arm, to serve as arm rests. In placing a patient in this position the nurse must be sure that the pillows do not crowd against the chest or shoulders, and that the arms are evenly supported. The knees should be in a flexed position with a support provided (knee roll or Gatch bed), to prevent the patient from slipping down in bed. A variation of this arrangement, and one which is restful for any patient who must remain in a sitting position, involves placing one or two pillows on an overbed table which can then be lowered into position in front of the patient. He may lean forward to rest on the padded table; several pillows may then be put at his back for support. In this position there is no pressure from the mattress against the posterior chest and the patient can breathe with less discomfort.

To Change Linen without Turning the Patient. The nurse may need to change linens on the bed without turning the patient if he is not permitted to turn, or if doing so is difficult or painful for him. The nurse may accomplish this alone by placing one arm under the shoulders of the patient to support his shoulders and head and the other arm under the upper part of the back, and then gently moving the upper part of the patient's body toward herself. In successive movements she should bring the upper and middle portions of the body and then the lower extremities to the side of the bed near where she is standing. Since it is important that the body remain in a straight line, the entire procedure should be repeated until the patient is lying on the mattress well toward one side of the bed. With the patient in this position clean linen may be applied to the opposite side of the bed. When the foundation of the bed has been completed, the patient, without being turned (by action just the reverse of that outlined above) may be moved by degrees until he is resting on the clean linen on the opposite side of the bed.

To Turn Mattress with Patient in Bed. The patient should be moved to one side of the mattress before beginning the procedure. Bed linens should then be loosened and rolled up close to the patient, with the foundation sheet forming the outer portion of the roll. The mattress should be moved so that it extends half its width over the edge of the bed, with the patient resting on that half of the mattress which is still on the springs. Three large pillows should be placed on the exposed springs and the patient lifted or rolled onto the pillows. With the help of a second person, the mattress may be turned and put back into place, extending across the springs to the center of the bed. The patient should be lifted or rolled back onto the mattress. The three pillows may then be removed and the mattress restored to its proper position on the springs.

To Change Mattress with Patient in Bed. This procedure is done in the same manner as that described above, except the new mattress instead of three pillows is placed on the exposed springs. When the patient has been lifted or rolled to the new mattress it may be placed in proper position on the bed and the mattress just removed may then be taken from the room.

To Change Patient's Gown. Because the regulation hospital gown may be changed readily, without disturbing the patient, most hospitals require that the very ill and the newly operated patient wear a hospital gown.

If it becomes necessary to change the gown the nurse should bring a clean one to the patient's bedside. The neck strings of the soiled gown should be untied and the gown sleeve removed from the arm at the side opposite where the nurse is standing. The clean gown, fan-folded lengthwise, is then placed at the patient's side (opposite the nurse) and the arm put through the sleeve of the clean gown. The soiled gown should be rolled across the patient's chest (this is done with top covers remaining in place so the patient is not exposed) and by withdrawing the other arm from the sleeve the gown can be removed. The clean gown should be brought across the patient's chest, his arm placed through the sleeve, the gown adjusted to correct position and, without moving the patient, the neckband strings tied so the gown will remain in place. The soiled gown should be discarded into the linen chute.

MOVING, TURNING, OR LIFTING THE PATIENT

The first factor to be considered in moving, turning, or lifting a patient is the use of good body mechanics on the part of the nurse and any other person who may assist her. During the procedure the nurse should avoid unnecessary strain or injury to herself, as well as to the patient. She should not hesitate to ask for help if the weight to be lifted, whether of patient or equipment, is too heavy to be handled properly alone. Most back injuries caused by lifting are due to an attempt to lift a load that is too heavy or to incorrect body mechanics. To lift a weight correctly the nurse should stand with feet planted firmly on the floor and rather wide apart. She should stand close to the weight to be lifted, lift close to the body, and flex her knees in order to use the large, strong, leg muscles. The nurse who keeps her knees stiff and bends at the hips to lift a patient, or a heavy weight, is using incorrect body mechanics and is subject to injury from lifting. When several persons are lifting and moving a patient it is necessary to avoid quick jerky motions which may injure the patient or the persons doing the lifting. The best means of developing a rhythm of motion is that of using the counting technique or of working in unison to the very simple and effective pattern of "one-two-three—*lift.*"

Moving the patient or merely changing his position slightly is often a means of providing more comfort. By moving an arm or leg to a different position on the bed discomfort caused by inactivity may be temporarily relieved.

To Move Patient from One Side of Bed to Other. This procedure, which is one of the simplest, is often effective in relieving discomfort. If the patient is not permitted to turn, or finds turning painful, movement across the bed affords the best method of relief from strain caused by prolonged stay in one position. To accomplish this the nurse places one arm under the patient's head and neck, the other under his shoulders, and moves the upper part of his body slightly toward herself. Movement of the middle portion of the body and of the extremities should be accomplished by degrees, since the body of the patient must be kept in correct alignment. If additional movement is required the entire procedure should be repeated until the desired position has been attained.

To Move Patient Upward or Downward on Bed. To move the patient upward on the bed, if he has slipped down, the nurse places

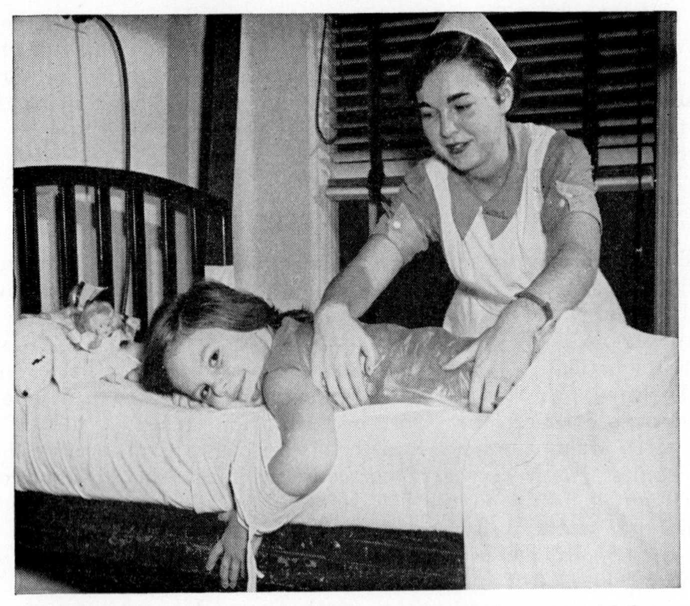

Fig. 69. The hands of the nurse should firmly support the patient while turning. (Evanston Hospital School of Nursing, Evanston, Illinois.)

one hand and forearm under the patient's shoulders, the other hand under his thighs. The patient, with knees flexed and feet set firmly on the bed, helps raise and move himself as the nurse helps to lift and move him upward.

If the patient needs to be moved downward in the bed the procedure is the same with the movement toward the foot of the bed rather than the head.

If the patient is unable to assist in these movements, a second person will be required to help the nurse. The second person stands at the opposite side of the bed. The nurse places one hand and arm under the patient's shoulders, the other under his lower back. The second person places one hand and arm under the patient's hips, the other under the lower thighs. Working together, both raise the patient and move him to the desired position on the bed.

To Turn Patient on Side. Turning the patient on his side affords rest and relaxation for back and legs. A very weak or very ill patient should be assisted so he need not exert himself. Before turning the patient the nurse should move him to one side of the bed so he is slightly off center on the mattress. To get the patient in position for turning, the nurse should reach across him to grasp the opposite hand and bring his arm across his chest. The knee of the leg farthest from her should be slightly flexed. She should then place one hand on the

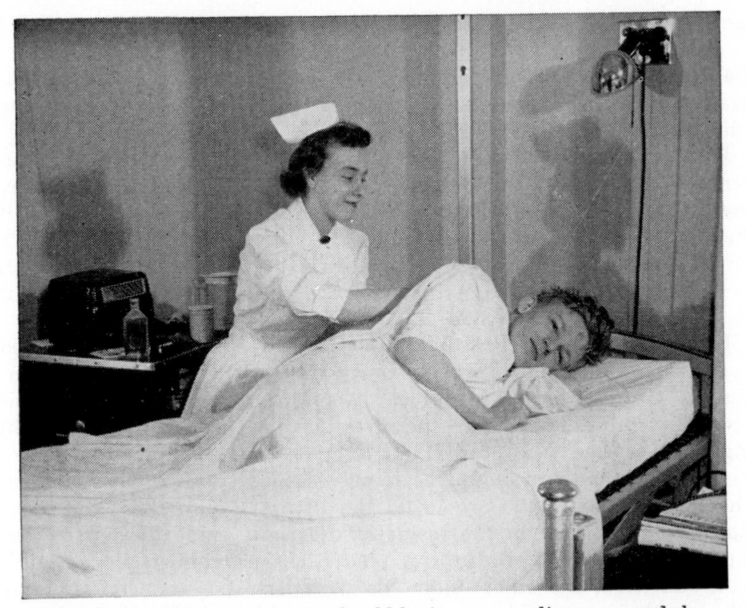

Fig. 70. When on his side the body should be in correct alignment and the arms in a comfortable position. (Presbyterian Hospital, Chicago, Illinois.)

patient's shoulder and the other on his hip and gently roll him toward her to turn him to his side and into proper position on the bed. With her hands cupping his shoulder and hip, she has complete control of his movement and can turn him only slightly or completely to one side, depending on the position desired.

To turn the patient away from her, he should be placed first in a horizontal position on his back. In preparation for turning him she will need to place one arm under his back to the far shoulder and slide the other under his hips. Then, by gently lifting and moving the patient toward her, his body will be moved slightly off center on the mattress.

From this position on the bed he may be gently rolled and turned to his side, facing away from her. When the patient has been turned on his side the nurse should see that his body (head, shoulders, hips, and legs) is in proper alignment and that the arms are not cramped or left in an uncomfortable position. Legs should be flexed, with thighs and knees in a position so that the upper leg is more acutely flexed and extends above and beyond the lower one. The upper leg may rest against a pillow placed between the legs to prevent weighing against the lower leg. A pillow that has been rolled lengthwise should be pushed firmly against the back for support. A small pillow placed snugly against the patient's abdomen may add to his physical comfort. The pillow beneath the head of the patient should be grasped by the nurse and drawn into place so that the corner fits snugly into the space between the patient's chin and shoulder. This prevents strain on the neck muscles and is an important factor in providing relaxation for the patient.

To Turn the Patient with a Half Sheet. A completely helpless patient, or one who is disoriented or irresponsible, may be turned by one nurse if assistance isn't readily available. She should place a half sheet or drawsheet under his body from neck to thighs then reach across him, grasp the sheet and, pulling it evenly and firmly, roll the patient (his body kept in perfect alignment) toward her until he comes to rest on his side.

To Lift Patient from Bed to Stretcher. Three persons will be needed to lift a patient of ordinary size and weight from bed to a stretcher. Usually two nurses and an orderly work together in performing this particular procedure. After the stretcher has been placed at right angles to the bed (the head of the stretcher just touching the foot of the bed), the patient should be loosely covered with a bath blanket. The three persons who are to do the lifting should then take their places side by side, on the inside of the right angle formed by bed and stretcher. One of the nurses places one arm under the patient's head and neck, the other under his shoulders. The orderly, standing between the nurses, places one arm beneath the patient's back and the other beneath his hips. The second nurse places one arm beneath the patient's thighs and the other under his lower legs, about midway between knees and ankles. The three, lifting in unison at a signal given by one of them, slowly raise the patient from the bed and turn him toward them so that he rests within the bend of their elbows and against their chests. Moving carefully, in step, they walk to the side of the stretcher and gently lower the patient, bending their bodies above him, until he is in the proper position on the stretcher.

A patient may be moved to the stretcher from the bed by placing the stretcher parallel to the bed and using the draw sheet to help lift him directly to the stretcher. This method is not as satisfactory as the foregoing one, since the patient is forced to exert himself to help with the lifting and is much more apprehensive about falling. Moving the patient in this manner is usually a distressing experience for him as movements are more jerky and uncertain and may result in pain and discomfort, especially if the patient has recently undergone surgical treatment.

If the patient is able to move or turn himself in bed he should be permitted to do so even though the process may seem exceedingly slow and painful. He will instinctively know the manner in which he can move or turn which will cause him the least amount of pain or discomfort.

To Lift or Move an Extremity. An extremity to be lifted or moved should be well supported and moved slowly and evenly to the desired position. Both hands should be used by the nurse, with support being given at two points of contact. If there is an injured or infected area on the extremity being lifted, care should be taken so that the involved area is not touched by the hands of the nurse. She should never try to move or lift an injured hand or arm by grasping the fingers, nor lift or move a leg by holding the toes. Inadequate support is given, in either case, and may cause pain to the patient. If an extremity is to be elevated on pillows it should be well supported. A leg needs support at knee and ankle. An arm should be supported at elbow and wrist. Pillows or other support should be arranged so that the highest elevation is provided for the part of the extremity most distant from the body. An extremity supported in an elevated position should be protected from top bed linen by use of a cradle.

MECHANICAL COMFORT DEVICES

The use of pillows in various arrangements for bringing increased physical comfort to the patient has already been discussed. Numerous other available devices help relieve discomfort and maintain correct posture of patients in standing, sitting, or reclining position.

A patient who is being cared for at home by members of the family may not be provided with the recent, mechanical devices or equipment available to hospital patients, but can be given adequate care by the use of improvised equipment. Often an enterprising member of the family can devise a piece of equipment that will closely approximate or surpass the manufactured product, offering even more comfort for the patient. Many of the available mechanical devices help keep the body in correct position so strain and fatigue may be avoided.

The Backrest. The standard hospital bed provides a suitable backrest for the patient in a sitting position. In the home, a backrest may have to be improvised. Canvas covered, adjustable backrests, available for home use, are inexpensive yet provide needed support for the patient in a sitting position.

The Knee Rest. A knee rest is required to relieve strain on abdominal muscles and on tendons beneath the knees. The hospital bed provides a suitable knee rest, although a rolled blanket or pillow may be used for that purpose. Change of position at frequent intervals is necessary, so the legs are not kept in a flexed position too long. Flexion deformities or contractures too often result from poor bed posture and may require weeks of time and treatment to correct.

The Foot Rest. The foot rest is a device so placed that the feet rest firmly against it when the patient is in a sitting position. It is used for comfort and to provide protection against the condition known as "foot drop." Normally the foot is at right angles to the leg; if it is pushed down by bed clothes or pulled down by its own weight, when the patient must remain in bed over a long period of time, deformity may result. The foot rest also aids in maintaining correct posture, since it prevents the patient from sliding down in bed.

Sandbags used to immobilize a part and relieve discomfort may also be used to provide needed support to prevent foot or wrist drop.

Bed Cradle. Bed cradles vary widely in size and in materials used for their construction. However, they always serve the same purpose, that of supporting the weight of the top covers to prevent them from coming in contact with the patient. Small cradles are used for one or both extremities; large cradles are available for use over the entire body. Cradles are used also in protecting wet dressings, applications of certain drugs, and drying casts. For application of heat, a cradle equipped with electric lights, in number and arrangement to supply the desired warmth, is used.

Rubber and Cotton Rings. Rubber and cotton rings are used to relieve pressure on certain body parts. The rubber ring (made of foam rubber or hollow to be inflated) is placed under the buttocks to relieve pressure on the region of the coccyx. Cotton rings, made of absorbent cotton to fit the part to which they are to be applied, are used to relieve pressure on smaller areas, such as elbows and heels.

Air and Latex Mattresses. Air and latex mattresses are useful for very thin or very obese patients and for those who must remain in bed for long periods of time. The principle on which the use of such mattresses is based is that pressure of air within a closed or confined space is exerted equally in all directions; thus pressure against bony prominences or areas subject to the development of pressure sores would be reduced, making the mattress an important factor in the prevention of pressure sores.

Footstool. The footstool is used to assist a patient getting into and out of bed. It should be placed so the patient steps near the center and there will be no danger of its moving or overturning.

Towels and Blankets. Folded towels and small rolled blankets are often used as substitute kneerolls or pillows. When pillows are not available a folded towel will offer needed support to the part.

POSTURE AND POSITION

To provide physical comfort through rest and relaxation, good posture (the proper relative arrangement of body parts) is essential, whether it be in the standing, sitting, or reclining position. Good posture helps to promote normal functioning of all parts and organs of the body. Good posture is needed for the patient confined to bed, to allow for maximum comfort and rest, to provide for adequate lung expansion in respiration, and to prevent muscular deformities. Posture denotes "characteristic position in which the body is maintained."

In a standing position correct posture is achieved when the body is balanced on the balls of the feet with weight placed on the outer side. The various parts of the body must be in normal alignment so that the chest is up and forward, the abdomen retracted, knees are slightly flexed, and the curve of the spine follows the normal line of the long axis of the body.

In a sitting position the body should be held erect from neck to hips, with both feet resting firmly on the floor. When sitting in bed knees should be flexed at an angle to correspond with that of the hips. The trunk of the body should be straight, with head and shoulders supported. Support should also be provided for flexed knees.

In a reclining position, the extremities should be flexed and support given where needed to keep the body in correct alignment.

Any position that may be comfortable for the patient will become exceedingly uncomfortable if maintained for a prolonged period of time so frequent change of position is necessary. The patient's position should be changed often enough to prevent undue pressure on certain body areas, to prevent fatigue, and to prevent development of posture abnormalities or deformities.

POSITIONS FOR COMFORT OR CARE

When being examined or treated the patient should be placed in the position best adapted for the procedure.

Position differs from posture in that the latter is position assumed by the patient, as the placement of body parts for relief of pain (for example, the characteristic position, right leg flexed and brought up tightly against the abdomen, of appendicitis).

The patient who is ambulatory may choose a wide variety of positions and is free to change from one to another at will. The very ill or helpless person is restricted in the number of positions available to him.

Some of the most commonly used positions for bringing increased comfort or to facilitate giving a treatment are:

Anatomical Position. The normal standing position, with body erect and arms extending downward at sides. Used for examination, to aid in making diagnosis.

Dorsal Position. The patient rests flat on his back with legs extended and with arms alongside the body. Used for general physical examination, various operative procedures, and for comfort by providing change of position.

Dorsal Recumbent Position. The patient lies on his back with head and shoulders slightly elevated. The knees should be slightly flexed to avoid strain on the tendons of the leg, and legs should be rotated slightly outward. The feet should be held in proper position by a foot rest or other similar support. When used for examination or treatment the knees are acutely flexed, with feet resting on the bed or supported in stirrups. The position is used for catheterization, pelvic examination, and operative procedures on the vulvar area.

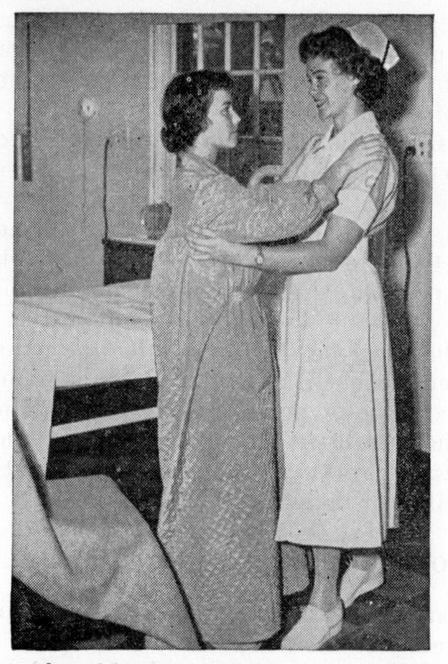

Fig. 71. A variety of positions is restful for the patient, even though it is merely from a sitting to a standing position. (Good Samaritan Hospital School of Nursing, Phoenix, Arizona.)

Fowler's Position. A partially sitting position with backrest elevated to approximately a 45° angle, knees slightly flexed and supported by a knee roll or by adjustment of the hospital bed. Used to maintain a comfortable sitting position, to relieve dyspnea, to facilitate drainage after surgery, and as a preliminary procedure to allowing the patient to sit up in a chair.

Horizontal Position. Same as dorsal position.

Jackknife Position. The patient lies on his back with shoulders slightly elevated, thighs brought up to form a right angle with the anterior part of the trunk, and knees flexed so lower legs rest against the thighs. Used in cystoscopy and for the passing of a urethral sound.

Knee-Chest Position. The patient is in a kneeling position with thighs extending upward. The head and upper part of the chest rests on the bed and arms are crossed above the head. Used as part of the treatment for displaced uterus, as a means of exercise following delivery and in the delivery procedure when indicated, as in transverse presentation.

Lateral Position. The patient is placed on his side with line of hips slightly back of the line of shoulders. Knees are flexed, one being more acutely flexed than the other. Used as a position of comfort for the patient and for special care or treatment of the back.

Lithotomy Position. The patient is placed on her back, head and shoulders resting on the bed (not elevated). Knees are acutely flexed so that the thighs are brought up against the abdomen. Thighs are abducted and lower legs are brought back against the thighs. Leg supports are necessary if the position is to be maintained for more than a very short time. Used for gynecological examination and treatment and for some surgical procedures involving the genitourinary system.

Prone Position. The patient is placed on his abdomen with arms at sides or flexed at the elbows and extended upward, and head turned to one side. Used in examination or treatment of back and spinal column, and as a change of position for comfort and rest. The position is not often used, but is desirable to relieve tired back muscles. In this position a small pillow should be placed beneath the waist and a larger one under the lower legs so the feet can hang over the edge in their natural position. No pillow is needed for the head.

Semi-Fowler Position. A semi-sitting position with head and shoulders only slightly elevated (backrest at 25–30 degree angle) and knees only slightly flexed. Used as a modification of Fowler's position. Used in treatment of minor respiratory diseases and for change of position to secure comfort.

Semi-Prone Position. Same as Sims' position.

Sims' Position. The patient lies on the left side, left arm extended along the back and upper part of the body turned forward so the chest rests on the bed. The left leg is flexed slightly toward the right, which is drawn up, with knee flexed, so that it extends approximately to waistline level. The left knee rests on the bed, extended outward away from the body. Pillows should be used to support the patient in this position. The Sims' position is generally accepted as the one permitting maximum relaxation and many persons assume this position in more or less modified form while sleeping. It is also used for comfort, to relieve pressure on the back, for various examinations and treatments (as for enemas), and for some surgical procedures on the perineal region.

Trendelenburg Position. The patient is placed on his back with the foot of the bed elevated (on shock blocks) so that legs extend upward at a 45 degree angle. Head and shoulders are lower than hips and legs. Used in treatment of shock or decreased blood pressure and for surgical procedures on the abdomen. When the patient is placed in this position on the operating table the legs are allowed to hang downward over the end of the table.

Walcher's Position. The patient lies on her back with hips brought to the edge of the bed. The knees are flexed and thighs are rotated outward, so the legs are separated. Feet are placed on supports (chairs

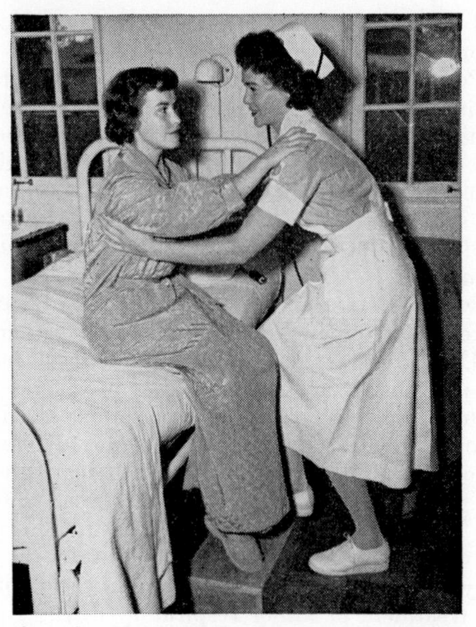

Fig. 72. The patient should "dangle" prior to being assisted to her feet when preparing to stand. (Good Samaritan Hospital School of Nursing, Phoenix, Arizona.)

or stools) so the legs hang down over the edge of the bed. Used for some examinations and treatments on the genital and vulvar areas.

VARIOUS ACTIVITIES OF THE PATIENT

One of the greatest satisfactions in nursing is watching a patient who has been critically ill respond to medical and nursing care by gradually recovering from the illness. Invariably, during convalescence, the patient reaches the stage of progress where he begins to take an active role in activities that help to bring about normal functioning of the body as a whole. Among the first such activities for the convalescent patient is that of "dangling."

Dangling. This term describes an important part of the necessary preparation for getting out of bed for the first time after a prolonged illness. Although the patient may have been permitted to sit up in bed with the help of backrest and knee roll, he must become accustomed to maintaining a sitting position more nearly like that the body assumes when seated in a chair. Dangling is a means of approximating that position by the patient who does not actually leave the bed to carry out the activity.

The nurse assigned to assist the patient in dangling should under-

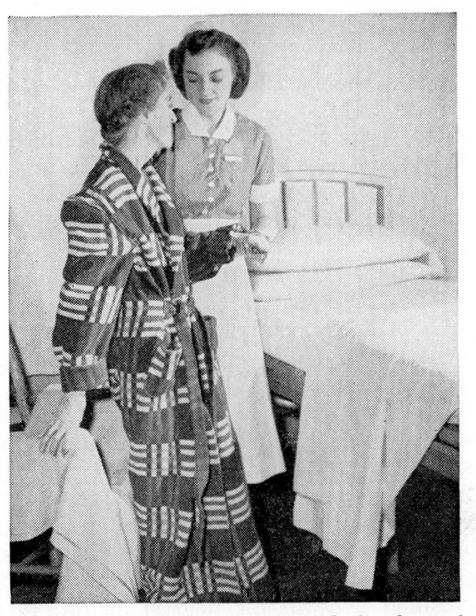

Fig. 73. A straight chair with arms is comfortable for the patient allowed to sit up at intervals. (Massachusetts General Hospital School of Nursing, Boston, Massachusetts.)

stand the importance of carrying out the procedure in a slow and deliberate manner. She should move the patient's feet and legs toward the side of the bed where she is standing and then slowly bring the patient into a sitting position by firmly supporting back and head. Raising him to a sitting position suddenly may cause him to faint, since the brain may thus be deprived momentarily of its normal blood supply. The patient should be allowed to remain in the upright position for the short time required for symptoms of dizziness or faintness to disappear. Supporting the back with one arm and placing the other beneath the patient's knees, the nurse should gradually bring feet and lower legs off the bed while turning the patient so that he is sitting upright on the side of the bed with lower legs and feet hanging free. In this dangling position circulation in feet and legs approximates that of the normal sitting or standing position. Through dangling the patient gradually overcomes weakness imposed by illness and is soon better able to attempt the activity involved in getting out of bed.

Assisting Patient into Chair. Sitting in a chair at intervals during the day will help the convalescent patient regain strength and will promote rest and comfort when he returns to bed. Before helping the patient to a sitting position on the bed, in preparation for sitting in a chair, the nurse should see that the chair is ready to receive the patient. A straight chair with arms is usually most comfortable for the patient. The seat and back of the chair, if it is not upholstered, should be padded with pillows, and blankets should be arranged to protect the patient from drafts. The chair should be brought close to the bed so the patient need not exert himself by walking toward it.

With the patient in the position of dangling, a footstool should be placed directly beneath his feet. He should be assisted into robe or dressing gown, so that both arms are in the sleeves and the robe is drawn around his upper body. No attempt should be made to put the lower part of the robe in position so long as the patient is seated on the bed. Folds of the robe should be allowed to fall into place around the patient. As the top covers are thrown back from across the front of the patient the robe should be brought across so he is not exposed.

With the patient resting in a sitting position on the edge of the bed his pulse should be counted. If pulse rate is normal and he is not pale or dizzy, the nurse may assist him to a standing position on the footstool. Movements should be slow to permit the patient to readily adjust to each new position. The hold on the patient (the nurse stands close beside him with one arm around his waist and one hand placed crutch fashion beneath his nearest armpit to help bear his weight) should be strong and firm so he feels secure in the support given him. Supporting the patient thus the nurse should instruct him to step down from the footstool and come to a standing position on the floor. (For a tall patient the footstool will not be needed, since the patient's feet will be only a very short distance from the floor when he sits in the dangling position.) Without taking steps the patient may be turned and slowly lowered into a sitting position in the chair. If allowed to grasp the arms of the chair the patient may help support himself so the nurse need not bear his entire weight as he is seated.

Pulse rate should be checked frequently while the patient is sitting in a chair for the first time, and his color should be closely observed. If he seems exceptionally weak or shows signs of fatigue or exertion, the nurse should remain at his side while he is in the chair. If no ill effect is noted he may be left alone with a book or magazine, *provided the signal bell is placed within easy reach* so he may summon the nurse if necessary.

Assisting Patient into a Wheelchair. This procedure is carried out in essentially the same manner as described for assisting him to sit in an ordinary chair. However, two nurses should help with the wheelchair procedure. It is most important that the wheelchair be held securely in place so there is no likelihood of its moving as the patient is being helped into it.

Returning Patient to Bed. Whether being moved from wheelchair or ordinary arm chair, the patient should be held securely and move-

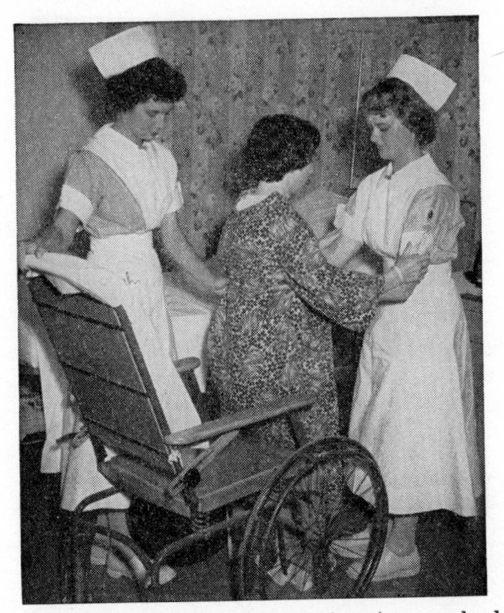

Fig. 74. Two nurses are needed to assist a patient into a wheelchair. (Baylor University School of Nursing, Waco, Texas.)

ments should be slow and smooth. He should be placed first in a sitting position on the bed, then with legs and back supported he should be pivoted onto the bed, with feet and legs brought up and placed in proper position. If he shows signs of exertion from the activity of being returned to bed he should be allowed to rest for awhile in a horizontal position. The robe and other clothing used while out of bed can be removed after he has rested a few minutes. After the patient has been returned to bed the nurse should make sure that he is comfortable, that personal necessities are within easy reach, that reading and other materials for recreation are at hand, and that the signal bell is again placed so that it is convenient for his use. Fresh water or nourishment should be offered him, and assurance given that he will again be permitted out of bed after a suitable interval of time. The effect of the activity of being out of bed should be observed and recorded.

Assisting Patient To Walk. If only one nurse is to assist the patient to walk she should place one hand, crutch fashion, under the arm nearest her, place her other arm securely about his waist and help him to a standing position. Allowing him to stand a moment to be sure of balance, she should move close to him so that her hip is firmly against his. By bending very slightly away from the patient and holding him securely against her as they stand side by side, she

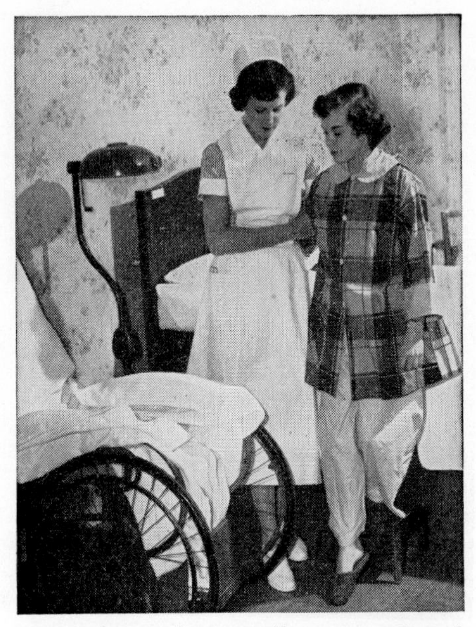

Fig. 75. One nurse may assist a patient to walk or to step down from the footstool. (Delaware Hospital School of Nursing, Wilmington, Delaware.)

will be able to bear much of his weight without throwing either of them off balance. The steps in walking should be taken slowly and in unison. The first few times at walking should be in the room, as the patient should never be more than a few steps from bed or chair so he could make use of either if necessary. The nurse should permit only a few steps at a time and the patient should be encouraged to pause frequently to rest. Walking should be discontinued at the first sign of weakness or faintness. If the patient suddenly becomes faint one nurse may not be able to bear his weight and thus cannot prevent his sinking to the floor. If she is supporting him properly she *can* prevent his falling. By maintaining a secure hold on him she can make the fall a slow and gradual sinking to the floor. When the patient is on the floor and in no further danger of falling she can then summon help to return him to bed.

If the patient is very weak two nurses are required to assist him in walking. One nurse at each side will assure him of adequate support should he be unable to maintain a standing position.

Assisting Patient To Walk with Crutches. Walking with crutches requires learning a new skill, that of using the crutches as a means of keeping the body in balance. If the lower limbs are incapacitated or unable to balance the body properly, crutches may be necessary for the patient to move about in an upright position.

Measurement for crutches for each individual is vitally important, as crutches of improper length greatly interfere with teaching a patient how to use them. Several means of measuring for crutch length have been devised. The method most commonly used is that of measuring from the axilla to the heel and adding four inches.

The armpiece of the crutch should be padded, although it is essential that the patient understand that much of his weight should be carried by the arms and borne on the handpiece of each crutch.

The nurse should demonstrate the proper use of the crutches by allowing the patient to observe her use of them as she slowly and carefully walks back and forth across the room. As she walks correctly with the help of the crutches she should point out to the patient every phase in their handling and the timing of the movements made. She should explain the necessity of rubber tips on each crutch to prevent sliding on smooth floors or surfaces. She should teach him to avoid small rugs or mats on the floor, caution him to be constantly alert for changes in floor level, for doorsills, or for other impediments to crutch walking.

When the patient is finally ready to try walking with crutches, practice should be for only a very short period of time at first. As he gains strength and confidence in his ability to handle the crutches, practice periods may gradually be lengthened and scheduled at more frequent intervals.

If the patient's physical condition is such that improvement in crutch walking occurs he may soon be able to walk with one crutch and a cane. Further progress may lead to the use of the cane alone to help in balancing the body. Eventually the cane too may be discarded, and the patient once more be able to walk about in a normal manner.

RESTRICTION OF MOVEMENT FOR THE PATIENT

Many states have passed laws designed to protect the patient from injudicious or unnecessary restraint. Devices used for restraining a patient cannot be used legally without having been ordered by a physician. In general hospitals, as well as in those caring for the mentally ill, members of the medical and nursing staffs attempt to gain the cooperation of the patient and avoid the use of protective or limiting devices if it is at all possible.

In hospitals the term "restraint" is seldom used because of its effect on the patient. Even though a patient does not physically resist, or is unable to do so, the word, and its unpleasant implication of limited movement, causes mental frustration and subsequent undesirable emotional reaction.

The natural reaction to restriction of movement is one of immediate resistance. Having the movement of a limb or a part of the body restrained in any way causes the conscious person, whether child or adult, to struggle to free himself. This obvious dislike of restricted activity is clearly indicated in the very young child if arms or legs are held immobile. The child so restrained will violently resist. The adult, unless he clearly understands and accepts the need for restraint, will react in a similar manner and may resist to the point of causing injury to himself or to those in attendance.

Despite the normal reaction against limitation of body movement there are times when the safety of the patient, or successful treatment, makes restricted motion essential. In some instances a patient will impose limitation of body movement on himself in an effort to overcome pain or discomfort. Whether limited movement is self imposed or ordered by the physician, the restricted activity may result in physical and mental strain for the patient. Conditions that require limitation of body movement as a part of the necessary medical or surgical treatment are not at all uncommon and include the following:

Skin conditions, in which severe itching occurs and the patient, especially a child, may need to have his hands restrained to prevent scratching of the involved area. Danger of secondary infection from rubbing or scratching in a primary skin condition is a matter of grave concern to the dermatologist and makes restraint of the patient mandatory.

Surgical conditions, such as eye surgery or plastic surgery of the face, require restraint of the patient's hands if there is any indication that dressings would be disturbed or removed, either consciously or during sleep.

Fractures and areas of localized infection may require immobilization of the affected part to promote healing.

Paralysis of a part of the body may make some limitation of movement necessary since the patient may more easily fall from the bed.

During the time a patient is *recovering from the effect of a general anesthetic* it is often necessary to restrain motor activity to prevent him from falling out of bed or from causing injury to himself or to others.

Any condition in which the patient is in a highly emotional or irrational state, such as that seen in functional mental diseases, may be cause for needed restraint to prevent self harm.

Devices Used To Restrict Movement of the Patient. Numerous devices are available for use in restricting movement of the patient, ranging from the very simple, only slightly restrictive, to the completely limiting body pack or stout restraining sheets. The most commonly used restraints are:

The clove hitch, made of soft, triangular bandage. It is effective as a restraint to prevent the hand from reaching the face or from reaching and scratching an involved skin area.

The top covers, tucked securely under the mattress, may serve as partial restraint for the patient who has a tendency to roll or fall out of bed.

Side rails placed on the bed protect the patient from falling. The rails are made of wood, canvas, or metal. It may be necessary to use pillows or padding to protect the patient if he bumps or struggles against the side rails, to prevent abrasions or bruises on his person.

Anklets or wristlets of leather effectively restrain arms or legs of the patient. Care must be taken to pad the leather well so the restraints do not cause injury to ankles or wrists.

Strait-jackets, which restrict movement of the arms, are especially distasteful to patients, and their use should be avoided if restriction of motion can be effected in another way.

Splints, sandbags, and plaster casts are used in immobilizing a part for the treatment of fractures, dislocations, and inflamed or infected areas.

The nurse caring for a patient who is in any way restrained should be aware of the need for constant vigilance to safeguard the patient from injury caused by the restraining device. Any device used for restraint tends to irritate the skin, and resistance by the patient will increase that danger. A device that causes pressure on underlying tissues should be removed at frequent intervals to re-establish normal circulation to the part and to prevent the formation of a pressure sore.

Devices likely to be soiled by body excretions must be kept thoroughly clean and dry so excoriation of the skin will be prevented.

The nurse should be cognizant of mental unrest caused the patient by a restraining device and should use her knowledge of psychology to minister to his mental as well as physical needs. By her own attitude of calm acceptance of the device as part of the necessary treatment and her frequent reference to the fact that its use is only temporary, she may help to counteract the undesirable effect it exerts on the mind and body of the patient.

After the student nurse learns the various means of making the patient comfortable and has become skillful in performing procedures related to comfort, she should practice the small, extra procedures which may not have been demonstrated in the classroom, yet add so much to the patient's comfort.

She should see that the bedside table, which contains personal belongings and equipment necessary for daily care, is always within easy reach of the patient, whether he is confined to bed or allowed to be in a chair. She should see that fresh drinking water is on the table, that books and magazines are there, that the patient is consulted as to personal belongings to be kept on top of the table and in the drawer. She should make certain that personal belongings are not crowded into hard-to-reach corners or removed from the table to make room for more and more hospital equipment.

By her attitude, tone of voice, and manner in which she carries out nursing procedures she should let her patient know that she is eager to render the service she gives and that her interest in his progress toward recovery is second only to his own. In providing for the com-

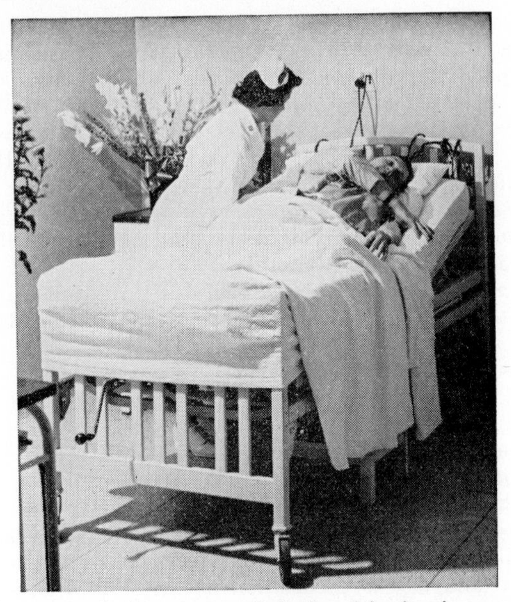

Fig. 76. The nurse obtains a great deal of satisfaction in providing for the comfort of the patient. (Bureau of Medicine and Surgery, Navy Department, Washington, D.C.)

fort of the patient the nurse is indeed putting into practice that part of the Florence Nightingale pledge which states, "I will do all in my power to aid the physician in his work and devote myself to the welfare of those committed to my care."

PROVIDING FOR MENTAL COMFORT

Mental comfort for the patient may be provided by allaying fear and worry, helping him adjust to the hospital environment and performing procedures with tactfulness and consideration. The factor of mental comfort as related to the various procedures in nursing is considered in the discussion of those procedures in succeeding chapters.

Chapter 37, on Spiritual Needs of the Patient, treats of various factors related to providing for the patient's spiritual comfort.

Care of Equipment after Use

Equipment used in comfort measures is the same as that used in giving daily routine care to the patient. Instructions for its care have been presented in detail in the chapters on the various nursing procedures.

Summary of Important Factors

The patient cannot be comfortable and cannot rest unless both body and mind are "at ease."

Some causes of physical discomfort are unclean or wet bed, lack of support to the body, noise, glaring lights, treatment devices, and inadequate nursing care.

Some causes of mental discomfort are fear and worry about illness, family, or finances, lack of understanding on part of the nurse, tension, and boredom.

Correct methods should be followed in moving, turning, or lifting the patient.

Some mechanical devices used for patient comfort are pillows, backrest, knee rest, foot rest, bed cradle, rubber and cotton rings, air mattress, footstool.

Close observation of the patient (counting pulse before and after) is necessary when assisting him up to chair for first time after prolonged illness.

Adequate support should be provided in assisting the patient to walk.

Demonstration is an excellent means of teaching crutch walking.

Conservative use of devices to restrict movement is essential to prevent undue resistance on the part of the patient.

Thoughtfulness on the part of the nurse is essential if the patient is to be made comfortable.

Factors To Teach the Patient

The importance of maintaining good posture in a sitting or lying position to prevent deformity from prolonged bed rest.

Ways of cooperating in the various procedures of turning, lifting, and moving him.

Ways of improvising mechanical devices to promote greater comfort for him at home.

Various positions that may be used to make him comfortable.

Cooperation in helping to prevent or treat pressure sores.

The way to correctly measure for crutches.

Safeguards in crutch walking: rubber tips to prevent crutches from slipping; support of weight at hand bar rather than at top of crutch; avoidance of small rugs or mats on floor; close watch for doorsills, steps, differences of floor level.

Reasons for restriction of movement.

Necessity for accepting illness and adjusting to hospital environment.

Value of recreation as means of obtaining mental rest.

Purchase or rental of hospital equipment and supplies is possible and adds greatly to comfort of the patient in the home.

Scientific Principles

Anatomy and Physiology. Muscular activity has a marked effect on body activities, influencing circulation, respiration, elimination, appetite, and posture.

Muscle tone is the constant state of mild contraction which characterizes all properly functioning muscles. Muscle tone is maintained by movement and by exercise.

In correct posture very little effort is needed to keep the body in proper alignment, and when in correct posture the patient can be comfortable.

A firm mattress is needed for correct lying position.

In the back-lying position supports (small pillows) are needed at the head and neck, the lumbar region or small of the back, and at the back of the knees.

Relaxation is achieved through proper posture which is necessary to overcome some of the ill effects of bed rest. In correct posture a balance is maintained between antagonistic groups of muscles, only a minimum of effort is needed to keep the body in proper alignment, and comfort is obtained. No position will remain comfortable over a long period of time so it is necessary that the patient be turned or moved about in the bed.

The correct standing position may be used as a standard on which to base good posture in any position.

Whether the patient is standing, sitting, or lying down, the head should be on a straight line with the spine, there should be no exaggeration of the curves of the back, the chest should extend forward, the feet should be at right angles to the legs, and knees and elbows should be slightly flexed.

Chemistry. Muscle is approximately three-fourths water and one-fourth solid constituents. Myosin, a protein substance, is the contractile substance of muscle fiber. Active muscle is acid in reaction because of the accumulation of sarcolactic acid which results from muscle contraction. Resting muscle is alkaline in reaction. Insufficient oxygen supply to the muscle causes fatigue by producing sarcolactic acid.

Microbiology. Mechanical devices used for comfort must be clean. Wheelchairs and stretchers should be kept free of dust which tends to accumulate on them where oil is used for lubrication of moving parts. Resistance may be lowered if the patient is exposed to drafts or to cold air.

Pharmacology. Sedative drugs may cause dizziness, and the patient who has had such a drug may need support in walking to the bathroom or will need to be moved by wheelchair or stretcher from one department to another.

Narcotics are drugs given to relieve pain and discomfort.

Physics. Muscles and bones function on the principle of mechanical leverage in moving the body. Bones and cartilages are the levers and muscles supply the force for movement.

The center of gravity of the body is the point at which the whole weight is said to be concentrated (the level of the second sacral vertebra). The feet form the supporting area of the body and a wider area of support can be obtained by placing the feet farther apart. Center of gravity remains in same vertical line for standing or sitting.

Work is the overcoming of resistance and is done by push or pull. Lifting is moving upward. In lifting a patient resistance offered by the patient's weight must be overcome.

The closer a force is applied to the center of gravity of a body the better the control of it. For this reason, the patient should be held close to the chest of those lifting and carrying him so his weight is exerted against the vertebral axis.

In the horizontal position, less strain is put on the spine and pelvic bones, so that position is one often assumed by the patient.

Psychology. Worry and fear cause much of the patient's discomfort, and the understanding nurse may help by listening to expression of that worry or fear and by offering reassurance.

Boredom may be a major factor in unrest and discomfort. If the patient must remain in bed throughout the day a special effort must be made to stimulate mental activity and interest through the use of various means of entertainment and of diversions.

Discomfort may be more readily accepted by the patient if he is encouraged and made to understand that present discomfort may be the means of attaining future comfort or proper functioning of an impaired organ or part.

Sociology. In health the individual is responsible for his own comfort. In illness the patient is dependent on hospital personnel to provide facilities or activities which promote physical and mental well being.

Members of the patient's family should be encouraged to contribute to his care by helping to provide means to avoid boredom and loneliness.

As the patient becomes physically able to do some things for himself, as care of teeth and taking a bath, the nurse should encourage him to do what he can. By being responsible for part of his own care, he feels less dependent and helpless.

As the patient becomes ambulatory, he may find interesting and enjoyable social contacts with other patients.

If confronted with social problems the patient may be greatly helped by the nurse who has some understanding of the problem. The Social Service Department in the hospital should be notified of the patient's need, since that department is best qualified to refer the patient to the proper agency.

Problems pertaining to family members in foreign service are handled largely by the American Red Cross.

Problems caused by the physical condition which may result in impairment of function may be referred to such organizations as the Blind Service Association, National Foundation for Infantile Paralysis, National Society for Crippled Children, and many others.

Problems pertaining to family relationships are handled by the Family Service Bureau or National Institute of Family Relations.

Situation Type Problems

1. A very short, very thin, very old, and very confused male patient was admitted to the hospital because of injury to a knee which resulted from having fallen in the bathroom at a home where he had long been provided board and room.

He resisted all efforts on the part of hospital personnel to remove a suit of long underwear which he was wearing. Two orderlies had to give up their combined efforts because the patient resisted so violently that he was in danger of increasing the injury which had been the cause of hospitalization.

Sandbags were placed at each side of the injured leg and the patient was given a sedative. Next morning the student nurse assigned to his care was instructed to try to remove the underwear so the patient could be properly cared for and the injured leg given suitable treatment. What would you have done?

2. In a semi-private room the patient nearest the window liked fresh air and adequate ventilation. She asked that the window be opened part way and the door to the room left open. The patient in the bed nearest the door wanted the door closed because the room was located near the kitchen and utility rooms and elevator. Noise from the corridor was always present and very annoying. Each patient complained to the nurse about the other. Neither patient would consider changing the bed location assigned to her and there were no vacant rooms available. What would you have done?

Suggested Reference Reading

"Posture and the patient," Katherine Allen; American Journal of Nursing, October, 1941.

"Preventing backstrain," Kathleen Newton; American Journal of Nursing, October, 1943.

"Floating words," Carol Lynn Gilmer; Coronet, August, 1948.

"The Invalift," Helen C. Anderson; American Journal of Nursing, March, 1952.

"Anxiety, a factor in nursing care," Dorothy E. Gregg; American Journal of Nursing, November, 1952.

CHAPTER 12

Exercise—Recreation—Rest—Sleep

TOPICAL OUTLINE

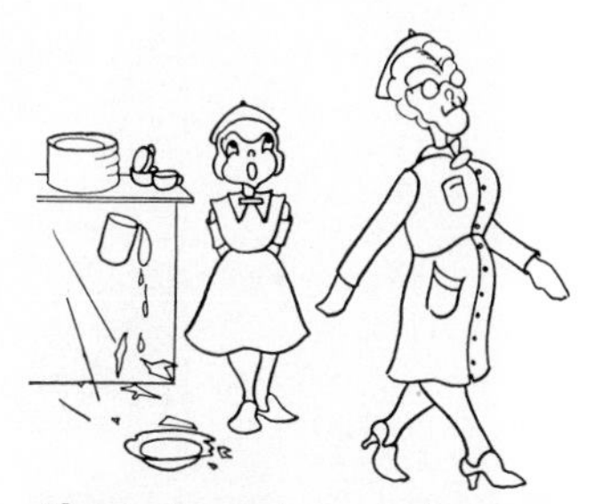

About the only exercise some people get is jumping to conclusions.

The therapeutic value of rest has long been recognized. Some diseases are treated chiefly by means of bed rest, yet prolonged inactivity may be dangerous for the patient. The slowed circulation at complete bed rest, with constant pressure of legs against the mattress, may cause thrombosis of the veins of the legs. Inactivity tends to weaken muscles and cause them to lose tone. Continued pressure on bony prominences may cause impaired circulation to the part and subsequent development of a pressure sore. Restricted body activity may also cause congestion in the lungs and predispose to pneumonia.

To overcome the ill effects of bed rest, exercise and recreation now form an important part of the planned care and treatment for the patient.

Exercise

Exercise is a normal activity and the vital organs need the stimulus that muscular activity provides. Muscle tone, the state of slight contraction present in all healthy muscle, is maintained through movement or exercise of the muscles. Even in sleep the muscular activity, although lessened, does not entirely cease, as is evidenced by the fact

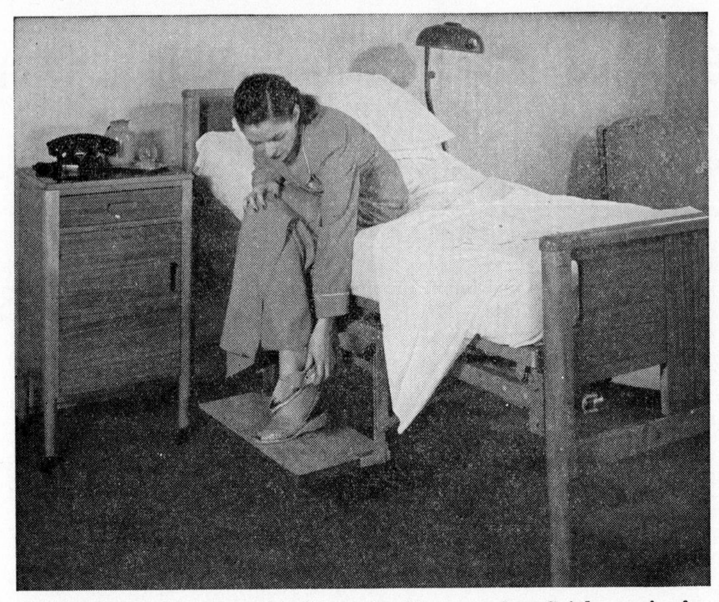

Fig. 77. Preparing to get out of bed unassisted becomes beneficial exercise for the patient. (Hill-Rom Co., Inc., Batesville, Indiana.)

that persons change their position frequently during the night and may turn from side to side without wakening. The functioning of different parts of the body, as heart, lungs, and brain, is improved by daily exercise.

TYPES OF EXERCISE

Exercise may be of two general classifications—active and passive. Active exercise is that which the patient does for himself by moving about in bed or by changing his position. Passive exercise is that produced in the patient by another person. For most patients exercise is usually restricted to that required in performance of routine daily procedures involved in personal care.

Active Exercise. Active exercise may consist of turning and moving from one position to another, reaching for objects that have been placed nearby, or performing definite prescribed exercises which can be done while remaining in bed.

Even if the patient has been critically ill, a certain amount of physical and mental exercise is needed. Exercise during convalescence helps to maintain general muscle tone, strengthens the body, and boosts the morale of the patient.

Simple exercises performed in bed are very worth while in helping the patient to overcome disabilities that may result from illness and prolonged bed rest.

If the student nurse understands that the patient will benefit by doing for himself anything which requires movement of muscles and joints that need exercise, she will encourage him to wash his own face during the bath procedure, to feed himself, to move about in bed, and to be as active as his physical condition will permit so long as such activities are not forbidden by the doctor or contraindicated by the treatment being given.

Passive Exercise. For the patient not permitted to exercise actively, passive exercise may be used. In passive exercise the movement or activity is carried out by another person (nurse or physical therapist), and the patient makes no voluntary effort to assist or resist the action.

Passive exercise is involved in such procedures as the bed bath, turning the patient from side to side, moving arms and legs, alcohol rubs, and massage. Postural exercises may also be ordered by the physician. The amount and kind of exercise will vary, depending on the needs of the patient.

Exercise in the form of muscle re-education plays a major role in helping prepare the patient for the time when he is permitted out of bed and may, with gradually returning strength, take part in an increasing number of activities. If the patient understands that increased body activity leads to improved body functioning, his wholehearted cooperation may be elicited, with the result that his physical condition improves and his hospital stay may be shortened.

Recreation

Providing the patient with suitable recreational activity will prevent him from dwelling too much on his own particular problems. For convalescent patients it should produce sufficient physical exertion to cause fatigue so rest and relaxation may be obtained and more sound sleep will result.

The psychological needs of the patient who has long been hospitalized may be very pronounced. Such patients may frequently experience marked lowering of morale which impedes progress toward recovery and often greatly interferes with desired results of surgical or medical treatment.

The many aspects of recreational therapy may do much to relieve the monotony of long days of convalescence. Occupational therapy will help stimulate anticipation of the day when the patient can once more resume the activities of normal daily routine.

The kind of recreational activity most beneficial to the patient will depend on his physical condition and his fields of interest. Established interests may provide a ready choice of diversional activity, or a new interest may need to be developed.

Most patients, relieved of physical discomfort and given an interest

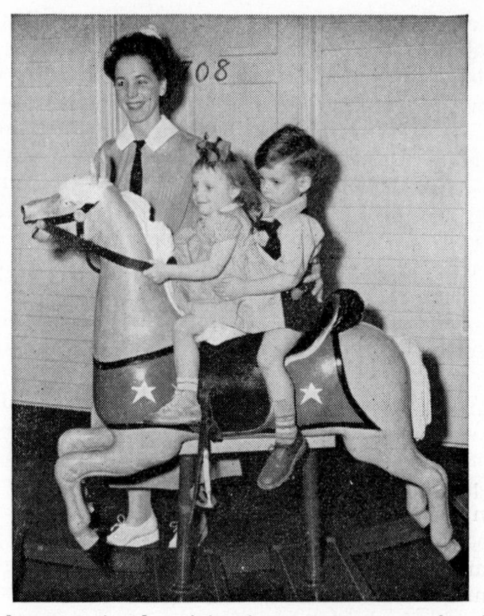

Fig. 78. Suitable recreational activity is necessary even for the very small patient. (Cook County Hospital School of Nursing, Chicago, Illinois.)

so that a desirable mental outlook is promoted, will progress at a normal rate toward complete recovery. A few may be overzealous in their desire to resume normal activities and will need to be restricted somewhat until they are sufficiently recovered to become quite active. Still others may tend to be overcautious and avoid activity, with a tendency to develop an unwarranted state of invalidism. Unless constantly reassured and encouraged by understanding nurses and recreational workers such patients may retard their recovery indefinitely.

The most common forms of recreation open to hospital patients include reading, projected books, radio, motion pictures, television, music, and art.

READING

Books and magazines of all types are usually available through the library in the hospital and are supplied to hospital patients by a library service. A person who has not previously become acquainted with the interesting personalities found between the covers of a book may be introduced to a few by the nurse who knows the enjoyment of spending leisure time in reading.

Books are friends who come to the patient when he is unable to go to them.

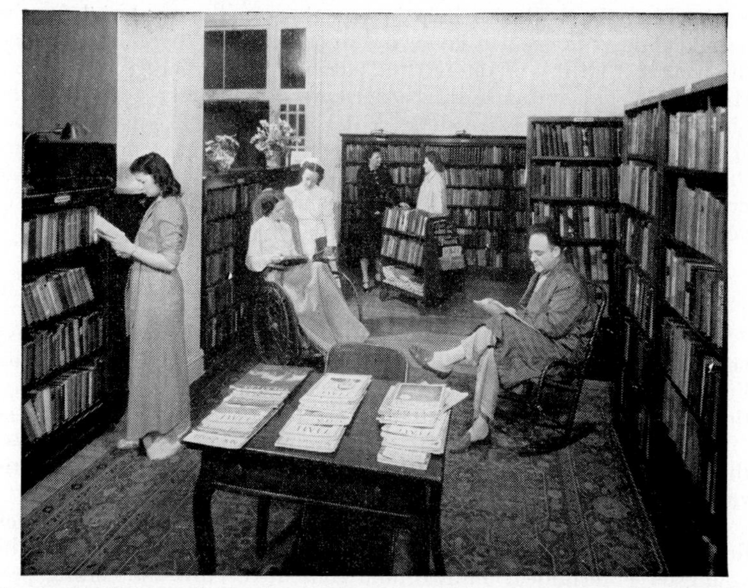

Fig. 79. Reading is a form of recreation enjoyed by most patients. (Presbyterian Hospital, Chicago, Illinois.)

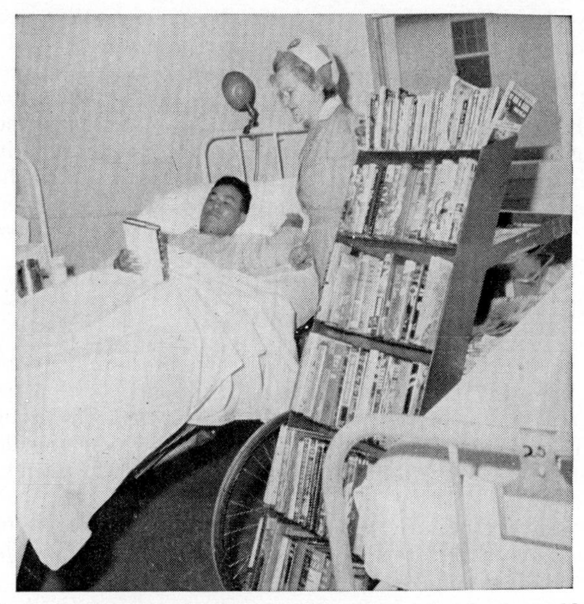

Fig. 80. Books are friends who come to the patient when he is unable to go to them. (Veterans Administration, Denver, Colorado.)

The librarian will also help in selecting reading material for the patient. She will need to know the importance of carefully choosing the book so that it will interest the patient and be readily understood. His educational and cultural background will largely determine the kind of book he enjoys reading. A day laborer who left high school at the age of fifteen to begin work may need books or magazines that are quite different from those likely to be chosen by a college professor or a person who has been an avid reader for a number of years.

PROJECTED BOOKS FOR PATIENTS

Patients too ill to sit up and those too weak to hold a book have been able to enjoy books through the use of the ceiling projector. Films used in the ceiling projector are carefully chosen with consideration of the condition of the patient as well as his reading level.

This means of entertainment contributes greatly to the morale of the helpless patient and is recognized as having definite, therapeutic value for patients whose conditions necessitate prolonged bed rest.

Projected books are especially of benefit to the sick child. When first put into use their sole purpose was that of helping to keep the youngster entertained, amused, and contented. Now the ceiling projector is being used extensively to enable the child of school age, who is completely helpless or partially handicapped, to continue with school work while in the hospital. Textbooks in history, geography, arithmetic, science, and social studies have been microfilmed and can be used with the ceiling projector. The use of the ceiling projector is confined to the child or adult patient who is able to punch the control button that operates the projector. Patients unable to push the control button by hand have operated it with the heel, or, in some instances, with the elbow. The many hours of enjoyment furnished by the ceiling projector have materially aided in producing a desirable mental attitude in the patient who would otherwise be subject to great discouragement and depression.

RADIO

Radio has long been an important field of entertainment and education for "shut-ins" at home or in an institution. At the present time few patients who enter the hospital for other than emergency treatment fail to bring a small, table model radio which provides entertainment and keeps them informed of happenings of local and national interest.

The radio is especially beneficial to the patient who is unable to read or enjoy other forms of recreation requiring sight. Those who have lost their vision, whether temporarily or permanently, may de-

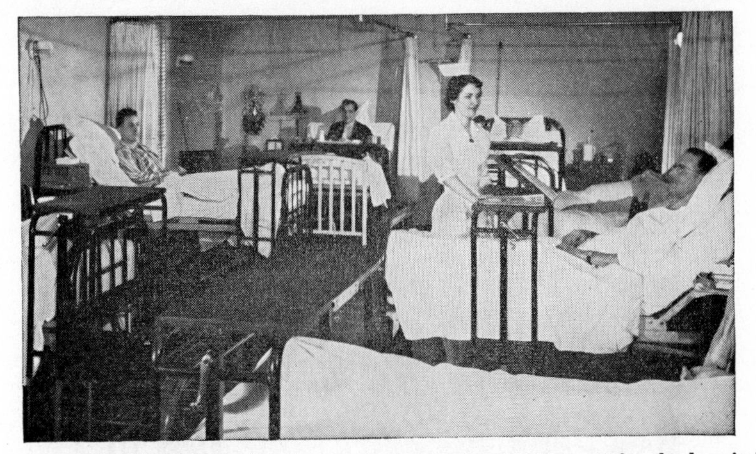

Fig. 81. Small, table-model radios are a source of entertainment for the hospital patient. (Presbyterian Hospital, Chicago, Illinois.)

pend almost entirely on radio for entertainment and for relief from mental strain and spiritual doubt and misgiving.

MOTION PICTURES

Many hospitals now provide movie programs for patients at regular intervals. Those confined to bed and those in wheelchairs may be transported to the ward or room where the movie is being shown.

Ambulatory patients usually are much interested in such programs and may operate the movie projector, help transport bed or wheelchair patients, and by their own appreciative evaluation of the film add to the pleasure other patients derive from this particular form of diversional activity.

TELEVISION

The use of television as a medium of entertainment for patients is somewhat limited, as other electrical appliances in the hospital tend to interfere with reception and many so-called "fringe areas" do not yet have television available. In areas where television *is* available it may be supplied to a group rather than to an individual patient. It is particularly suitable, and valuable, for the patient whose recreation must be of a passive type.

Just as good judgment must be shown by nurse or librarian in helping the patient choose books for reading enjoyment, the selection of programs to be viewed on television may also need to be supervised.

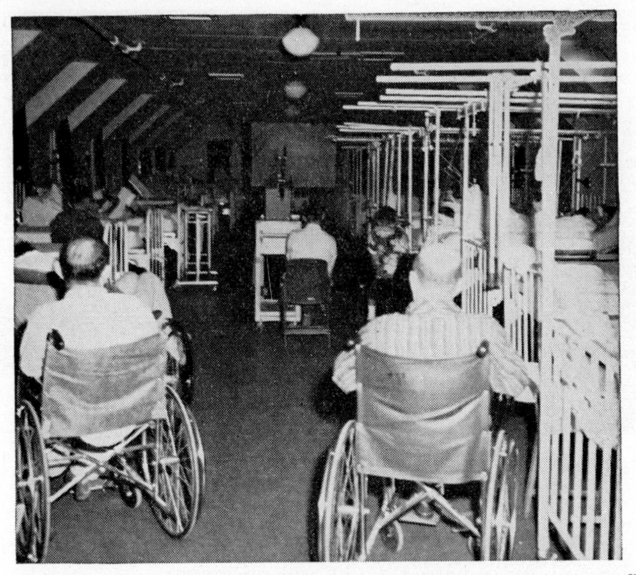

Fig. 82. Movies are a favorite form of diversional activity for patients confined to bed or wheelchair. (Veterans Administration, Denver, Colorado.)

Patients with a tendency toward depression and discouragement should be encouraged to choose light or comedy type programs and to avoid the intensely emotional drama type play which may be somewhat morbid and depressing.

MUSIC

Hospital recreational rooms are not complete without a well tuned piano and other popular musical instruments. Patients who can play the piano will find relaxation and enjoyment in being permitted this form of self entertainment while in the hospital.

Besides providing instruments which patients may play, music may be made available through different means. Radio has already been mentioned as an outstanding form of entertainment. Another method of providing music is having it piped to the various clinical departments by means of the paging system in use in the hospital.

If an audible paging system is used in the hospital a record player can be attached to it. Paging can be done when the music is on without interruption of the musical program. The music can be played approximately five hours each day, with long-playing records being used. Vocal recordings would not be included in the program, except on holidays or Sunday. Each program could be started with a subdued selection and only records with satisfactory arrangements used.

The volume can be under control at all times so the music can be low in tone and sound.

Since the loud speakers of the paging system are located in the halls or lobbies the music would not be directed to the bedside. Most patients and hospital personnel react favorably to soft music and may make special requests for favorite tunes or orchestras. Records could be arranged in the library so no one recording is played too frequently on the program.

ART

Wall Pictures. Art, through pictures selected for use in the patient's room, can be made available to all interested hospital patients. Through the Department of Public Interest one large hospital evolved the unique scheme of supplying a bedside picture service. A collection of pictures, each one mounted, covered with sheets of acetate, and bound with black tape which served as a suitable frame, was assembled as the first step in starting the picture service.

The patient was allowed to choose a picture to be hung on the wall of his room. Over a period of time the three most popular categories, reflected in the choice made by patients, were religious pictures, animal or bird pictures, and pictures of floral arrangements. No attempt was made to educate the patient with reference to art, the chief purpose of the plan being to satisfy his interest in and desire for the picture which appealed most to him.

Patients introduced to this particular service have expressed enthusiasm for the idea and spend a much longer time in selecting a picture and having it hung to their satisfaction than they usually spend in choosing a book for reading enjoyment.

Painting of Pictures. The painting of pictures, in oil or in water color, has been of benefit to many chronically ill patients. It is not unusual for a patient who has never attempted to paint before, and who was unaware of any talent, to become vitally interested in painting and to make it his chosen avocation. In some instances the efforts have been very successful, and painting has become a vocation rather than a pleasurable pastime.

Finger Painting. Finger painting is one of the most light hearted, relaxing pastimes that could be chosen by a patient and is ideal for one who must remain in bed. Commercial finger paints are available. However, it is relatively simple for the patient to make his own paint from laundry starch, soap flakes, and poster paint. The beginner should be encouraged to work with only one color at first and to gradually progress to the use of additional colors.

OTHER PASTIMES FOR PATIENTS

Patients often find that illness has provided them with time for a hobby or for a pastime which they have long wanted to pursue, but

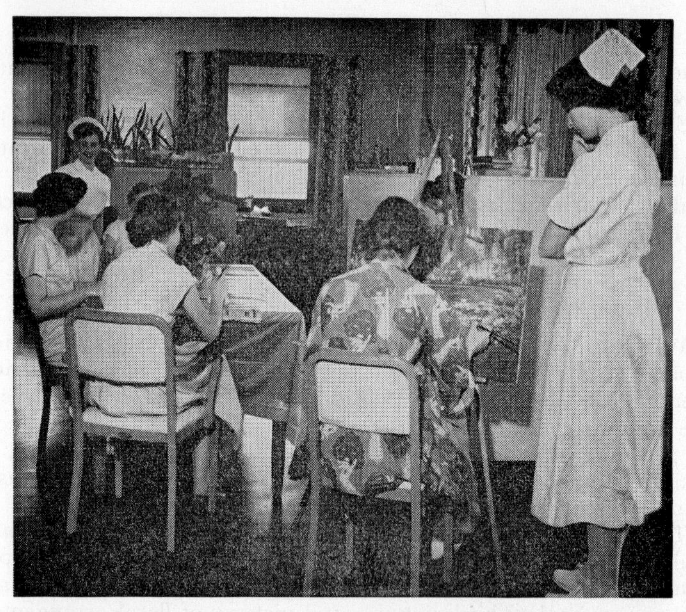

Fig. 83. Hospitalization sometimes causes hidden talent to be recognized. (University of Tennessee School of Nursing, Memphis, Tennessee.)

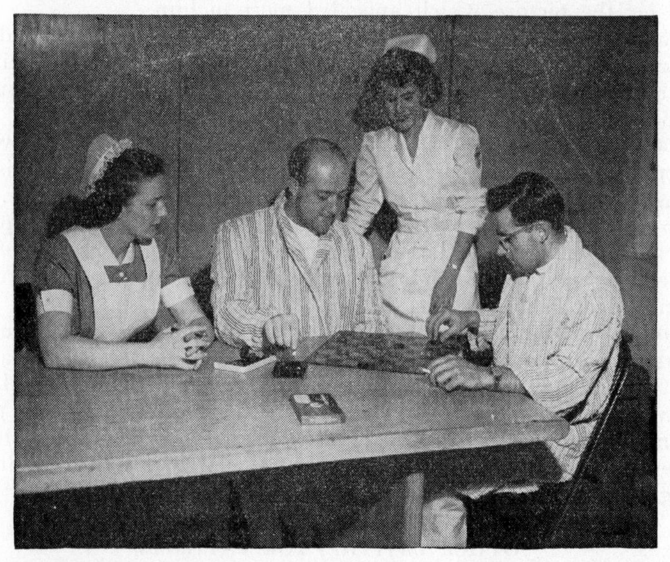

Fig. 84. Sometimes helpful suggestions from the sidelines turn out to be not so helpful. (Massachusetts General Hospital School of Nursing, Boston, Massachusetts.)

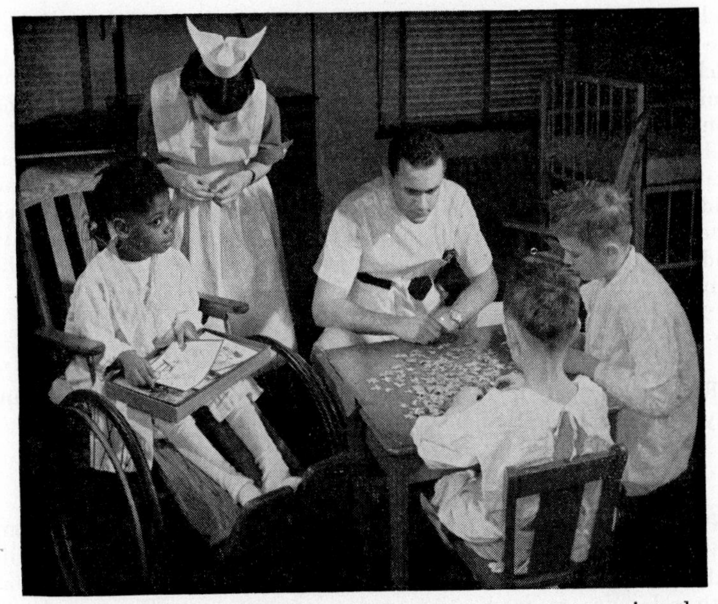

Fig. 85. When a jigsaw puzzle is in evidence everyone wants to get into the act. (Presbyterian Hospital School of Nursing, Chicago, Illinois.)

have been unable to fit into their previously busy days. Those patients should be encouraged to become actively engaged in a hobby and to try several different ones, if necessary, to find one which will be of real interest to them. The hobbies or recreational activities frequently chosen by patients include miniature gardening, sketching, adding to a collection of articles (stamps, coins, picture post cards, etc.), playing games or working puzzles, and making scrapbooks.

For the patient who must remain at complete bed rest, or who is unable to actively participate in the above types of recreation, there is still available to him the recreation of observation. Such recreation, for the patient unable to engage in any form of physical activity, should include the opportunity to watch ever-changing scenery from a nearby porch or from a window of the room. During convalescence, when even slight physical exertion may cause fatigue and the patient must sit quietly, he may, without any special effort on his part, become an interested audience for nature's panorama of color and activity. Days go more swiftly and are made more interesting if the growth and development of a nest of birds should become a matter of daily observation by the patient. A bush or tree that gradually changes from the lush green of summer to the multicolored loveliness of autumn may afford pleasure for many days. In the winter, the window in the hospital room may frame a scene of beauty made fresh and clean by softly falling snow. If the bed or wheelchair is placed near the window, the patient may benefit by the quiet restful feeling such a scene produces, and he is more apt to develop the cheerful, amiable attitude which leads to progress in achieving recovery from illness.

The type of diversional activity in which a patient actively participates is unimportant, so long as it serves to relieve mental strain and to help him adjust to the situation in which he finds himself. The nurse who is resourceful in helping the patient find an interesting and worthwhile pastime is rendering nursing service "above and beyond the call of duty."

Rest

Rest for the patient is twofold, and must include both mental and physical rest if the patient is to benefit.

PHYSICAL REST

Physical rest depends almost entirely on the nurse's ability to anticipate the patient's needs and to perform nursing procedures skillfully. If rest is to be obtained the orders of the attending physician with reference to medication and treatment must be carried out, proper postural position should be maintained, and the immediate surroundings of the patient should be quiet, clean, and comfortable.

All routine nursing procedures, as bath, back rub, and change of linen, are done to bring physical rest and comfort to the patient. Constant observation of symptoms or change in condition, and the use of available devices for lessening discomfort or pain also provide for rest and relaxation.

Other aids to rest include a well balanced diet, proper elimination, protection from disturbing noises or other sensory stimuli, and adequate ventilation of the room or unit.

"Complete bed rest" may be ordered for a patient by his attending physician. Such an order indicates the patient is to remain in bed and is not permitted to exert himself, even to the small extent of changing position, feeding himself, or reaching for an article on the bedside table. When complete bed rest is ordered, the nurse should explain to the patient that he should refrain from even slight physical exertion. He will be dependent on hospital personnel to care for all his physical needs until such time as he can again perform personal services for himself.

For some patients bed rest may necessitate remaining in bed but permit freedom of movement. Some form of exercise is usually indicated. Such patients should be encouraged to do much of their own personal care, as taking baths, combing hair, and caring for teeth and nails.

A convalescent patient may require rest periods during the day,

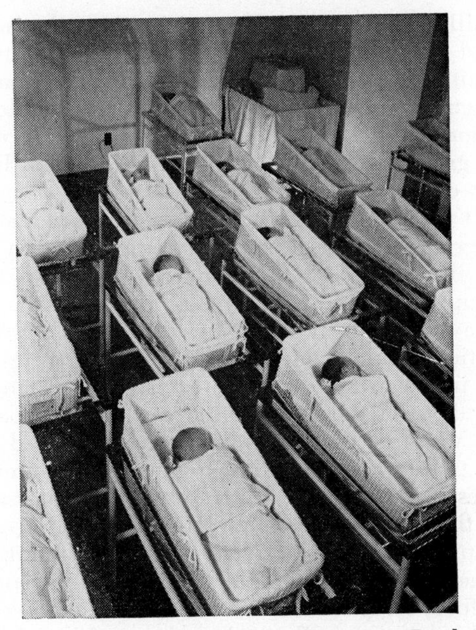

Fig. 86. A large number of patients at complete bed rest. (Presbyterian Hospital, Chicago, Illinois.)

intervals spent in sleep or relaxation. For the remainder of the day he may be up and about as he desires.

Procedures which make the patient feel refreshed and comfortable are effective in promoting physical comfort and rest. In addition to giving the routine care, including daily baths, oral hygiene, proper positioning of the patient, and provision of a pleasant and orderly environment, the nurse helps the patient achieve physical rest by administering drugs to relieve pain or discomfort and by assisting with treatment to combat physical ailments.

MENTAL REST

There are several ways in which the nurse may help the patient to gain mental rest. By explaining the basic principles of nursing procedures, or of treatments and examinations, she may banish much of the fear and worry with which the patient anticipates them. If he understands what to expect and what is expected of him and just how he may be helpful to the doctor or nurse, he is apt to be more cooperative and to benefit more by the treatments.

The patient will be relieved of mental anxiety, too, if the persons providing care to him perform their duties in an efficient and understanding manner. His confidence in the nurse's ability to carry out procedures skillfully is directly proportional to the amount of self-confidence and assurance she displays in giving nursing service.

If the patient is worried about finances, the nurse may help relieve subsequent mental stress by suggesting that the problem be brought to the attention of the local or state social welfare department. If the patient is greatly disturbed by the possibility that his illness may jeopardize his employment status, the nurse or a social worker may need to contact the employer and obtain information about the amount of sick leave granted to the hospitalized employee, the amount of insurance that will be available to him during his illness, and the length of time the employer may "hold" the job so that, after convalescence, the patient may return to it.

Rest is practically impossible if the patient has not learned to accept the illness or injury which necessitated hospitalization. The average person, whose days have been balanced with definite periods of work, play, and rest, will find that when he is confined to bed and must give up familiar activities he must adjust to a new environment and a new set of activities. Anxiety, fear, frustration, and depression may occur as a result of the needed adjustment. He may deeply resent having to accept the ministrations of the nurse who does for him the very personal things he has long done for himself. Being dependent on others for intake of food, for personal cleanliness, and for needs of elimination is disturbing emotionally and may interfere with rest and relaxation.

The nurse should understand that in adjusting to new environment and activities the patient undergoes great emotional stress. By careful explanation of the daily routine care, by expression of confidence in the doctor, and by cheerful reference to his expected and eventual recovery she can often reassure a discouraged and apprehensive patient. By diverting his mind from fear and worry she can help him make the adjustment which is essential if he is to get the physical and mental rest necessary to regain normal health.

Rest and relaxation, so essential to ultimate recovery of the patient, are possible only when the patient is free of physical discomfort, mental disturbances, and spiritual unrest. To insure physical comfort but permit the patient to remain in an apprehensive or fearful state of mind will not accomplish the benefits usually associated with nursing care.

In addition to the above measures which promote mental rest, the patient should be informed of the many financial plans that are available for the payment of hospital and medical expenses if he is concerned about the mounting expenses of doctor and hospital bills. He should know that administrative officers of a hospital will usually accept a method of payment that is consistent with the patient's financial status and can be met by him without undue hardship. Given this reassurance, the patient will be relieved of mental strain and will be better able to achieve physical rest and relaxation.

Persons not considered to be deeply religious may turn to religion when they are ill and the nurse should be able to tell them of the spiritual help which is available. She could provide them with a copy of the Bible, ask if they would like to be visited by the chaplain, or take them for a short time to the chapel. Any measure which provides for spiritual rest or aid will help the patient to overcome physical disability.

Sleep

Sleep is defined as "a state of unconsciousness, or of partial consciousness, with the body and mind at rest and body functions suspended." The cause of sleep is not yet definitely known, although a number of theories have received careful consideration. A prevalent theory is that sensitivity of sensory receptors is lessened, with increased resistance at the nerve synapses, so the mind is not disturbed by ordinary sensory impressions.

Approximately one third of the normal life span of the individual is spent in sleep. Refreshing slumber renews health and vigor, restores a frayed temper, and helps produce the pleasing personality so necessary to harmony and success in life. Sleep is necessary to the hospital patient if normal body functioning is to be restored.

It has been estimated that approximately half the population of the United States have trouble falling asleep all or part of the time. It is, therefore, not surprising that large numbers of hospital patients require special nursing care to promote sleep, and may require a physician's order for sedatives.

Prolonged illness compels thousands to spend long periods of time in bed, and the hours seem long and monotonous. If the patient can sleep eight or more hours each night and for an hour or two during the day, the remaining hours will not seem so long and so lacking in activity or interest.

During sleep vital involuntary activity of various organs of the body continues. The respiratory and circulatory systems continue to function much the same as during waking hours. The digestive system also continues functioning, although digestive processes may be slowed during sleep.

SLEEP REQUIREMENTS

The hospital patient, in need of the healing benefits of sleep, requires more sleep than the average well person. Eight or nine hours is generally accepted as the amount of sleep required by the average adult patient each night.

It is not essential that all persons sleep eight hours each night. Broken periods of sleep, even long periods of wakefulness, are not unusual for hospital patients who may nap during the day and seem to require less sleep at night. The elderly patient may sleep only for

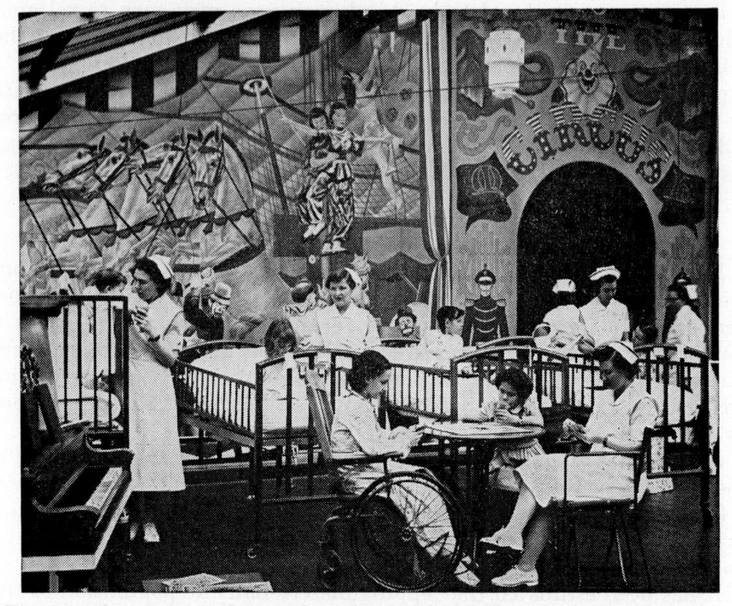

Fig. 87. The circus background is fine for the children's recreation room; it would not be desirable for the room where rest periods or nap times are observed. (Methodist Hospital School of Nursing, Indianapolis, Indiana.)

short periods of time during the night and seemingly suffers no ill effects from lessened hours of sleep.

Children require more sleep than adults. The sick child should sleep approximately 10 to 12 hours out of each 24.

FACTORS THAT MAY DISTURB OR PREVENT SLEEP

To help the patient get sufficient sleep the nurse should guard against any condition or factor which may disturb or prevent sleep.

A change in external conditions may rouse a person from sleep as resultant nerve impulses are transmitted to the sensory area of the brain. Thus one may be awakened by an unusual sound, a bright light, a drop in room temperature, or other external phenomena. A state of mental excitement or nervous tension may prevent sleep, and for that reason it is necessary to limit visitors and the time they spend with hospital patients. Loneliness, worry, and apprehension may cause sleeplessness. If the patient is unduly concerned about his physical condition and fearful of needed treatment procedures, he may be unable to sleep. Even the fear of being unable to sleep may become a direct cause of wakefulness. Noise or light may produce stimuli

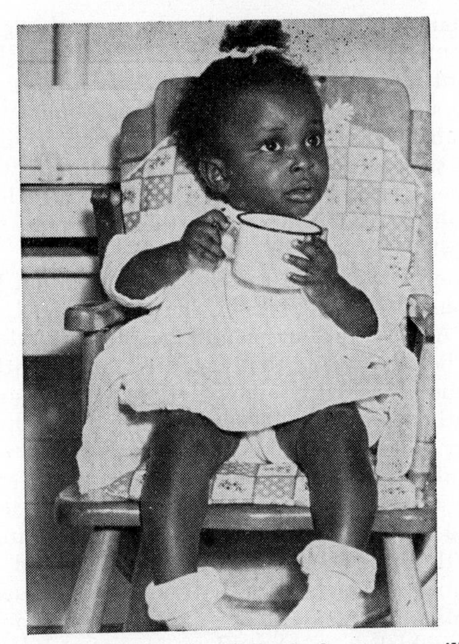

Fig. 88. A small pre-bedtime snack of light food or warm milk induces physical relaxation and sleep. (Presbyterian Hospital School of Nursing, Chicago, Illinois.)

which send nerve impulses to the brain and thus prevent sleep. Physical discomfort or pain will prevent rest and sleep and will need to be overcome if sleep is to be obtained.

Too much fresh air, especially cold air, may cause wakefulness. If the window is open a few inches sufficient fresh air will be circulated to properly ventilate the room without disturbing the patient's rest.

PREPARATION FOR SLEEP

To prepare the patient for sleep, whether for an afternoon nap or for sleep at night, the nurse should practice the following routine:

1. Establish a regular hour when the patient is to be made ready for sleep. Habit formation plays an important part in inducing sleep.
2. Eliminate, as much as possible, distractions caused by noise, light, and improper ventilation. Noise may cause a patient to be restless, even though it may not actually prevent sleep.
3. See that the patient's room is darkened. Light from a lamp in the room or from a street lamp or from a flashing sign outside may cause a patient to be restless at night. Early morning sunlight may rouse a patient from deep sleep much earlier than is desired.

4. Give a small pre-bedtime snack to prevent hunger contractions of an empty stomach. A glass of warm milk or a small serving of hot broth is sufficient.

5. Induce physical relaxation by means of a warm bath. If the patient is up and about a hot tub bath before he retires will help to loosen and relax tired, stiff, and sore muscles. The bed patient may have face and hands washed and, if time permits, his back may be bathed. After the bath, a soothing back rub will further relax the patient so that sleep is practically assured.

6. See that the patient is in a comfortable position for sleep. If he is lying on his back, a small pillow should be placed under his head and shoulders. Another pillow should be placed under his knees or the bed should be adjusted so that the knees are slightly flexed. Arms should be at the sides with elbows slightly bent and hands held loosely or slightly closed. If the patient is lying on his side, support should be given where needed to make his position comfortable. So far as possible all joints should be in a position of semiflexion.

7. Encourage mental relaxation. Worry, nervous tension, and an over-active mind is not conducive to sleep. The nurse may help relieve anxiety and restlessness by determining its cause and trying to overcome it. She can suggest that the patient replace unpleasant or distracting thoughts with pleasant ones. Calm, roving reminiscences of past experiences which have been pleasant or satisfying will decrease mental stimulation, as will daydreaming or giving attention to the procedure for obtaining physical relaxation.

OTHER FACTORS PERTAINING TO SLEEP

If the patient has not already developed good habits of sleep the nurse may explain the important function of sleep and encourage better sleep practices.

Patients who seem inclined to worry or to remain mentally alert when trying to sleep should be tactfully informed of a beneficial rule for sleep which can be stated briefly, "Never try to solve a problem after dark."

A patient should not be disturbed at night or roused from sleep to have temperature, pulse, and respiration taken or to be given a medication or treatment unless the doctor has specifically ordered that the patient be awakened.

An excellent means of inducing children to sleep is reading from a book which they enjoy. If conditions of environment are right for sleep and the reader promotes the idea of sleep by tone of voice and manner of reading, the child will usually fall asleep in a relatively short time.

Reading, if the book is light and entertaining, may also be a means of inducing sleep for the adult patient if he ordinarily enjoys reading.

The patient who does not sleep soundly during the night and who seems not to require the usual number of hours of sleep should be encouraged to rest even if he doesn't sleep. The nurse should inform the patient that lying awake at night is in no way harmful so long as he doesn't worry or become emotionally upset by wakefulness. He should know that the body rests just as effectively when he lies quietly awake as it rests during sleep.

Summary of Important Factors

Inactivity of "complete bed rest" can weaken muscles and cause impaired circulation.

Exercise and recreation help overcome harmful effects of bed rest.

Two general classifications of exercise are active and passive. In passive exercise the movement is carried out by another without effort by the patient.

Recreational activity helps boost morale of the patient. The kind of recreation depends on age, interests, and physical condition of the patient. Common forms of recreation are reading, radio, television, music, art, conversation, collections, and games.

Rest, to benefit the patient, must be mental as well as physical. "Complete bed rest" requires that the patient remain in bed and not exert himself.

Nursing procedures promote physical rest. Reassurance and referral of problems to the proper agency promotes mental rest.

Sleep is a state of complete or partial unconsciousness. Most patients require eight to nine hours of sleep each night.

Factors that prevent or disturb sleep include: noise and light, change in temperature, nervous tension, pain or discomfort, fear and worry.

Factors that promote sleep include: elimination of distractions, prebedtime snack, warm bath with back rub, comfortable position and relaxation, freedom from worry, reading.

Factors To Teach the Patient

Necessity for exercise, even though bed rest is ordered.

Beneficial exercises that may be done in a sitting position in bed.

Advantages of certain types of recreation for him: pleasure to be derived from recreational activity; interest grows as the activity continues; interesting personalities are to be met in books.

Need to keep books, games, and toys clean and free from pathogenic microorganisms.

Fear and worry can interfere with recovery from physical impairment.

Meaning of term "complete bed rest."

Importance of rest and sleep in recovery.

Rest may be obtained without sleep.

Means of relaxing tense muscles.
Means of promoting sleep.

Scientific Principles

Anatomy and Physiology. Muscle tone is maintained by active or passive exercise.

Exercise is needed to stimulate activity of the vital organs, but should normally be limited to suit the particular needs of the individual.

Exercise affects circulation, respiration, appetite, and elimination. The more vigorous the exercise the more rapid the circulation and the greater the increase in appetite and in respiration.

Exercise usually produces a feeling of well-being in the patient, although it may have an adverse effect if it is overdone.

The orders of the doctor control the amount of exercise the patient may have.

Relaxation is obtained when the body is in a reclining position. It produces rest and lessens fatigue, and enables the body to function at low capacity so tissue damage can be repaired.

Recreation may provide for exercise or for relaxation, and the choice of recreational activity for the patient should be made according to his needs.

During sleep the body continues to move and turn and muscles continue to be activated. Vital body functions also continue during sleep, although their rate may be considerably slowed in comparison with that which occurs during waking hours.

Chemistry. The reaction and oxygen requirement for muscle tissue differs in the resting and the active state. Resting muscle is slightly alkaline and requires approximately 250 cc. of oxygen per minute. Activated muscle is acid in reaction and during vigorous exercise may require as much as 4,000 cc. of oxygen per minute. Because more oxygen is needed during exercise, the rate of respiration is increased.

Microbiology. Recreational supplies such as books, games and toys for children should be looked upon as potential carriers of disease and provision should be made for cleanliness, sterilization or fumigation.

Pharmacology. Sedatives are given to promote rest and sleep for the patient. Before giving the patient a sedative drug the nurse should see that other factors such as a quiet room, shaded light and comfortable position are assured the patient.

All other measures for inducing or promoting sleep should be taken before the sedative drug is administered.

Physics. Heat causes acceleration of muscular contraction. Cold has the opposite effect.

During rest and sleep the temperature of the body is lower than when the patient is awake and is active. For that reason additional blankets are needed at night to keep the patient warm.

Psychology. The strangeness of the hospital environment and the worry or concern caused by illness may produce restlessness and wakefulness at night.

By repeated assurance of her presence and of her intent to be always near or within call, the nurse can lessen the emotional strain of the patient beset with worry and fear.

Persons not considered deeply religious may turn to religion when they are ill and the nurse should be able to inform them of the spiritual help which is available. She should provide them with a copy of the Bible, ask if they would like to be visited by the chaplain, or take them for a brief period to the chapel.

Sociology. The relationship of patient to nurse is characterized by marked dependence. The patient looks to the nurse for his physical and mental needs which he formerly actively controlled for himself.

The nurse may need to confer with members of the patient's family so that they too may help provide for his comfort and care.

If relaxation or sleep is prevented by worry or fear the nurse should enlist the help of qualified social workers and social agencies where help may be obtained when needed.

The nurse may need to acquaint the family with the importance of rest and sleep for the patient and ask their cooperation in providing freedom from worry and from physical disturbances for him.

Situation Type Problems

1. On the third night of her night duty term the student answered a light for a patient who had p.r.n. order for a narcotic to be given for rest and sleep. The patient complained of wakefulness and the student obtained the narcotic from the night supervisor. When the student returned to the patient's room to give the medication she found the patient fast asleep. Thinking the patient would awaken again and ask for the medicine the nurse placed it, clearly labeled, in the pocket of her uniform.

Next morning the nurse removed her uniform in preparation for retiring and found the narcotic which had not been used the previous night for the patient with the standing p.r.n. order. What would you have done?

2. A student nurse who had been assigned to night duty found it very difficult to sleep during the day. She asked the doctor in the Student Health Service office to prescribe sleeping pills. He refused, stating that she would make the adjustment from day to night duty without the use of drugs. He pointed out to her that because of classes during the morning it would be unwise for her to resort to drugs in order to sleep.

The student asked her roommate, who was on duty in the pharmacy department, to bring her a few sleeping pills. The roommate did not refuse but failed to comply with the request. The student had borrowed $1.00 from her roommate the week before. She now informed her that the dollar would not be repaid, but would be used to *buy* sleeping pills. If you were the roommate, what would you have done?

Suggested Reference Reading

"Librarians bring projected books to rescue of patients," Ruth Jane McNutt; Hospital Management, March, 1950.

"Sleep and how to get more of it," Robert Coughlan; Reader's Digest, August, 1950.

"Television helps patients," Rudolf Leiser; Hospital Management, January, 1952.

"Others sleep—why can't you?" Registered Nurse, April, 1952.

"They shall have music," Charles A. Turner; Modern Hospital, June, 1952.

"A combination T.V.-radio system for patients," Jay W. Collins; Hospitals, November, 1952.

"Sleep tight," Joyce Newton, Ruth C. Ross, and Gloria Brown; American Journal of Nursing, December, 1952.

CHAPTER 13

Admission of the Patient

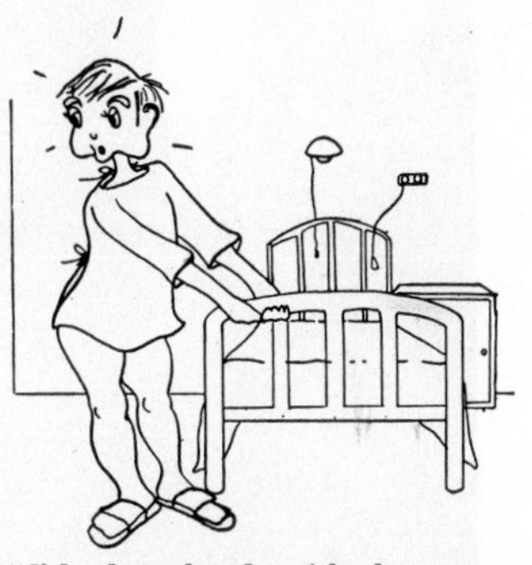

"I'd heard there'd be some changes made in men's clothing, but this is ridiculous!"

TOPICAL OUTLINE

Admission of the Patient

Usually the patient has complete confidence in the ability of the physician he has chosen for medical or surgical treatment and because of that confidence results of treatment are even more likely to be effective.

When the patient is admitted to a hospital he tends to accept all members of the hospital staff and to have confidence in the hospital itself largely because of the relationship that exists between his doctor and the institution. At the time of admission hospital personnel must establish a desirable relationship with the patient and give nursing and medical care that will maintain that desirable relationship and promote the feeling of confidence and security needed for his recovery.

Some patients may have had preliminary tests or treatment before hospitalization was required and not only have known that they were to be sent to a hospital but have been permitted to choose the date and time for their admission. Other patients may become ill suddenly or meet with an accident which requires immediate hospi-

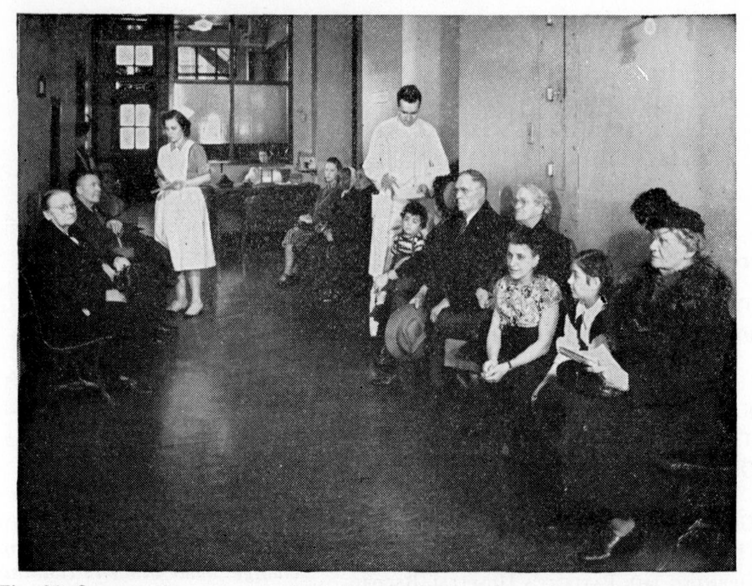

Fig. 89. Some patients are admitted from a clinic or from the out-patient department of the hospital. (Presbyterian Hospital School of Nursing, Chicago, Illinois.)

talization. Under such circumstances the patient has little or no choice in regard to his admission to the hospital.

Whether the experience of hospitalization is approached gradually or encountered suddenly, whether it is a new or an old experience, the admission procedure is apt to be difficult for the patient, and hospital personnel should make a special effort to be friendly and courteous and to make him feel that they are sincerely interested in his welfare.

THE PATIENT'S EMOTIONAL REACTION

The nurse should have a basic and real understanding of the various probable reactions which the patient may experience if she is to satisfactorily meet his needs during admission.

If he is entering a hospital for medical, surgical, or emergency treatment, he may be in a highly emotional state of mind. Because of unvoiced fear and worry or because the experience is new to him, his reaction to all hospital personnel concerned with the procedure of admission may be quite different from his usual or normal reaction to a new experience.

The extent of fear and anxiety which the patient may feel when being hospitalized for the first time will depend on many factors.

His age, occupation, and financial status may largely determine the manner in which he reacts. Family relationships, educational background, and the duration and severity of the illness requiring hospitalization may also influence his reaction to the admission procedure.

If he is an adult male, in all probability he is the sole wage earner for his family and may be deeply concerned about the cost of medical or surgical care. He may fear that enforced absenteeism from his work will bring about the possibility of losing his job. He may be apprehensive in regard to his recovery. He may be extremely fearful of surgical treatment or of medical procedures which can cause physical pain and discomfort. He may be resentful of the fact that his physical condition makes it necessary for him to enter the hospital, and because of that resentment he may be morose, uncooperative, and disagreeable.

If he is uncertain as to the nature of his disease, and ignorant of the kind and amount of medical treatment that will be required, his feeling of strangeness and insecurity will be increased. And when he is expected to answer questions of a very personal nature put to him by a person he may never have seen before, it is little wonder that he reacts emotionally.

With these factors in mind, the nurse will readily understand that the admission routine can be a trying ordeal for the patient. His background may include racial and family superstitions and beliefs which influence the way in which he reacts to this new experience of hospitalization. Under such circumstances, it is not at all unusual for the behavior pattern of the newly admitted patient to be quite different from his normal behavior. His reaction to hospital personnel when he first meets them may largely determine if a satisfactory adjustment to hospital routine will be made or if he will remain throughout his hospital stay a hypercritical and difficult patient.

If the patient is an adult female, especially if she is the mother of young children, added to the pain or other physical symptoms of illness and the anxiety as to the outcome of the proposed treatment may be the worry of submitting her children to the care of another person. She knows that her absence from home disrupts the daily routine there and may be hazardous to the welfare of her family. She knows that her mother, or sister, or the helpful neighbor with whom she left the children will do their best to properly care for the youngsters, but she will be quite certain that they will forget to add the few drops of vanilla extract to the glass of milk for Johnny, who won't drink it without the flavoring, and that Susie will manage to remove essential scarf and mittens while playing outside and will catch a cold. Although she is sure of her husband's understanding and sympathy, she may feel that she is failing him. She knows there will be little chance of adding to their savings account when hospital and doctor bills must be paid.

Admission to the hospital may be a trying experience too for the single, adult patient (a high school or college student). Although exempt from the worry of providing for a family he may have the substitute worry of missing classes and school activities. Long-continued absence from class can result in failure to maintain a suitable scholastic record or to complete the course of study.

Admission for the young child, who may be surprised and frightened by his first experience with illness and pain, may cause an even more severe emotional upset. Taken from his familiar home surroundings to the unfamiliar environment of the hospital room or ward, he may feel unwanted and neglected by his family, especially when they leave him alone in an environment to which major adjustment must be made. He is apt to mistrust the nurse and other hospital personnel first because they are strange to him and second because the treatment and care given him may include such procedures as a hypodermic injection or the withdrawal of blood for laboratory tests, procedures which he cannot understand, but is forced to endure.

With the knowledge that the patient being admitted is undergoing severe mental and emotional strain, as well as suffering physical pain or impairment, the nurse should make a special effort to reassure him. She should try to gain his cooperation and to merit the trust and confidence which forms the basis for the most desirable nurse-patient relationship.

FIRST IMPRESSIONS ARE IMPORTANT

The Admission Clerk. As a rule the admission clerk is the first member of the hospital staff to see and talk with the patient on his arrival at the institution. The manner in which she greets him and the relatives or friends who may have accompanied him can largely determine the immediate reaction of all of them. She should convey to them, by tone of voice, by gracious manner, and by tact and understanding, that the chief aim of all hospital personnel is to make the patient's period of hospitalization as pleasant as possible.

It is the admitting clerk who serves as the liaison officer working with patients and their families and with doctors, interns, nurses, social workers, and others to effect a smooth and pleasant entrance into the hospital for the new patient. She becomes the effective means of establishing rapport between the patient and hospital staff.

The well trained admission clerk has usually been instructed in the importance of treating all persons with kindly interest and respect. She can do irreparable damage to the institution by treating the patient in a brusque or disinterested manner. It is essential that she understand the significance of the patient's social, economic, and financial standing as factors that influence his mental reaction to the injury or illness which brings him to the hospital.

She must be constantly aware of the fact that the majority of patients who come to her office for the admission routine are experi-

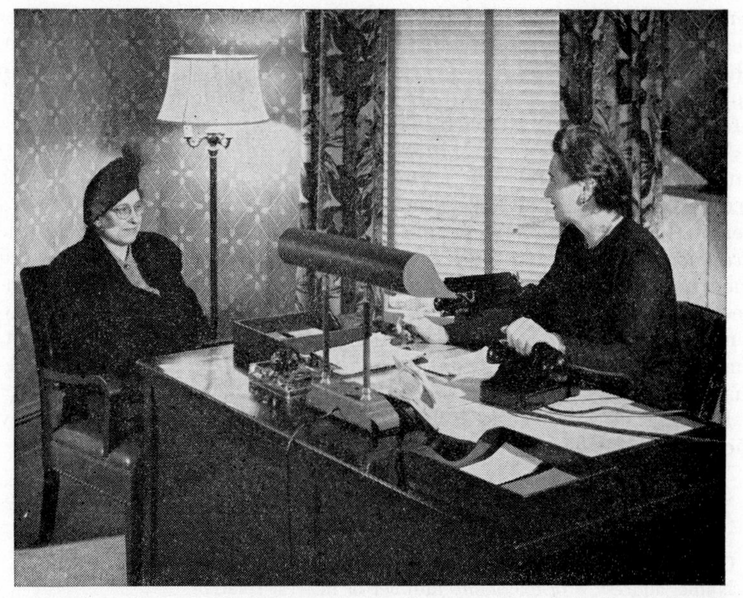

Fig. 90. The admitting clerk is usually the first member of the hospital staff to see and talk with the patient. (Presbyterian Hospital, Chicago, Illinois.)

encing mental conflict, with feelings of insecurity, dread, and apprehension which may cause even more discomfort than that produced by their physical condition.

The admitting officer must understand that a patient may be irritable, confused, aggressive, or suspicious, and that he may withdraw into himself and answer questions reluctantly or not at all because of fear and anxiety.

Whenever possible, as soon as the patient enters the hospital building, he should be taken at once to the admitting office and the admission routine started. If he is forced to wait, even a relatively short period of time, he is made to feel that the hospital is not prepared to receive him as a patient. He will also be convinced that his presence is probably unwelcome to the staff of workers who are obviously too busy to take on the additional duties his admission imposes upon them.

Only by establishing a friendly relationship between herself and the patient can the admitting clerk win his confidence and gain his cooperation. She should be sincerely interested in him as a person and should ask the necessary questions simply and without any perceptible desire to hasten the interview in order to attend to other duties. She should realize that a quick and sure way of stopping the patient from adequate expression of his physical and mental problems is to interrupt his conversation by answering the telephone or beginning a conversation with another worker in the department. She should be continually aware of the fact that the patient forms an opinion of the hospital and its personnel as he talks with her, the first person on the staff with whom he comes in contact.

While being questioned in regard to pertinent information that must be obtained for the admission record, the patient should be accorded absolute privacy. Much of the information needed is of a personal nature and few people like to speak of such matters in the presence of others. If others are waiting their turn to be interviewed they may seem to derive some measure of relief from their own undesirable situation by becoming interested spectators and avid listeners to the conversation of the admitting clerk and the patient. For the latter, such a situation may be disconcerting and embarrassing.

Leading questions asked during the admission interview usually include the following:

Age — date of birth — place of birth
Address — telephone number
Nationality — race — religion
Occupation — marital status
Name, address, and telephone number of nearest relative
Name and address of employer
Date of previous hospital admission

Information given to the admission officer should be considered confidential by that person and the patient should be informed that such is the case.

Other information needed for the admission record pertains to the size of the family, number of wage earners, number of dependents, the salary being earned by the patient prior to his illness, type of work he was doing, name of bank where he may have a checking or savings account, whether he is entitled to the benefits of health insurance, and the effect of his present illness and subsequent hospital costs on the family finances.

The admitting clerk should attempt to relieve anxiety in regard to financial obligations of the patient and bear in mind that many patients, fearful of not being granted admission, may profess to greater incomes than they actually possess, while others, anticipating a larger bill than would otherwise be presented, will disclaim a large part of their savings or of their earned income.

In many hospitals an advance payment, usually a small per cent of the estimated total bill, is required at the time of admission. This procedure should be explained to the patient in such a way that he will understand it to be a policy of the institution, applicable to all patients and not merely a request that he supply proof of his ability and intent to pay hospitalization costs.

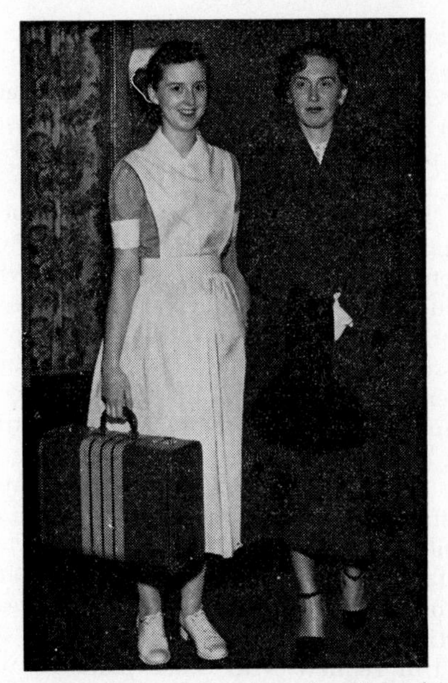

Fig. 91. The nurse who admits the patient should be friendly and cheerful and reassuring. (Birmingham Baptist Hospital School of Nursing, Birmingham, Alabama.)

Many patients are reluctant to speak of some of the factors which are necessary to include in the admission interview. Tactfulness and understanding on the part of the clerk who asks the questions can accomplish a great deal in overcoming the tendency of the patient to give false or incomplete answers, merely because of his desire to terminate what has become for him an unpleasant experience.

Information regarding the financial status of the patient determines whether he should be assigned to a private room or ward, unless he is critically ill or is admitted as an emergency measure. For the patient who is very ill or seriously injured the admission information must be obtained from another member of the family. Another person will need to supply admission information when the patient is physically unable to take part in the interview or is reluctant to answer the questions.

As soon as the patient is assigned to a room or to ward accommodations the admission clerk should notify the nurse in charge of that particular department so the unit he is to occupy can be made ready for his arrival. He should then be taken to the department by the clerk, who introduces him to the head nurse and to the second phase of the admission procedure.

The Nurse Who Admits the Patient. The nurse assigned to admit the patient, if she has not been introduced to him, should introduce herself and make a special effort to make him feel at ease. Her friendly manner, her own self-confidence, and her interest in his welfare can soon dispel the feeling that he has lost his identity by becoming one of a large group of patients being cared for at the hospital.

If the patient has not met the head nurse before he is taken to his room, he should be introduced to her soon after his admission. Such a meeting enables him to become acquainted with another member of the nursing staff and promotes a willingness on his part to place himself in the care of personnel that make up a well organized team. He is reassured by the knowledge that the head nurse, a mature and experienced member of the staff, is overseeing the work done by the younger nurse or student and is taking responsibility for insuring him correct and adequate nursing care.

It is necessary for the nurse who admits the patient to listen attentively to his statements in regard to his illness and events leading up to his admission to the hospital. It is essential, too, that she treat members of his family with courtesy and consideration. Although it is always desirable to have accompanying relatives remain outside the room, or patient unit, during admission, this should be accomplished by a tactful request with the explanation that only a relatively short time is required and that they may then return to be with the patient again.

The nurse who curtly asks the family to leave, her tone of voice rather than the spoken words implying that they are a nuisance and a problem, invariably causes them to experience doubt and concern regarding her treatment of the patient. Fearing that she may be ungracious and not at all sympathetic toward the patient, they want to remain with him longer than would be the case if they could feel that he was being cared for with kindness as well as efficiency.

The thoughtful nurse, anxious to make the patient feel that he is welcome and that she is desirous of helping him, should begin at once to carry out the necessary procedures of taking temperature, pulse, respiration, and blood pressure. She should work quietly and smoothly to give him the feeling of assurance he needs. By accurate and skillful nursing she can earn the patient's respect and establish confidence in her ability to help him regain health and normal activity.

She should be aware of the patient's unexpressed fear of being left alone and carefully explain to him the need for going to and from the room to obtain necessary supplies or equipment, although each time she leaves the room she should mention her intent to return "very soon."

The head nurse or the nurse admitting the patient, or both, may have ample opportunity to mention that they are acquainted with the patient's doctor and have helped in the care of other patients referred by him. The confidence which the nurse has in the physician, whether it be actually expressed in words or only implied, will serve to renew the patient's faith and confidence, a most important factor in his ultimate recovery.

During the admission procedures, the nurse may have an opportunity to relieve mental strain for the patient. If, for instance, he is worried about his family's financial status, she can tell him of the various local social workers and welfare agencies which are eager to help in providing financial aid or material assistance to his family during the time he is to be away from home.

FACTORS TO OBSERVE ON ADMISSION

While admitting the patient, the nurse may, by tactful questioning, learn much regarding his family, social background, and educational and occupational experiences, as well as his greatest fear or worry regarding his present physical condition.

By observation alone, if the patient seems reluctant to answer questions or to volunteer information, much can be learned about him. His preference in reading material which he may have brought with him furnishes an excellent key to his educational background. His taste in music, as evidenced by his choice of radio or television programs, will reveal a great deal regarding his social standing and may be indicative of his financial situation.

A brief examination of the admission record on the chart will give enough information regarding family, cultural background, religion, etc., so the nurse may form an accurate mental image of the patient in relation to his experiences and habits prior to his entrance into the hospital.

OTHER ADMISSION PROCEDURES

Nursing procedures used in admitting the patient to the hospital are chiefly those used in giving routine nursing care.

The room should be in order when the patient arrives on the clinical service department. All needed equipment, supplies, and linen should be on hand and an "open bed" should be made ready for the patient.

If the patient is able to undress and get into bed without assistance, he should be provided privacy and sufficient time to do so. If he is in a weakened condition or confused state of mind, the nurse will need to assist in getting him to bed.

As soon as the patient is in bed, temperature, pulse, respiration, and blood pressure should be taken and recorded. He should be given the urinal with explanation as to its use and asked to void so a urine specimen can be sent to the laboratory.

Clothing and valuables should be checked and listed, and the proper

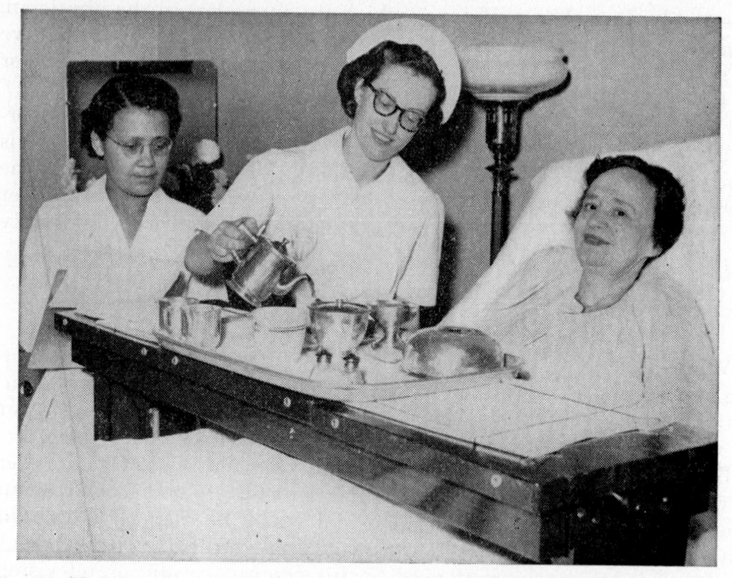

Fig. 92. If the patient is admitted at mealtime, a light lunch should be served. (Mercy Hospital School of Nursing, Denver, Colorado.)

forms signed by both patient and nurse. Clothing should then be sent to the clothing room to be properly stored until needed at the time of the patient's dismissal.

If the patient is admitted about mealtime and has not eaten, unless there are orders prohibiting food intake, a light lunch should be served.

An admission bath should be given to prepare the patient for the physical examination which he will undergo soon after admission.

ORIENTATION TO HOSPITAL ENVIRONMENT AND ROUTINE

While carrying out admission procedures, the nurse should inform the patient in regard to the established daily routine at the hospital. She should explain each of the admission procedures just before it is performed. Mention should be made that within a short time the intern or resident doctor will appear to perform the admission physical examination and to obtain information for the record of personal history. With a few words of explanation she can show the relationship which previous history may bear to the present illness and thus gain a willingness on the part of the patient to answer questions and to submit to the various measures employed by the intern or physician in giving him a complete physical examination.

The Patient Unit. To further inform the patient as to his new hospital surroundings, he should be introduced to the intricate mechanism of the hospital bed. Unless contraindicated, he may be placed in semi-Fowler's position while he learns that the backrest can be raised or lowered, and the lower part of the bed can be adjusted to permit greater physical comfort as well as more efficient treatment and nursing care. In many hospitals at the present time there are hospital beds which can be raised and lowered at will. They are raised to the required height for the performance of nursing duties and then lowered to regulation height while the patient is resting or sleeping. Side rails may be applied to the hospital bed to prevent the patient from falling.

If the patient is to remain in bed he should be shown the compartment in the bedside table where the bedpan and urinal are stored. Other articles kept in the bedside table, such as the emesis basin, mouthwash cup, and supplies for his personal toilet should be brought to his attention. At this time, too, the nurse should mention that the unit which the patient occupies can be screened to provide absolute privacy, not only for procedures relative to elimination, but for the treatments and nursing procedures which his condition may require. While explaining the use of various articles provided for his care the nurse should assist the patient in putting away personal articles which he has brought to the hospital. He should be permitted to choose the most convenient location for such articles as spectacles, cigarettes, comb, shaving equipment, and other items that will be used daily.

The Admission Bath. In spite of the fact that most patients prepare for hospitalization by taking a tub bath and wearing clean clothing to the hospital, the admission procedure requires that the patient be given a bath. There are several reasons for strict adherence to this regulation, few of which are not at all concerned with his cleanliness.

While bathing the patient the nurse is given an opportunity to carefully observe his general physical condition. Any abnormality of physical structure that might be present can be noted. His general appearance can be observed, whether he seems well nourished or shows symptoms of emaciation. Extreme pallor or other abnormality of skin coloring can be observed. The general condition of hands (well kept or showing signs of neglect) should be noted. During the bath procedure the mental attitude of the patient will become apparent and if he seems extremely nervous or restless that fact should be noted on his hospital record and the nurse should attempt to reassure him. Learning the cause of anxiety or apprehension may provide the means of overcoming those emotional factors and help the patient to make a good adjustment to the hospital environment.

The presence of a pressure sore, a bruise, or an abrasion may be

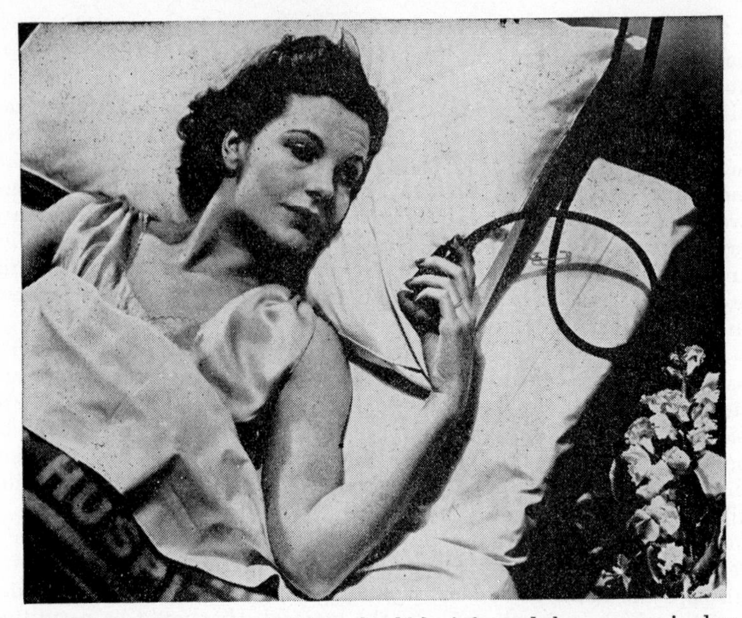

Fig. 93. The newly admitted patient should be informed that a nurse is always as near to her as the signal call bell. (Parke, Davis & Co., Detroit, Michigan.)

noted during the admission bath and the fact duly recorded on the chart to prevent confusion at some later date as to the exact time which the pressure sore or injury occurred.

If pediculi are present they may be discovered during the bath and proper steps can be instituted at once to correct the condition.

During the admission bath, the nurse should carefully drape the patient for each phase of the procedure, to demonstrate that it is possible for him to be bathed and cared for by nurses without being exposed or subjected to embarrassment.

The Signal Bell. All patients, on admission, should be given careful instruction in manipulation of the call bell or signal bell used to summon a nurse. The signal bell, always within easy reach of the patient, is his assurance that at any time, day or night, he may call a nurse to his bedside merely by flashing the signal. Because this method of gaining the attention of the nurse is an excellent means of gaining absolute confidence of the patient in the hospital and in hospital personnel, all nurses, students and graduates, should make a special effort to answer promptly all call lights which flash on in the corridor or on the board at the nurses' station. If a patient is forced to wait a long period of time for his call to be answered when his needs are routine and quite unimportant, he may become appre-

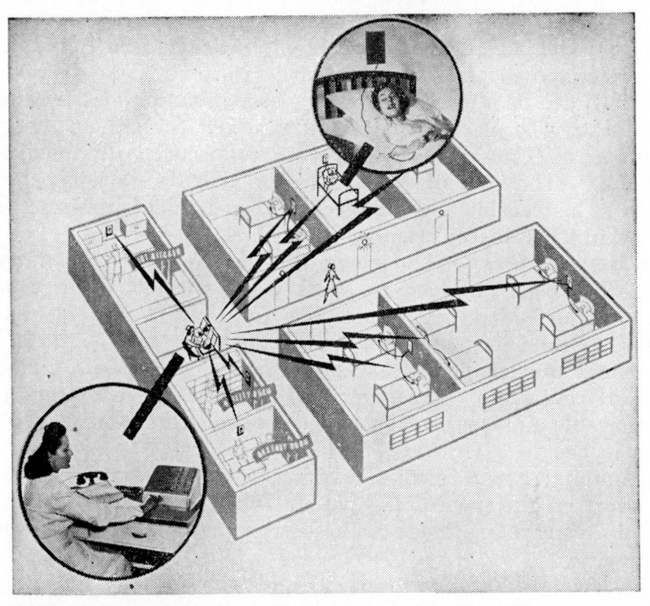

Fig. 94. The Executone Nurse Call System provides immediate communication between nurse and patient. (Executone Company of Chicago, Chicago, Illinois.)

hensive as to serious consequences that could result from delay in answering the signal bell if his need should be of an emergency nature and immediate medical care might be required.

The signal bell, probably more than any other device in the hospital, serves to reassure the patient that he is under constant surveillance and care; it helps him to overcome the fear and dread of being left alone in unfamiliar hospital surroundings.

The Nurse Call System. The Executone audio-visual nurse call system is another device which insures prompt and careful attention to the patient. By means of this system of communication the nurse and patient may converse while the nurse remains at her desk. The nurse can "listen in" to each patient's room at regular intervals and quickly locate and attend to a patient in distress. The patient benefits from a new feeling of security when he knows that he can speak to the nurse immediately by merely depressing the bedside call button.

Bedside Telephone Service. One of the important factors in the adjustment to hospital environment that must be made by the patient is that of being separated from family and friends. If the patient is given an opportunity to keep in touch with members of his family by telephone he is much more apt to accept hospitalization without complaint.

Bedside telephone service may be made available to patients by plug-in telephone in their room or by means of the Telecart, a portable pay-station telephone. This ingenious device is a coin collector telephone mounted on a movable cart with a long plug-ended cord attached. It can be plugged in where a corresponding jack is installed, and jacks may be placed in strategic positions throughout the hospital, although Telecart circuits are not connected with the hospital switchboard. The patient who wishes to make a call has the cart brought to his bedside and plugged in, then by depositing the proper coins he can obtain the number wanted.

The Hospital Gown. The gown provided for the patient by the hospital has been designed for long wear, without thought of the esthetic factor. Made of serviceable (able to withstand repeated launderings) and inexpensive material, the gown is large, short, open at the back and shapeless, except for rounded neckline and set-in sleeves. It covers only the upper two thirds of the body, but is not uncomfortable and is especially suited for use of the patient who must remain in bed.

The hospital gown permits easy access to dressings and requires little effort on the part of the patient when it must be changed or removed during a treatment or the carrying out of a routine nursing procedure.

Patients who are not seriously ill and who do not require special treatments or nursing care should be encouraged to wear their own gowns or pajamas. Their own garments are much more attractive and are an effective means of creating a desirable mental attitude through the knowledge of improved personal appearance.

The Ambulatory Patient. If the newly admitted patient is permitted to be out of bed and is free to walk about, the nurse should see that he knows the location of the bathroom, the nurses' station, and toilet facilities on the department. He should also be told the location of the telephone booth if he wishes to communicate with relatives or friends by telephone.

The Serving of Food. While admitting the patient the nurse should inform him of the designated times at which meals are to be served. The patient soon learns to adjust to a mealtime which may at first seem to vary greatly from the time at which meals are served at home. If the bedpan or urinal is offered to him before mealtime the explanation should be made that such an offer is routine and made so that the meal need not be interrupted by physical demands related to elimination. He should be advised that a part of the preparation to receive his tray is washing of face and hands if he so desires.

If the hospital provides a selective diet a brief explanation as to how to mark the menu will suffice until such time as is required for the dietitian to pay him a visit, so he may express to her his likes and dislikes regarding food.

During admission, if the patient is informed of many of the routine nursing duties which are carried out each day, he will not be placed in the position of being constantly taken unaware when he is expected to do certain procedures for himself or to participate in their performance.

Available Spiritual Aid. Most patients will appreciate being informed of religious services that are available at the hospital. The amount of service will vary greatly in different institutions. In some a chapel is provided for use of patients and hospital personnel and a resident chaplain or a member of his staff may be called to see a patient at any time during the day or night. Other hospitals may not have a chapel or the full-time services of a chaplain, but will impart to the patient the information that a minister or clergyman will be asked to visit him if he so wishes.

CARE OF CLOTHING AND VALUABLES

Care of Clothing. Patients being admitted to private rooms will usually have sufficient space in clothes closet and dresser drawers to provide for suitable care of clothing which was worn or brought to the hospital. Patients admitted to wards or semi-private rooms should have their clothing sent to the central clothes room for care and storage.

The nurse who admits the patient is responsible for properly filling out the clothes list, in the presence of the patient. Both their signatures on the list attest to the accuracy of the listing. Clothing that is soiled or in need of repair should be sent home with the family. That to be stored should be placed on suitable hangers and put into a dustproof bag to be hung in the clothes room. It will be necessary to advise the patient as to the care which will be given the clothes before they are removed from his presence. If he understands that the clothes will be properly cared for and made available to him at any time he may need them he will probably be satisfied that they will not be lost or improperly handled during the time he remains in the hospital.

Provision should be made for the patient to have his own dressing robe and bedroom slippers so he may use them when permitted out of bed.

Care of Valuables. If the admitting officer has not provided for the care of valuables by suggesting that large sums of money and valuable jewelry be placed in the hospital safe, the nurse, who admits the patient to his room or ward bed, should remind him that there is no provision made to insure the safekeeping of such articles if they are kept at the bedside.

A small sum of money to provide for the purchase of newspapers, magazines, cigarettes, or other personal articles required for daily comfort should be kept by the patient, but he will have no need for large sums of money during his hospital stay.

Patients who had planned to keep valuable jewelry in their own possession when admitted should be encouraged to send it home with a responsible relative. Jewelry remaining in the patient's possession will need to be placed in the hospital safe should he be required to submit to surgical treatment or to a medical procedure which may temporarily prevent him from being entirely responsible for keeping the articles safe. While undergoing the effects of a general anesthetic or the administration of a narcotic, the patient is unable to protect his belongings for long periods of time because of complete or partial unconsciousness.

HOSPITAL VISITORS

An important part of the admission procedure is the establishment of a desirable relationship between relatives or friends of the patient and hospital personnel. Most visitors are eager to cooperate with members of the nursing staff in securing for the patient the rest and care which is needed, and they will welcome advice or instruction from the nurse as to what is desired of them.

Visiting regulations should be fully explained to family and friends and they should be made to realize the importance of being governed by those regulations so they can help rather than hinder progress of the patient toward recovery. They should be encouraged to send mail to the patient since letters or cards are always gratefully received. Mail furnishes an excellent means of communicating to the patient their interest and best wishes for his welfare without subjecting him to the emotional tension or exhausting experience of having them appear in person at a time when he should be resting or is undergoing a distressing medical or surgical procedure.

Relatives who are anxious to do something for the patient will be grateful to the nurse who is sympathetic enough to understand that their desire to be of help stems from a recognition of their inability to perform the services for him which the nurse has been trained to do. She should suggest that they express their feeling for him by sending flowers, by making certain that he has such necessities as toothbrush, razor, or comb, and that he is supplied with some of the articles that formed part of his daily routine when he was at home—articles such as newspapers, magazines, a radio, and/or a television set if he is able to enjoy them.

For the female patient numerous toilet articles such as perfume, face tissues, soap, talcum, nail polish, and lingerie aid materially in helping her to accept the experience of hospitalization.

A new book, one on the current best-seller list, has been the means of offering encouragement and entertainment to many patients and is appreciated even more when it comes as a message of good will from a friend or family member.

Visitors should be discouraged in the practice of bringing candy and other edible gifts to patients. Many times the patient is forbidden candy or is restricted from eating certain types of food. When he receives such foods from well meaning friends he is placed in an embarrassing position having to decide whether to accept the food, giving the false impression that he will eat and enjoy it, or to refuse it and perhaps cause hurt and embarrassment to the giver. If the food is left in his room he is subjected to the temptation of secretly partaking of it, especially since it seems all the more appetizing because it has been restricted or withheld from his diet.

Although as a rule visitors should not bring food to the hospital, an exception is made for the patient who is permitted practically all types of food and who needs to eat well, yet has no appetite. If food is prepared at home, and thus seems more palatable, it may be wise to have such food made available to the patient. For a child, the nurse may suggest that certain foods which he likes especially well may be brought to the hospital for use at mealtime.

OPENING THE PATIENT'S HOSPITAL RECORD

The nurse who has completed the procedure of admitting the patient and has attended to all the requirements incidental to his physical comfort and peace of mind has a final responsibility which concerns opening the chart or hospital record of the patient.

To open the chart it is necessary to have all the required forms, such as doctor's order sheet, graphic sheet, nurses' notes, etc. Headings will need to be filled in giving such information as patient's name, hospital number, name of doctor, room number, and the date. Temperature, pulse, respiration, and blood pressure should be recorded on the graphic sheet and the opening remarks should be placed on the first page of nurses' notes. In addition to T.P.R. and B.P., all data pertinent to the admission procedure for the patient should appear on the nurses' notes. Such data should contain the following information:

Date and time of admission
Manner of arrival (ambulatory, per wheelchair or stretcher)
Objective symptoms, as noted during the admission bath
Subjective symptoms, as related by the patient
The admission bath
Information in regard to specimens sent to the laboratory
Visits of the attending physician or intern
All medications and treatments given during the admission procedure.

When the admission procedure has been completed the nurse should make certain that the patient is in a comfortable position in bed, see that the room is neat and orderly, eliminate glare from lights by turning out lamps and adjusting window shades to the proper height. She should place stationery and articles for entertainment, as books, magazines, and radio, within easy reach of the patient. Unless contraindicated, a small tray with pitcher of water and a clean glass should be placed at the patient's bedside.

Through measures described above the nurse can greatly facilitate the adjustment which the patient must make to his new environment and she will experience the satisfaction that comes with knowledge of having helped to make the admission procedure a more pleasant experience for him.

Care of Equipment after Use

The thermometer is kept in the patient's room if individual thermometer technique is used. If thermometers are used for the entire department from a thermometer basket, the thermometer should be cleaned, allowed to stand for at least twenty minutes in an antiseptic solution, and then placed in a clean container along with other thermometers used in the department.

The sphygmomanometer should be returned to its proper storage place after use.

Bags used by the patient to bring personal articles and clothing to the hospital should be placed in the clothes closet in a private room and in the patient's locker in a ward.

Clothing should be checked and sent to the clothing room for proper handling and care during the time the patient is in the hospital.

Equipment used for the admission bath should be cared for as described in Chapter 9, on Cleansing Baths—Personal Hygiene—Routine Care.

Summary of Important Factors

The patient may be experiencing fear, worry, depression, and resentment, and his behavior is apt to be quite different from normal.

The nurse should be introduced or should introduce herself to the patient.

Relatives should be treated with kindness and consideration—An explanation in regard to visiting regulations should be given to them.

The nursing procedures required for admission of a patient include: recording temperature, pulse, respiration, and blood pressure; collection of urine specimen; admission bath; care of clothing and valuables; opening the chart; providing fresh water at bedside, and making patient comfortable.

Cooperation of the patient may be gained by explaining each procedure before it is performed.

The patient should be informed in regard to his immediate surroundings (bedside table and its equipment), use of the signal bell, the time meals are served, and the various nursing procedures that make up the daily routine. The nurse should mention religious service that is available but should not urge her own religious belief on the patient.

To open the patient's chart recording should include: proper headings for all forms used in the chart; date and time of admission; manner of arrival; objective and subjective symptoms; medications and treatments; specimens to laboratory; visits of attending physician or intern.

Factors To Teach the Patient

The value of cooperating with doctors and nurses to gain the utmost benefit from medications and treatments.

The mechanism of the hospital bed.

Where articles used in daily care are kept and use of unfamiliar articles.

The use of the signal bell.

Reason for wearing the hospital gown.

Daily routine of nursing procedures, as serving of meals and nourishment, bath, care of mouth, and provision for elimination.

Best method for caring for clothes and valuables during his stay in the hospital.

How to obtain available religious services or activities.

Scientific Principles

Anatomy and Physiology. Medical terms should be used in describing complaints, location of pain, or abnormalities of appearance or action.

Microbiology. Cleanliness of the patient unit should be checked before the patient is admitted.

A cleansing bath should be given as part of the admission procedure.

Disinfection of the patient's clothing may be necessary if vermin are found on the patient or on the clothing.

Treatment for pediculosis should be given if the physical examination reveals the presence of pediculi in the hair.

Pharmacology. The nurse who admits the patient is responsible for administering medications which may have been ordered for him. She should understand the relationship of drugs that are ordered to the diagnosis and condition of the patient.

Physics. The newly admitted patient should be placed in a room where the temperature is about 72° F. The room should be adequately ventilated.

Psychology. The psychological needs of the newly admitted patient should receive careful consideration from the nurse. The adjustment to the hospital environment may not be easy. An effort should be made to relieve his mind of fear and worry. Hospital routine and nursing procedures should be explained. Serving of meals, visiting regulations, and time for delivery of mail are matters about which the patient should be informed. The patient should be prepared psychologically for the physical examination and for subsequent treatments which may be ordered for him.

All actions and words of the nurse should be such that the patient will have confidence and trust in her.

Sociology. The patient is dependent on the nurse for care and attention. He looks to her for guidance in the matter of being informed as to how he can cooperate to help in his recovery.

Social problems of the foreign-born or the physically handicapped patient may become barriers to recovery and will need to be solved.

Social agencies that may be helpful to the patient or to his family can be informed of his need through the social service department at the hospital. The nurse should see that the social service worker visits the patient soon after his admission if there is indication that her services may be needed.

Situation Type Problems

1. A patient, being admitted for surgery, was assigned to a semi-private room. The other patient in the room was seriously ill following thoracic surgery. He was being given oxygen by nasal catheter, but had marked dyspnea with stertorous respiration. The newly admitted patient asked to be transferred and learned that the only other available bed was one in a 10-bed ward where there were two patients in equally serious condition. He requested that the nurse bring his clothes so he could dress and leave the hospital. What would you have done?

2. When checking the clothes list with a newly admitted patient the student nurse learned that he had a large sum of money in a wallet which he had placed in the bedside table drawer. She suggested that he might wish to have the money placed in the hospital safe and was told by the patient that "If I had wanted the money in the safe I would have put it there before coming to the department." When she asked that the amount of money be listed along with other valuables and his clothing, he refused to count the money and told her to list it as "approximately $300." What would you have done?

Suggested Reference Reading

"The patient's first hour," R. D. Yaw; Hospitals, September, 1939.

"The psychology of admission and discharge," W. N. Miller; Canadian Hospitals, July, 1946.

"The patient and his family," E. W. Hard; American Journal of Nursing, January, 1948.

"Patients are people," Editorial, American Journal of Nursing, April, 1949.

"Portrait of a patient," M. H. Saeger; American Journal of Nursing, October, 1949.

"A new admitting system," Frank A. Lynch; Hospital Management, April, 1952.

CHAPTER 14

Observation of Patient—The Hospital Record

TOPICAL OUTLINE

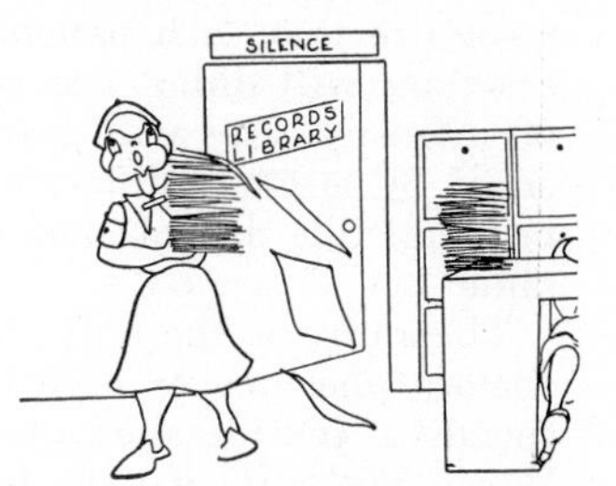

Work is a fine way to escape being bored.

Observation of the Patient

A vital factor in nursing care is intelligent observation of the patient by the nurse. Each nursing procedure performed by her is much more than a step-by-step performance of a learned technique to accomplish a particular task. It is, in reality, an opportunity for her to observe the patient, to ascertain if he reacts to medication, to treatment, or to a situation, as he is expected to react. It is a chance for her to learn to know the patient, to understand the condition of his physical, mental, and spiritual being. Through observation any change in condition (improvement or regression) may be detected, specific information that will help in diagnosis may be obtained, and results of treatment, medication, and nursing care may be determined.

If the patient's condition is undiagnosed the nurse should be informed of the suspected or probable diagnosis so she will be able to anticipate the symptoms which are apt to appear.

OBSERVATION–THE NURSE'S RESPONSIBILITY

To observe is "to watch carefully"—and careful watching of a patient is one of the nurse's chief responsibilities. The many hours of classwork included in her course of study are meant to give her the knowledge required for meaningful observation.

Experience in methods of observation may be gained by the student nurse through hours spent in clinical practice. Performing nursing procedures, under supervision, provides her with an opportunity to gain skill in observing, in accurately interpreting that which is observed, and in knowing the proper course of action to follow.

Because "no two patients are alike," the nurse cannot learn from a book all the observations which can and should be made. She must recognize that each patient is different from all other patients, that reactions will differ, and symptoms will vary in kind and in degree of intensity. She will learn that the patient may be greatly influenced by so many different factors that observation one day may not be at all like that of another day, although the situation may be the same.

The nurse is the only member of the health team, including the doctor, pharmacist, dietitian, social worker, and technician, who spends a considerable amount of time with the patient each day. While with the patient for prolonged periods of time she is in a position to observe, to report her observations, and thus to aid the doctor in making a diagnosis. Accurate observations made by the nurse are needed in planning the course of treatment and preventing complications. Such observations may also play an important part in the prevention of disease.

To observe intelligently the nurse must learn to know her patient as a person, to recognize the individual as a characteristic product of his own particular family background, education, and experiences. She must have a thorough knowledge of the usual signs and symptoms of disease and know what to expect or "watch for" in closely observing each patient.

When a nurse is assigned to give care to a patient she assumes responsibility for his welfare. By promptly reporting symptoms to the doctor she may prevent the development of undesirable complications and may even save the life of the patient.

By keen observation and accurate reporting of her observations she may aid in making a diagnosis and in determining the best course of treatment. If she is observant of the convalescent patient she may prevent undue fatigue or strain and be the means of greatly reducing the time which must be spent in regaining health and vitality.

Responsibility for observation on the part of the nurse is not confined entirely to concern for a hospital patient. She should be taught to use her powers of observation to promote health and prevent disease in her own immediate surroundings of home and community. She should be aware of early signs or symptoms of physical or mental impairment in those with whom she comes in contact and encourage them to secure needed medical treatment to prevent spread of dis-

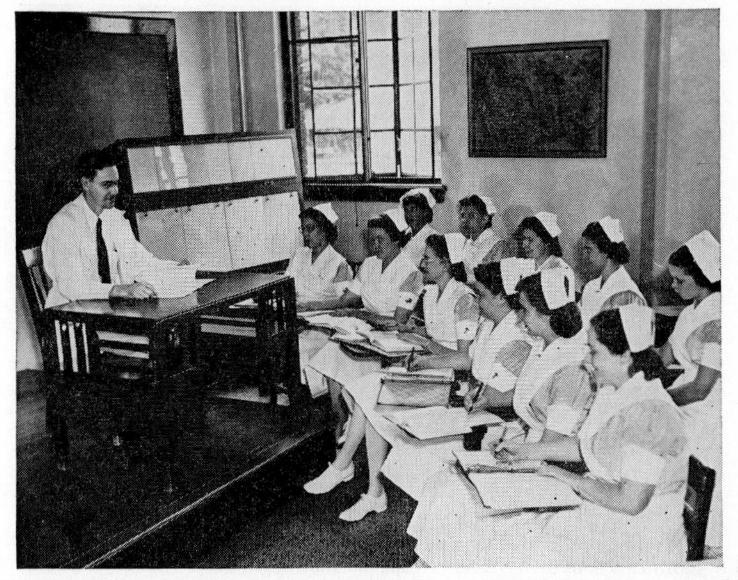

Fig. 95. To be of value, observation must be considered with reference to information obtained in the classroom. (Methodist Hospital School of Nursing, Indianapolis, Indiana.)

ease. She should know and practice good health habits for herself and be a teacher of health and of personal hygiene for others.

In addition to knowing the general effects of the disease, she should know the kind of person the patient is and the effect, mentally as well as physically, the disease may have on *him*. To assist the physician in effective treatment she must keep him informed of signs of improvement or of complications. She must be continually aware of symptoms and be able to describe accurately certain definite characteristics of those symptoms. She will need to recognize signs or symptoms that may appear unexpectedly and require immediate treatment to avoid serious developments.

The nurse is responsible, too, for advising the patient of the inherent danger of self-medication. Pain and discomfort are often the first warning signs of a beginning disease process. Taking drugs without seeking advice from the doctor may relieve the pain or undesirable symptoms temporarily, but will do nothing to check the disease or to overcome the condition producing the symptoms.

Observation is of value only when considered with reference to background information and knowledge of what to expect as the disease progresses and therapy is continued. To give intelligent nursing care the nurse must have information which will help her to understand the patient and to better interpret that which she observes.

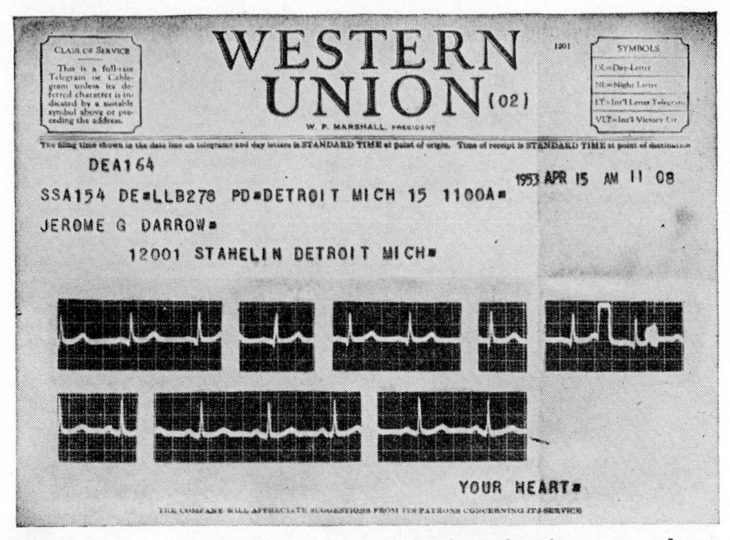

CLASS OF SERVICE
This is a full-rate Telegram or Cablegram unless its deferred character is indicated by a suitable symbol above or preceding the address.

WESTERN UNION (02)

W. P. MARSHALL, PRESIDENT

SYMBOLS
DL=Day Letter
NL=Night Letter
LT=Int'l Letter Telegram
VLT=Int'l Victory Ltr

The filing time shown in the date line on telegrams and day letters is STANDARD TIME at point of origin. Time of receipt is STANDARD TIME at point of destination

DEA164

1953 APR 15 AM 11 08

SSA154 DE=LLB278 PD=DETROIT MICH 15 1100A=

JEROME G DARROW=

12001 STAHELIN DETROIT MICH=

YOUR HEART=

THE COMPANY WILL APPRECIATE SUGGESTIONS FROM ITS PATRONS CONCERNING ITS SERVICE

Fig. 96. The student who knows the normal values of various tests understands the significance of a deviation from normal. (Parke, Davis & Co., Detroit, Michigan.)

SOURCES OF INFORMATION

The information necessary to understanding of a patient and giving intelligent nursing care may be obtained largely through definite procedures set up routinely in most hospitals. Sources of information concerning the patient include:

The Patient's Chart. The admission record, which is part of the patient's chart, is always a valuable source of information, giving such vital statistics as age, nationality, race, religion, marital status, and occupation. The patient's chart also contains the social history record, which provides detailed information regarding family, financial standard of living, and the patient's interests and activities when in normal health.

The medical history gives information on the health of the family in general and the patient in particular. If present illness is related to past illnesses or to a previous hospitalization, that fact will be noted.

Laboratory reports are an important source of information for the nurse. If she knows the normal values of tests that have been made, and the significance of deviations from normal, she will know the symptoms that may be expected to appear and will be better able to help prevent undesirable complications.

Progress records containing notations made by the attending physician and the nurses' notes, notations made by all nurses caring for

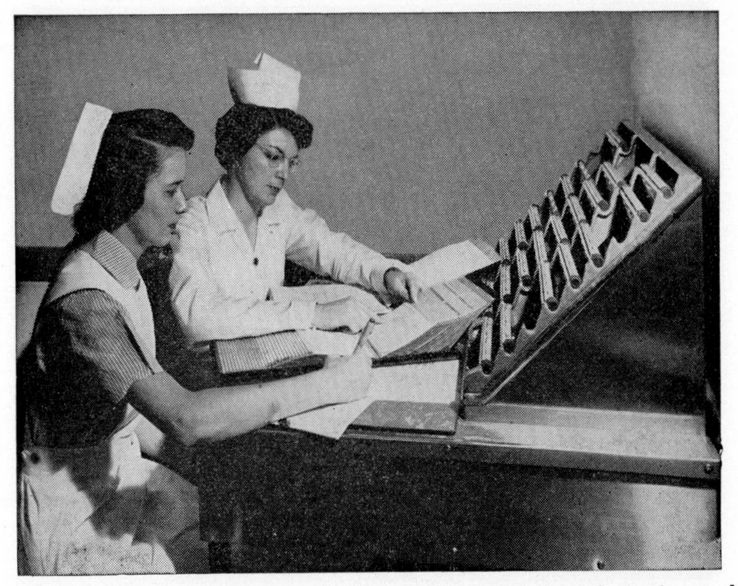

Fig. 97. Each order written by the doctor gives additional information to the nurse which helps her to observe the patient intelligently. (Presbyterian Hospital School of Nursing, Pittsburgh, Pennsylvania.)

the patient, including her own as well as those of the night nurse and others, keep her well informed as to changes in the daily condition of the patient.

Doctor's Orders. Each new order for medication or treatment provides further information helpful to the nurse in observing the patient. If she knows the expected result of therapeutic measures that are ordered she can watch the patient closely for indications of that result or for symptoms that would indicate deviation from the expected or usual effect of treatment or medication.

Information Obtained from the Patient. By tactfully questioning the patient with reference to information already known about him and his condition the nurse may make important additions to knowledge already obtained. It is largely through conversation with him that she may more accurately interpret indications of fear, worry, pain, restlessness, and other characteristic signs and symptoms worthy of note.

SIGNS

Although the term "sign" may be used interchangeably with "symptom" it usually denotes objective symptoms that are made apparent by special methods of examination. Vital signs, so called

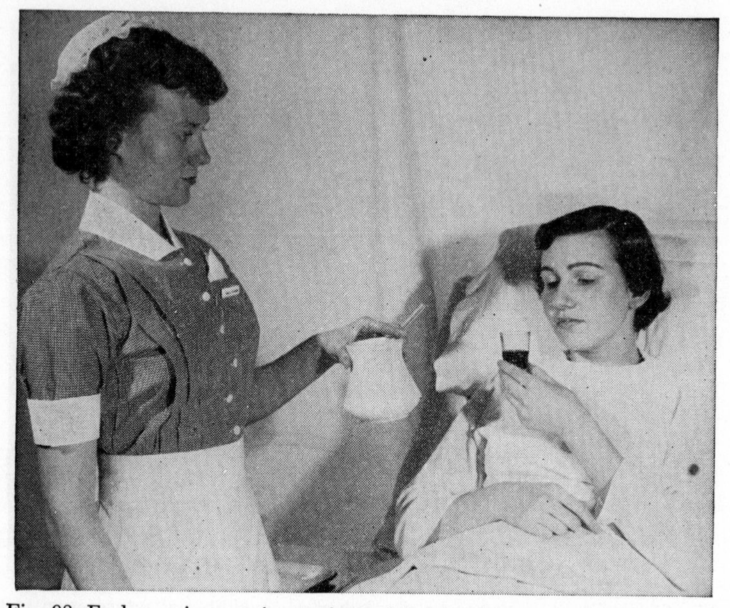

Fig. 98. Each nursing service performed for the patient provides opportunity for observation. (Massachusetts General Hospital School of Nursing, Boston, Massachusetts.)

because they have a significance in health as well as in sickness, include temperature, pulse, respiration, and blood pressure. These signs are discussed fully in Chapters 21 and 22. Vital signs may vary only slightly in health. In sickness, marked variation of any one of these signs becomes an important factor in diagnosis and in determining progress made by the disease process or effectiveness of treatment and medications being used to combat the disease.

SYMPTOMS

A symptom may be defined as any disorder of appearance, sensation, or function experienced by the patient. It may be indicative of a certain type of disease, or of a certain phase of a disease.

The nurse needs to be constantly observant as to symptoms in order to detect, and to report to the physician, any change in condition of the patient. Through experience the student nurse learns to anticipate certain signs and symptoms in observing a patient and to recognize the symptoms which are related to the disease and which may be of importance from the standpoint of medication and treatment.

Classification. Symptoms are classified in a number of different ways and are often grouped according to their relationship to a cer-

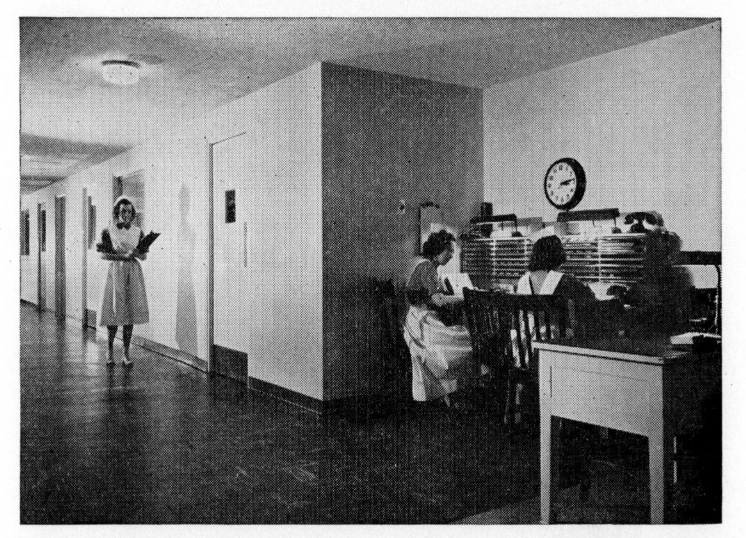

Fig. 99. Cardinal symptoms should be recorded immediately after temperature, pulse, respiration, or blood pressure has been taken. (Presbyterian Hospital School of Nursing, Chicago, Illinois.)

tain phase or stage of disease, the organ or part of the body affected, or as they pertain to treatment and nursing care.

Symptoms may be classified into three main groups as objective, subjective, and cardinal symptoms.

Objective Symptoms. Objective symptoms are those readily observed by the nurse or doctor, symptoms that are perceptible to others as well as to the patient (as pallor of the skin).

Subjective Symptoms. Subjective symptoms are those apparent only to the patient, which are made known to the nurse and doctor only through complaints of the patient (as pain or discomfort).

Cardinal Symptoms. Cardinal symptoms are variations from normal in temperature, pulse, respiration, and blood pressure.

Another classification is that which would include Familial Symptoms and Social Symptoms.

Familial Symptoms. Familial symptoms are those peculiar to a certain family and may indicate a definite predisposition toward a certain physical condition (as a cough or tendency toward or susceptibility to tuberculosis).

Social Symptoms. Social symptoms are those which result from social standing of the family and are concerned with environmental factors (such as poor housing, lack of proper food, etc.).

Symptoms may be classified according to the extent of the body which they involve.

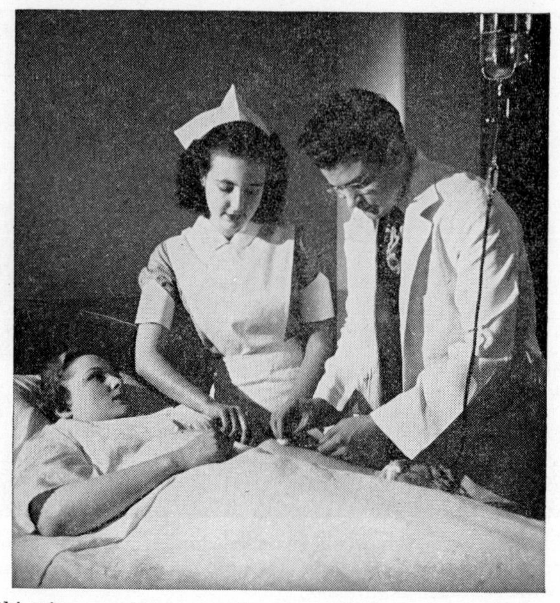

Fig. 100. Objective symptoms, as pallor, are readily apparent to the doctor and the nurse. (State University of Iowa College of Nursing, Iowa City, Iowa.)

General Symptoms. General symptoms are those affecting or pertaining to the whole body (as fever).

Local Symptoms. Local symptoms are those affecting or confined to one certain part or area of the body (as swelling).

Symptoms may also be classified as *physical,* those pertaining to the physical condition of the patient (as hunger), and *mental,* those originating in disorders of the mind (as fear and worry).

Other classifications of symptoms are concerned with certain characteristics of the disease process and are described by the term used in identifying them. Such symptoms are termed "Characteristic symptoms."

Descriptive Terminology. A few of the most common types of symptoms are listed and defined in the following paragraphs.

Characteristic Symptom. One which indicates the presence of a certain disease or is usually made apparent by administration of a certain drug.

Induced Symptom. One produced intentionally to aid in diagnosis or treatment.

Premonitory Symptom. A sensation which gives warning of the approach of a morbid condition, as of an epileptic seizure.

Presenting Symptom. The symptom, or group of symptoms, of

which the patient complains most often, or which is the immediate cause of his seeking medical advice.

Prodromal Symptom. One which indicates oncoming disease.

Withdrawal Symptom. The manifestation produced by sudden removal of a customary stimulant.

Other descriptive terms used to indicate types of symptoms are usually self-explanatory and used for the purpose of differentiation in speaking of several symptoms or groups of symptoms.

Objective Symptoms. Objective symptoms, which are readily observed by the nurse and doctor, are directly related to the physical appearance and condition of the patient, to variations from normal values in regard to secretions and excretions, and to positions of the body which have come to be characteristic of certain diseases.

Symptoms related to physical appearance and condition are usually noted by the doctor during physical examination and are apparent to the nurse as she performs routine nursing procedures.

Pertinent items of appearance and physical condition which should be observed, and recorded are discussed in the following paragraphs and include factors listed below.

Head and Face. Position, size, and shape, especially if there is variation from normal; skin coloring (pale, cyanotic, flushed, jaundiced); presence of swellings, abrasions, contusions, or lacerations; ease of movement of the head; muscle spasms or paralysis; facial expression—fear, anxiety, worry, pain, fatigue, and other subjective symptoms may be made apparent by expression on the face of the patient. Lack of expression may be equally significant as an indication of attitude or of the presence of a brain lesion.

The Eyes. Sensitiveness to light, puffiness, presence of dark circles beneath the eyes; vision—lack of vision, or blurring of vision; movements of the eyeball, and whether it appears to be sunken or protruding; if lids are drooping, swollen, reddened, or show tremor; condition of the pupils, whether contracted or dilated, equal or unequal accommodation; degree of lacrimation or of discharge, if present; color of the conjunctiva and sclera.

The Ears. Pain, tenderness, or swelling in or about the ears; complaints of tinnitus (ringing in the ears); presence of discharge from the ears.

The Nose. Any abnormality of shape (enlarged, deformed, edematous) or coloring (reddened); difficulty in breathing; impairment in sense of smell.

The Lips. Coloring (pale, cyanotic); appearance (dry, cracked, edematous, presence of lesions).

The Breath. Odor (sweet, ammoniacal, sour, fetid, alcohol—characteristic of certain disease conditions); type of respiration.

The Teeth. Whether in good condition or loose, decayed, showing lack of care; presence of partial or complete denture.

Mouth and Gums. Presence of sordes, ulceration, infection, edema,

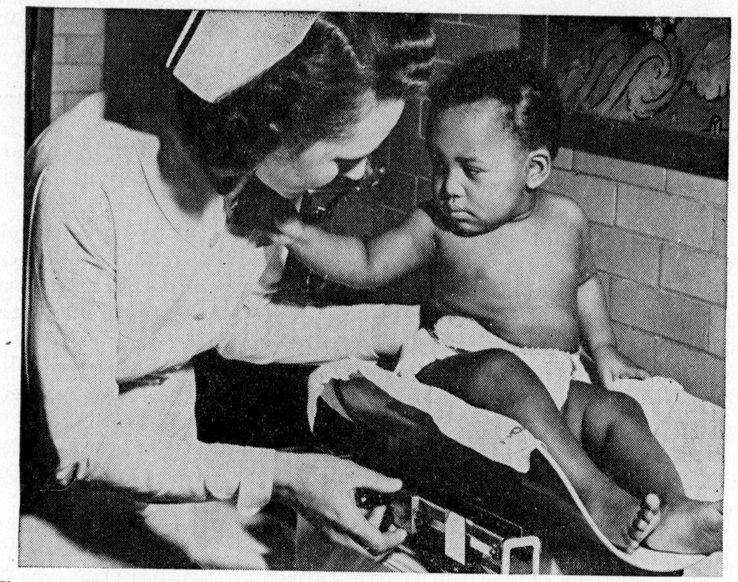

Fig. 101. Odor of the breath, easily detected by the nurse, may be a very important symptom. (Rochester General Hospital, Rochester, New York.)

bleeding; color (pale, highly inflamed); any unusual abnormality or marking.

The Tongue. Color (normal or pale, brown or gray with furred appearance); note if coated; presence of patches, fissures, scars.

The Throat. Presence of redness, swelling, ulceration, discharge; hoarseness or difficulty in swallowing; note if tonsils are present and whether diseased or healthy.

The Neck. Abnormalities (swellings, growths); restricted movement.

The Chest. Abnormalities of size, shape; presence of coughing or expectoration; abnormalities of breathing.

The Breasts. Abnormalities of size and shape; presence of undiagnosed lumps or growths; nipples (normal or inverted).

The Abdomen. Whether distended, rigid, soft, enlarged, or bulging in certain areas; appearance of skin (marked, discolored, shiny); emesis—associated with abdominal disturbances.

The Extremities. Shape of fingers (long, tapering, clubbed); nails (pale, cyanotic, brittle, broken); if hands are restless, trembling, fat, or extremely thin; condition of joints (enlarged, swollen, deformed); legs (varicosities, deformities, edema); feet (deformities, presence of corns, symptoms of circulatory disturbances).

Condition of the Skin. Presence of abrasions, ulcers, scratches, wounds, scars, rashes; edema—pressure areas; whether warm, dry, hot, cold, clammy; abnormal color (pale, cyanotic, reddened, jaundiced).

Reflexes. Common reflex actions, motor responses to stimulation, tested during physical examination, indicate to the physician disturbances of nerve function or of muscular activity. The nature of the disturbance and possible cause may be largely determined by deviation from normal reflex action.

Posture. Postures which the body may assume in various diseases, usually to afford relief from pressure or pain, may be important in diagnosis and should be observed by the examining physician or by the nurse in giving routine care to the patient.

Some of the commonly noted postures are: *coiled posture* (on one side, with legs drawn up against the body in a rigid position for relief of pain, as in renal colic); *dorsal inertia posture* (on back, slipping down in the bed, showing great weakness, as in typhoid); *dorsal rigid posture* (on back with both legs drawn up tightly against the body, as in peritonitis; right leg drawn up to relieve pain on right side, as in appendicitis); *orthopnea posture* (sitting upright with hands or elbows supported by table or pillows—a position made necessary by dyspnea or other conditions, as late stages of heart disease).

Other postures have been noted and classified so that posture is an important objective symptom and often one of the first to indicate a probable diagnosis. Any unusual posture or attitude of the body should be observed by the nurse and reported to the physician if he is not already aware of it.

Discharges and Excretions. Certain characteristics of discharges or of normal body excretions should be noted, as: *vaginal discharge* (amount, color, odor, and consistency); *vomitus* (amount, color, odor, and consistency; presence of undigested food); *urine, perspiration, sputum, feces* (amount, color, odor, and consistency; pain on urination or defecation; presence of foreign matter or parasites in feces).

Subjective Symptoms. Subjective symptoms, felt or perceived only by the patient and not apparent to the observer except through the facial expression or complaints of the patient, may usually be classified into two main groups according to cause. The first group includes feelings or sensations produced by physical causes within the body, physical causes not known or observed by the doctor. The second group includes symptoms produced in part or wholly by the patient's imagination.

Subjective symptoms are also classified into three groups, as: (1) pain and tenderness; (2) other sensations; and (3) emotions.

Pain and Tenderness. Pain is the most important of all subjective symptoms. It is an indication that normal body functioning is disturbed and corrective measures may be necessary. Pain may often indicate the location of the affected organ or part. In some instances,

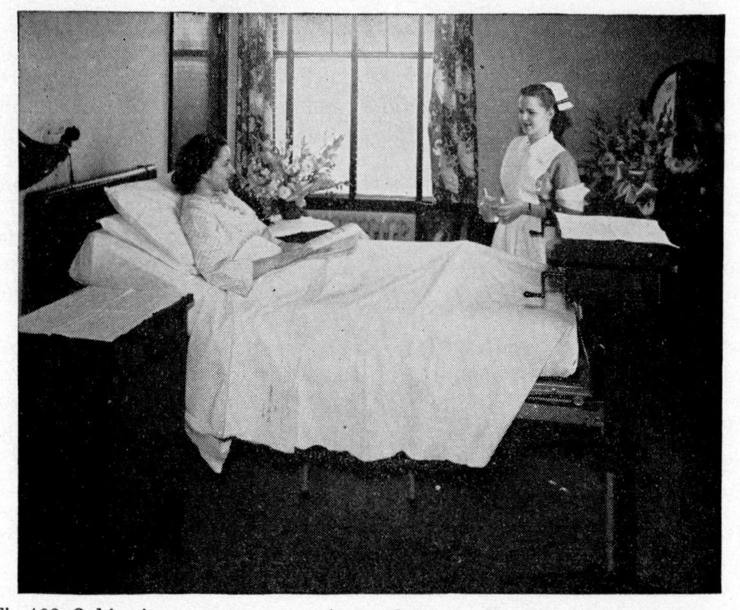

Fig 102. Subjective symptoms, as pain, are known only to the nurse if the patient complains. (Norwegian American Hospital School of Nursing, Chicago, Illinois.)

however, pain may be a misleading symptom, because it can be referred or felt in an area located some distance from the affected region or part.

Pain is the sensation produced by stimulation of certain special nerve endings or by overstimulation of a sensory nerve. The immediate reaction on the part of the patient is desire to escape from the pain. Because of the intensity of that desire, the patient will dread or fear any procedure which is likely to produce pain.

Pain may vary in intensity from slight to excessive. It may be variable in nature from dull and aching to acute or sharp. It may be continuous or occur only in paroxysms. In reporting pain the nurse should accurately describe its character, duration, location, and intensity.

Tenderness is a form of pain and soreness elicited by contact or pressure. The patient may be unaware that a part is tender until sharper pain is produced by the examining hands of the doctor or by pressure from appliances or from his own body weight.

Other Sensations. Sensation is a mental impression or perception produced by stimulation of certain nerve endings. The most important sensations, beside pain and tenderness, and the five senses of sight, taste, smell, hearing, and touch and pressure, are those of temperature, hunger and thirst, weight resistance or muscle sense, equilibrium, and those concerned with visceral and sexual sensations.

To understand subjective symptoms the nurse must recognize that such symptoms depend largely on the patient's ability to feel or to perceive and recognize the many different sensations. The nurse needs to know that afferent or sensory nerve fibers convey impulses from sense organs to the reflex centers or to centers in the brain. She should know, in a general way, that stimulation of fibers of the sympathetic nervous system usually results in constriction of blood vessels in the part, a rise in blood pressure, dilation of the pupils, secretion of small amounts of thickened saliva, increased heart activity, and decreased activity of the gastrointestinal tract. Stimulation of fibers of parasympathetic nervous system causes dilation of blood vessels in the part, lowered blood pressure, contraction of the pupils, copious secretion of thin saliva, increased gastrointestinal activity, and decreased heart activity. The action of the nervous system as a whole is preservation of the needed balance of nervous activity within the body, stimulation by one part being accompanied by inhibition of another.

Any distortion of the sensations listed above should be reported, in the patient's own words, so that his description of symptoms may be understood and evaluated in relation to his own personality—the kind of person he seems to be and whether he tends to exaggerate or minimize subjective symptoms.

Various instruments used in physical examination, as the stethoscope, ophthalmoscope, and sphygmomanometer, supplement the work of the senses of the examiner and give more accurate findings. The thermometer accurately measures the degree of fever for the patient who experiences the sensation of increased body temperature but is unable to accurately determine the extent of increase.

Emotions. "Emotion" is a term used to denote a "disturbance of feelings," or "a form of mental excitement." Emotions have a marked effect on mental powers, often interfering with judgment or reasoning and resulting in great exaggeration of symptoms. The nurse must recognize the temperament of the patient and evaluate subjective symptoms accordingly.

Symptoms frequently occurring in association with a mental state and not originating from known organic lesions or abnormalities include hysteria, delirium, delusions, hallucinations, illusions, and phobias.

Various phobias are given names which indicate that of which the patient is afraid, as claustrophobia, an unreasonable or unnatural fear of being in a closed room.

Symptoms That Require Reporting. Reporting of symptoms is just as important as to be aware of them. Through observation, the nurse must understand and recognize those symptoms that should always be reported. Only when the doctor learns of a symptom can the way be opened for action or treatment which is the primary purpose of intelligent observation.

Any abnormality of activity or function must be reported as should conditions marked by all symptoms: (1) that are severe or marked by great degree of intensity; (2) that persist over a long period of time; (3) that indicate a change in the condition of the patient; (4) that indicate an impairment in, or loss of, function of an organ or part; (5) that result from lack of health practices or from faulty health habits; (6) that are deviations from normal; (7) that recur at regular or stated intervals; (8) that become progressively more severe; (9) that are known to be present at the onset of certain diseases; (10) that indicate development of complications; (11) that show fear, anxiety, or other form of mental disturbance which the doctor may be able to help overcome; (12) which require treatment beyond that provided by ordinary nursing procedures.

The Patient's Hospital Record

Many articles and books have been written on the subject of the patient's hospital record and on charting, especially with reference to "Nurses' Notes." The pages on the chart that bear the heading "Nurses' Notes" contain notations relative to observations made by the nurse as she gives nursing care to the patient.

Nurses' notes are only a small part of the over-all record compiled for the patient during his stay in the hospital, and to properly evaluate their importance the nurse must understand the chart as a complete record. She should know the chief purposes for maintaining a hospital record for each patient, in order to grasp the importance of the notes which she may add to that record.

PURPOSES SERVED BY THE PATIENT'S CHART

The patient's chart serves the following purposes: to provide an accurate and detailed account of treatments and care given the patient and to furnish a guide for future care.

In event of transfer to another department or institution, or of change of doctors, the chart provides a complete record of past medical findings and the kind of treatment given.

Patient charts furnish the hospital with needed vital statistics and give information needed to evaluate the service it renders the community in which it is located.

The chart provides an accurate record of the results of medication and treatment and keeps the physician informed as to the patient's condition.

The chart furnishes reference material for research work, for ad-

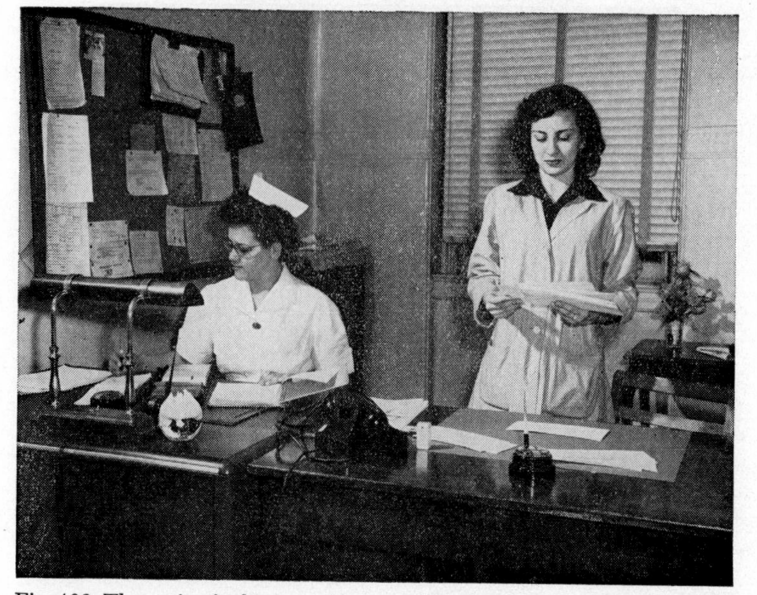

Fig. 103. The patient's chart provides a needed record from which assignments may be made to non-professional nursing personnel. (Presbyterian Hospital, Chicago, Illinois.)

vancement in methods of diagnosis and treatment, and for teaching of doctors, nurses, and other hospital personnel.

It provides important evidence in legal matters, as for litigation arising from malpractice.

Patient charts furnish a means for the community to be advised of its own public health problems and to help point the way to a solution of such problems.

Although the patient's hospital chart is made up of many different records, such as the record of personal history, of medical history, of results of diagnostic tests, and of findings in physical examination, the record of nursing care is of utmost importance.

Because the notations made by the nurse are of help in making the diagnosis and in evaluating treatment, their significance and value to the doctor has long been recognized.

In an effort to make nurses' notes complete and meaningful, student nurses have been instructed, in previous years, to make notations that are complete and detailed. As a result, nurses' notes have sometimes grown to great volume in a single chart and have contained detailed information in regard to routine nursing procedures such as bath and backrub, which are important in providing comfort

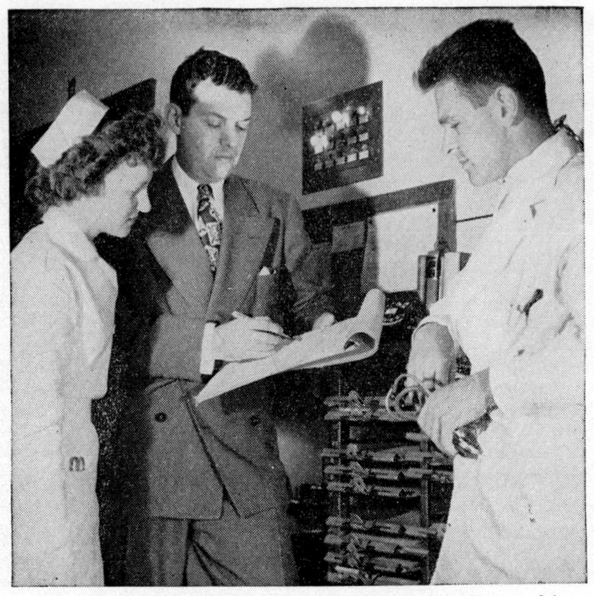

Fig. 104. The patient's chart furnishes material for the teaching of doctors, nurses, and other hospital personnel. (Michael Reese Hospital School of Nursing, Chicago, Illinois.)

for the patient, but should not be considered important enough to be given a great deal of space on the chart.

The phrase "Routine Care" takes little space in the nurses' notes, requires only a few seconds of time for recording, and includes all routine daily procedures. Doctors and nurses and other members of the hospital staff should be advised as to the specific procedures, as bath, backrub, care of unit, etc., which the term "Routine Care" would include. And all personnel should understand that any unusual reaction to a treatment or change in symptoms or condition of the patient would not be "routine" and should be recorded fully.

Some hospitals have evolved their own method of simplifying nurses' notes and have developed suitable records for their own use. Whatever the method used to reduce charting time and charting notations, it should be flexible enough to permit detailed and accurate recording of all procedures or treatments necessary for the care of the critically ill patient or the patient who has undergone major surgery and whose medical and nursing care for the first few postoperative days cannot be termed "Routine Care."

Regardless of the kind of nurses' notes record in use, whether it be very brief and used only for special care, or consists of detailed and sometimes unnecessary notations, there are a few basic rules that apply to charting. The student should be familiar with the basic requirements of charting and should be guided by the basic rules of charting. An effective means of teaching the student the fundamentals of charting is through the use of a charting manual which not only gives charting rules and requirements, but shows sample pages of correctly recorded notations for most nursing procedures.*

Summary of Important Factors

The nurse must watch the patient closely for symptoms she may need to report which will be helpful in diagnosis and in planning treatment.

Observation is primarily the nurse's responsibility, since she spends more time with the patient than do other personnel of the hospital.

The patient's chart, doctor's progress notes and orders, and laboratory reports furnish information that will help the nurse to know the patient better and to observe him with more intelligence and understanding.

Tactful questioning of the patient is another means of gaining information.

Subjective symptoms are those apparent only to the patient.

Objective symptoms are those observed by doctor or nurse.

Cardinal symptoms are those pertaining to temperature, pulse, respiration, and blood pressure.

Symptoms originating in emotional disturbances are just as real to the patient as those produced by organic disorder.

The chief purpose of observation is recognition of symptoms so that action may be taken to prevent greater disorders or disturbances which might be disastrous for the patient.

Factors To Teach the Patient

The importance of accurate description of subjective symptoms, since they help in making a diagnosis and may largely determine the kind of treatment given.

Dangers involved in self-medication, which may serve only to disguise warning symptoms of disease.

Correction of faulty health habits which may produce undesirable symptoms.

Advantages of cooperation in furnishing information which will help the nurse to interpret observations accurately and help to assure correct diagnosis or treatment.

* "A Handbook of Charting for Student Nurses," by A. L. Price, C. V. Mosby Co., St. Louis, Mo.

Scientific Principles

Microbiology. Observation should include awareness of the patient's surroundings. Cleanliness of furnishings and equipment used in the care of the patient is essential.

Pharmacology. The use of drugs to relieve distressing symptoms can be effective only if the nurse has accurately observed and reported those symptoms.

Physics. Awareness of patient's environment should include careful observation to insure correct ventilation, lighting, and temperature of the room or unit.

Psychology. Recognizing symptoms of mental stress and interpreting them accurately enables the nurse to understand the patient's behavior and to give more intelligent nursing service.

The depressed, apathetic patient may need some form of recreation which could be supplied by the nurse. A patient may be irritable and complaining only because of worry and anxiety which could be relieved by an understanding nurse.

Observation of the immediate surroundings of the patient may furnish a clue to his mental outlook. The patient in isolation may need special attention from the nurse, since he is subject to loneliness and a feeling of being neglected or rejected by friends and family.

Sociology. The patient's educational and cultural background are major factors in planning his recreational activities.

Patients who speak a foreign language and have difficulty understanding, or being understood, may be unable to describe subjective symptoms adequately.

Patients who have similar occupations may find they have many interests in common and can be benefited if an observant nurse makes an effort to see that they become acquainted.

Situation Type Problem

1. A student nurse who had just completed the Nursing Arts assignment which dealt with Observation—Signs—Symptoms made a special effort the following day to become very well informed about a patient assigned to her care so she could more accurately interpret observations. She questioned him about his family life, his educational background, and his religious beliefs. She asked about his financial situation, and if there was a possibility that he might lose his job as a result of his present hospitalization.

The patient became alarmed, thinking that the nurse implied his absence from work would be a prolonged absence. Convinced that the doctor had not been frank with him in suggesting that he need stay only a few days in the hospital, the patient felt that the true diagnosis of his condition was being withheld and he demanded that the attending physician be asked to visit him immediately, in spite of the fact that it was several hours before time for the physician's daily call at the hospital. What would you have done?

Suggested Reference Reading

"Training the senses in clinical observation," Agnes Barrie Meade; Trained Nurse and Hospital Review, December, 1936.

"Background of symptoms," Arlie V. Block; American Journal of Nursing, July, 1941.

"Streamlining the nurses' notes," Marion J. Wright and Donald McKinley; American Journal of Nursing, February, 1949.

"The nurse and the medical record," Betty Wood McNabb; American Journal of Nursing, February, 1949.

"Visible card file," Sister Mary Coletta, American Journal of Nursing, February, 1952.

"Simpler and better nurses' notes," Patricia Brandt; American Journal of Nursing, October, 1952.

CHAPTER 15

Physical Examination

TOPICAL OUTLINE

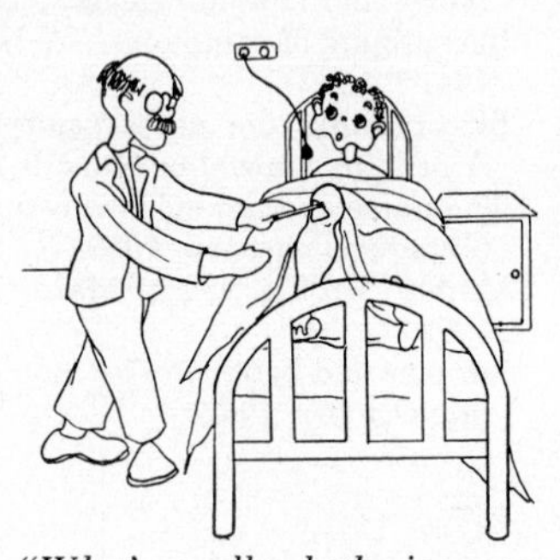

"*What's really bothering me, Doc, is a pain in the neck—but I guess there isn't much you can do about* her!"

Each person seeking hospital care usually does so on the recommendation of a physician he has consulted because of some illness or injury. He may be sent to the hospital for diagnosis, treatment, or nursing care. He may be acutely ill or experiencing only a few symptoms of beginning illness. The disorder causing the symptoms may be of mental or physical origin, or it may result from involvement of both mind and body.

The cause of the disorder may have been determined before the patient was sent to the hospital, or it may be unknown and the laboratory facilities and other diagnostic aids will be needed to identify the disease and find the causative agent.

Because of uncertainty as to what the diagnosis may be and of what may await him in the form of medical or surgical treatment, the patient is apt to be apprehensive and nervous. He may experience real fear at the possibility of diagnosis revealing a condition which could indicate only slight chance for relief of symptoms and return to health and normal living. He may be experiencing physical pain or discomfort which is augmented by mental distress at the prospect of having to undergo painful examinations or equally painful treatment procedures. His anxiety may produce such symptoms as excessive perspiration, headache, diarrhea, a need to void frequently, and cold hands or feet.

The attitude of the nurse should be that of friendly understanding and reassurance. By showing a real interest in the related account of symptoms and his complaints of pain or discomfort without displaying surprise or great concern, she can do much to allay the patient's fear. Her self-confidence and the efficiency and skill with which she performs admission procedures promote a feeling of confidence on the part of the patient and help to put him at ease.

PERSONAL AND MEDICAL HISTORY

Very soon after the patient is admitted to the hospital he will be interviewed by the attending physician or by an intern or resident physician who is a member of the hospital staff. The interview usually is carried out in a routine and orderly manner with the doctor questioning the patient so that a complete personal and medical history can be recorded.

Factors related to personal history of the patient include age, address, occupation, marital status, religion, and family history. Factors pertaining to medical history include habits of eating and sleeping, previous illnesses, operations, or accidents, chief complaint of present illness, time and description of onset of symptoms, height, weight, habits of elimination, habits of drinking or smoking, and physical activities other than those of occupation. The patient's interests, family relationships, and daily health practices are also important because of their relationship to his medical history.

Because the personal or medical history often furnishes the basis for provisional diagnosis, the interview between doctor and patient is a very important diagnostic measure. If the patient is too ill to be interviewed, much of the needed information may be obtained from a member of his family or from a friend interested in the patient's welfare.

The doctor may learn through the patient's history that he comes from a family whose members are subject to such disorders as nephritis, diabetes, tuberculosis, hypertension, allergy, or emotional instability. He may observe that the patient is subject to such occupational hazards as inhalation of dust particles, improper lighting or ventilation, abnormal temperatures, lead poisoning, or mental strain. The doctor may find by questioning the patient that he has just experienced profound emotional shock because of loss of employment, loss of a loved one, financial reverses, or failure in achievement. Such information may lead to an accurate diagnosis of the patient's physical disorder and indicate the kind of treatment and nursing care that will be most effective in bringing about recovery.

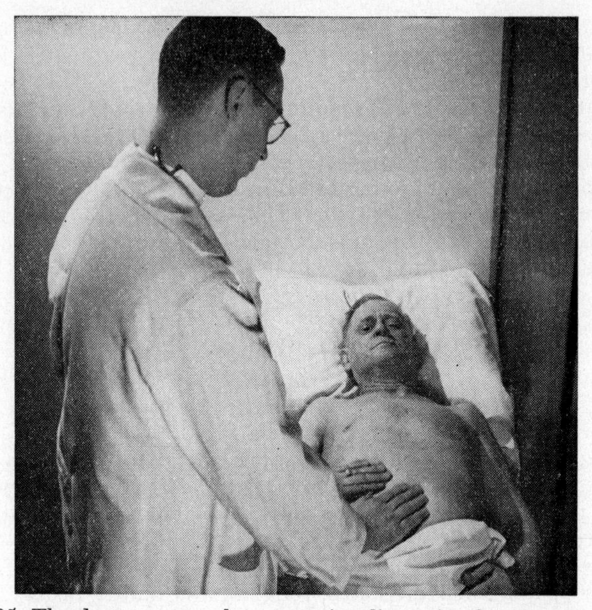

Fig. 105. The doctor may make a tentative diagnosis when interviewing the patient and through physical examination confirm that diagnosis. (Presbyterian Hospital, Chicago, Illinois.)

PREPARATION FOR EXAMINATION

Several of the nursing procedures performed during admission furnish the background of information needed for a complete physical examination. The nurse should always take and record temperature, pulse, and respiration before the doctor begins the physical examination. If the weight and height of the patient can be obtained it should be included on the physical record. The nurse should also take and record blood pressure.

A bedpan or urinal should be offered to the patient just before the physical examination. If the bladder is empty the patient will not be uncomfortable during the examination and the doctor will be better able to determine the condition of the abdomen and pelvic organs.

In addition to these procedures, the nurse should assist the patient to undress and get into bed so that the examination can be done without the interference of unnecessary articles of clothing. Even if the patient is not to be admitted to the hospital, if he is to be given an examination the preparation as described above will need to be carried out.

After the patient has been undressed he should be helped into a hospital gown or into a special examining gown provided by out-patient departments and should then be put to bed or placed on an examining table. Sufficient covers for privacy and protection from cold or drafts should always be provided.

While assisting him to undress and while performing the various other procedures related to preparation for physical examination, the nurse should advise the patient that the examining doctor will question him in regard to personal history and past medical history. She will greatly foster cooperation on the patient's part if she explains to him that such questions are a necessary and important part of the total examination. The key to diagnosis may be found in the history.

The nurse should explain just what will be done and how the doctor will go about the process of examining the patient so the latter will be more at ease, less apprehensive, and in a much better position to cooperate so the examination is conducted in a minimum amount of time and with the greatest efficiency.

When the nurse has adequately prepared the patient for examination the doctor will find that there is little need for explanation on his part as the examination progresses, and that the patient responds intelligently to suggestions in regard to positions he will need to assume and activities, such as coughing, deep breathing, and giving of verbal responses, which he will be asked to do. In some instances the doctor may examine a male patient without the assistance of the nurse. For a female patient it is essential that a nurse be present during the physical examination. The nurse serves as a necessary chaperon, as well as assistant, when a female patient is being examined.

ARTICLES USED FOR EXAMINATION

All patients on admission to the hospital are given a general physical examination and equipment for the procedure should be kept in readiness at all times. An examining tray or basket may be kept in each clinical service department, or a number of such trays may be available from a central supply service.

Each nurse should be thoroughly familiar with the contents of the examining tray so that a quick glance will assure her that all needed articles are present when the tray is taken to a room or unit for examination of a patient. Failure to check the tray may result in unnecessary delay of the procedure. An article missing from the tray when it is needed will force her to search for it in her own department or go to an adjoining department to "borrow" while doctor and patient wait for her to return.

Although examining trays or baskets may vary somewhat in different hospitals they will be basically the same, usually including the following articles: flashlight, ophthalmoscope, skin pencils, tuning

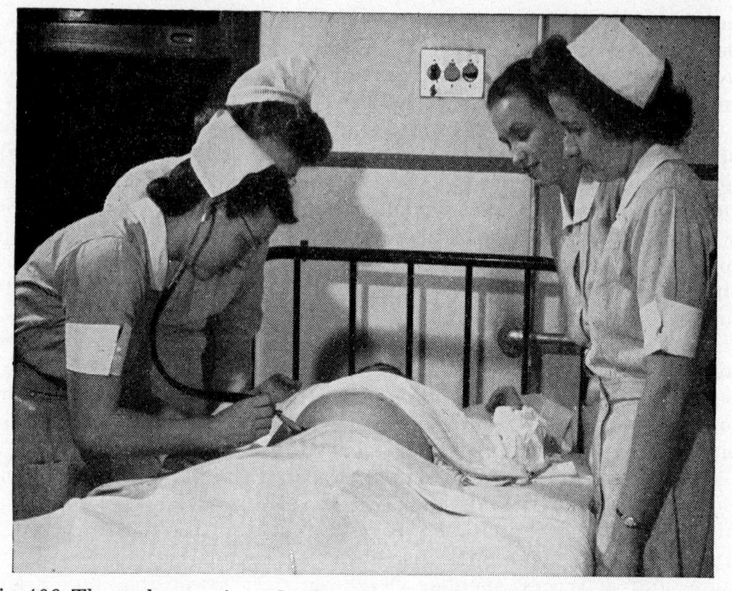

Fig. 106. The stethoscope is used to listen to sounds not readily detected by the ear alone. (Johns Hopkins Hospital School of Nursing, Baltimore, Maryland.)

fork, tongue blades, paper towels, mouthwipes, stethoscope, sphygmomanometer, percussion hammer, tape measure, small paper bags, 2 by 2 gauze sponges in antiseptic solution, safety pins.

In addition to these articles, which should be kept in the examining basket or on the examining tray, the nurse will need to see that the following articles are placed conveniently ready for use: bath blanket, emesis basin, face towel, waste basket.

METHODS USED IN EXAMINATION

Examination of the patient is usually accomplished in order, from head to foot. The doctor uses different methods of examination to determine the general condition of the patient and of various parts or organs. Several methods may be used to examine one particular part of the body, or one method may serve for examination of several parts. Methods of examination include:

1. Inspection: observation by looking closely to determine general appearance and characteristics or to detect abnormalities of structure.

2. Auscultation: listening to sounds from within the body, as a means of examining various internal organs or parts. The stethoscope is used to listen to sounds not readily detected by the ear alone.

3. Palpation: examination by feeling; use of the hands to feel or

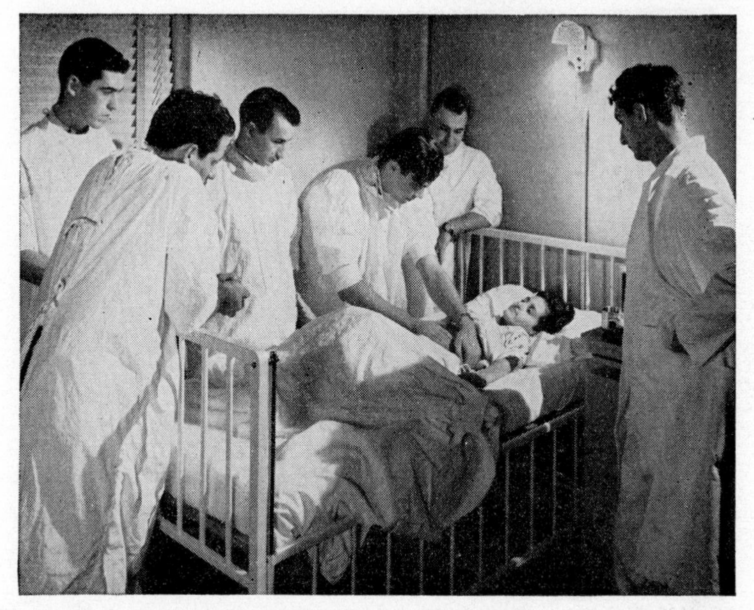

Fig. 107. Palpation is the method used to examine soft parts of the body. (Presbyterian Hospital, Chicago, Illinois.)

examine soft parts of the body and to determine relative size and condition of many glands of the body.

4. Percussion: examination by tapping with the fingers; by placing a finger of the left hand firmly against the part to be examined, as chest or abdomen, and tapping it smartly with finger tips of the right hand various resonant sounds are produced. Variation in sounds suggest different conditions that may exist in the affected area.

5. Manipulation: by moving or attempting to move the part being examined; limitations of movement are discovered by this method.

6. Testing of reflexes: considered part of a neurological examination, the testing of some reflexes is often included as part of the general physical examination. A safety pin is used to elicit abdominal and plantar reflexes; for deeper reflexes, such as that of the knee, the reflex or percussion hammer should be used.

GENERAL PHYSICAL EXAMINATION

In assisting with the examination of a patient the nurse should know whether it is to be limited to the general physical examination or is to include other specific examinations, such as the pelvic examination. She is held responsible for explaining the procedure to the patient, for

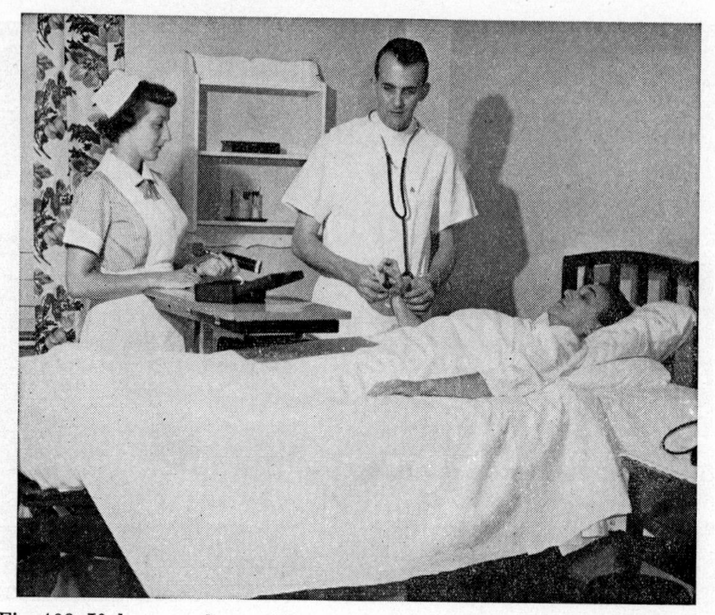

Fig. 108. If the nurse knows the procedure of physical examination she is able to anticipate the needs of the doctor. (Grant Hospital School of Nursing, Chicago, Illinois.)

assembling all the needed articles of examination, and for seeing that the patient is in the correct position and properly draped.

Although the doctor will perform the actual procedure of examining the patient, the nurse will play an active part as assistant. She should know the order of procedure so that she can anticipate and supply the needs of the doctor without undue delay.

If the patient is not in a private room the unit occupied should be screened to afford privacy during the examination. Prior to the examination, top covers should be folded to the foot of the bed, the patient should be covered with a bath blanket and gown or pajamas should be removed. At the beginning of the examination, the patient should be lying on the back in a horizontal position.

The doctor may first observe the patient's general physical condition, noting color and texture of skin, color and amount of hair, body build, and state of nutrition.

As the doctor examines the head he will need the ophthalmoscope. This particular instrument is adapted for use in examining eyes, ears, and nose, and if the nurse needs to do so she may quickly change the end pieces or specula provided as attachments and used in examination of each of the three organs named. Eyes are examined for reaction to light and accommodation, as well as for abnormality of structure or appearance. The condition of the ear drum and of the external auditory canal is noted. In examination of the nose the presence of any unusual excretion would be significant.

For examination of the throat the doctor will need the flashlight and a wooden tongue blade. Since one end of the tongue blade will be inserted into the patient's mouth and the doctor will grasp it at the opposite end the nurse should always hand it to the doctor by holding it between thumb and finger at the center. The flashlight should be turned on, then handed to the doctor so that he takes hold of it at the end opposite the lighted bulb. The used tongue blade should be discarded into the paper bag, the emesis basin, or the wastebasket. If the doctor returns the used tongue blade to the nurse she should again grasp it at the center so she need not touch the part which was in the patient's mouth.

For examination of the chest the bath blanket should be turned back exposing the patient from the waist up. For the female patient a face towel should be placed across the chest. The doctor can move it about at will so that it does not interfere with the examining process. Breasts are also examined at this time. It is not necessary that both breasts be exposed to view at the same time. Both the patient and doctor will prefer that the examination be performed with a minimum of exposure. Breasts are examined by palpation to detect abnormal growths or areas of tenderness.

If the posterior chest is examined the patient should be helped to a sitting position. The pillow should be moved down so the lower back is not exposed to view. A face towel may be held to cover the anterior chest. The head should be turned away from the doctor if the patient is asked to cough. If necessary, a paper towel may be used to prevent cough droplets from being sprayed on the doctor and nurse.

Percussion of the chest may produce sounds of dulness or other symptoms of an abnormal condition. Auscultation, with or without the stethoscope, may determine the presence of rales or other abnormal breath sounds. The size and location of the heart may be noted at this time, and skin pencil and measuring tape may be needed to outline the area.

The heart is examined by means of the stethoscope to detect murmurs or arrhythmias.

Inspection of the back for proper alignment is very quickly and easily accomplished while the patient remains in a sitting position.

When the abdomen is being examined the patient should be in a dorsal recumbent position and draped so that other parts are not unnecessarily exposed. By palpation and percussion the doctor may detect growths, tenderness, presence of fluid, and other abnormalities.

The lower extremities are examined with both being exposed to view at the same time so observation may be done on a comparative basis. Examination is made for deformity, for muscular atrophy, or for

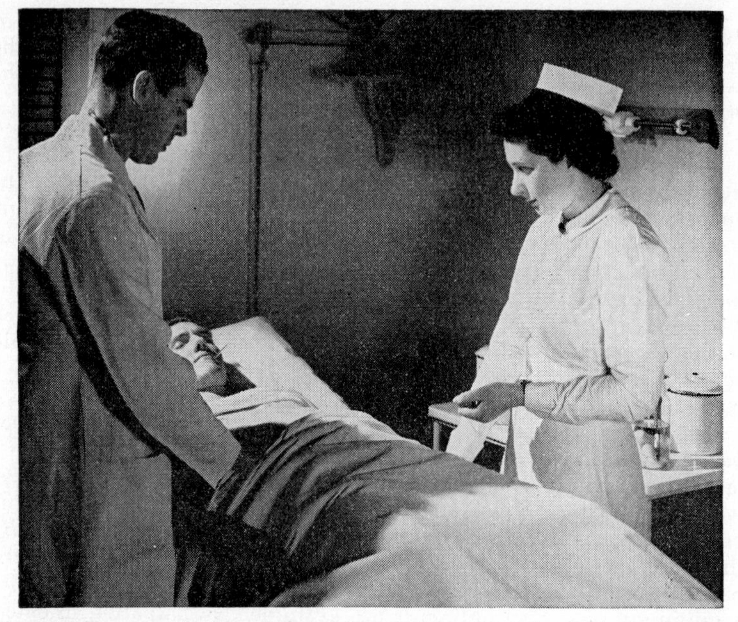

Fig. 109. For examination of the abdomen the patient should be in the dorsal recumbent position. (Presbyterian Hospital, Chicago, Illinois.)

limitation of movement. Manipulation is used in examining for joint limitation. Observation for circulatory disturbances is also a part of the examination. If reflexes are to be tested the percussion hammer will be needed.

If the doctor wishes the patient to stand for examination of the feet the nurse should see that the patient is properly draped and should place a paper towel on the footstool or on the floor so the patient's bare feet will not come in contact with an unclean surface.

PELVIC EXAMINATION

When the general physical examination is being made the doctor may often request that the patient be prepared too for a special examination, such as pelvic, which is then done as a part of the total examination.

One of the special examinations frequently included for the female patient is the vaginal examination.

Vaginal Examination. In this examination the doctor examines vulva, vagina, and various pelvic organs by observation and by digital palpation. Although the examination is not painful it may be a source of embarrassment for the patient. The nurse should explain what will be done during the examination, why it is necessary that the examination be performed, and how the patient may best cooperate so the results will be helpful in making a diagnosis or in planning treatment and nursing care.

Articles Needed for Vaginal Examination. If a vaginal examination is to be performed, a tray should be available, containing rubber gloves, powder, lubricant, vaginal speculum, and emesis basin.

Just before the examination the patient should be asked to void. The bladder must be empty to prevent discomfort to the patient and interference with the examining procedure by the doctor. The patient should be placed in the dorsal recumbent position and should be properly draped for a pelvic examination.

If the vaginal speculum is to be used, adequate lighting must be available. The light will need to be directed into the vaginal orifice to enable the doctor to satisfactorily observe the condition of the vagina and cervix. The glove which the doctor will wear should be well powdered and held properly for him. When the glove is in place, lubricant should be applied in a generous amount to the finger or fingers which will be used in doing the examination. When the examination has been completed, the glove should be removed and placed in the emesis basin until it can be properly washed and sterilized.

Rectal Examination. Examination of the rectum is usually done as a diagnostic procedure.

The patient should have a cleansing enema before examination so the rectum will be free of fecal material.

Articles Needed for Rectal Examination. The articles which should be available for rectal examination include rubber gloves, powder, lubricant, proctoscope, emesis basin, cotton balls and applicators.

The patient should void just before examination. He should be placed in the dorsal recumbent or Sims' position, and should be properly draped. If the proctoscope is to be used, it should be warmed so there will be little chance that it will cause discomfort to the patient. An adequate light must be provided for the examination. A rubber glove will be worn by the doctor to perform digital examination, and a sufficient amount of lubricant should be applied. After the examination the soiled glove should be placed in the emesis basin until it can be properly washed and sterilized.

PRIVACY FOR THE PATIENT

One of the chief responsibilities of the nurse in caring for the sick and injured is that of insuring privacy at times when privacy is indicated, and she should recognize situations in which privacy is required. An important factor in providing privacy is avoidance of embarrassment to the patient by the use of drapes to prevent unnecessary exposure of parts or of all the body.

When Privacy Is Indicated. The need for privacy depends on many variable factors, such as age, physical condition and temperament of the patient, or the treatment or procedure being done.

Growth and development of the student nurse is characterized by her increasing awareness of patient needs and her ability to recognize situations requiring her to provide or to help provide privacy. Some of the most obvious situations requiring privacy for the patient are: *during the admission procedure, during collection of a urine specimen,* or *while temperature is being taken rectally,* and *after the bedpan or urinal is given.*

Other situations in which privacy should be accorded the patient include when *giving an enema* and when doing *daily nursing procedures* of an intimate nature.

Procedures related to personal hygiene (as mouth care, baths, back rub) should not be done with visitors in the room or with other patients in a ward able to watch from their beds. Too often beginning student nurses are reluctant to ask a visitor to leave a hospital ward or room and will attempt to do routine nursing procedures with the visitor as an interested onlooker, causing needless embarrassment for the patient. The nurse should simply state to the visitor, "It is time now for Mrs. Jones to have her bath. Will you please wait in the room at the end of the corridor?" Visitors are usually eager to cooperate and will not object to being asked to leave for a short while. The nurse should be sure to let the visitor know when the procedure has been completed and she is free to return again to the patient's room.

If the patient is able to perform some daily nursing procedures for himself, such as *taking a bath,* he should be screened from view and be assured of privacy while the procedure is in progress.

For any physical examination by doctor or intern, such as *general physical examination, pelvic examination,* or *examination of any other particular organ or part,* the patient should be afforded privacy.

During examination of a male patient the doctor may be left alone with the patient unless he specifically requests the nurse to assist with the examination. If the nurse does not assist she should be sure that all needed equipment is at hand before she leaves the room.

The nurse must remain in the room or unit when the doctor is examining a female patient. Even if the patient should request that the nurse leave the room, she is obliged to stay unless dismissed by the doctor. Doctors have been embarrassed and in some instances involved in legal proceedings by the accusations of unscrupulous women who have been alone with the doctor during examination.

When treatments are being given (as change of surgical dressings), or *medical, surgical, or nursing procedures* (as catheterization) *are being performed,* the patient should be given privacy. The chief nursing duty in relation to preparation for such treatments or procedures is the placing of screens so privacy will be assured.

Privacy should be accorded the patient who has requested it in order to remain alone and undisturbed for a time, or to be with a particular person without unwanted interruption by others. *If the patient has requested that the Chaplain visit him,* he should be accorded privacy for the visit.

The patient who wishes, or needs, to rest or sleep at intervals during the day should be made comfortable, have window shades lowered, the door closed and a "NO VISITORS" sign placed on the door so he will not be disturbed.

The extremely nervous patient, especially if he is annoyed by noise or confusion, should be protected from too many visitors and from unnecessary noise.

Patients who are emotionally disturbed may be in need of privacy or may require almost continuous companionship and observation. The nurse must learn by experience when it is best to leave the patient alone and when it is essential that she remain with him.

The unconscious, the delirious, the critically ill patient requires close attention and attendance by the nurse, but should be shielded from persons not members of his immediate family or concerned with medical and nursing care.

The newly handicapped patient, one who has lost sight or hearing, who may be without hands or has suffered other physical impairment will, for a time, need the privacy which helps him to make gradually the adjustment to a radical change in his life. If he is not placed immediately with others who are handicapped in a similar way he should be protected from those who are merely curious. He needs to be given time to regain self-confidence through repeated successes in relearning simple skills required for routine daily activities. The patient who must adjust to a physical handicap should very gradually resume social activities before being released from the hospital to return to his place in the family and in the community to which he belongs.

DRAPING FOR EXAMINATION

Draping which is correctly and adequately done will add much to the comfort of the patient by preventing unnecessary embarrassment through needless exposure.

Articles used for draping for routine procedures include the bath blanket, bath towel, face towel, and sheet. For operative procedures special drapes made of cotton, of a size to be especially suitable for their purpose and sterilized and handled with sterile technique, are used. Sterile towels are used extensively, too, in draping for operative procedures.

Care must be taken in draping the patient to prevent exposure and to apply the drape so that it will not interfere with the examination or treatment to be given.

Proper draping for various positions is outlined below.

Dorsal Position. A bath blanket or sheet is spread across the patient, covering the body completely from neck and shoulders downward.

Dorsal Recumbent Position. A folded bath blanket or bath towel is placed across the patient's chest. A bath blanket is placed diagonally over the patient, so that one corner extends over the far leg and foot, another corner extends upward on the chest, the third covers the near leg and foot, and a corner lies on the bed between the legs of the patient. The far leg and foot is covered with the blanket, the corner being wrapped firmly about the foot, which is then placed flat on the bed so the blanket is held in place. The near leg and foot is covered and wrapped in the same manner. Corner four is then drawn under the rest of the blanket toward the chest, while corner two is drawn downward over the blanket to cover the perineal region. When the doctor is ready to examine the patient corner two may be lifted or drawn upward, so that the part to be examined is exposed to view.

Knee-Chest Position. A bath blanket is placed over the patient as for the dorsal recumbent position. A special treatment sheet should then be placed over the buttocks so the opening exposes the external genitalia and perineal region.

Sims' Position. The upper part of the body is covered with a folded bath blanket or bath towel. The bath blanket is placed over patient, covering the entire body from neck and shoulders downward. The upper part of the bath blanket is folded across the lower half, making the fold at lower edge of the drape covering upper part of the body. Fold upper left corner of the blanket diagonally across the patient, so that lower thigh and perineal region is exposed.

For Patient in Wheelchair. A bath blanket is folded in half and placed across the chair so that the folded edge is at the juncture of seat and back of the chair, and the blanket extends up and over the arms of the chair and downward across the support for the legs. A second bath blanket is folded and placed across the chair back so that the folded edge hangs over the back and the opposite edges reach the juncture between back and seat of the chair. When the patient is placed in the chair the lower blanket may be draped across the legs and lap of the patient, and the upper blanket over the upper part of the body, with the folded edge brought round the neck and down the front so the blanket covers shoulders and arms.

With practice the nurse soon learns to apply drapes skilfully and quickly. She should see that patients are properly draped for any procedure which requires draping, following the general rule which is applicable to all situations, that "drapes should be applied so as to keep the patient covered, yet permit a clear view and easy access to the part being examined or treated."

Care of Equipment after Use

Flashlight. Cleanse the glass end of the flashlight with a damp cloth and remove fingerprints from the body of the flashlight. Check to see that batteries are strong enough to give a good light. Be sure the light is turned off when the flashlight is no longer in use.

Ophthalmoscope. With a cotton pledget dampened with alcohol cleanse all specula or parts used with the ophthalmoscope.

Skin Pencil. See that the pencil is ready for use again.

Stethoscope. With an alcohol sponge cleanse the ear pieces and the bell part which comes in contact with the patient.

Other Equipment. The examining tray should be checked. All equipment should be ready for use, and all supplies that were used, such as paper towels, tongue blades, paper bags, safety pins, etc., should be replaced so the tray is complete when needed for another examination.

Articles used in pelvic examination should be washed, rinsed, and dried, and returned to Central Supply. Rubber gloves should be washed clear of all lubricant and of body discharge.

Summary of Important Factors

The nurse, by her manner and conversation, may do much to relieve the patient of fear and anxiety caused by hospitalization.

The physical examination for a female patient always requires the presence of a nurse. The nurse acts as chaperon as well as assistant to the doctor during the procedure.

The nurse should explain to the patient the important part personal and medical history plays in helping the doctor to make an accurate diagnosis. The patient then may be more cooperative in answering questions.

An explanation as to what the general physical examination consists of should be made to the patient by the nurse.

The nurse should be sure that all needed articles are on the examining tray before taking it to the room to assist with a general physical examination.

The female patient's reaction to the pelvic examination will depend largely on the way the nurse explains the procedure to her.

Before a pelvic examination the patient should be asked to void so the bladder will be empty.

The nurse should know the various positions used for examination or treatment, and know the correct way to drape the patient for each position.

Privacy is needed for patients in various stages of physical disorder and of mental or emotional upset.

The responsibility of properly draping the patient rests with the nurse and she should consider draping an important part of any nursing procedure which may be embarrassing to a patient if part of the body is unnecessarily exposed to view.

Factors To Teach the Patient

That a complete personal and medical history may be very helpful to the doctor in making an accurate diagnosis.

That cooperation during physical examination assures the best results.

That examination or treatment of the perineal or vulvar region need not cause a great deal of embarrassment since with the use of drapes exposure is limited.

That pelvic examination need not be painful and is a matter of daily routine for the doctor; that the examination need not cause undue embarrassment and may often help to prevent serious disorders of the genitourinary system.

That various positions may need to be assumed as a part of their treatment or care. The way to assume a necessary position.

Scientific Principles

Anatomy and Physiology. A knowledge of normal anatomy and physiology is needed for examination to discover abnormalities that may be present.

In order to help the doctor efficiently, the nurse will need to know the routine manner in which physical examination is performed so she can anticipate the doctor's needs and supply them without delay or hesitation.

The order of procedure is usually as follows: observation of general physical condition—followed by examination of head, eyes, ears, nose, throat, mouth, chest, breasts, abdomen, arms, back, lower extremities.

An understanding of the effect of various positions on different organs of the body will help the nurse to explain the need for assuming such positions for diagnostic examination or for treatment.

Chemistry. A history of dislike for milk may indicate a condition of calcium deficiency. Other factors brought out in examination or observation of the patient may bear similar relationship to diagnosis and treatment.

Microbiology. All articles used in examination must be clean.

Various parts of the ophthalmoscope should be cleansed with an antiseptic sponge immediately after use.

In examination of the chest, if the patient is instructed to cough, a paper towel should be held as a shield to prevent the spray of microorganisms from his throat.

Pharmacology. Quiet and privacy should be provided, along with the use of sedatives for rest.

Physics. Injury to tissue may be caused by pressure. Greatest pressure is made at points of bony prominences and where the greatest weight of the patient is borne, as on the buttocks in the dorsal position.

Psychology. Fear of the examination can be relieved by an understanding nurse who explains the procedure to the patient. Careful draping for examination and for procedures requiring privacy will prevent undue embarrassment to the patient.

Sociology. If physical examination reveals a condition that requires referral to an organization for further examination or continued treatment, the nurse may need to offer explanations and reassurance.

If physical findings indicate that an impairment, such as loss of vision or hearing, is apt to occur, the nurse may need to enlist the aid of the social service worker who can consult organizations such as a Blind Service Organization or similar organizations for aid to the hard of hearing.

Situation Type Problem

1. A patient who had been admitted to a medical service department for observation was given a complete physical examination by the attending physician. A senior student assisted the doctor. She had to leave the room several times to secure various articles needed for the examination. She left the room the first time to get a bulb for the flashlight which had burned out. The second trip was for a test tube, and the third for adhesive tape to reinforce a dressing which had been applied over a superficial wound by the patient prior to admission to the hospital.

When the doctor had completed the examination he angrily informed the nurse that hereafter when she assisted him in a physical examination he would expect her to have in readiness, before beginning the procedure, all the necessary articles that would be used in doing that procedure. What would you have done?

Suggested Reference Reading

"Self-examination of the breasts," American Cancer Society; American Journal of Nursing, April, 1952.

"What is a routine physical examination?" Arthur N. Jay; American Journal of Nursing, March, 1953.

"Heartburn, strange deceiver," John L. Springer; Coronet, August, 1953.

CHAPTER 16

Food Requirements and Food Service

TOPICAL OUTLINE

NORMAL NUTRITION
CLASSIFICATION OF FOOD
BASIC FOOD REQUIREMENTS
CALORIC VALUES AND REQUIREMENTS
NUTRITION IN ILLNESS
FOOD ALLERGY
STANDARD AND SPECIAL DIETS
THE NURSE'S RESPONSIBILITY IN FOOD SERVICE
- General Customs and Dietary Regulations
- To Prepare the Patient for Food Service
- Serving the Tray
- Feeding the Helpless Patient
- Feeding Infants and Children

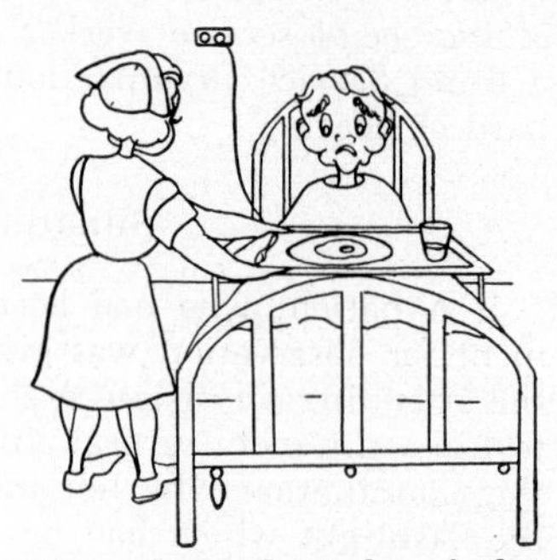

The real tragedy of ulcers is that you can have them and still not be a success!

Food has been defined as "any substance, taken into the body, that is capable of producing heat and energy, building and repairing body tissues, or regulating body processes." Nutrients or foodstuffs are chemical compounds which in various combinations make up food.

Anatomists have frequently compared the human body with its complex system of related parts and their various functions to that of the automobile, a man-made machine also of complex design and make-up. To continue such comparison, food serves as fuel to keep the machinery of man running just as certainly as gasoline serves as the energy-giving fuel for the auto. But, unlike the man-made machine whose parts must be replaced by factory-made new parts, the body of man is capable of promoting its own growth through properly balanced proportions of various food elements and, to a certain extent, of furnishing its own repairs.

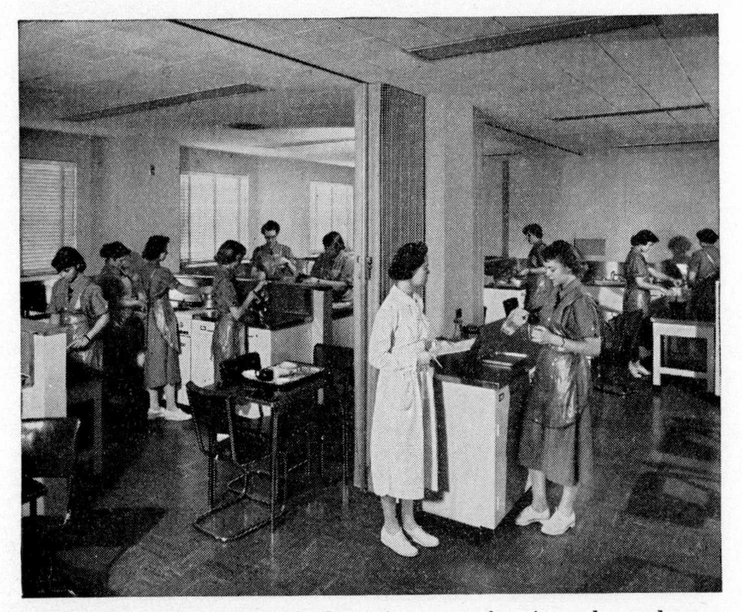

Fig. 110. To understand the food requirements of patients the student must first learn of normal nutrition. (Presbyterian Hospital School of Nursing, Chicago, Illinois.)

NORMAL NUTRITION

Nutrition, defined as "the process of nourishing or of being nourished," refers to the processes of digestion, absorption, and assimilation of food which supplies the elements necessary for growth, repair, and maintenance of healthy body tissue. Digestion is the process by which food is converted into simple substances which can be absorbed or assimilated and used by body tissues, or stored as reserve material for later use. Food taken into the body supplies energy for body activity, rebuilds body tissue, and helps to regulate all body processes.

Total nutritional needs of the body are adequately met only when the food is of sufficient quantity and proper quality (containing all essential food elements in the proper amount). Instances of inadequate nutrition or evidences of malnutrition are found in the homes of the wealthy, as well as of the poor, since food inadequacies may relate to either quantity or quality.

Health problems associated with nutritional deficiency manifest themselves through such symptoms as undue fatigue, lack of energy, nervous irritability, depressed mental state, impairment of vision, edema, poorly formed bones and teeth, and various skin diseases.

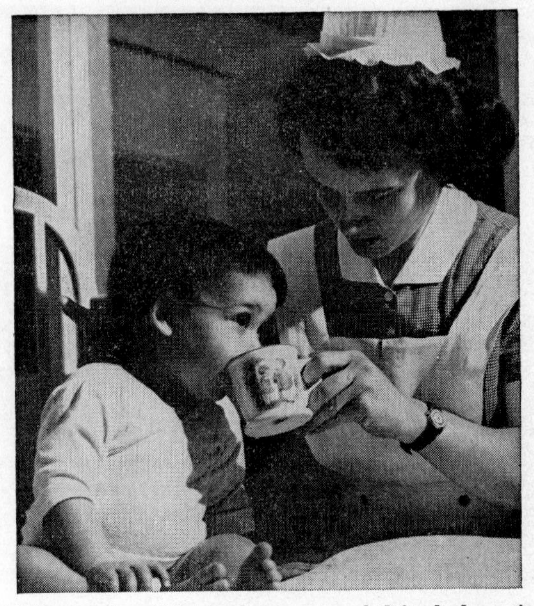

Fig. 111. Milk contains all food substances needed for body maintenance and growth. (Massachusetts General Hospital School of Nursing, Boston, Massachusetts.)

Careful attention to diet, with correction of any deficiencies, is an important factor in the treatment of many diseases.

CLASSIFICATION OF FOOD

Food may be classified in several ways: according to its chemical nature, according to its function in the body, and according to its role in regulating body processes.

According to Chemical Nature. Food is obtained from both the animal and vegetable kingdoms, and all food contains, in varying amounts, one or more of the six classes of nutritive substances, namely: carbohydrates, fats, proteins, vitamins, minerals, and water.

According to Function. Some foods contain nutritive substances in such variety that they provide for all the body needs. Milk is such a food, since it possesses needed elements for all body functions. Most foods contain only one food element in sufficient amount to answer body needs, and it is therefore necessary to eat a variety of foods regularly to supply food elements in the proportion needed each day.

Foods Which Supply Heat and Energy. Carbohydrates and fats are the two classes of chemical compounds which serve as the main sources of heat and energy. Both yield energy when oxidized in the

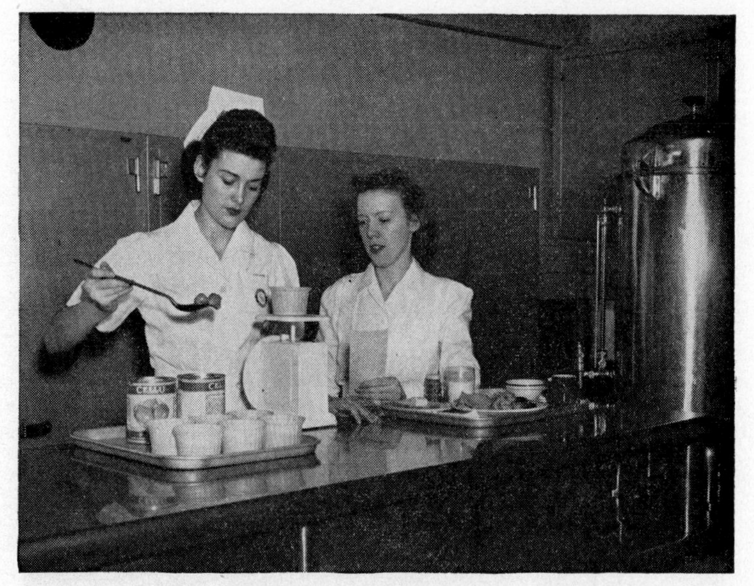

Fig. 112. Fruit is added to the diet to supply needed carbohydrates. (Charity Hospital School of Nursing, New Orleans, Louisiana.)

body, and both may be stored as reserve fuel and used or burned at a later date. Oxidation is the term used to describe the chemical process that takes place in the burning of food—the adding of a sufficient amount of oxygen to break up the compound and produce combustion or burning.

The chief sources of carbohydrates are cereals, vegetables, and fruits. The process of digestion changes the carbohydrates to simple sugars, and in that form they are taken by the blood to the liver to be stored as glycogen. With sugar always present in the blood it is readily available when needed by muscle cells for burning and for producing the energy needed in carrying out muscular activity.

So long as a balance is maintained between intake of carbohydrates and fats on the one hand and energy output on the other, a constant weight will be maintained. If more energy is expended than is provided for by intake, the individual will lose weight. If the intake of carbohydrate and fat exceeds the amount used to supply energy, they will be converted into fat and stored as adipose tissue, and the individual will gain in weight.

The chief sources of fats are milk, cream, butter, vegetable oils, and nuts. During digestion fats are split into fatty acids and glycerol. If not used as an immediate source of energy, they are stored in the liver and in various other parts of the body.

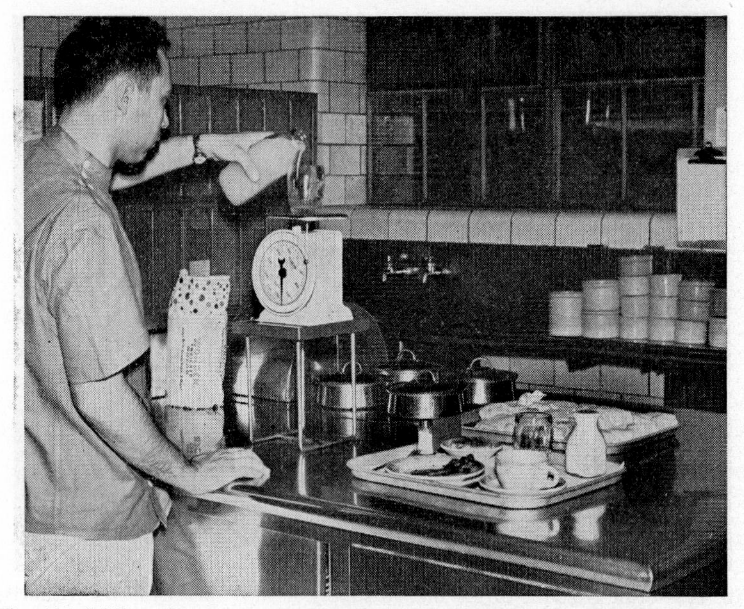

Fig. 113. Milk and meat are two chief sources of protein. (Kansas City General Hospital School of Nursing, Kansas City, Missouri.)

Carbohydrates and fats each contain varying proportions of carbon, hydrogen, and oxygen. The final products, after oxidation, are carbon dioxide and water. Fats differ from carbohydrates in that they contain more carbon and hydrogen and less oxygen. (The formula for glucose, a simple sugar, is $C_6H_{12}O_6$; a typical formula for a fat is $C_{57}H_{110}O_6$.)

Fats, when burned, produce more heat and energy, and burn more slowly and with more difficulty. Carbohydrates need little oxygen for combustion and are easily burned. In illness, when vitality is low, glucose and other forms of simple sugars are used freely, since they can be easily digested and assimilated. Excess amounts of fat should be avoided since it serves to increase body weight to the point where health is threatened and the life span may be shortened.

The amount of carbohydrates and fats needed in the diet will depend on such factors as age, sex, occupation, exercise, recreation, and general physical condition. Children need energy foods in amounts sufficient to provide for increased growth as well as for muscular activity. Adults need only sufficient energy foods to maintain proper body weight. An inadequate supply of carbohydrates and fat for either child or adult will result in loss of weight, loss of physical power, and decreased mental alertness or activity.

Foods Which Provide for Building of Body Tissue. Protein is the food element which is needed to build and maintain body tissue. In addition to carbon, hydrogen, and oxygen, proteins contain nitrogen which is an essential constituent of protoplasm and is needed not only for tissue growth and repair but for life itself. Some proteins also will provide varying amounts of sulfur, phosphorus, and iron for the body.

The chief sources of protein are meat, eggs, milk, fish, cheese, grains, and vegetables. Animal proteins are more easily digested than are vegetable proteins. In digestion proteins are changed into chemically more simple substances, termed amino acids.

Amino acids are absorbed into the blood stream and carried to tissue cells throughout the body. In addition to their function of building and repairing body tissue, they are used in the formation of hemoglobin, they help to regulate water distribution within the body, they aid in forming fibrinogen, which is needed in the clotting of blood, and by creating antibodies they help to bring about resistance or immunity to disease.

Amino acids not used by tissue cells of the body are not stored for future use. If the intake of protein is greater than needed, the carbon and hydrogen are oxidized as a source of heat and energy and the nitrogen is excreted through the kidneys as a waste product.

A diet with increased protein content is needed for growing children, pregnant women, persons engaged in heavy muscular work, and patients convalescing from prolonged illness. An inadequate amount of protein in the diet will cause malnutrition, interference with tissue growth and repair, functional nervous diseases, and lowered vitality.

Foods Which Help To Regulate Body Processes. In addition to the nutrient elements of proteins, carbohydrates, and fats, there are substances associated with them that are essential not only to their proper utilization in the body but to the growth and functioning of the body itself. These necessary elements are minerals, inorganic salts, and vitamins.

Many *minerals* are needed for proper body functioning, but are readily available in foods which supply the two essential minerals which must be made available through proper diet.

Calcium occurs in the body in greater quantity than any other mineral and is essential to the formation of bones and teeth. In combination with other minerals it serves other important functions in the body, such as aiding in muscle contraction and in blood coagulation. Milk is the chief source of calcium and at least a pint of milk a day is needed to provide half the needed calcium intake. The other half can be obtained from foods in the diet which are necessary to supply other food elements.

Iron is an essential constituent of hemoglobin found in the red cells of the blood and is needed to prevent anemia. Liver is the chief source of iron, although appreciable amounts may be found in raisins and other fruits and in lean meat, egg yolks, and whole grain cereals.

Sodium, potassium and magnesium salts help to maintain a normal water balance in the body. Iodine is needed to prevent the formation of a goiter. Other salts, sulfur, chlorine, phosphorus, and copper are essential for normal growth and functioning of the body.

Vitamins are unrelated organic substances existing in small quantities in natural foods, or produced synthetically, which are essential to proper metabolism, nutrition, growth, and reproduction. Large numbers of vitamins have been named, the best known and those most often prescribed include vitamins A, B, B_1, B_2, C, D, E, and K. The term B complex includes a number of soluble substances generally occurring together, but further investigation has resulted in isolation and identification of several separate components, such as thiamine hydrochloride, nicotinic acid, riboflavin, and pyridoxine.

Although vitamins are needed in the diet only in very small quantities, a total lack of them may cause specific deficiency diseases. An inadequate vitamin intake may result in fatigue, apathy, poor appetite, and general poor health.

Water. Water makes up approximately two thirds of the total body weight and is even more essential to life than is food. It forms a large part of the digestive juices, bile, and the blood and lymph, which serve to transport nutritive substances to body cells, and it makes up part of the urine, feces, and perspiration, which are waste products of body metabolism. Water plays an important part in the exchange of substances between the blood and cells of the body. With proteins and minerals it helps to regulate fluid balance of the body.

Water is available to the body from three sources: fluids, water contained in foods, and water produced when foodstuffs are oxidized in the tissues. In health there is usually a balance between intake and output of fluid for the individual.

One to three liters of fluid is needed each day for the average adult. In hot climates and in some disease conditions the intake of fluid needs to be substantially increased; in other diseases fluid intake may need to be restricted. Water or other fluids may be taken with meals but should not interfere with proper chewing of solid foods.

BASIC FOOD REQUIREMENTS

Knowledge of the basic principles of good nutrition makes the feeding of a well person a relatively simple matter. When the needed food elements and the sources from which they may be obtained are known, the dietitian or other person responsible for diet planning need only select proper amounts of the seven basic foods and encourage the patient to eat the adequate diet.

Basic foods for normal nutrition and the estimated amounts needed each day include: *Meat-fish-fowl,* 1 to 2 servings; *vegetables,* 2 or more servings—1 vegetable should be raw, 1 should be of green or yellow variety; *fruits,* 2 or more servings, 1 citrus fruit or tomato; *cereals,*

4 servings—bread, natural or whole grain cereal; *egg*, 1 egg, or another protein food substituted; *milk*, at least 1 pint—other milk products, cream, cheese; *butter*, 1 tablespoon; *water*, 1000 to 2000 cc.

CALORIC VALUES AND REQUIREMENTS

Oxidation of food taken into the body produces energy which is measured in terms of heat units or Calories. A Calorie is the amount of heat required to raise the temperature of one kilogram of water one degree centigrade.

Caloric Values. By use of the calorimeter caloric values have been determined for the various foodstuffs. The body receives approximately 4 Calories in a gram of protein, 4 Calories in a gram of carbohydrate, and 9 Calories in a gram of fat. Handbooks containing information as to the number of Calories in various food products are available for guidance in supplying the right amount of Calories and proper nutritive elements in the diet.

Caloric Requirements. The basal metabolic rate of the individual is determined by measuring the amount of oxygen required to sustain life when the body is at as near complete rest as possible. The amount of energy expended under such conditions has been standardized at one Calorie per hour per kilogram (2.2 pounds) of body weight. Thus a man of average size would need, merely to sustain life, about 1700 Calories per day. The woman of average size would require approximately 1400 Calories per day for the same purpose.

Such factors as age, sex, occupation, body build, climate, and physical condition must be considered in determining true caloric requirement. The kind of work the person does, light desk work or heavy manual labor, has marked influence on energy output and caloric requirement. A man of average size doing office work may need approximately 2500 Calories per day. The same man working at hard labor would need about 4200 Calories each day.

Exercise increases basal metabolism rate and caloric requirement. Rest will decrease both. An increase in body temperature will increase metabolic rate, as will eating a large amount of food. If a person eats more than is required for normal body activity, he will gain weight; if he eats less than is required, he will lose weight. Weight control, then, is not difficult for the person who knows the caloric value of foods and his own personal caloric needs.

Many factors affect dietary habits of the individual. The amount of income, knowledge of nutrition, geographic location, race, and customs may influence to a marked degree the choice of food for a family. Inadequate diets may be found most frequently as a result of ignorance and of poverty. Food patterns are determined by family or community practices and those associated with religion. For this reason the nurse must take advantage of the opportunity to teach good food practices to patients. If poor eating habits are to be changed the

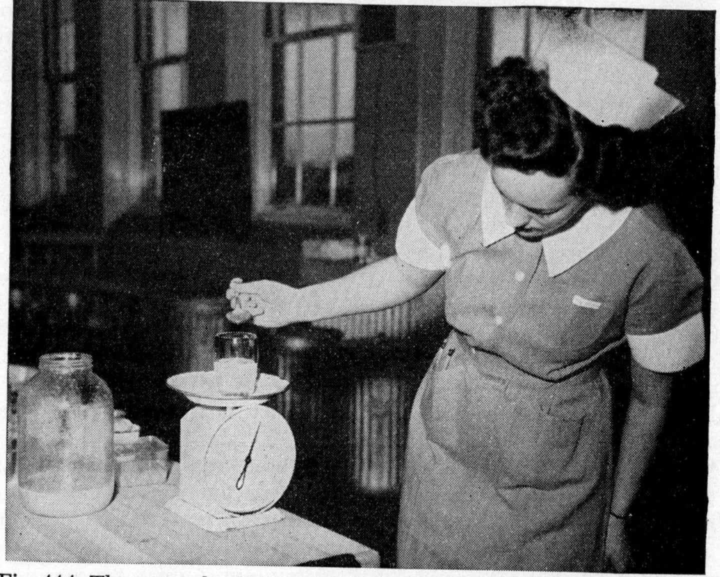

Fig. 114. The nurse should explain to the patient the significance of a special diet and the reason for weighing the food. (Presbyterian Hospital School of Nursing, Denver, Colorado.)

person concerned must be made to understand the reason for change and the importance of proper diet in promoting good health.

If the nurse has a good understanding of dietary needs it will not be difficult for her to explain to the patient why a variety of foodstuffs should be included in his diet—why such foods as milk, meat, eggs, fruit, and vegetables are important, and why the correct number of Calories should be determined.

Patients who are served a special diet as a part of their medical treatment often have little understanding of why certain foods are selected for their diet. Because they fail to understand the significance of the selected foods, they may have little interest in observing diet restrictions. Explanation by the nurse will often result in complete cooperation on the part of the patient who understands the necessity for eating the foods selected for him. Many illnesses are treated largely by modification or restriction of diet, and the nurse should consider guidance in nutrition an important part of her responsibility in giving nursing care to the patient.

NUTRITION IN ILLNESS

With an understanding of food requirements for the well person the nurse is in position to understand how to modify or alter those requirements to meet the needs of the person who is ill. To determine dietary needs for the patient, the doctor, dietitian, and nurse will need to take into consideration various factors which influence choice of diet in illness. Such factors may include lessened activity because the patient is confined to bed; increased body temperature which affects total energy requirement; impaired circulation and its effect on digestion; the disease condition, which may disturb digestion and other body processes; loss of appetite which so often is a part of the syndrome of disease; mental and emotional disturbances that may accompany a physical injury or illness.

In planning the treatment and nursing care of a patient, much thought needs to be given to diet. In addition to providing a diet that would be adequate and well balanced, provision must be made, and changes effected, which will meet additional requirements that may be produced by the condition that caused hospitalization of the patient.

FOOD ALLERGY

Allergy is an unusual or exaggerated reaction to a substance which in similar amounts is harmless to most persons. Food substances are often the cause of allergic reactions in some individuals. If the food concerned is one that may readily be omitted from the diet, as strawberries, or for which substitutes are available, the solution to the problem is not difficult.

Milk, eggs, and wheat products are the most common allergens and are essential food elements in nutrition. Diagnosis of food allergy is made by the use of elimination diets and may be a prolonged and expensive undertaking for the patient. If the food is one which is needed in the diet, an attempt may be made to desensitize the person. The substance causing the abnormal reaction is thought to be some form of protein substance. Treatment of the condition is based on the food concerned, the condition of the patient, and the extent to which the allergic reaction may interfere with proper nutrition.

STANDARD AND SPECIAL DIETS

Diets ordered for hospitalized patients have been standardized to meet the needs of large groups who require little or no change in daily menus except that of progressive change from liquid to the general or normal diet.

The most commonly used diets may be classified into five groups, supplying the required foodstuffs in increasing amounts and consistency, and ranging from the inadequate, wholly liquid, very easily digested diet, to the regular diet with solid foods which closely approximates the well balanced diet of the well and active person. The patient's likes and dislikes of various foods should be considered when possible; preferred foods should be in the diet prescribed for him. For certain conditions special diets may be necessary.

Doctors and nurses are familiar with the content and purposes of the different diets and make intelligent use of them in the treatment and care of patients.

Standard Hospital Diets. The five standard hospital diets are clear liquid, full liquid, soft, light, and regular, also termed "general" or "standard." (See Table 3.)

Clear Liquid Diet. A diet of limited fluids for surgical patients and those with marked impairment of digestive processes. The diet is not an adequate diet, and should be used only for short periods of time. Liquids which may be given in this type of diet are tea, coffee (without milk or cream), lemonade, ginger ale, Jello, and broth with all fat removed.

Full Liquid Diet. A diet for those who cannot be given soft foods, but are permitted to have foods in fluid form. Such a diet is easily digested and can be made to meet nutritional needs adequately. It is used in cases of acute infection, severe gastrointestinal disturbances, and prolonged fever, and as an introductory diet for the patient soon to receive foods of more solid consistency. Foods supplied by this diet include milk and various milk beverages, eggnog, broth, strained cereal gruels, strained vegetable juices, strained fruit juices, soups, Jello, cream, butter, ginger ale, tea, and coffee.

Soft Diet. Foods of soft consistency are used and the diet may be nutritionally adequate. It is used as an intermediary diet between liquid and light diets. Patients unable to take regular food or unable to chew foods of a more solid nature are given soft diets. Foods supplied by the soft diet are milk, eggs (not fried), meat, fish or poultry (ground, chopped, scraped, or by other means made easy to masticate), cheese, toast, crackers, cooked cereals, potatoes (not fried), puréed vegetables, strained or cooked fruits, soups, puddings, sauces, and frozen desserts.

Light Diet. A diet used intermediately between soft and regular diets. It is the same as the regular diet without fried meats, raw fruits, or raw vegetables.

Regular Diet. An adequate diet for the convalescent patient. Foods supplied by this diet are those of the well proportioned diet of the well person, except for omission of fresh pork, fat meats, highly spiced meats and gravies, fried foods, gas-forming vegetables, rich pastries, and alcoholic beverages.

Special Diets. Many pathologic conditions such as ulcers, diabetes, anemia, hypertension, and malnutrition bring about changes in body processes which make it necessary that certain foods be in the diet. Such diets are termed "special," and are made up of foods that are necessary for treatment of the patient.

Although the nurse may not be responsible for diet calculation, which rests with the specially trained dietitian, she should be able

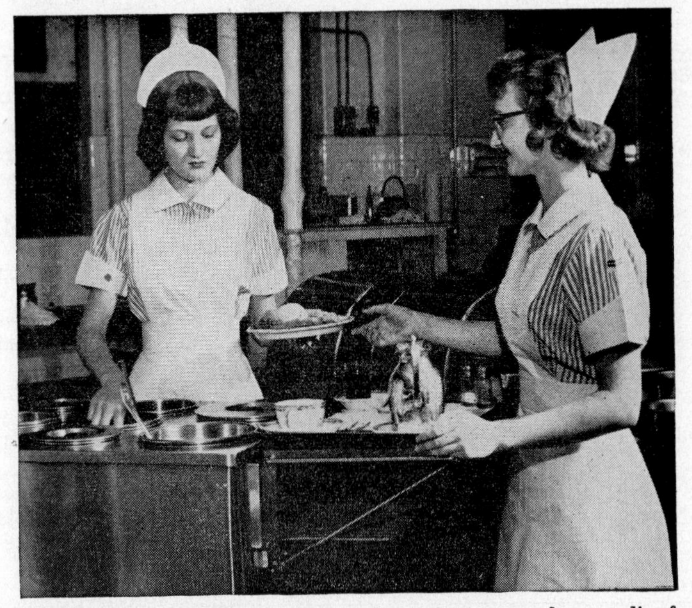

Fig. 115. The nurse should know how to plan and serve an adequate diet for the patient. (Allentown Hospital School of Nursing, Allentown, Pennsylvania.)

to interpret the diet intelligently for the patient and should see that he understands the importance of eating required foods and of omitting all foods that are forbidden him. The nurse should work in close cooperation with the dietitian in planning and carrying out all dietary measures.

Commonly used special diets include low-calorie diet, high-calorie diet, low-residue diet, bland diet, diabetic diet, Sippy diet.

Many other "special diets" in use bear names that are usually self-explanatory, as the salt-free diet, low-protein diet, and low-fat diet.

NURSE'S RESPONSIBILITY IN FOOD SERVICE

In the hospital the dietitian assumes the responsibility for planning the meals for the patient. The nurse, however, should be well versed in such planning since she needs to interpret dietary restrictions or modifications to the patient. She may be required to plan adequate diets when the services of a dietitian are unavailable, as in a private home.

The nurse is responsible for observing and reporting conditions of appetite. If the patient has little or no appetite the nurse should try to determine the cause and to correct it, if possible. She should keep the doctor and dietitian informed as to the patient's appetite and as

Table 3. Standard Hospital Diets

FOOD ITEM	CLEAR LIQUID	FULL LIQUID	SOFT	LIGHT	REGULAR
Meats	Albumen water Broth	Clam broth Beef tea Broth	Cheese Chicken breast (grd) Baked fresh fish Creamed tender grd. beef Eggs	Cheese Calves' liver Lamb chop Chicken Fish Steaks Sweetbreads Scraped beef Bacon Eggs	All meats—fried foods to be avoided: highly seasoned meats should not be included
Cereals	Cereal water	Gruels	Cereals (well cooked) Toast Crackers	Soft and prepared cereals Graham bread Toast Crackers	All cereals
Vegetables and Potatoes	None	Strained vegetable juice	Puréed vegetables Baked or mashed potatoes	Cooked bland vegetables Potatoes Celery hearts Lettuce	Gas-forming vegetables to be avoided; all others may be included
Soups	Clear broth Beef tea	Cream soups (strained)	All soups	All soups	All soups
Fruits	None	Fruit juices (strained)	Fruit juice Cooked bland fruits	Liquid and cooked fruits	All fruits
Desserts	Jello	Ices Jello	Strained or cooked fruits Custard Gelatin Frozen desserts	All desserts, excluding pastries	All desserts, excluding pastries

Table 3. STANDARD HOSPITAL DIETS (*Continued*)

FOOD ITEM	CLEAR LIQUID	FULL LIQUID	SOFT	LIGHT	REGULAR
Beverage	Tea (clear) Coffee (clear) Lemonade Ginger ale	Cocoa Chocolate Milk Tea Coffee Eggnog	Milk Coffee Tea Eggnog	All beverages, excluding those of alcoholic nature	All beverages, excluding those of alcoholic nature
Frequency of Feedings	Every two hours	Every two hours	Three meals; with liquids between	Three meals; extra nourishment as ordered	Three meals
Quantity	6 ounces	6 ounces	Small servings	Average servings	Average servings

to the success or failure of her attempts to persuade the patient to eat.

She will be expected to know the patient's likes and dislikes concerning food and to give them consideration when discussing with the doctor or dietitian plans for changing or modifying the diet. If the patient has certain food allergies the nurse should be informed and should report to persons responsible for diet planning. If the patient is governed, to some extent, by religious or racial influences in regard to food, the nurse should be aware of this and should inform the doctor and the dietitian.

For all patients who have received special dietary consideration the nurse should be sure that the patient, or a responsible member of his family, is fully informed as to correct dietary procedure to be followed after he leaves the hospital.

General Customs and Dietary Regulation. Volumes have bees written on racial and national habits of eating and the nurse should know in a general way some of the well established practices in regard to food for persons of foreign birth. If she has knowledge of general customs, such as that of Italian mothers who use olive oil in place of lard or butter in cooking, and of Chinese families who expect to be served rice and tea rather consistently, she will avoid embarrassment to herself and to the patients.

She should know that the orthodox Jewish patient will refuse to eat dairy products and meat in the same meal, and that there are laws governing the preparation of certain foods which he will not wish to eat unless they have been prepared according to those laws.

The Roman Catholic patient will abstain from meat on Fridays and Fast days, and some religious services of the church require total abstinence from food and fluids for several hours before participation.

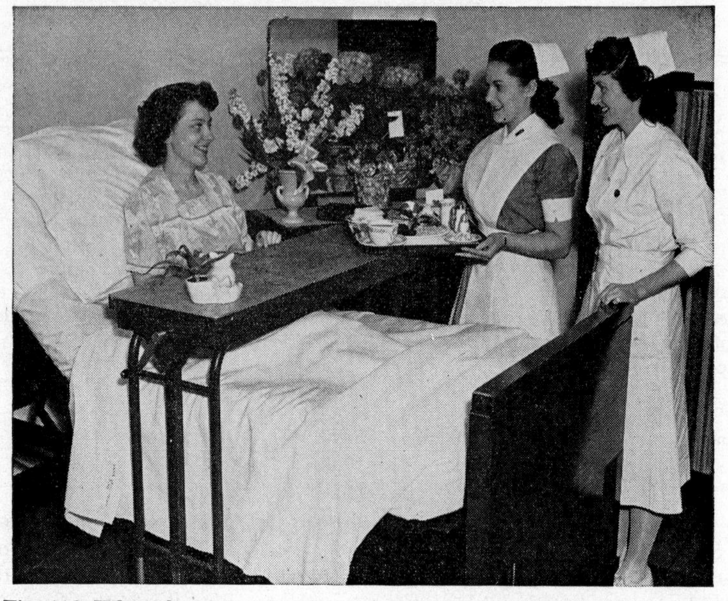

Fig. 116. When the patient has been properly prepared for mealtime, serving the tray will be a pleasure. (Lutheran Deaconess Hospital School of Nursing, Chicago, Illinois.)

If the dietary restrictions interfere with medical treatment or nursing care of the patient the nurse should consult the rabbi or priest and, if necessary, have them confer with the patient in regard to being released from strict observance of such regulations.

To Prepare Patient for Food Service. The nurse who is to serve the tray to a patient at mealtime will need to attend to details of preparation so the patient will be ready to receive the tray and to enjoy the food provided.

The patient confined to bed should have the bedpan or urinal offered to him 15 or 20 minutes before mealtime and should be permitted to wash his hands and face and, if he wishes, to comb his hair and attend to other details of grooming. Bed linens should be straightened, pillows arranged, and the backrest elevated if the patient is allowed to sit up. The overbed table should be cleared of books, magazines, and such articles and put into place to receive the tray.

For the patient who must remain in a horizontal position, if he feeds himself, he may prefer to be turned to his left side and to have the tray placed beside him on the bed or on the bedside table.

An ambulatory patient may sit in an easy chair or wheelchair while eating his meal.

If visitors are present in the room when the tray is served the nurse may need to tactfully suggest that they withdraw to let the patient eat his meal in an atmosphere of quiet relaxation. If the patient specifically requests that a visitor remain in the room during mealtime the nurse should readily grant permission. Digestion may be stimulated by a pleasant companion and interesting conversation.

Before the meal is served all equipment used in carrying out medical treatments or nursing procedures should be removed from the room or from sight of the patient. All lights except those needed for indirect lighting of the room should be turned off. Shades should be adjusted, and the room should be made as neat and attractive as possible. Serving of the meal should be made as pleasant for the patient as possible. If the nurse's manner is cheerful and she shows an interest in the choice of food that has been made for this particular meal, the patient may show more interest, his appetite may be increased, and the digestive processes stimulated.

If the nurse is present in the room during mealtime she should be guided by the wishes of the patient in regard to conversation. By permitting the patient to take the lead in conversation, to select the topic or topics, and to carry most of the responsibility for their discussion she will avoid long, detailed accounts of her own experiences or opinions which may become tiring and interfere with his enjoyment of the meal.

Serving the Tray. Meals should be served at a regular hour each day and effort should be made to avoid undue delay in serving a tray at any meal. The patient usually looks forward to mealtime as a welcome break in the long day of inactivity. Disappointment when a meal is late may not be quite reasonable but may nevertheless cause loss of appetite and lack of interest in the food.

The tray should be attractive in appearance. The tray cover and napkin must be spotlessly clean. China, glassware, and silver should be attractive in appearance. Containers for sugar, salt, pepper, and cream should be filled, and the contents of the tray arranged as for a normal table setting. If water is permitted with the meal a glass of fresh water should be provided.

Small servings of food will tempt the appetite of most patients more effectively than will too generous servings. Hot foods should be covered and should be hot when the tray is placed before the patient. Cold food or beverage should be cold. If ice cream is served for dessert it should be brought to the patient after the rest of the meal has been eaten. Butter should be soft enough to spread easily but should not be melted out of shape. A single flower, small greeting card, or other slight memento placed on the tray may make it more inviting to the patient.

When the nurse serves the tray she should hold it at each side and carry it at waist level, with the base of the table setting away from her, it will then be in correct position as it is set in place before the patient on overbed table or tray table.

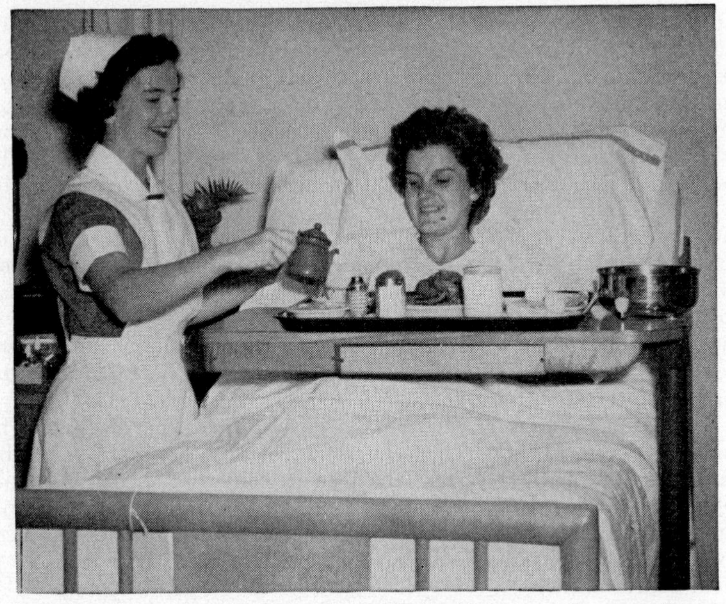

Fig. 117. The nurse who serves the tray should remove the cover from the main dish and pour coffee or tea for the patient. (Jackson Memorial Hospital School of Nursing, Miami, Florida.)

The nurse should remove the cover from the hot food, lift the napkin from the tray, and hand it to the patient or place it in position across his lower chest. This should be done even if the patient is to feed himself. If the patient wishes her to do so, or needs assistance, she should spread butter on toast or bread, cut the meat into bite-size pieces, and arrange all dishes on the tray so they are in easy reach.

The patient should never be made to feel that he should hurry in eating a meal, and the serving of food should not be subject to unnecessary interruptions, as by conversing with another patient or nurse before placing the tray in position.

If the patient appears displeased by any one of the foods offered, the nurse should remove it from the tray. When on a special diet the patient is expected to eat all food contained on the tray. Complaints concerning food or food service should be given prompt attention, and if necessary arrangements should be made for the patient to discuss the matter with the dietitian.

If a patient refuses to eat or eats very sparingly, it may be necessary to explain to him the important part the diet plays in helping to hasten recovery.

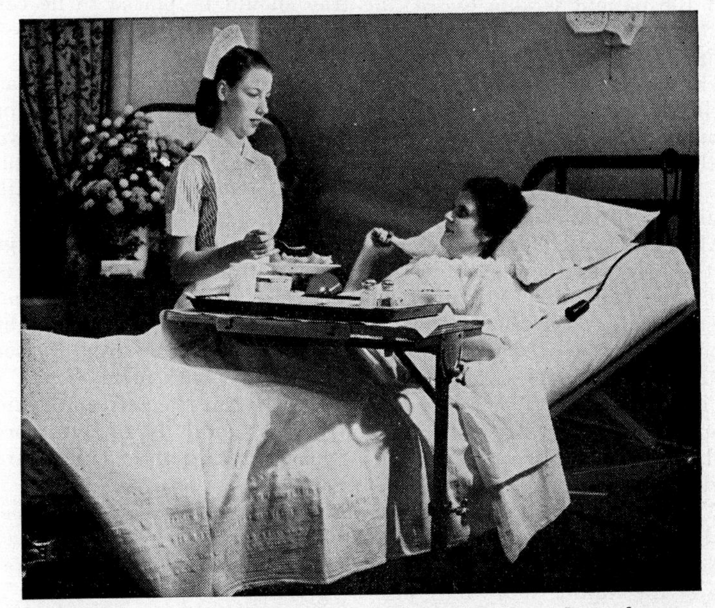

Fig. 118. The patient who is unable to feed herself depends on the nurse for that particular service. (Allentown Hospital School of Nursing, Allentown, Pennsylvania.)

When the patient has finished eating the tray should be removed at once. The nurse should observe the amount and kind of foods eaten and, if necessary, report such observations to the dietitian.

The table should be reconverted to a useful bedside table and the patient made comfortable. Provision should be made for the patient to brush his teeth. If he is in need of rest and quiet after the noon meal he should be encouraged to sleep for a while.

Feeding the Helpless Patient. The patient who is unable to feed himself must be fed by a nurse or other member of the nursing staff. If the patient is being cared for in the home a member of the family may feed him. In some instances family members are permitted to feed the patient in the hospital. It gives them the satisfaction of being able to help the loved one and is helpful to the busy nurse who may thus be freed for other duties.

Under no circumstances should a nurse endeavor to hurry a patient who is being fed. Most helpless patients are deeply regretful of the necessity for being fed, and mealtime is not a pleasant experience for them. A helpless patient, though still hungry, is apt to refuse food if it is being fed to him by a nurse who is obviously in a great hurry to be doing something else.

If the patient is able to see, the tray should be placed so he can see the food that is to be offered him. If he is unable to see, the nurse should inform him as to the various foods that are on the tray.

The patient should be placed in a comfortable position with head slightly forward and supported by a pillow. In this position swallowing is made easy. He is apt to be more relaxed if the nurse sits down while feeding him. A high stool placed close to the bed will enable her to reach the food on the tray and give it to the patient with minimum effort.

After the patient has been informed as to the food and beverage on the tray the nurse should offer the food in small amounts and in much the same order in which she would eat it herself. After he has eaten several portions of food from a spoon or fork, he should be offered a drink of water or other beverage. No one dish of food should be fed to the patient without alternating with other dishes.

The spoon or fork should be placed firmly on the lower lip and tongue when the patient slightly opens his mouth to receive more food, and by raising the end of the spoon or fork the contents are easily deposited in the patient's mouth.

Water or other liquid should be given through a drinking tube. If the liquid is hot, as coffee or tea, the patient should be warned and told to take only small sips until he is accustomed to the temperature of the liquid. Soups may also be given to the patient through a drinking tube.

When changing from solid to liquid food the patient should be informed. It is embarrassing to him to shape his mouth for receiving another spoonful of food only to find that he must alter the position of his lips to grasp the end of a drinking tube.

If the patient has use of his hands he should be given a small portion of bread or toast to hold for himself and to eat as he desires along with the food being fed to him.

The nurse should not carry on a continuous conversation as she feeds the patient, but a few well chosen remarks, along with information as to the food being given to him, will help to convey the impression that she is pleased at being able to help him and that she is not bored or impatient with the task.

Part of the unpleasantness of being fed by another is in the unhappy experience of having food spilled about the mouth or chin. The nurse who understands the patient's feeling of helplessness and dependence will make a special effort to avoid spilling food or beverage and will use the napkin frequently to keep the patient's mouth and chin dry and free of food.

Patients who need to be fed should be served later than other patients so the nurse will be free to feed them without interruption to attend to the wants of the others.

Feeding Infants and Children. Infants are fed from a bottle and are held by the nurse for the 15 to 20 minutes required for each feed-

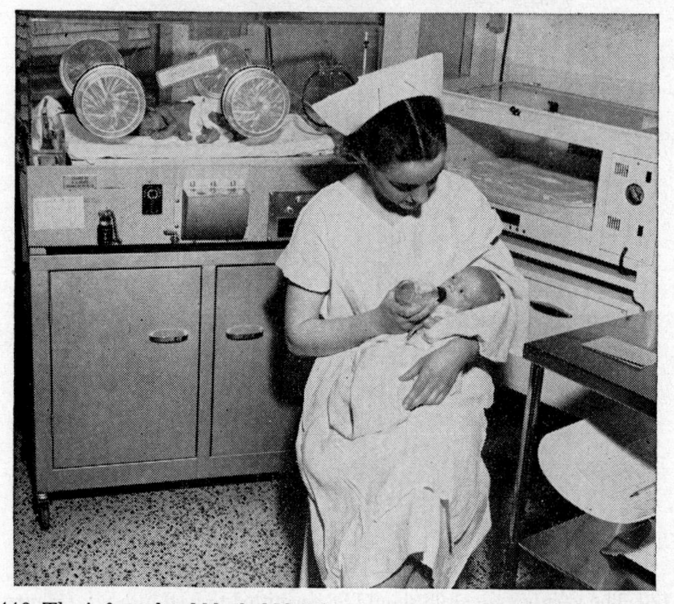

Fig. 119. The infant should be held by the nurse for a bottle feeding. (North Carolina Baptist Hospital School of Nursing, Winston-Salem, North Carolina.)

ing. Before taking the baby from the crib the nurse should place the bottle in a water bath and heat it to body temperature (pleasantly warm when tested on the inner wrist). While the feeding is being warmed, the baby's diaper should be changed. The nurse then washes her hands, puts on gown and mask, and takes the baby on her lap and sits comfortably in a chair to hold him during the feeding. Nipples should be carefully checked at intervals to make sure the openings have not enlarged, permitting the formula to be swallowed too quickly by the baby.

After the formula has been taken, the baby should be held upright against the nurse's shoulder and gently patted on the back to encourage eructation.

The very young child should be allowed to feed himself if he is able to do so. Before the tray is brought to the child his face and hands should be washed and his hair combed. Linen on the bed should be straightened and the room or unit put in order.

The nurse will need to spread butter on bread or toast, remove shells from soft boiled eggs, and assist in many ways so the child finds it easy to feed himself. If an unfamiliar food is served to the child he should be encouraged to taste it but should not be made to feel that he must eat it. The child should be taught to eat slowly,

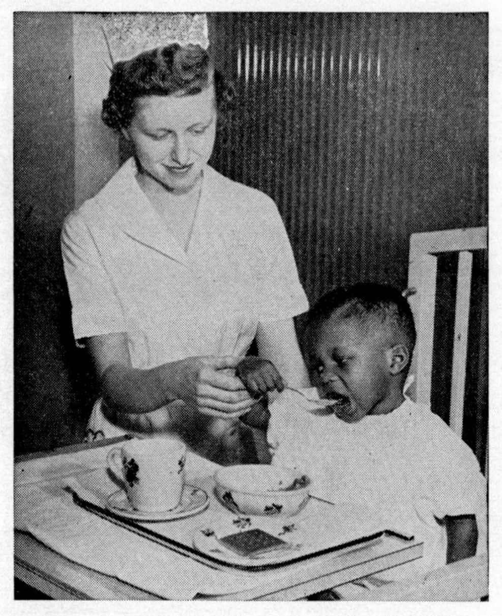

Fig. 120. The very young child should be permitted to feed himself. (Henry Ford Hospital School of Nursing, Detroit, Michigan.)

to chew food thoroughly, and to feed himself in a neat and orderly manner.

The clothing of the child should be covered with a bib so it is fully protected if food should be spilled.

The ill child should never be forced to eat; no rewards should be offered or threats made in an attempt to get him to eat. If he refuses food the refusal should be accepted as a matter of course so it does not assume importance in the mind of the child.

By encouragement and reassurance the nurse may be successful in getting the child to eat the food, but he should be allowed freedom as to his choice of food from the tray and the amount he wishes to eat.

The attentive nurse will be able to observe when the child is managing very well for himself and when he may need assistance in order to prevent fatigue or exertion. Emotional disturbances should not take place at mealtime. Irritability, excitement, or crying will interfere with digestion, and no food should be offered a child who is exhibiting such signs of emotional unrest.

Care of Equipment after Use

The tray and all dishes should be removed from the patient's room or unit as soon as the meal is over.

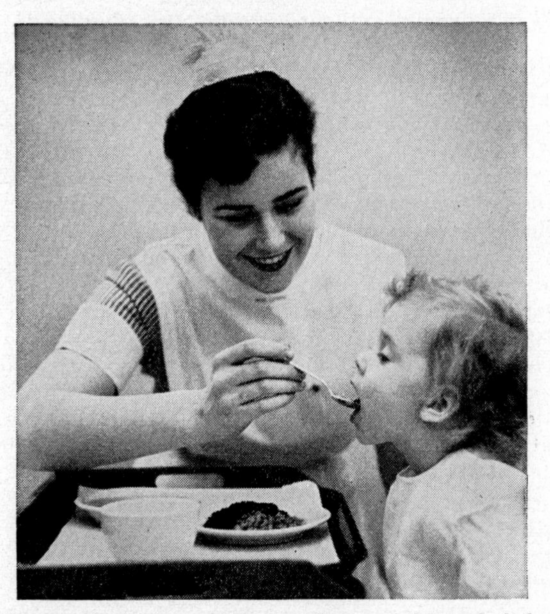

Fig. 121. The attentive nurse will know when a child needs help in feeding himself. (Lenox Hill Hospital School of Nursing, New York, New York.)

Care of equipment will depend on the serving practices in the hospital. If trays are set up in a central serving kitchen the entire tray is sent back to the kitchen. If trays are set up in the kitchen of the clinical department, salt and pepper containers, tea pots or coffee pots, and sugar containers should be removed before the tray and dishes are sent to the central kitchen to be washed.

After use sugar, salt and pepper containers should be refilled and made ready for use again.

Summary of Important Factors

Food supplies energy and material needed for rebuilding body tissue, and helps to regulate body processes: carbohydrates and fats supply heat and energy; proteins build and repair body tissue; minerals and vitamins help regulate body processes.

Water makes up about two thirds of the body weight and is even more essential to the body than food.

Basic food requirements are meat, vegetables, fruits, cereals, egg, milk, butter, water.

Caloric requirements depend on age, sex, occupation, body build, physical condition, and the climate in which the individual lives.

Modification of an adequate diet for a well person is needed for a person who is ill.

Standard hospital diets are *clear liquid*, *full liquid*, *soft*, *light*, and *regular*.

The nurse is responsible for interpreting diet to the patient, for teaching good dietary practices, observing and reporting conditions of appetite, and knowing general customs and regulations concerning diet.

The patient should have his hands washed and be made comfortable for receiving the tray.

Trays should be clean, attractive, and pleasantly served.

Patients who must be fed need understanding and consideration and should never be hurried.

Infants should be held when fed from the bottle and should be "burped" after each feeding.

Young children should be taught good eating practices and should be encouraged to feed themselves when possible.

The child's actions at mealtime should be accepted casually. Refusal to eat should not create a situation whereby the child feels he is the center of attention.

Factors To Teach the Patient

Importance of washing hands before meals or before handling food.

Need for balanced diet so that body receives all requirements in regard to foodstuffs.

Seven basic foods, and part they play in promoting health.

Chief sources of iron and calcium—part vitamins play in helping to regulate body processes.

Importance of fluid to the body and how to supply body needs.

How to control weight by understanding of caloric value of foods.

How adequate diet of well person may be modified to meet needs of person who is ill.

Relationship of special dietary treatment to medical treatment of the patient.

Important factors in serving of food to the sick.

Best method of feeding the helpless patient.

Basic concepts for successful feeding of infants and children.

Scientific Principles

Anatomy and Physiology. Organs of the digestive system are the mouth, esophagus, stomach, and small and large intestine.

In the mouth, food is ground by the teeth. The enzyme ptyalin (from saliva) converts the starch in food to sugar.

Food remains in the stomach about one to four hours. It is changed, chemically, by the action of enzymes in gastric juices. The sight, taste, and odor of food stimulate secretion of gastric juice.

Digestion prepares the food for use in the body. The end-products of digestion are absorbed into the blood stream and then assimilated by the body cells.

Residue or waste expelled from the large intestine is made up of cellulose, connective tissue, and undigested fats.

Chemistry. In the mouth, ptyalin (an enzyme) acts on starch.

In the stomach, pepsin and rennin (enzymes) act on protein in the presence of hydrochloric acid.

In the intestines, trypsin, steapsin, and amylopsin (enzymes) act on carbohydrates, proteins, and fats.

Carbohydrates and fats contain carbon, hydrogen, and oxygen and furnish heat and energy.

Carbohydrates are eventually changed to glucose to be used in the body. Insulin, a secretion from the pancreas, regulates the blood sugar level.

Fats yield fatty acids and glycerol to be used in the body. Fats are hard to digest so are given sparingly to patients.

Proteins contain carbon, hydrogen, oxygen, and nitrogen, and serve to rebuild body tissues. Proteins are broken down into the amino acids of which they are composed.

Minerals needed for the body are calcium, iron, iodine, sulfur, phosphorus, sodium, potassium, and chlorine. They help to maintain the acid-base balance in the body.

Vitamins are needed for growth and nutrition, to build up resistance to disease, and for normal body functioning.

The absorption of food is by osmosis. Because of the large surface area of the intestinal tract rapid absorption of food is possible.

Microbiology. Organisms enter the body through the mouth in food and drink. The hydrochloric acid in the stomach destroys many microorganisms taken into the body through the mouth.

Many kinds of bacteria normally inhabit the intestines; they cause putrefaction, fermentation, and disintegration of food stuffs.

Washing hands frequently is a means of preventing the spread of disease. The nurse should always wash her hands before handling or serving food.

Bacteria may be transferred from one patient to another by unclean dishes and other food containers and utensils. Drinking tubes should be washed and sterilized after use.

Pharmacology. Various pharmaceutical preparations are available to supply mineral and vitamin deficiencies.

When the body fails to manufacture its own insulin, it may be administered in dosages needed to maintain correct blood sugar level.

Physics. The nurse has better control over the tray if she carries it in front of and close to her body.

The patient who sits up in bed while eating should have his head and back well supported.

Differences in pressure forces liquid to move. This helps the patient in the use of the drinking tube. As air is drawn from the tube, liquid from a glass or cup is forced into the tube by the air pressure above the liquid.

Psychology. The mental state of the patient has a marked effect on digestive processes.

The patient's surroundings should be quiet, pleasant, and attractive when the tray is served.

Worry, fear, and anxiety inhibit normal digestive processes. Food should not be served to a patient who is mentally distressed. With relief of mental anxiety or discomfort, the patient will be able to enjoy the food served to him.

When possible, the patient's likes and dislikes concerning food should be considered in planning meals for him.

Food well prepared and served in small portions will be more appetizing to the patient.

The feeling of dependence and embarrassment by the patient who must be fed can be overcome by an understanding nurse who lets the patient know that she is pleased to be of assistance.

Sociology. Customs attendant on the eating of food have made of that activity a socializing event. Enjoyable companionship adds to the pleasure of eating a delicious meal. The nurse is often called on to converse with the patient during mealtime.

Eating habits are greatly influenced by racial and religious practices, and the nurse should know those in common usage.

Federal, state, and local governments have food laws designed to protect the general public as the consumer of foods. The Pure Food and Drug Act prohibits adulteration of foods and the use of misleading labels. Other laws provide for the inspection of meat.

Poor nutrition, caused by economic situations, misinformation about food, and undesirable food habits, is one of the major public health problems. Most communities have a program of free school lunches, agencies that supply food to poor families or provide money with which to buy food, and a program to educate the homemaker in regard to food requirements and good food health practices.

Situation Type Problem

1. A student nurse, who was to report for ward class at 1 o'clock, learned at 12:45 P.M. that a patient who had to be fed had not received a tray at the time other trays had been served on the department. She found the patient's tray in the diet kitchen where it had obviously been overlooked.

The patient informed her that she had not yet eaten and that she had hoped to be fed early because she expected a daughter who visited her frequently to arrive within a very short time.

The food on the tray was cold. The patient was notoriously slow in eating. The student would not have time to heat the food and feed the patient before time to attend the 1 o'clock class.

The only other nursing personnel on the department were busy with their assignments and would not have time to feed the patient without negelecting their other duties. What would you have done?

Suggested Reference Reading

"Dietary patterns and food habits," M. Mead; Journal of American Dietetic Association, January, 1943.

"The emotional factor in nutrition," T. B. Rice; Hygeia, February, 1944.

"Well fed but ill nourished," Lois Mattox Miller; Hygeia, July, 1949.

"The fat and the lean," J. John Henry; American Journal of Nursing, October, 1949.

"Establishing good food habits," Lorraine Weng; American Journal of Nursing, March, 1950.

"Hot weather diets," Julia Ord King; American Journal of Nursing, July, 1950.

"Streamlining tray service," Mary M. Northrop; American Journal of Nursing, November, 1950.

"Be smart—eat a good breakfast," M. Estelle Ingoldsby; American Journal of Nursing, September, 1951.

"Why be fat?" Herbert Pollack; American Journal of Nursing, December, 1952.

CHAPTER 17

Elimination

TOPICAL OUTLINE

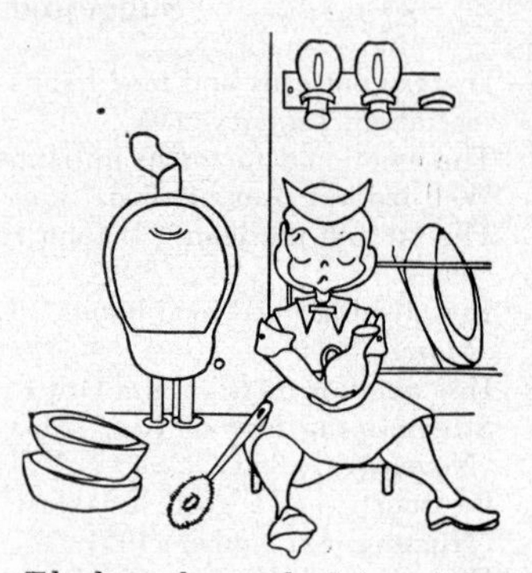

The best place to look for a helping hand is at the end of your arm!

ELIMINATION FROM THE KIDNEYS

The kidneys serve as an organ of elimination by excreting body wastes in the form of urea, uric acid, creatinine, phosphates, and various other salts.

For the average adult, the normal kidney output may range from 1500 to 2000 cc. daily. Urine, which contains the waste products from the kidney, is secreted by the kidney and passed through the ureters into the urinary bladder. The bladder, a hollow, highly elastic, muscular organ in the pelvic cavity, serves as a reservoir for the urine and retains it until it is expelled through the urethra.

Because of its elasticity the bladder is able to change its shape as well as its position in the pelvic cavity to accommodate an ever-increasing amount of urine which is collected there between voidings. Although the bladder is capable of holding several thousand cubic centimeters of urine the amount usually retained in that organ varies from 250 to 500 cc. If the bladder is functioning normally, an accumulation of 250–300 cc. of urine causes a desire to void. This desire to empty the bladder is created by stimulation of sensory nerves when the intravesicular tension has reached a certain point determined by the amount of urine contained within the bladder.

Voiding is accomplished by the simultaneous action of the sphincter muscle and of the three layers of muscle which make up the bladder wall. The sphincter muscles of the bladder relax at the same time the muscular wall of the bladder contracts, thus expelling the urine from the bladder through the urethra.

Some patients may find it difficult to use the bedpan or urinal when forced to remain in bed. An understanding nurse sees that the patient is given an opportunity to respond promptly to the impulse to void and makes it her business to provide the patient with adequate amounts of fluids so there will be normal elimination from the kidneys.

For the patient who is unable to void, even though the bladder may be distended and the desire to void present, there are several things which the nurse may do to help.

The sound of running water when the patient is in position to void may help stimulate the process; this can be accomplished by allowing a nearby faucet to run or by pouring water from one container to another. Pouring warm water over the patient's perineum, encouraging the patient to drink large quantities of water or lemonade, and allowing the patient to stand beside the bed may be other successful means of helping to start the process of voiding.

For the patient who is unable to be out of bed the bedpan may be placed near the edge of the bed and the patient so placed on the bedpan that his feet rest on a chair beside the bed. This position is more nearly that assumed by patients who are granted bathroom privileges for the benefit of encouraging proper elimination. Assuring the patient of absolute privacy when he is on the bedpan or attempting to use the urinal may help to start the process of voiding.

Many patients become quite tense and are somewhat nervous if another person is present when they are trying to void. For many such patients the nurse should leave the room for a few minutes.

If a patient finds it difficult to void while remaining in bed, the nurse should determine the cause. Factors that may cause difficulty in voiding may include the unnatural bed position, inadequate privacy, lack of familiarity with the bedpan and the way in which it should be used, and fear and tension which accompanies illness and hospitalization.

The well qualified nurse will know the normal fluid intake and output for the average patient. She must accept the responsibility of notifying the patient's doctor if any discrepancy should occur between fluid intake and urinary output.

She should know that in some disease conditions, such as diabetes mellitus, an unusually large amount of urine is expelled, and that in diabetic acidosis the urine has a characteristic fruity odor. She should

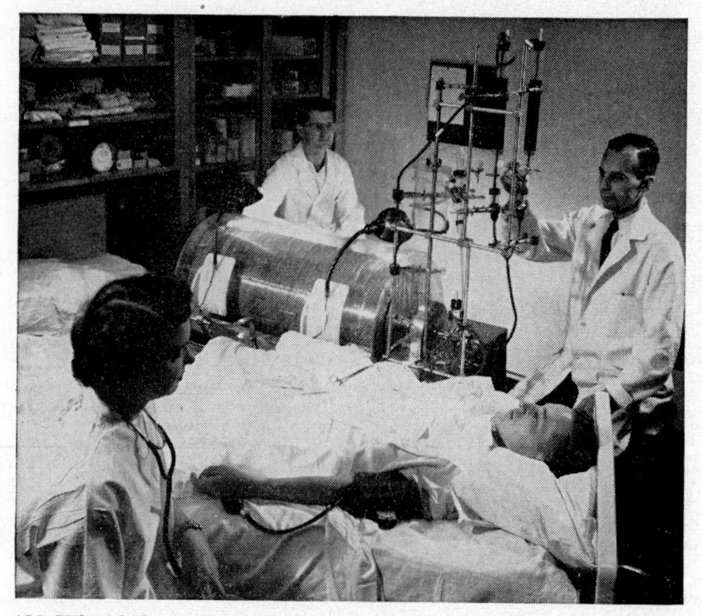

Fig. 122. When kidneys do not function normally use of the artificial kidney may be indicated. (Presbyterian Hospital, Chicago, Illinois.)

know that conditions which impair circulation in the kidneys, such as heart disease, may decrease urinary output.

She will need to know, besides the amount normally voided, the character, color, and consistency, and even the odor of normal urine. Urine normally is light amber in color, is clear, and does not have an offensive or unpleasant odor. Normal specific gravity of urine is 1.015 to 1.025. Normal reaction of urine is acid. Albumin and sugar are not found in normal urine, except in very small quantities and for short periods of time.

If kidneys are functioning normally the patient may need to void every four to six hours during the day. The amount voided each time is usually 200 to 300 c. Approximately 1500 to 2000 cc. is voided each day.

Usually the bedpan should be offered the patient just before he is made comfortable and ready for sleep at night. One of the first responsibilities of the nurse when the patient wakens in the morning is to see that proper provision is made, at that time, for elimination of urine from the bladder.

The nurse should feel responsible for making sure that the patient voids several times during the day, and in sufficient quantity, so that normal urinary output is maintained.

ELIMINATION FROM THE INTESTINES

Waste products of metabolism are eliminated by the intestines as well as from the kidneys and the skin. The solid waste material eliminated from the intestines is known as feces and consists chiefly of dead bacteria and undigested food materials. It also contains indigestible substances such as cellulose, various secretions from the intestinal tract itself, and some inorganic salts. The large intestine is approximately five feet in length and is divided into three parts—the ascending colon, transverse colon, and descending colon.

The terminal portion of the large intestine, known as the rectum, is six to eight inches in length; its opening on the body surface is known as the anus. Elimination from the intestinal tract is controlled by the two sphincter muscles of the anus. The internal sphincter muscles act involuntarily; the external sphincter muscles can be somewhat controlled.

The small intestine is much longer than the large intestine and is connected to the latter by the ileocecal valve, which acts in such manner as to prevent fecal material that has passed into the colon from returning to the small intestine.

Material contained in the intestinal tract is propelled slowly along from the small intestine into the larger portion of the intestinal tract by what is known as peristaltic movement. This movement of intestinal contents is brought about by alternate contraction and relaxation of the walls of the organ. When feces have accumulated in the intestinal tract in an amount to cause intracranial pressure the patient experiences the desire to defecate. The urge to have a bowel movement is closely related to the action known as mass peristalsis which is a movement that occurs in the intestine at regular intervals during the twenty-four hour period. Mass peristaltic action usually occurs soon after an intake of food. It is this action which causes the patient to feel the desire for defecation. Establishment of a regular time each day for defecation is possible because of mass peristaltic action.

Elimination of waste material from the intestines may vary for different individuals; some people require or need to defecate once each day; others may normally eliminate waste products from the intestinal tract several times a day; still others may have normal defecation only once in several days.

The rectum does not serve as a reservoir for waste material of the intestinal tract and when it is filled with feces the individual experiences the desire to defecate. The desire for defecation may last only a very few minutes. If for some reason the patient does not respond by use of bedpan or toilet, the desire soon ceases. Failure to respond to the desire for defecation usually results in failure to establish a regular time for defecation or good elimination habits.

Proper elimination is one of the most important aspects of personal hygiene. The nurse is expected to know the elimination habits and activity of all patients in her care. She should know, and should teach the patient, if necessary, that a well balanced diet, adequate fluid intake, sufficient exercise, and freedom from worry or anxiety are definitely related to good elimination habits. The establishment of a regular time for elimination is also of major importance in establishing proper elimination routine. By offering the bedpan at regular intervals and at the same time each day the nurse may help the patient to establish a satisfactory routine for intestinal elimination.

Patients whose condition permits should receive green vegetables and varieties of raw fruit, to provide bulk in the form of undigested food and indigestible cellulose.

Encouraging the patient to drink a sufficient amount of fluids is also the responsibility of the nurse. Exercise is necessary for proper elimination even for patients confined to bed, and the nurse should encourage the patient to move about in bed, to turn from side to side, and to be active without actually getting out of bed, unless such activity has been restricted by the attending physician.

Constipation. Constipation is present when bowel movements are delayed and symptoms of discomfort are experienced. The usual symptoms of constipation, caused by distention of the rectum with fecal material, include loss of appetite, headache, distention of the abdomen (caused by accumulation of gas in the intestinal tract), and unpleasant breath. The very severe form of constipation may result in complete stoppage of elimination and cause what is termed "intestinal obstruction." In most cases faulty habits of elimination are the chief cause of constipation.

The desire to defecate, produced by passage of feces into the rectum, is of very short duration and if defecation does not take place the desire is lost. More water is absorbed from the feces and the mass then becomes hardened, making defecation at a later time more difficult. Frequent distention of the rectal wall will result in loss of muscle tone, and the rectum becomes less sensitive to distention so that desire for defecation at regular intervals may not be felt. When this condition exists the rectum, which normally is empty except at short intervals before evacuation, contains feces most of the time and the individual is constipated, to some degree, at all times.

While a patient is confined to bed it is necessary that proper habits of elimination be established and maintained. The nurse should explain the basic concepts of digestion and elimination and in this manner make sure the patient understands the need for certain foods in the diet, for taking a sufficient amount of fluids, and for evacuation of feces each day, shortly after the breakfast tray has been served.

Many factors may interfere with normal elimination. Those which represent the most common causes of constipation include:

A diet without roughage—with very little roughage in the diet there is little residue available to form the bulk of fecal material.

Lack of exercise—when exercise is restricted normal peristaltic action may be decreased and the muscles of the digestive tract may lose their tone.

Nervous tension and worry—an undesirable mental state may depress vital physical functions so that digestion and elimination are adversely affected.

Confinement to bed—the position in which the patient is placed on a bedpan is not that usually assumed for elimination, and many patients find it difficult to maintain good habits of elimination when they are not granted bathroom privileges.

Abdominal surgery involving the intestines—trauma that results from handling of the intestines during the operation may cause interference with elimination.

The presence of tumors—tumors or other disease condition in the intestinal tract may interfere with elimination.

Insufficient fluid intake—when fluids are restricted the fecal material may lack sufficient fluid content to permit of easy passage through the lower intestinal tract.

Neglect in establishing a regular time for defecation—without the habit formation needed to insure elimination of feces at the same time each day, the desire to defecate will not be strongly felt and constipation may result.

Various means of overcoming constipation include: (1) a sufficient amount of water intake each day; (2) roughage in the diet; (3) establishment of a regular time each day for defecation; (4) muscular exercise; (5) freedom from mental stress or worry.

The nurse should remind her patient of the dangers of self-medication in an effort to overcome constipation. Many drugs are on the market and are highly advertised. The claims of manufacturers of such drugs are very apt to be misleading. Practically all such medications are habit forming and their continued use will cause the intestinal tract to become less and less able to function normally. The regular use of enemas will also become habit forming, and after a period of time the enemas will become less effective.

In addition to the elimination of waste products from the intestinal tract, a patient must also eliminate toxins which may be present in the body. For the average patient daily elimination from the intestinal tract would amount to approximately 100–250 grams.

GIVING AND REMOVING THE BEDPAN

In giving and removing the bedpan the following factors are of primary importance.

The patient should have absolute privacy during the procedure. There should be no inhibitory condition which would affect the desire to defecate or to void.

The patient should be placed on the bedpan in the position that is most comfortable for him.

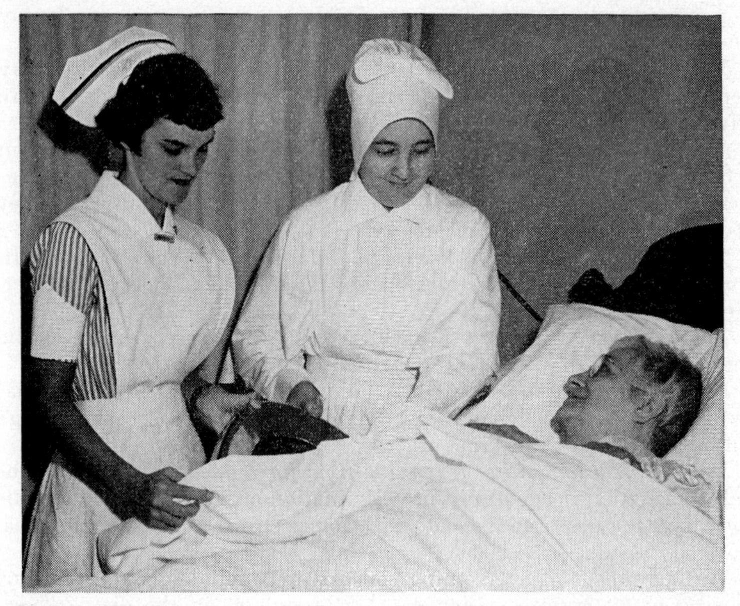

Fig. 123. For using the bedpan the patient should be placed in a semirecumbent position. (Georgetown University Hospital School of Nursing, Washington, D.C.)

The equipment used for this nursing procedure should be in good condition. Usually the bedpan should be warmed before being placed under the patient. For the patient who is in a semi-reclining position, giving the bedpan may be a very simple procedure. The nurse should first make certain that the patient's gown is folded back out of the way, and ends of the gown must not be allowed to fall into the bedpan. By folding back top covers on the bed, the nurse can place the bedpan on the bed beside the patient. The pan should be placed with the wider, deeper end toward the foot of the bed, the side of the pan being parallel to the side of the bed. By placing her left hand under the small of the patient's back the nurse can give support to the patient as he raises his buttocks in position for resting on the bedpan. The patient should be instructed to flex his knees and to set his feet firmly on the bed. By bearing part of his weight on his feet, and with the help of the nurse whose hand is properly placed at his back, he can raise his buttocks so the pan can be moved into place beneath him.

After placing the patient in correct position on the bedpan the nurse should make sure that he is comfortable and firmly supported. If the patient is able to care for himself after using the bedpan, a roll of toilet paper should be put within easy reach.

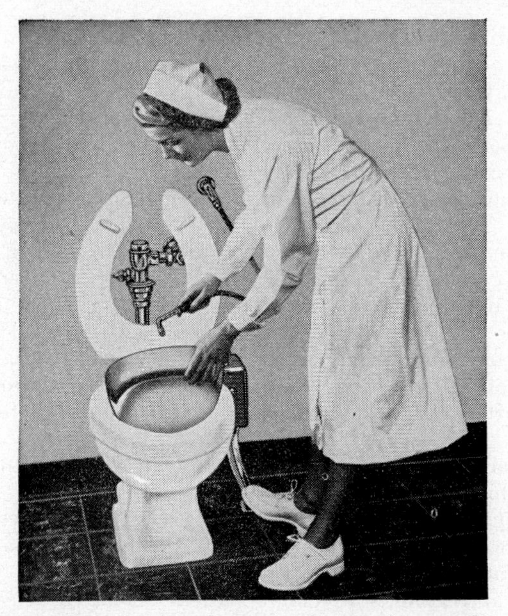

Fig. 124. If the toilet adjoining the patient's room is properly equipped, the bedpan may be emptied and cleaned there and returned to the bedside table. (Crane Company, Chicago, Illinois.)

If he seems to be so weak that assistance is needed, the nurse may ask another nurse or a nurse aide to help her in lifting him and adjusting the bedpan to the proper position.

Unless it is unwise to leave the patient alone the nurse should then leave the room or ward so the patient may use the bedpan in privacy. The signal cord should be placed within reach of the patient before he is left alone in the room.

If the patient's condition is such that the nurse must remain in the room, she should make the situation less embarrassing by being busily engaged in some other activity which will permit her to carefully watch the patient without seeming to do so.

To remove the bedpan the nurse should again instruct the patient to help in raising his buttocks from the bedpan. By firmly grasping the bedpan, at the side, with her right hand, using her left to help support the patient, she may move the bedpan and its contents to the side of the bed, then assist the patient to lower himself to the bed.

Beginning student nurses sometimes need to be reminded that they should not grasp the bedpan by curving their fingers around its upper edge. It is not necessary to touch the inner portion of the bedpan, and to do so results in needless contamination of the nurse's hands.

If the patient has voided only, removal of the bedpan is a simple procedure. Should the bedpan contain fecal material care must be taken so that bed linens are not soiled as the pan is removed. If the patient has had an enema the bedpan will also contain the large amount of solution that was used. The nurse should remove a bedpan that contains a large amount of fluid and waste material carefully, since it is not easily balanced in one hand and the contents may be spilled.

After Care. An integral part of giving and removing the bedpan is adequate care to the patient after the procedure has been completed.

Patients able to care for themselves after use of the bedpan will prefer to do so. Such patients, after the bedpan has been removed from the room, should be given a basin of warm water, soap, towel, and washcloth. The patient should be permitted to thoroughly wash his hands, after which the nurse should remove and care for the equipment used.

For the very ill patient, or for one who may be unable to give proper after care to himself, the nurse will need to carefully and gently give the required care. After the bedpan has been removed the nurse should thoroughly wash and dry the perineal region and lower back of the patient.

The vulvar region of a female patient should be cleansed while the patient is lying on her back. The patient should then be turned to her side while the perineum and area adjacent to the anal region is thoroughly washed and dried. It is most important that the patient's skin be absolutely dry when the cleansing procedure has been completed.

Helpless patients are often embarrassed because someone else must give them this care after use of a bedpan. By her actions and manner in carrying out the procedure, the nurse can relieve such patients of unnecessary embarrassment. Regardless of the kind of procedure being done the nurse should let the patient know that she is glad to be of service to any patient who is unable to help herself. Embarrassment and humiliation can be lessened, also, if the nurse is thoughtful in draping the patient and exposes only that part which is made absolutely necessary to carry out the proper cleansing procedure.

Patients confined to bed usually receive special and frequent care of the skin of the back. This care includes washing and drying the back, and rubbing it with alcohol or a specially prepared lotion. Such special care should also be given after use of the bedpan.

GIVING AND REMOVING THE URINAL

An important factor in giving the urinal to the male patient is to do the procedure without embarrassment to the patient.

When a male patient is admitted to the hospital, if he is not to be permitted bathroom privileges, an explanation should be given him so that he will understand the term "urinal" and its purpose as a part of the necessary equipment for his care.

Many patients have undergone the discomfort of bladder distention because of their hesitancy to ask for information and their lack of knowledge in regard to the name of the article needed if they are to empty the bladder.

In giving the urinal to a male patient who is able to place it in position for use without assistance, the only requirement of the nurse is that she bring the urinal to the patient's bedside and place it on the bed, beneath the top covers, in such position that the patient may readily grasp the handle of the urinal.

If the patient is unable to use the urinal without assistance, an orderly or a nurse must place the urinal and assist in holding it in position so that the contents will not be spilled in the bed. In doing this, the nurse should fold back the top covers, then fold the patient's gown upward, taking care that the patient is not needlessly exposed. The patient's legs will need to be slightly apart so the urinal can be placed on the bed between them. The open end of the urinal should be directed toward the patient and should be held close to the scrotum. Holding the urinal in her right hand, the nurse should gently raise the penis in her left hand and direct it into the opening of the urinal. The urinal will need to be held in position as the patient voids, and the upper portion of the urinal should be held higher than the body or lower portion. Care should be taken so that no pressure is exerted on the scrotum while the urinal is held in position. After the penis has been placed inside the urinal it will remain in the desired position without being held in place while the patient voids.

The urinal may be removed by withdrawing it from between the patient's legs, being careful to keep the top of the urinal directed upward so the contents will not be spilled.

The patient who is able to place the urinal for himself will, after using it, remove it from beneath the covers and hand it to the nurse, who should cover it and take it from the room.

Bedpans and urinals are usually made of monel metal or of enamel. If the bedpan or urinal is enamelware, care should be taken that the article has no jagged edges where the enamel has been chipped. Such rough edges might injure the patient.

Many hospitals which have long been equipped with bedpans and urinals in enamel finish are gradually replacing them with articles made of monel metal. Monel metal offers a very smooth finish, and there is no danger of chipping or of roughened areas in the finish of the article.

Urinals are made of glass as well as of enamel and monel metal. The glass used for these articles is quite heavy, and there is little danger of a patient being injured by chipped places since any unevenness along the edge or mouth of the urinal would be easily detected by an observant nurse.

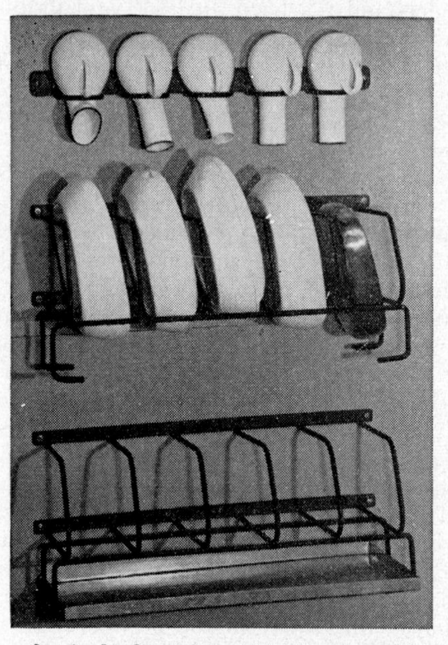

Fig. 125. Bedpans and urinals cleaned, sterilized, and ready for use again. (Wilmot Castle Company, Rochester, New York.)

Urinals are available with a specially constructed opening which makes them adaptable for use by the female patient. Such urinals are particularly useful for patients who must wear certain orthopedic appliances or who are placed in body casts and find it difficult to use the ordinary bedpan.

Muslin bags are used in many institutions so that urinals may be kept at the patient's bedside. If the urinal is kept in such a bag, the patient may reach it without assistance. The bag, with handles of proper length, also serves as a convenient carrying case when the urinal is being emptied.

For the patient who remains at home for nursing care the urinal bag is a definite asset. If the urinal is kept in the bag at the bedside, the patient is able to use it without the need to wait until another person brings it to him.

MEASURED INTAKE AND OUTPUT

Although the actual procedure of measuring intake and output is discussed in another part of the text, it is well to mention here that the nurse who is responsible for emptying a bedpan or urinal should know if the contents of either should be measured.

If the nurse is in doubt as to whether or not urine should be measured, it is much better to measure the urine, and find out later it was unnecessary, than to discard the urine without measuring and then find that the patient is on measured output.

Graduate containers are kept in all hospital utility rooms so that urine from either bedpan or urinal may be quickly measured before being emptied into the hopper. These graduate containers are marked in pints and cubic centimeters. Usually the amount of urine as measured is registered in cubic centimeters.

For the patient being cared for at home, if a graduate container is not available, a pint milk bottle could be used for measuring the urine. The amount of urine thus measured would necessarily be an approximate amount, although the average person would soon be able to estimate almost within 100 cc. the exact amount of urine voided.

INVOLUNTARY URINATION AND DEFECATION

Most patients maintain control of urination and defecation, but some are unable to control elimination from the urinary tract or from the intestines. Involuntary urination or defecation may occur in patients who are very ill, very young, very old, or in a comatose condition. Patients not included in any of the above categories may have involuntary urination or defecation for a short time following surgical treatment, especially if the surgery involved portions of either the urinary or intestinal tract.

For involuntary urination, in some instances, a catheter may be left in place in the bladder. The catheter may be opened and the bladder drained of its accumulation of urine at stated intervals during the day. Leaving a catheter for a prolonged period may tend to produce cystitis, so the treatment is usually continued only a few days.

For the chronically ill patient, subject to involuntary urination, the nurse will need to be vigilant in keeping bed linens dry to keep the patient comfortable. The patient should be placed on the bedpan at regular intervals and special care is needed to keep the skin dry and in good condition. Pads of cellucotton, which are highly absorbent and helpful in keeping the patient dry, should be used.

For the comatose patient the perineal region should be cleansed after each involuntary urination or defecation. The patient, even though not conscious of his surroundings, may often be induced to use the urinal or bedpan if it is placed in position at a time when elimination is apt to occur. The unconscious patient grows restless and moves about in bed if the urinary bladder is distended or if there is an accumulation of feces in the rectum and the desire for defecation is present.

For the involuntary patient who is conscious the nurse must be aware of the psychological effect of the patient's condition. The thoughtful nurse will not show by action or words that the task of cleansing the patient or of changing the bed is in any way distasteful to her. Nor will she indicate to the patient that inability to control either urination or defecation is subject to criticism and a condition which he should attempt to correct.

The bed of an involuntary patient should be protected with additional rubber sheets, and specially prepared pads of absorbent material that can be placed under the patient's hips.

ELIMINATION FROM THE SKIN

Although the amount of waste products eliminated from the skin is not large in comparison with that eliminated by kidneys and intestines, the skin also is an important excretory organ of the body.

The nurse should understand the composition of the skin and its functioning as an excretory organ. She should know changes that may occur in the skin and in its functioning in the event of disease.

The skin forms a surface covering for the entire body and has nerve fibers of pressure, temperature, and pain distributed over its surface. Perhaps one of the most important functions of the skin is that of helping to regulate body temperature. Through perspiration the skin acts to stabilize or to regulate body temperature so that it remains fairly constant under varying circumstances.

By keeping the skin or body surface clean the accumulation of perspiration, dirt, and oil from the glands of the skin may be completely removed.

The patient confined to a hospital bed usually will have decreased circulation in the skin and, therefore, a diminished amount of elimination of waste products through the skin. In contradiction to this fact, it has been noted that patients who are acutely ill or have a highly elevated temperature may have increased skin perspiration and elimination.

The amount of fluid normally excreted through the skin in the form of perspiration is more than most persons are aware of, largely because evaporation occurs so rapidly. As much as a quart of such fluid may be eliminated within a period of 24 hours.

Although perspiration occurs over the entire body surface, it is much more prevalent in areas of the body where two skin surfaces may be in contact. The regions under the arms and at the groin are especially prone to perspiration. In these particular regions evaporation is less apt to occur, and the unpleasant odor associated with perspiration is likely to be present.

Patients who are fearful or anxious about their physical condition may have increased perspiration. Frequent bathing may be required to prevent unsightly manifestations of excessive perspiration likely to appear on gown or pajamas in the underarm region. Only through proper cleansing is it possible to secure normal skin functioning and to prevent the accumulation of waste products which cause offensive odor.

Use of Deodorants and Antiperspirants. Since the skin serves as an excretory organ and helps to eliminate waste products from the body, the use of an antiperspirant, especially for a patient in the hospital, is usually contraindicated. Antiperspirants are designed to prevent or decrease the amount of perspiration. Normally the body will react so that when an antiperspirant is applied to one area, such as the axilla, perspiration from another area of the body will be increased and the total amount of perspiration kept fairly constant. A person who finds it necessary to use an antiperspirant to check underarm perspiration will usually find perspiration of the feet or some other body region is increased. Instead of using antiperspirants for hospitalized patients, there should be more frequent bathing or cleansing of the areas involved. If the underarm area is washed with warm water and mild soap, carefully rinsed, and dried, excessive perspiration need not be a distressing problem, and the unpleasant odor of underarm perspiration can be effectively avoided.

Deodorants, designed to remove unpleasant odors, may be used for the hospitalized patient, although with thorough cleanliness a deodorant is usually not needed. The psychological effect of the use of a deodorant, especially for a patient who may have an unpleasant odor from dressings or from a certain area of the body, will be beneficial. Knowledge that the unpleasant odor has been removed by use of a deodorant helps the patient maintain a desirable mental attitude in regard to the physical condition that caused hospitalization.

Many deodorants are now available, in liquid or cream form, and most of them have a pleasing odor and are easily applied. The wise nurse will encourage the use of deodorants for her hospital patient. The explanation that thorough cleanliness eliminates the need for antiperspirants may be required for the patient whose daily routine has long included use of an antiperspirant and who is unwilling to risk offending hospital personnel. Re-education of such a patient and the assurance that she can resume the use of an antiperspirant on dismissal results in cooperation in the substitution of frequent underarm bathing as a means of protection from perspiration odor.

Care of Equipment after Use

Whether the equipment to be cared for is bedpan or urinal, it should always be thoroughly cleaned after use. The best method is rinsing it first in cold water. This is necessary because hot water tends to coagulate protein materials that might be contained in the waste products of the body.

After the equipment has been rinsed well in cold water it should be washed, preferably with a stiff brush, in hot soapy water, rinsed again, and allowed to dry. If the bedpan or urinal is not kept in the patient's room and used only for the individual patient, it should be sterilized before being placed in use again.

Summary of Important Factors

The bladder normally holds 300–500 cc. but can expand to hold 1000–1500 cc.

Privacy should be provided for any procedure involving elimination from the bladder or intestines.

Normal urine is light amber in color, acid in reaction, clear, and free of albumin or sugar.

Waste products from the intestines consist chiefly of dead bacteria and undigested food materials.

Feces are moved along the intestinal tract and finally eliminated by means of peristaltic action.

Proper diet, exercise, adequate water intake, and establishment of a regular time for evacuation will prevent constipation.

The skin acts as an excretory organ, eliminating waste products through perspiration.

The signal bell should be placed within easy reach of a patient who is left alone on the bedpan.

The use of deodorants for the hospitalized patient has a desirable psychological effect.

The nurse should never indicate to the patient, by word or manner, that after care following elimination is distasteful to her.

If individual bedpans and urinals are not provided, they should be thoroughly cleaned and sterilized after use.

Measured intake and output may be an important part of the patient's treatment. All such measurements should be accurate and should be correctly recorded.

Involuntary urination or defecation usually occurs in the patient who is very old, very young, or very ill, and all such patients should be given special care to prevent pressure sores.

Factors To Teach the Patient

The importance of adequate fluid intake to promote normal functioning of the kidneys.

Means of overcoming dislike and difficulty of using bedpan or urinal.

Means of preventing or overcoming constipation.

Danger of habit formation in use of laxatives and of enemas.

Importance of cleanliness in promoting elimination through the skin.

Necessity for washing hands after giving own care following elimination.

Benefits to be derived from use of deodorants and antiperspirants.

Improvised equipment for use in measuring intake and output for the patient cared for in the home.

Desirable mental attitude with reference to involuntary urination and defecation.

Scientific Principles

Anatomy and Physiology. Understanding of the anatomy of the intestinal tract is necessary to understanding of the process of elimination of waste from the intestines. Walls of the large intestine are composed of involuntary muscular tissue. Contraction and relaxation of involuntary muscles produces peristalsis which propels the contents of the intestinal tract from stomach to rectum.

Muscle tissue reacts to irritation by contracting. Food bulk or gas may cause irritation to the walls of the rectum and thus help in waste elimination.

When an accumulation of fecal material passes into the rectum, sensory nerve endings are stimulated and the patient experiences the desire for defecation. If defecation does not occur, water may be absorbed from the fecal matter, and constipation results because of increased difficulty in evacuation of feces.

Frequency of evacuation is controlled somewhat by the kind of food eaten and the amount of fluid taken into the body.

The three chief functions of the intestine are: (1) continuation of the process of digestion; (2) absorption of water and of drugs; (3) the elimination of waste products.

The urinary bladder is elastic and can expand to accommodate an accumulation of urine up to approximately 2000 cc.

Chemistry. Urine contains water, urea, inorganic salts, pigment, and other end-products of protein and mineral metabolism.

The specific gravity of normal urine may vary from 1.015 to 1.025.

Feces contain indigestible material, intestinal secretions, products of bacterial decomposition, purine bases, pigment, and inorganic salts.

Protein putrefaction takes place normally in the large intestine. The odor of feces is due to substances produced by the action of bacteria on amino acids.

The normal color of feces is due to presence of undigested food and metallic compounds as well as to a pigment derived from bile.

Microbiology. Specific organisms may be found in a urine culture test. The colon bacilli are found normally in large numbers in feces. The colon bacillus, by contamination of the opening to the urinary tract, is a common cause of urinary infections.

Because intestinal wastes contain large numbers of pathogenic bacteria, the nurse must wash her hands thoroughly after emptying a bedpan or urinal. She should keep her hands from her face and mouth (avoid the habit of biting her nails) to protect herself from infection. The mouth is a channel of entrance for intestinal infection.

If patients are not provided individual bedpans and urinals, these articles should be sterilized after each use.

Pharmacology. Diuretics are drugs given to increase the secretion of urine. Those most commonly used are aminophylline, ammonium chloride, and various mercurial diuretics.

Drugs may be given by rectum to be absorbed. Sedatives administered rectally include such drugs as sodium bromide and chloral hydrate. Drugs given rectally are given in larger doses than when administered orally.

Disinfectants commonly used in cleansing bedpans and urinals are Lysol and chlorinated lime.

Physics. Pressure increases as urine accumulates in bladder and initiates nerve impulses which cause the desire for urination.

Pressure of gas against intestinal walls can cause pain and discomfort to the patient.

Pressure against small veins in the anus results in the formation of hemorrhoids.

After use of the bedpan, the room should be ventilated to remove the odor caused by feces and by the expulsion of gas which often accompanies defecation.

Psychology. Excitement, fear, or other emotional stimulus may cause frequent urination. The nurse should attempt to relieve the emotional tension of the patient in order to relieve the urinary symptom.

Providing privacy and adequate draping for use of the bedpan or urinal helps to prevent embarrassment to the patient.

Sociology. The attitude of the nurse in carrying out procedures such as giving the bedpan and urinal influences the patient's attitude toward these essential hygienic measures.

A very ill patient is dependent on the nurse for the very personal services related to elimination, the attitude of the nurse should be such that the procedure becomes merely a part of the daily routine.

Situation Type Problems

1. A student nurse was asked by a graduate nurse to assist in changing linen on the bed of a patient who was subject to involuntary urination.

After much effort on the part of the two nurses (the patient was not at all cooperative and weighed approximately 200 lb.), the bed was made clean and dry.

As the nurses started to leave the room the patient remarked in a most regretful tone of voice, "I'm afraid I just did it again." The graduate nurse voiced the utter dismay she felt by exclaiming to the patient, "Oh, NO! That was the last clean draw sheet from the linen closet." and to the student, "She'll just have to stay wet until they bring up additional linen." What would you have done?

2. A preclinical student, who had just been instructed by the supervisor to take fresh drinking water to all patients in the men's ward, was busily engaged in performing the assignment when one of the patients asked her to bring him a urinal. She complied with the request and several minutes later answered the signal light and emptied

the contents of the urinal into the hopper in a nearby utility room. When she returned to the room to continue taking fresh water to the patients the man said, "Aren't you going to write down the amount?" and explained in answer to her inquiry, "They're keeping a record. All the other nurses write down the amount of urine on this record." The record was that used for recording measured intake and output. What would you have done?

Suggested Reference Reading

"Diets to secure proper elimination," Henrietta Jessup; Trained Nurse and Hospital Review, July, 1936.
"Constipation," Eileen McLaughlin; American Journal of Nursing, March, 1936.
"The artificial kidney," Barbara K. Coleman and John P. Merrill; American Journal of Nursing, March, 1952.

CHAPTER 18

Enemas—Other Rectal Treatments

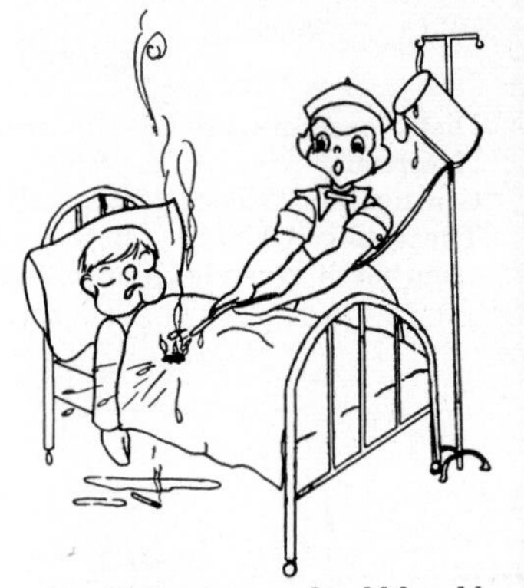

An efficient nurse should be able to improvise equipment when the occasion demands.

TOPICAL OUTLINE

About four hours after food has been taken into the stomach waste material begins to appear in the cecum, that part of the large intestine into which contents from the small intestine are emptied. Most of the absorption of food occurs in the small intestine, so that which is passed into the large intestine by peristaltic action ordinarily contains very little nutrient material. In the cecum much of the water is absorbed from the waste, leaving it a soft mass, termed "feces."

By an occasional strong peristaltic wave fecal material is moved into the descending colon, where it remains until it is moved into the rectum just prior to elimination from the body. Normally the peristaltic wave is set in motion by the intake of food. Through peristaltic action fecal material enters the rectum and acts as a stimulus to nerve endings in that organ to produce the desire for defecation. Most persons have one bowel movement each day; some may have more than one daily movement, and others normally defecate only once in two or three days.

The Enema

The term enema is defined as "an injection into the rectum of a solution to cleanse the lower intestine or to provide nutrients or administer medications."

Although the number of enemas used in treatment of patients is quite large, the kind most commonly used is the cleansing enema. Because of the frequency with which it is used, the term "enema" has come to mean "cleansing enema," and this is the kind given unless another type is specifically indicated.

The purpose of the cleansing enema is to remove feces from the rectum and lower colon. It is used to aid in elimination when that process has been disturbed or interrupted. Cleansing enemas are given when the patient may be unable or unwilling to take a laxative by mouth. Before an operative procedure involving the intestinal tract a series of cleansing enemas may be given to remove fecal material from the intestines.

Other enemas may be given for expulsion of gas from the colon and rectum, expulsion of intestinal worms, to relieve intestinal pain and discomfort, to soothe irritated intestinal walls, to help in providing nutrients for a patient who cannot take food orally, and to apply medication to the anal canal.

POSITION OF THE PATIENT

In preparing the patient for an enema the nurse should make sure that he is in a comfortable position, with body relaxed. If the patient has not had an enema previously, the procedure should be explained so that complete cooperation may be had. Part of the effectiveness of the procedure depends on the amount of solution the patient is able to take and the manner in which the enema is given.

The patient should be placed on the left side in a horizontal position, with not more than one pillow under the head. The arms should be away from the anterior surface of the abdomen so as not to interfere with expansion of the intestine as the solution is introduced. The left side position is preferable since in that position the anal canal is somewhat higher than the rectum and descending colon, and the solution flows readily into the lower intestinal tract.

If the patient is instructed to breathe deeply the inflow of solution will be facilitated. The nurse should have informed the patient that the solution flowing into the colon will cause some spasmodic contractions of the intestinal tract and may produce some slight abdominal pain. When such spasmodic pains occur the nurse should stop the flow of solution until they subside. Assurance that the flow of solution will be regulated so that the procedure is not painful will enable the nurse to gain the confidence of the patient. By reducing the flow of solution to relieve the spasmodic contractions, the full amount of solution may usually be given without undue discomfort to the patient.

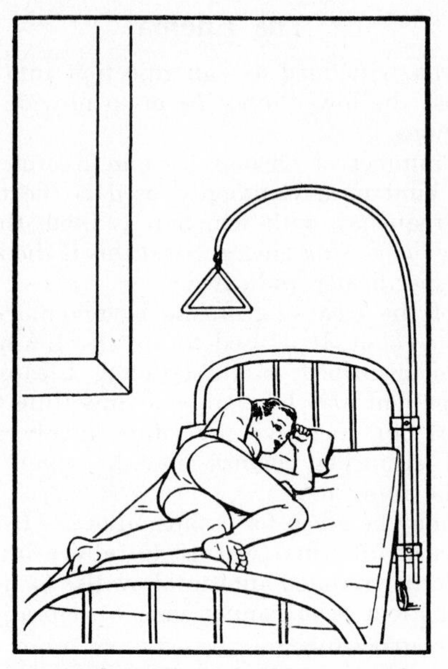

Fig. 126. For an enema the patient should be turned to her left side with knees flexed. (M. C. Winters, Protective Body Mechanics in Daily Life and in Nursing.)

If the enema cannot be given with the patient on his left side, he may be permitted to lie in the dorsal recumbent position with buttocks slightly elevated on a rubber covered pillow. An enema should not be given with the patient in a sitting or standing position, since such a position would necessitate that the solution flow against, rather than with, the force of gravity.

TYPES OF ENEMAS

Enemas may be classified into two general types, according to the purpose for which they are given, those to be expelled and those to be retained. The most commonly used therapeutic enemas are summarized in Table 4 and discussed in the following paragraphs.

The Cleansing Enema. The cleansing enema is an injection of water, or other solution, into the rectum and colon for the purpose of washing out that part of the intestinal tract and to stimulate peristaltic action to help promote evacuation.

The cleansing enema is contraindicated in conditions of abdominal pain, the cause of which has not been determined. The cleansing enema should not be given without a written order from the physician.

Solutions usually used for a cleansing enema are tap water, normal saline, sodium bicarbonate, and a rather weak solution of soap suds.

Table 4. Commonly Used Therapeutic Enemas

Enemas To Be Expelled		
KIND	PURPOSE	SOLUTION COMMONLY USED
Cleansing	To wash or cleanse the colon	Soap suds
Anthelmintic	To expel worms	Quassia
Astringent	To contract tissue To check bleeding	Solution of alum
Carminative	To expel flatus	Milk and molasses

Enemas To Be Retained		
KIND	PURPOSE	SOLUTION COMMONLY USED
Diagnostic	To outline colon for X-Ray	Barium sulfate
Emollient	To coat the mucous membrane of the intestinal tract	Starch solution
Lubricating (oil retention)	To soften feces	Olive oil or sweet oil
Nutrient	For nourishment	Dextrose solution
Sedative	To induce sleep	Paraldehyde
Stimulating	To stimulate body processes	Coffee

The amount of solution used ranges from 500 to 1000 cc., depending on the age and physical condition of the patient. The temperature of the solution should be approximately 105° F. A bath thermometer may be used to check the temperature of the solution.

Equipment used in giving a cleansing enema includes an irrigating can, a bath thermometer, lubricant, and a small rectal tube (22–24 French with opening at the end and at one side). Sufficient tubing will be needed so the lower edge of the can is about 12 inches above the insertion level of the rectal tube as it is held in position at the anal sphincter. At this level, pressure exerted on the solution in the can is great enough to cause it to flow rather slowly into the rectum, yet is not so great as to cause stimulation of the defecation reflex.

The bed should be protected with a small rubber pad and cover and the bath blanket is used to drape the patient. If the irrigating can is not used the solution, kept in a pitcher until time for the enema to be given, may be poured through a funnel attached to the tubing and rectal tube.

If the irrigating can or funnel is elevated to a higher level pressure is increased, the solution will be rapidly injected and stimulate expulsion from the rectum before all parts of the colon can be "cleansed." Given under low pressure and at a fairly slow rate, the cleansing enema requires approximately 6 to 10 minutes for injection.

Method of Administering the Enema. With the patient lying on the left side, with knees flexed, the bath blanket drape should be turned back so that the patient is exposed as little as possible to avoid embarrassment. The rectal tube should be well lubricated and inserted very carefully into the anus. The nurse will need to see the anal opening if she is to insert the tube properly, so it is necessary that she raise a portion of the upper buttock so it does not interfere with a clear view of the anal region.

Before inserting the tube into the anal opening, enough solution should be allowed to run through it so that all air is expelled. The tube should be inserted about four inches into the rectum, which is about five to six inches in length. The tube does not pass through into the sigmoid, so if it is inserted beyond four inches it only tends to turn back on itself inside the rectum. If introduction of the rectal tube causes pain rather than the usual slight and temporary discomfort, it should be withdrawn. Conditions such as hemorrhoids, a stricture of the rectum, or rectal abscess may contraindicate the giving of an enema.

The solution should be injected slowly and the flow discontinued entirely at intervals when beginning peristaltic action may produce abdominal cramps. Instructing the patient to breathe deeply during the procedure will also help to reduce discomfort.

At no time during the procedure should air be allowed to enter the tubing. If a funnel is used it should always be about two-thirds filled with solution.

When an adequate amount of solution has been given the tubing should be clamped off and the rectal tube removed. The patient should be encouraged to retain the solution for a short time (5 to 10 minutes in order to soften feces in the colon) before being placed on the bedpan. After the patient has been placed on the bedpan, the back rest should be elevated and the signal bell placed within easy reach. The very ill patient or one with cardiac disturbance should not be left alone while the enema is being expelled.

If the patient is able to properly cleanse herself after an enema she should be permitted to do so; if she is too weak to care for herself the nurse should see that the perineal area is clean and dry. After the enema has been given the patient should be permitted to wash her hands. The room should be thoroughly aired to remove any unpleasant odor that may have resulted from the enema procedure.

The bedpan and all equipment used in giving the enema should be removed from the room to be thoroughly washed and cleaned. The rectal tube, after being cleaned, should be boiled for five minutes.

The patient who has taken an enema each day over a long period of time may be helped to overcome the habit by use of a smaller amount of solution each time an enema is given, and by being instructed to eat a well balanced diet, drink a sufficient amount of fluids, and establish a regular time for elimination.

If the patient is unable to expel an enema soon after it has been given, it may be necessary to siphon off the solution. To do this the rectal tube is inserted again into the rectum and the free end of the tube is placed in the bedpan. The solution will then flow from the rectum into the bedpan.

The Retention Enema. The solution used for a retention enema is given in a small amount and at a very slow rate. Retention enemas are used as a means of supplying fluid or of administering a medication rectally (medicinal enema). Stimulation of peristalsis and of the desire to defecate should be avoided so the solution may be retained for several hours.

Normal saline and tap water are the solutions commonly used for supplying fluids rectally. Anesthetic agents and sedatives are medications sometimes given as retention enemas. The patient should be given a cleansing enema about one hour before rectal administration of a drug, so the intestinal tract will be clear and the drug can be absorbed. For a medicinal enema (1) the rectum must be clear of feces; (2) the drug used must be soluble; (3) the solution should be of the consistency of thin starch water; (4) the temperature of the solution should be 100° F.; (5) the enema must be given slowly. Drugs which might irritate the intestinal mucosa or stimulate peristalsis cannot be given by this method.

Corn oil or cotton seed oil may be administered rectally and retained for two or three hours to soften feces so that a cleansing enema will be more effective.

The equipment needed for a retention enema consists chiefly of an 18–20 French catheter, a funnel, and a small length of rubber tubing.

The amount of solution is limited to 3 to 6 ounces, so the rectum will not be distended. The temperature of the solution should not exceed 105° F. Air should be expelled from the tubing and the solution given slowly. The bed should be protected and the patient draped as for a cleansing enema.

The procedure should be explained to the patient so her cooperation is gained and she understands the necessity for retaining the solution.

After completing the procedure, the equipment should be thoroughly washed in soap and water and boiled for 10 minutes so it will be ready for use again when needed.

Enema for the Child. The procedure of giving an enema to a very young child (under 6 years of age) differs somewhat from that of giving an enema to an adult. The child is usually unable to retain the solution, which may be expelled as it is being given. The container for the solution should not be more than 15 to 18 inches above the level of the child's buttocks, thus limiting the amount of pressure exerted against the intestinal walls.

A catheter should be used instead of the rectal tube. The catheter should be well lubricated and inserted into the rectum approximately three inches.

The temperature of the solution should be 100° F., and the amount should depend on the results being obtained. Usually 500 cc. will be sufficient. The amount may be increased to 1000 cc. if necessary, although only small amounts should be injected at one time.

The child should be given an explanation as to what is expected of him so he can cooperate during the procedure and good results will be obtained. The procedure should be discussed in terms familiar to the child and understood by him.

If it is necessary to restrain the very young child, a bath blanket wrapped securely around the upper part of his body so that the arms are held close to his sides will usually suffice. If possible, another nurse or the mother of the child should be asked to help with the enema. Restraint for such a nursing procedure may cause the child to react violently not only against the enema procedure but also against any other treatment or nursing procedure his physical condition may require.

Enema Self Administered by the Patient. It is often necessary for the patient to continue taking enemas after leaving the hospital, and in such cases the nurse should instruct the patient as to the correct technique for taking an enema at home.

Instruction should be given on how to prepare the solution. By permitting the patient to prepare solution for an enema to be given in the hospital, the nurse can supervise the preparation and the patient can learn to do by doing. She should note the appearance of the solution and so learn to know when the solution she may prepare at home has attained the right degree of soapiness.

She should be taught to test the temperature of the solution by pouring a small amount across her inner wrist. If the solution is just pleasantly warm on the wrist, the temperature will be about 105° F.

The way in which the height of the container of solution governs the rate of flow, pressure being increased or decreased as the container is raised and lowered, should be explained.

The patient should be told the reason for lying on the left side during the procedure. She should be taught that the treatment will be more effective if approximately 10 minutes is utilized for the inflow of solution.

The habitual use of enemas should be discouraged, and the dangers of such use discussed with the patient. If she understands that frequent and regular enemas accustom the lower intestine to the stimulus of distention much greater than that caused by normal accumulation of feces she will understand that the more the treatment by enema is used the more necessary it tends to become. Understanding of this principle will lead to better cooperation in the matter of giving less solution in each enema and giving the enema at gradually increasing intervals so that the procedure may in time be discontinued.

While being instructed in regard to taking an enema, the patient should be fully informed as to the important part played by diet, habit formation, and other health measures in overcoming constipation and in correcting the enema habit. Instruction in regard to self-administered enemas is not complete without detailed information on the dangers involved in taking an enema in certain conditions affecting the abdomen, as in appendicitis.

If the patient does not know of the services of the Visiting Nurse Association and that those services are available in her community, she should be informed. The public health nurse will give an enema to the patient at home or assist in giving further instruction if it is needed.

REMOVAL OF FECAL IMPACTION

In some instances it may be necessary to forcibly remove an impacted fecal mass from the rectum before an enema can be administered. Fecal impaction, or the presence of a hardened mass of fecal material in the rectum, may prevent the entrance of the rectal tube or catheter tip so that not even an oil retention enema can be given.

The nurse or intern who is to remove the impacted mass should wear a rubber glove, see that the index finger is well lubricated, gently insert the gloved finger into the rectum and, without causing discomfort to the patient, forcibly break up the mass so that it can be removed in small parts. A fecal impaction is formed by addition of small nodules or particles of fecal material which are tightly pressed against other particles to form the whole mass. As the fluid content is absorbed from the mass while it remains in the rectum, the particles of material tend to become hardened and form into many separate sections rather than combining into one complete formation. Because the mass is made up of tightly compressed small sections, it is relatively easy, by finger manipulation, to break it up and remove it. By extracting the broken sections the entire mass which blocked the entrance into the rectum may be removed in a short time.

FORMULA, METHOD OF ADMINISTRATION, PURPOSE OF SPECIAL ENEMAS

The formula, method of administration, and purpose of the various other kinds of therapeutic enemas listed in Table 4 are discussed in the following paragraphs. The anthelmintic, astringent, and carminative enemas are to be expelled; the other enemas, with only small quantities of solution, are to be retained.

Anthelmintic Enema. Given to expel certain types of parasitic worms. A solution made by adding about 8 ounces of cold water to 1 dram of quassia chips is used. The solution should be left standing for two or three hours, then strained and used in treatment of pin or thread worms. The material expelled after an anthelmintic enema should always be examined closely (by microscope, if necessary) to determine if it contains worms.

Astringent Enema. Now used only on rare occasions to help in checking hemorrhage. The solution causes contraction of the tissues, and this type of enema may aid in the expulsion of worms and other parasites. The most commonly used solution is 16 cc. of alum in 250 cc. of water. To make the enema more effective, the temperature of the solution should be 110° F.

Carminative Enema. Given to relieve distention caused by flatulence and to stimulate peristalsis. Solutions most commonly used are milk and molasses, 180 cc. of each, or magnesium sulfate 1 ounce, glycerin 2 ounces, and water 3 ounces (the "one, two, three" enema). The temperature of the solution may be as high as 110° F. if the patient does not object.

The Diagnostic Enema. Given to aid in x-ray diagnosis. A solution of barium sulfate is given rectally so the walls of the colon will be clearly defined in the x-ray. One hundred to 150 grams of barium sulfate is dissolved in one pint of water. Temperature of the solution should be about 100° F.

Emollient Enema. Given to coat the intestinal mucous membrane and thus relieve local irritation. Starch solution is most commonly used. One dram of starch is added to a small amount of cold water to make a smooth paste, then 6 ounces of boiling water is added. The mixture is allowed to cool to 105° F. before being injected as a retention enema.

Lubricating Enema. Given to soften feces and to lubricate the anal canal so that evacuation of fecal material, following surgery on the rectum, will be less painful. Olive oil or sweet oil, 4 to 6 ounces, may be used. The temperature of the solution should be about 105° F. In case of fecal impaction a lubricating enema followed several hours later by a cleansing enema may be effective.

Medicinal Enema. Enema to which some drug or medication has been added. Drugs which cannot be given by mouth may be administered rectally. Corrosive drugs, of course, should not be given by enema as the irritation caused by the drug would produce peristaltic action and the enema would be expelled.

About one hour before the medicinal enema is to be given the patient should be given a cleansing enema so the intestinal tract will be clear and the drug can be absorbed. For a medicinal enema:

The rectum must be clear of feces.

The drug used must be soluble.

The solution should be of the consistency of thin starch water.

The temperature of the solution should be 100° F.

The enema must be given slowly.

Nutrient Enema. Since it is known that digestion cannot take place in the colon and that that organ is capable of absorbing only small amounts of water or weak solutions of dextrose, saline, and brandy, the amount of solution that can be utilized when given as an enema is restricted, but when other channels of administration cannot be used the rectal method may be extremely worth while. The solutions most commonly used are tap water, 5 per cent dextrose, and normal saline. The temperature should not exceed 100° F.

Sedative Enema. A retention enema containing a sedative drug, used when the drug cannot be given by mouth or by other methods. Three to 6 ounces of solution is usually used. The drug is dissolved in a small amount of hot water, then added to the required number of ounces of starch water. Temperature of the solution should not exceed 105° F. Drugs most commonly used for sedative enemas include chloral hydrate and paraldehyde.

Stimulating Enema. Given as a retention enema for stimulant effect. Six to 8 ounces of coffee was the solution usually used, at a temperature of 100° F. Other solutions used include saline solution, with addition of ½–1 ounce of spiritus frumenti, tincture of digitalis, and Lugol's solution.

Other Special Enemas. Other special enemas sometimes used include the egg and ether enema, Mayo enema, Nobel's enema, olive oil and turpentine enema, the purgative enema, normal salt solution enema, paregoric enema, and the SS. and P. (soapsuds and peppermint) enema.

Proctoclysis

Although not used at the present time, proctoclysis was formerly an important postoperative procedure. Commonly called "Murphy drip," after the well known Chicago surgeon who first used and described it, it consisted of introduction of a solution into the rectum at a very slow rate of flow. The inflow tube contained a device that provided for the escape of gas from the rectum.

The treatment was continued for several hours, or for several days, to supply fluids, dilute toxins, and reduce distention caused by gas in the colon and rectum.

Hypotonic sodium chloride was commonly used. The temperature of the solution was maintained near 98.6° F. by placing the inflow tube between two hot water bottles.

A cleansing enema was given before the treatment was started, if necessary, to insure that the rectum was empty of fecal material.

Protoclysis is not used at the present time because blood, plasma, and fluids can be supplied more effectively by intravenous injection.

Colonic Irrigation

Colonic irrigation, or enteroclysis, refers to the treatment of washing out the colon with large quantities of a solution. The irrigation may be given to cleanse the colon, to apply drugs locally to the mucosa of the colon, and to help neutralize and remove corrosive poisons.

Solutions commonly used are tap water, normal saline, sodium bicarbonate, or an astringent such as silver nitrate, 1:2000, or a weak solution of tannic acid. The amount of solution used may be 2 to 4 gallons, and the treatment may require 20 to 40 minutes.

A cleansing enema should be given an hour or so before treatment is started, so the rectum will be free of fecal material.

The irrigating can, tubing, and a small rectal tube (20–24 French) is used for the inflowing solution. A larger rectal tube (30–32 French) with connective tubing and a large pail are needed for collection of the outflow. A single rectal tube may be used with a glass Y connector which permits regulating inflow and outflow in the same manner as the two-tube method. If one tube is used, it is attached to one prong of the glass Y. The tube for outflow is attached to the other prong and the tubing from the irrigating can is attached to the base of the Y. Stopcocks on inflow and outflow tubes make it possible to introduce about 500 cc. of solution into the colon then close the inflow tube and open the outflow tube to drain the solution from the rectum.

The same procedure may be carried out if two tubes are being used. In the two-tube method the outflow tube should be inserted into the rectum about four inches. The inflow tube should extend further into the rectum, approximately five or six inches.

The irrigating can should be about 24 inches above the patient's hips so there will not be too much pressure exerted by the inflowing solution. The waste pail should be placed on a stool near the bed. If placed on the floor, suction that drains the solution from the rectum may be too great.

Cooperation of the patient is necessary if the treatment is to be effective, so the procedure should be explained to the patient. During the treatment the patient should be assured privacy by careful draping and screening.

After use, all equipment should be washed with soap and water, rinsed well, and the rectal tubes should be boiled for 10 minutes.

Anal Irrigation

Irrigation or washing of the anal region is the means of giving proper aseptic care to a hemorrhoidectomy patient after each defecation.

Solutions used are boric acid 5 per cent or sterile water. Equipment needed includes rubber bulb syringe, basin of solution, cotton balls, and emesis basin.

The bed should be adequately protected at the time the patient is placed on the bedpan. When the bedpan is removed the patient should be turned to her side. The emesis basin should be placed firmly against the lower buttocks and the solution should be gently expressed from the rubber bulb syringe to irrigate the anal region. Cotton balls should be used to gently pat dry the area after the irrigation is completed. After use, the irrigation tray should be made ready for use again, with needed supplies replaced. Used equipment should be washed and returned to the tray.

Rectal Suppositories

Rectal suppositories are cone shaped and made of a variety of substances, depending on the purpose for which they are to be used. They are used chiefly to promote evacuation of feces and to introduce a drug or medicine into the rectum.

Suppositories are made of soap, glycerin, or plain or medicated cocoa butter. They retain their shape at ordinary room temperature, but melt when subjected to body heat in the rectum. Drugs contained in the suppository are released when the suppository is dissolved.

The suppositories most commonly used are:

Soap or Glycerin Suppositories. Used to cause expulsion of feces from the rectum. Irritation caused by the suppository stimulates the rectum to expel its entire contents, including the suppository itself. Glycerin suppositories for children are long (three inches) and cylindrical in shape; those for adults are much shorter and larger in diameter.

Astringent Suppositories. Used to contract tissues and help check bleeding and diarrhea. Such suppositories may contain tannic acid, belladonna, glycerin, or bismuth.

Anodyne Suppositories. Used to relieve pain in such conditions as dysentery, diarrhea, rectal abscess, and hemorrhoids. The drugs most commonly used are cocaine, opium, and belladonna, added to cocoa butter. Opium suppositories are used also for a general sedative effect.

Specific Suppositories. Used to treat a specific disease, as the quinine suppository used in treatment of malaria.

For inserting a suppository, a rubber glove should be worn, so the suppository can be inserted as far as the finger can reach. Suppositories should be well lubricated before they are inserted. The ends of all suppositories should be well rounded so there is no danger of inflicting injury to the mucous membrane of the rectum as they are inserted. After the suppository has been inserted, pressure should be applied over the anus for a few moments until desire to expel the suppository has passed.

Suppositories should be stored in a cool place; glycerin suppositories should be kept in the refrigerator.

Care of Equipment after Use

The bedpan should be emptied of contents, rinsed well with cold water, washed with warm water and soap, rinsed and sterilized, then returned to the patient's bedside table.

The enema can should be rinsed with cold water, washed in warm soapy water, rinsed and sent to Central Supply to be boiled for 10 minutes before being placed in use again. The funnel and pitcher used in giving a retention enema should be cared for in the same manner.

Rubber gloves used in removing a fecal impaction should be washed thoroughly and sent to Central Supply to be sterilized.

Equipment used in proctoclysis and irrigation should be washed with soap and water, rinsed well, and sterilized. The irrigation tray should then be made ready for use again.

Summary of Important Factors

Enemas. Fecal material is moved through the intestinal tract by peristaltic action.

Symptoms of constipation: loss of appetite, headache, abdominal distention, depression, irritability, unpleasant breath.

To overcome constipation: drink plenty of fluids, get roughage in the diet, exercise, establish regular time for daily evacuation.

Position of patient for enema: left side, head low, knees flexed.

Explain procedure before it is started, to gain cooperation of patient.

Enemas to be expelled: cleansing, carminative, anthelmintic, astringent.

Enemas to be retained: diagnostic, emollient, lubricating, nutrient, sedative, stimulating.

Temperature of solution: 100–110° F. Amount: few ounces to 1000 cc.

Insert tube only about four inches into rectum.

Retention enema should be given slowly and in very small amounts.

It may be necessary to restrain a child to give an enema.

Very young children usually expel the enema as it is being given.

Proctoclysis. The introduction of a solution into the rectum at a very slow rate of flow.

Colonic Irrigation. Washing out the colon with large quantities of solution.

Anal Irrigation. Washing or cleansing of the anal area.

Rectal Suppositories. Cone-shaped substance inserted into the rectum to promote defecation or to introduce a drug.

Factors To Teach the Patient

The importance of proper diet, sufficient fluids, exercise, and habit formation in overcoming constipation.

That after use of bedpan or toilet, hand washing is essential to prevent spread of harmful microorganisms which may have contaminated the hands.

Instruction in regard to dangers of "straining" at stool when on the bedpan.

Proper terminology with reference to elimination, enemas, and rectal treatments.

How proper position of the patient aids in giving the enema more effectively and without undue discomfort.

The danger involved in taking an enema when undiagnosed abdominal disorder is present. Danger especially in appendicitis.

The dangers of frequent use of laxatives and enemas since either may be habit forming and both tend to increase rather than decrease tendency toward constipation.

The proper method of using toilet tissue so contamination from the anal region is not carried forward to the vaginal region.

How to obtain equipment for taking an enema at home and how to prepare the solution.

For taking an enema at home, (1) height of container should be not more than 2½ feet above bed; (2) temperature of solution should be checked by pouring on inner wrist; (3) about 10 minutes is necessary for giving the enema; (4) the proper position is lying on left side, knees flexed, head lowered. How to overcome the daily enema habit.

That services of the public health nurse, if they are available to him, include the procedure of giving an enema.

The method of inserting rectal suppository, if instruction is needed in that procedure.

Scientific Principles

Anatomy and Physiology. The large intestine in the adult is approximately five feet long and is made up of the cecum, colon, and rectum. The ileocecal valve, separating the small and large intestines, functions in one direction only, so that fecal material is moved always toward the large intestine. The colon is divided into ascending, transverse, and descending colon, and the sigmoid flexure. The rectum is about six inches long and terminates at the anal opening. The internal and external sphincter muscles, controlled by nerves from the central nervous system, govern the opening and closing of the anus.

Relaxation and contraction of involuntary muscle in the intestinal tract produces peristalsis, which moves the fecal material toward the rectum.

Hemorrhoids are dilated veins in the region of the rectum and anus.

Sensory nerve endings in the rectum are stimulated by fecal material there and the desire for evacuation is induced. Defecation is a voluntary process caused by contraction of abdominal muscles. Frequency of evacuation may be influenced by the kinds of food eaten.

Chemistry. Water is absorbed through the intestinal wall by osmosis. The speed with which water or drugs is absorbed when given rectally depends on the area of the intestinal tract reached by the solution.

Feces are made up of indigestible material, bacteria, intestinal secretions, products of decomposition of bacteria, purine bases, pigment, and inorganic salts.

Protein putrefaction is constantly occurring in the large intestine.

Solutions commonly used for cleansing enemas are soapsuds solution or a solution of sodium chloride or sodium bicarbonate.

Hot water causes protein to coagulate. Cold water should be used to rinse the bedpan to dissolve protein substances before the pan is washed in soap and water.

Microbiology. The colon and rectum provide favorable conditions for the growth of bacteria. Organisms found in the colon and rectum may be harmless or pathogenic. The colon bacilli make up about 70 per cent of all living bacteria found in feces. Common pathogenic organisms that cause intestinal disease are those of typhoid and dysentery.

When pathogenic organisms are present in feces, the stool should be disinfected before it is emptied into waste pipes.

All articles and equipment used for enemas must be thoroughly cleansed; rectal tubes should be boiled to destroy harmful bacteria.

After evacuation toilet tissue should be moved toward the back in cleansing the anal region to prevent contamination of the vagina and urinary meatus.

Cleanliness of the anal area is especially important after hemorrhoidectomy or perineorrhaphy, because such wounds provide a channel for the entrance of bacteria.

Contaminated hands of the nurse transfer disease organisms readily. For that reason the nurse should carefully wash her hands after caring for the bedpan or giving a rectal treatment.

Rectal tubes or tips should be boiled or subjected to steam sterilization after each use. Solutions used in enemas and rectal treatments need not be sterile.

Pharmacology. Drugs are given by rectum for their stimulating emollient, irritating, or sedative effect. For rectal administration, drugs should be well dissolved so absorption can take place readily.

Cornstarch solution is commonly used for its emollient action on the intestinal tract. It serves as a protective coating of the mucous membrane of the intestines and lessens irritation caused by drugs.

Larger doses of drugs are used for rectal than for oral administration, since absorption from the rectum is limited.

Lubricants for rectal tubes are of the water-soluble glycerin variety.

Disinfectants used for bedpans are of the cresol group.

Physics. Rate of flow in enemas depends on pressure, caliber of the tube, and the density of the fluid. To increase pressure and rate of flow, the container of solution will need to be raised. To lower the pressure and decrease rate of flow, the container should be lowered.

When the solution flows too fast, pressure is increased and causes contractions of the intestinal walls which may be painful to the patient. When the patient thus experiences pain, the solution is expelled and the total amount given may be inadequate.

If an enema must be siphoned off, the solution flows out through the inserted colon tube because pressure in the colon is greater than pressure at the end of the tube.

With the patient on the left side, gravity will aid the inflow of solution. By raising the backrest when the patient is placed on the bedpan, gravity will help in expulsion of the enema.

Psychology. Privacy, draping, and explanation of procedure help to lessen embarrassment of the patient who must use the bedpan. The signal bell should be placed within easy reach.

If the patient is relaxed and at ease during the giving of an enema, it will be more effective. If necessary, the nurse may divert the patient's attention by conversation in order to promote relaxation.

Prompt answering of lights lessens irritation or annoyance caused by waiting for or on the bedpan. Offering the bedpan before meals and before visiting hours may prevent embarrassment of the patient.

After an enema or other rectal treatment, the room should be well ventilated to make sure it is free of unpleasant odor.

Sociology. Patients are apt to be embarrassed when the nurse gives an enema or helps with other rectal treatments. The nurse should, by her attitude and manner of performing such services, let the patient know that the procedure is a routine part of her daily duties and not objectionable to her.

Patients requiring rectal treatments after dismissal from the hospital should be informed that such services are available through the Visiting Nurse Association or can be obtained at certain clinics or Out-Patient departments in local hospitals.

Situation Type Problems

1. A young student nurse had disregarded a regulation imposed on students in the school which prohibited social engagements with members of the opposite sex who were patients in the hospital. She felt justified in infringement of the rule since she had gone out with a patient from a department quite far removed from the one in which she was on duty. She assured herself that since she was not assisting in the nursing care of this particular patient there was no reason why she should not enjoy his company when she was free of classwork and duty and had time for recreational activities.

After several "dates" with the young man, she became very fond of him and was sure that he was equally fond of her.

In an unexpected and very sudden interruption to routine, she was relieved of the assignments in her department and sent to the department where the young man was hospitalized, to replace a student who had suddenly become ill.

The head nurse to whom she reported for duty gave her an assignment of patients that included "her young man" and she was to give him an S.S. enema as preparation for a scheduled examination by one of the doctors that morning. The student asked to be assigned to another patient instead of the young man. The head nurse refused. Then the student asked if she might have an orderly give the enema. The orderly for that department was off duty until after noon. The student felt she could not perform the nursing procedure without great embarrassment to herself and the young man, yet she could not explain to the head nurse without disclosing the fact that she had disobeyed regulations of the school. What would you have done?

2. The student in the above situation tried unsuccessfully to change assignments with one of the graduate nurses on the department. She then contacted a preclinical student who was on duty on the department for only a short period of time. The preclinical student had had the enema procedure in class but had not been supervised in doing the procedure in the hospital. At the insistence of the advanced student, the preclinical student gave the enema to the young man. She did the procedure accurately so that the patient suffered no ill effects, but the clinical supervisor came into the room just as the treatment was being completed. The preclinical student was severely criticized for doing the procedure without supervision and was taken from duty. She did not mention that the older student had insisted she do the procedure and could give no reason to the supervisor for her failure to observe the strict regulation of first performing each procedure under supervision. If you were the preclinical student, what would you have done?

3. The preclinical student who gave the enema without proper supervision was asked to appear before the judiciary committee of the school, because of her failure to observe the regulation in regard to supervision of procedures. The senior member of the judiciary committee was the student who had been assigned to give the enema. In *her* place, what would you have done?

Suggested Reference Reading

"Colonic irrigations," Walter A. Bastedo; American Journal of Nursing, June, 1936.

"About enemas," Walter A. Bastedo; American Journal of Nursing, April, 1937.

"Physics and pressure," Hessel Howard Flitter; American Journal of Nursing, January, 1948.

"Giving enemas to infants and children," Ruby Roberts; American Journal of Nursing, November, 1949.

CHAPTER 19

Collection of Specimens

TOPICAL OUTLINE

Containers for Specimens
Labels for Specimen Containers
Preservation of Specimens
Methods of Collecting Specimens
- Urine Specimens
- Specimens of Stomach Contents
- Sputum Specimens
- Specimens of Feces
- Blood Specimens
- Specimens of Spinal, Pleural, and Peritoneal Fluids
- Cultures from Nose and Throat
- Smears

Examination of Specimens as a Public Health Service

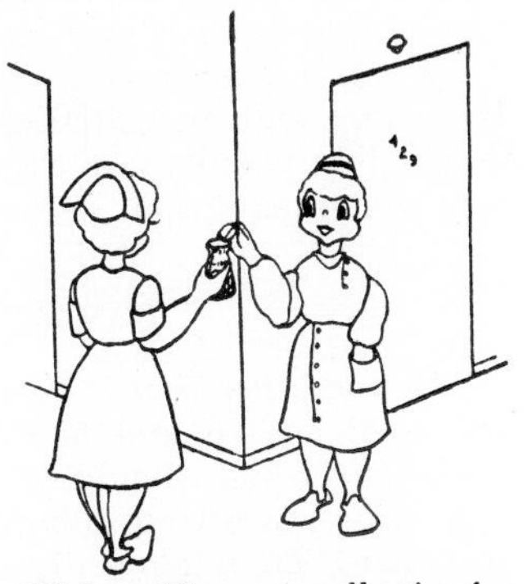

"We're taking up a collection for Miss Schmaltz. She isn't going to leave or be married, but feels she's stuck here for the rest of her life!"

A specimen is defined as "a small quantity of a substance or object which shows the kind and quality of the whole, as a blood or urine specimen."

Specimens sent to the laboratory are examined chemically and microscopically, to aid in making a diagnosis or in determining the course of treatment.

The collection of a specimen has come to be a very important responsibility of the nurse since the accuracy and reliability of laboratory findings may depend, to a great extent, on the way the procedure is accomplished. If the specimen is carelessly handled by the nurse before it reaches the laboratory, the results of the test done there may be inaccurate and may lead to a wrong diagnosis or method of treatment.

A specimen should always be collected according to instructions in the hospital's laboratory procedure book. All specimens should be properly labeled and sent to the laboratory in the best possible condition for the examination or tests which will be done there.

For the detailed method of collecting certain specimens, the nurse will need to consult the procedure book or be guided by the doctor's orders. General information in regard to collection of specimens can be obtained by an understanding of such factors as the kind of containers to use, the best method of collecting the specimen, information which should appear on the label, and proper care of the specimen after it has been collected.

By understanding the manner of test that will be done in the laboratory and by realizing the importance of following exactly the detailed instructions in regard to collecting the specimen, carelessness which may result in inaccurate laboratory reports can be avoided.

CONTAINERS FOR SPECIMENS

The container that is best suited to receive the amount or kind of specimen needed and best adapted to the requirements of the test is the one which should be used.

A wide variety of containers are available for use in collecting specimens. Those generally used include the following:

glass bottle with wide mouth—for routine urine specimen
large glass bottle (1 gallon)—for 24 hour urine specimen
sterile glass jar with cover—for sputum or stool specimen
wax-lined cardboard cup with cover—for sputum or stool specimen
sterile or unsterile test tube (various sizes)—for body fluids
sterile flask—for blood culture
slides—for smears

Glass petri dishes may be used for collection of specimens. Any variation of the containers listed above may be used, if large enough to hold a sufficient amount of the material needed for testing.

Specimen containers should be clean on the outside as well as on the inside. If a container is cracked, broken, or damaged it should not be used. The container should be such that it will not be contaminated on the outer surface when the material is placed within. For a specimen that is to be cultured for pathogenic organisms, the container must be sterile.

The nurse should know and use the type of container best suited for collection and testing of the specimen, and the proper size so that the container need never be filled to full capacity. If the amount of material needed for testing would fill the container more than three-fourths full, a larger container should be used.

LABELS FOR SPECIMEN CONTAINERS

Part of the proper procedure of collecting a specimen is proper labeling or identification. Even if the nurse does not deliver the specimen to the laboratory, she should fill out and affix the correct

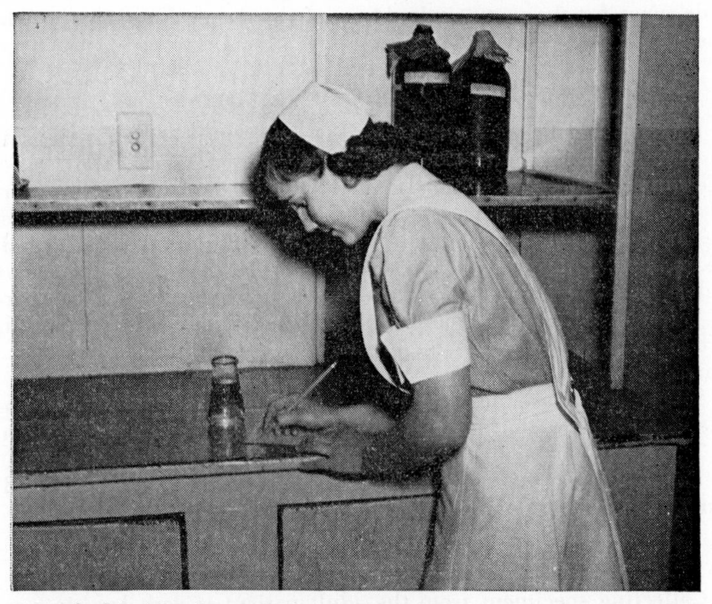

Fig. 127. The label for the specimen should be legible. (Crawford W. Long Hospital School of Nursing, Atlanta, Georgia.)

tag or label, bearing name of patient — ward bed number or room number, department in hospital (floor name or number) — date — kind of test desired — name of attending physician.

The label should be properly printed or written and attached to the specimen immediately after it has been collected. An unlabeled specimen should be discarded because of the obvious danger of a mistake in identification. If a specimen must be saved for observation by the doctor before it is placed in another container and sent to the laboratory, the container holding the specimen should be conspicuously labeled to the effect that the specimen is being saved for inspection.

The requisition for a laboratory test which usually precedes collection of a specimen should contain the information listed above and, in addition, should give age of patient, diagnosis (if definite diagnosis has not been made, the tentative diagnosis should be given), any important fact related to the test, and the name of the doctor requesting the test.

If there is more than one laboratory within the hospital, the label of the specimen should indicate the location of the laboratory to which the specimen is to be delivered.

Special containers for mailing specimens are provided by health department laboratories and are available for whatever type of specimen is collected for examination. Labels of these containers also provide space for the name and address of the doctor or agency to whom the laboratory report is to be sent.

PRESERVATION OF SPECIMENS

For best results in laboratory tests a fresh specimen is desirable; however, when it is impossible or impracticable to obtain a fresh specimen, certain specimens may be preserved for a limited period of time for examination at a later date. Some specimens will need to be placed in the refrigerator for preservation; others which need to be maintained at body temperature should be placed in an incubator.

Urine may be kept for 24 hours in a refrigerator, or 2 to 4 drops of a preservative (as formalin) may be added to each ounce of fluid, provided the examination requested does not include microscopic examination.

Sodium fluoride and thymol may be used to preserve a blood specimen and prevent clotting, if the specimen is kept in the refrigerator.

The laboratory will furnish detailed instruction if a preservative is to be used or the specimen must be kept for a definite period of time before laboratory examination can be made.

METHODS OF COLLECTING SPECIMENS

Collecting specimens from the adult patient is very largely a matter of explanation as to the kind of specimen needed and the purpose of its collection. The patient will usually cooperate to help obtain a satisfactory specimen for the tests to be done in the laboratory.

For collection of specimens of body discharges or body fluids the patient should be advised as to what is expected of him in the procedure.

Urine Specimens. The most common laboratory test is urinalysis, and quite often the diagnosis of disease has been made possible by the study of laboratory findings of such a test.

Complete urinalysis includes determination of the color, reaction, and specific gravity of the urine; chemical analysis for the presence of albumin or sugar, and microscopic examination for such abnormal constituents as pus, blood, and casts.

An "admission" urine specimen is obtained as part of the procedure for admitting a new patient to the hospital. It contains a portion of the routine urine specimen collected from the patient as described below. Ideally, the specimen for complete urinalysis should be part of a 24 hour collection. In most hospitals this is impractical, so the early morning specimen is used for complete urinalysis when possible.

The quantitative urinalysis is usually requested because single specimens may show a variation in specific gravity, pH, albumin, and sugar content. The specimen may be a sample of the total urine collected in 24 hours, or it may be a partitioned specimen collected

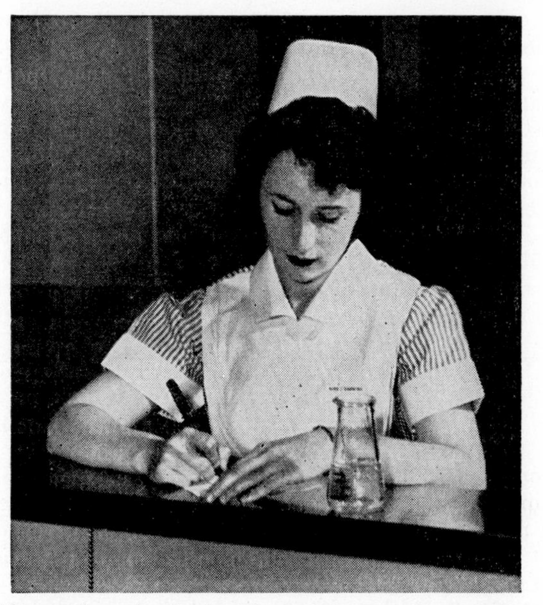

Fig. 128. The specimen bottle should contain an ample quantity of urine for the needs of the laboratory technician. (Delaware Hospital School of Nursing, Wilmington, Delaware.)

from the urine voided in certain specified periods of time during the 24 hour period. Specimens from a diabetic patient should be collected just before mealtime, to help the doctor regulate the insulin dosage by keeping him informed as to insulin-food balance.

Routine Urine Specimen. The female patient will need to be informed that routine urine specimens collected while she is menstruating are not satisfactory for examination. Both female and male patients may need an explanation as to use of bedpan or urinal in collecting the specimen. The patient should be instructed to void in bedpan or urinal or, if ambulatory, directly into the specimen bottle, taking care that the urine thus obtained is not contaminated by contact with outer surfaces of the body or the outer surface of the container.

The specimen bottle should be filled to about three-fourths its capacity, approximately 4 ounces, so there will be an ample quantity for the needs of the laboratory technician.

If a "clean" specimen is requested, the external genitalia should be washed with soap and water and rinsed with clear water. The female patient should wash her hands and hold the labia majora apart while voiding so the urine will not be contaminated by contact with those parts.

If an "early morning" specimen is desired, it should be obtained from urine voided when the patient wakens after a night's sleep.

To obtain a routine urine specimen from a baby it may be necessary to restrain its movements for the period of time required to get the specimen. A test tube or bottle may be used to obtain a specimen from the baby boy. The baby should be restrained, soon after feeding, and the test tube or bottle should be placed over the penis, and then held in place with strips of adhesive fastened over the buttocks on each side.

A specimen of urine may be obtained from the baby girl by use of a birdseed cup, fastened snugly against the vulva while the baby is restrained.

Twenty-four Hour Urine Specimen. The 24 hour specimen is made from the collection of the total amount of urine voided by the patient in a period of 24 hours, to determine the total output for 24 hours and for diagnostic purposes.

Collection of the specimen is usually begun at 7:00 A.M. one day and terminated the following day at 7:00 A.M. The first voiding should be made just before 7:00 A.M., and that urine discarded. All subsequent voidings should be measured and added to the glass bottle of 1 gallon capacity, used for the collection. At 7:00 A.M. the following day the patient should be asked to void. Urine voided then should be added to the collection. The urine should be kept in a cool place and, if ordered, a preservative is added to it.

The total amount voided should be recorded. The entire amount of urine should be thoroughly mixed and about 4 ounces of it placed in a specimen bottle (the wide necked glass bottle used for routine urine specimens), the label correctly filled out and affixed, and the specimen delivered to the laboratory.

For collection of a 24 hour specimen from a baby a small funnel may be attached over the vulva of a girl and the barrel of a 5 cc. syringe over the penis of a boy. A length of small rubber tubing is attached to the other end of the funnel or syringe to convey the urine to a collecting bottle fastened to the side of the crib.

It will be necessary to restrain the infant so that the collecting device will not be dislodged or other equipment interfered with. The nurse will need to be in almost constant attendance, because the restraints will have to be loosened frequently to prevent discomfort to the infant.

Sterile Urine Specimen. A sterile specimen of urine should be collected in a sterilized specimen bottle or sterile test tube. The cover for the container must also be sterile; a pledget of sterile cotton may be used for the test tube container.

The sterile specimen of urine is obtained by catheterization. After the catheter has been introduced into the bladder and 20–30 cc. of urine has been allowed to run through it into the collecting basin, the end of the catheter is held directly above the sterile specimen bottle until it is approximately three-fourths filled.

The label should indicate, in addition to the usual information, that the specimen was "obtained per catheter."

A male patient, after cleansing of the genitals, may void directly into the sterile container in order for a sterile specimen to be obtained.

Specimen for Renal Function Tests. Renal function tests are performed to determine if the kidneys are functioning properly to concentrate and secrete urine. The exact procedure of conducting the tests may differ according to the hospital, so definite instructions of the laboratory manual should be followed. The most commonly used renal function tests are the P.S.P. (phenolsulphonephthalein) test, and the dilution and concentration tests.

The P.S.P. Test. Before beginning the test the patient should be allowed to drink two glasses of water. After about 20 minutes he should be asked to void and the urine should be discarded.

The doctor then administers 1 cc. of phenolsulphonephthalein, a dye that can be given intravenously or intramuscularly.

The first specimen should be collected 15 minutes after the dye has been given. The second specimen should be collected 30 minutes after injection of the dye. The third specimen should be collected one hour after dye injection and the fourth specimen should be collected two hours after the dye was given. All specimens should contain the full amount of urine voided.

A glass of water may be given every half hour so each specimen will contain more than the minimum required amount of 80 cc.

Wide-mouthed glass specimen bottles should be used as containers and each specimen should be labeled to indicate the time of collection with reference to the time the dye was given. The specimens should be numbered "Specimen No. 1," "Specimen No. 2," etc. Specimens should be taken to the laboratory soon after they are collected.

The Urine Concentration Test. This laboratory test is done to determine the ability of the kidney to concentrate urine after food and fluids have been withheld.

All food and fluid should be withheld from the patient for a period of 18 to 20 hours, usually starting in the late afternoon. On waking next morning the patient should be asked to void and that urine discarded. Specimens should then be collected every hour for about four or five hours, to determine the specific gravity of each specimen.

The specimen may be collected in the standard glass specimen bottle and each collection may be a voided specimen. Successive specimens should be labeled "Specimen No. 1," "Specimen No. 2," etc. and the time of collection of the specimen should be indicated. Specimens should be taken to the laboratory soon after they are collected.

The Urine Dilution Test. This laboratory test is done to determine the ability of the kidney to form dilute urine when fluid intake is greatly increased.

The patient should be asked to void on awakening in the morning, and then should drink 1000 cc. of water within a half hour. He should be given no more fluid or food until the test is completed. Voided urine specimens are collected every hour for four or five hours. A record is kept of the amount voided, and the specific gravity of each specimen is determined.

The standard glass specimen bottle is used, and labels should indicate the specimen number and time of collection. Specimens should be taken to the laboratory soon after they are collected.

Urea Clearance Test. For this test, breakfast should be omitted.

Note time of first voiding after patient wakens in the morning. This urine is discarded.

Fifty-five minutes after first voiding, sample of blood should be drawn from the patient.

One hour after first voiding, the patient should be asked to void. This entire specimen, with notation of exact voiding time, should be sent to laboratory, labeled specimen No. 1.

Two hours after first voiding, the patient should be asked to void again, and again the entire specimen, with notation of exact voiding time, is sent to laboratory, labeled specimen No. 2.

The patient may have one-half glass of water between collection of the specimens, if he wishes.

The standard glass specimen bottles should be used. Specimens should be delivered to the laboratory soon after they have been collected.

Glucose Tolerance Test. The patient should be given no food after 7:00 P.M. In the early morning a specimen of blood is taken for a fasting blood sugar determination. About 100 grams of glucose is then given, usually in a glass of water flavored with lemon juice.

Specimens of blood and urine should be collected 30 minutes, and one, two, and three hours after the glucose was given.

The urine should be collected in the standard glass specimen bottle by having the patient void at the designated times. Labels should be numbered "Specimen No. 1," "Specimen No. 2," etc., and the time of collection, as well as other pertinent information, should appear on each label. The specimens should be taken to the laboratory soon after collection.

Hippuric Acid Test. The patient is not permitted to have breakfast and should void just before the test is started. This urine should be discarded.

Sodium benzoate, 1.77 gm., is then injected intravenously.

A urine specimen should be collected exactly one hour later, by having the patient void. If the patient is unable to void at the designated time, the urine should be withdrawn by catheter.

The standard glass specimen bottle should be used, and the total amount voided or obtained by catheter should be sent to the laboratory soon after it is collected. The label, in addition to the usual information, should indicate whether specimen was voided or obtained per catheter.

Specimens of Stomach Contents. If the stomach contents to be examined consist of vomitus, the specimen should be collected in a wax-lined cardboard container or in a glass jar. It should be transferred from the emesis basin into the specimen container and delivered to the laboratory soon after collection. The label should give the usual information in regard to patient's name, room number, etc.

If the stomach contents are for gastric analysis, the specimen should be collected about 40 minutes after subcutaneous administration of 0.5 cc. of 1:1000 solution of histamine. The drug stimulates gastric secretion. The patient swallows a Levin tube, and stomach contents are aspirated by means of an attached syringe.

The specimen should be collected in a sterile test tube, correctly labeled, and delivered at once to the laboratory. If necessary, more than one test tube may be used, in which case each tube should be labeled according to the sequence of collection, as "Tube No. 1," "Tube No. 2," etc.

Sputum Specimens. Sputum to be examined for tubercle bacilli, for spirochetes, or for tumor cells should be collected in a clean wide-mouthed glass jar which can be tightly covered. In some instances the sputum is collected in the wax-coated cardboard or paper sputum cup and, after being correctly labeled, is sent immediately for laboratory examination.

If sputum is to be collected for examination for pneumococcus, influenza, and other organisms, the patient should be instructed to expectorate into the container (a wide-mouthed glass jar or bottle which has been sterilized) only that sputum which is coughed up from the lower parts of the respiratory tract. Saliva and postnasal discharge should not be included with the specimen. To avoid having food particles in the specimen, the patient should be instructed to rinse his mouth with clear water after eating.

The label should include routine identifying information and the name of the organism for which the sputum is to be examined.

To obtain a sputum specimen from a very young child, a cotton applicator should be used. The child may be made to cough by titillation of the back of the throat with a piece of gauze. If sputum is coughed up, the applicator can be used to mop up the amount needed for a specimen. The applicator to which the sputum has adhered may be dropped in a sterile test tube. The tube should be closed with a sterile cotton pledget. It should then be correctly labeled and sent to the laboratory for examination.

Specimens of Feces. Examination of feces is usually done for diagnostic purposes, to discover the presence of parasites or of occult blood, or to detect certain metabolic disorders. Feces may be examined, too, for pus, worms, gallstones, shreds of membrane or mucus, and for foreign bodies.

For the routine examination a small amount of fecal material may be transferred from the bedpan to a waxed cardboard cup or to a wide-mouthed glass bottle or jar by means of a wooden tongue depressor.

If the examination is for typhoid, dysentery, or other bacteria, the bedpan must be sterilized and the container for the specimen must be sterile. The tongue blade used to transfer the specimen from bedpan to container must also be sterile. A sterile cotton applicator saturated with the feces may be placed in a sterile test tube, which is securely plugged with a sterile cotton pledget, and, with a proper label the specimen can then be taken to the laboratory.

If the examination is for a tapeworm, or for segments of a tapeworm, the entire stool should be sent to the laboratory in a wide-mouthed glass jar.

If the examination is for ameba, the stool should be kept at body temperature and sent to the laboratory immediately. The cysts of the parasite can be detected in routine examination but the developed parasites, characterized by their mobility, can be identified only when they are active, so the examination must be made when the stool is still warm and fresh. If fecal material is allowed to stand for even a short time the specimen will cool and the parasites will be immobile.

A wide-mouthed glass jar should be used. It should be tightly covered and partially immersed in a water bath of 110° F. while being transported to the laboratory.

The label for the stool specimen should indicate the type examination desired. If the specimen is to be examined for parasites, a laboratory technician should be previously notified that the specimen is being collected, so she can examine it immediately on delivery to the laboratory.

Blood Specimens. Blood specimens may be examined for many different purposes: to determine the number and character of red or of white blood cells, to learn the percentage of hemoglobin, to determine coagulation time, or to learn the amount of sugar, urea, urea-nitrogen, non-protein nitrogen, creatinine and uric acid present, and to detect certain bacteria.

To obtain a specimen for cell count and study the lobe of the ear or the end of the middle finger may be punctured. The skin is first cleansed with an alcohol sponge, the puncture is made with a sterile needle, and the blood is collected in a sterile pipette or sterilized tube. For counting of cells, the blood is placed directly on a slide and prepared for microscopic examination.

A larger amount of blood is needed for chemical analysis and for blood cultures. It is usually withdrawn from a vein, the median basilic, which is near the surface on the inner portion of the elbow. A sterile needle is introduced into the vein and the desired amount of blood withdrawn into a 5 cc. syringe. The blood is then carefully injected into a sterile test tube which is closed with a sterile cotton pledget.

The specimen is then correctly labeled and delivered to the laboratory.

Blood to be examined for sodium, chlorides, uric acid, or carbon dioxide–combining power must be taken under oil to avoid contact with the air. This is a special procedure and must be done by the trained laboratory technician.

Specimens of Spinal, Pleural, and Peritoneal Fluids. Specimens of spinal, pleural, and peritoneal fluids are obtained by lumbar puncture, thoracentesis, and abdominal paracentesis, respectively. The nurse must know, before the procedure is started, the number and type of specimens to be collected, so she can have the proper containers ready for use.

Spinal fluid specimens are collected in a sterile test tube which is held under the open needle until sufficient fluid has dripped into the container. About 8 cc. of the fluid should be collected in this manner. If more fluid is required, a sterile glass graduate container may be used. The specimens should be correctly labeled and delivered at once to the laboratory.

Pleural fluid for culture or guinea-pig inoculation should be collected in a sterile culture tube. Specimens of pleural fluid for cell count and specific gravity, which need not be sterile, may be collected in the standard glass specimen bottle. About 120 cc. is needed for such examination. If examination for tumor cells is ordered, an additional amount of fluid may be withdrawn and placed in a large glass bottle, correctly labeled, and sent to the laboratory.

A specimen of peritoneal fluid is obtained by holding the container under the trocar, during paracentesis, until the desired amount has been collected.

The type of container used and the amount of fluid needed are the same as described for pleural fluid.

Cultures from Nose and Throat. A bacterial culture may be made from a swab of infected material. To obtain the specimen, a sterile cotton swab is gently rotated over the infected area and then carefully inserted into a sterile test tube. For a culture, the swab must be thoroughly saturated with the exudate from the nose or throat. The specimen should be properly labeled and clearly marked as "Nasal" or "Throat" culture. The specimen should be delivered to the laboratory immediately, since it must be examined while still moist. If the specimen is allowed to dry, any bacteria that might have been present will have died before the examination is made.

The swab method may also be used to obtain cultures from the eyes and ears, as well as from wounds or from feces.

Smears. Examination for bacteria may be made of a smear on a glass slide. To make a smear, the material is taken from the affected area with a sterile cotton swab, which is then gently rolled across the surface of the glass slide. The slide should not be rubbed with the swab.

A smear for gonorrhea from an adult female is taken by the doctor, since the material must be taken from the cervix rather than from the vagina. Articles needed include a vaginal speculum, and a probe or long wooden applicator to which sterile cotton may be attached for swabbing.

If a smear is to be taken from a child suspected of having gonorrheal vaginitis, the nurse may carry out the procedure, since swabbing of the vaginal wall will be adequate and no special instruments are needed.

The slide which has been smeared for examination should be protected by being covered with a second slide. The slides must be kept apart; this can be done by use of a rubber band wound around each end of the smeared slide.

The specimen should be correctly labeled and delivered to the laboratory.

EXAMINATION OF SPECIMENS AS A PUBLIC HEALTH SERVICE

State and local public health departments have well equipped laboratories whose services are available to doctors, health officers, clinics, and hospitals.

The control of communicable diseases is a major responsibility of the health departments, and much of their work relates to that responsibility.

Blood may be examined for syphilitic infection or for the presence of typhoid bacilli. Sputum may be examined for the tubercle bacillus. Cultures of the nose and throat may be made to detect diphtheria.

Suitable containers are supplied by the health department laboratories for each kind of specimen to be collected. The method of obtaining the specimens is the same as in standard hospital or nursing practice.

The health department also supplies proper forms and labels for giving of all identifying information. Each label should give patient's name and address, date and time the specimen was collected, kind of material, type of examination to be made, and the name and address of the doctor or agency to whom the report is to be mailed.

Care of Equipment after Use

Glass containers for various specimens should be thoroughly washed and sterilized by boiling after use.

Test tubes can be washed and then sterilized by being boiled.

Waxed heavy paper sputum cups should be burned after use.

Tongue depressors, applicators, and cotton pledgets used in the collection of specimens should be burned.

Bedpans or urinals used for collecting specimens should be thoroughly washed and sterilized or disinfected.

Summary of Important Factors

A specimen is a small quantity of a substance that shows the kind and quality of the whole.

Carelessness in collecting or labeling a specimen may result in inaccurate laboratory reports.

The type of container best suited for the collecting and testing of a specimen is the one that should be used.

All specimens should be identified by proper labels.

The specimen container should never be filled to capacity.

The early morning specimen is usually the preferred urise specimen.

To obtain a urine specimen from a baby may necessitate restraining the child.

A sterile specimen of urine can be obtained from the female patient by catheterization.

Exact timing for the collection of specimens is important in renal function tests.

Sputum specimens should consist of "coughed up" material, not saliva.

A specimen of feces to be examined for tapeworm must contain the whole stool.

A specimen of feces to be examined for parasites must be warm and fresh so the parasites are mobile and can thus be detected.

A stool specimen for examination for bacteria should be collected by aseptic technique.

Blood for examination is obtained from a slight puncture wound or, if a larger amount is necessary, withdrawn from the median basilic vein.

Swabs may be used to obtain material for cultures or smears.

Test tubes should be provided with other equipment needed for lumbar puncture, thoracentesis, and abdominal paracentesis, to collect specimens of fluid if it is necessary.

Factors To Teach the Patient

How to handle specimen containers so the outside is not contaminated by specimen material being deposited in the container.

Explanation to the patient of the benefits to be derived from laboratory examination of the specimen will insure his cooperation.

Explanation of the proper method of procedure permits obtaining a sterile specimen of urine from the male patient without catheterization.

A sputum specimen should include only material which is "coughed up."

That state and local public health departments are equipped for laboratory testing, and the services are available to the public when needed.

Scientific Principles

Anatomy and Physiology. Normal and abnormal constituents are excreted in the urine so laboratory tests of specimens of urine are of material benefit in making diagnosis. Sputum usually contains material "coughed up" from the bronchial tubes and trachea.

Chemistry. Gastric juice is constantly being secreted but in such small amounts that when a specimen is desired stimulation by food or drugs is necessary.

Microbiology. Specimens to be examined for bacteria should be obtained under aseptic technique and should be collected in sterile containers. Sterile containers should be used for a urine specimen obtained by catheter. The outside of specimen containers should not be contaminated with the specimen material. If the outside of the container is not clean, persons handling it are exposed to infection.

Pharmacology. Water is a diuretic and may be given in rather large quantities so that an adequate amount of urine may be obtained for needed specimens. Phenolsulphonephthalein is a dye used to test kidney function. Glucose is used for testing tolerance for sugar. A mild laxative may be given if it is necessary to obtain a specimen of feces within a short period of time. Histamine is used to stimulate the flow of gastric secretions so an adequate amount may be obtained for examination.

Physics. To obtain specimens of body fluid, a needle or trocar is introduced into the cavity and the fluid flows out to an area of less pressure.

Psychology. When the collection of specimens requires that food and fluids be restricted for a period of time, an explanation should be made to the patient. When food and water may be had again, the delayed meal should be immediately served to the patient.

Sociology. Specimens may be sent by mail to state and local public health departments, and the mailing of specimens is under special regulations. Containers for mailing specimens are supplied by the health departments.

Situation Type Problem

1. In a morning report, all nurses on a certain department within the hospital had been informed that a 24 hour urine specimen was being collected for a certain patient.

The container for the specimen was clearly labeled and placed in the utility room. A notice was posted above the hopper in the utility room to the effect that a 24 hour urine specimen was being collected for the patient.

The student nurse assigned to give that patient care in the morning carefully measured and added to the collection the urine voided just before she gave the patient a bath.

As she was ready to report off duty she answered a call light signal from the patient, who had voided again and requested that the urinal be emptied. She was in a hurry to get off duty since she had made plans to meet some friends a little later at the public library. She hastily measured the urine in the graduate container kept on a shelf beside the hopper, then emptied the contents of the container into the hopper and flushed it.

As she was recording the amount that had been voided she realized she had discarded urine which should have been added to the 24 hour collection. What would you have done?

Suggested Reference Reading

"Urinalysis as an index of health," Robert A. Kilduffe; American Journal of Nursing, May, 1931.

"Collecting specimens," Ruth M. Bassett; American Journal of Nursing, November, 1933.

"Understanding the laboratory report," Margene O. Faddis; American Journal of Nursing, February, 1937.

CHAPTER 20

Diagnostic Tests

TOPICAL OUTLINE

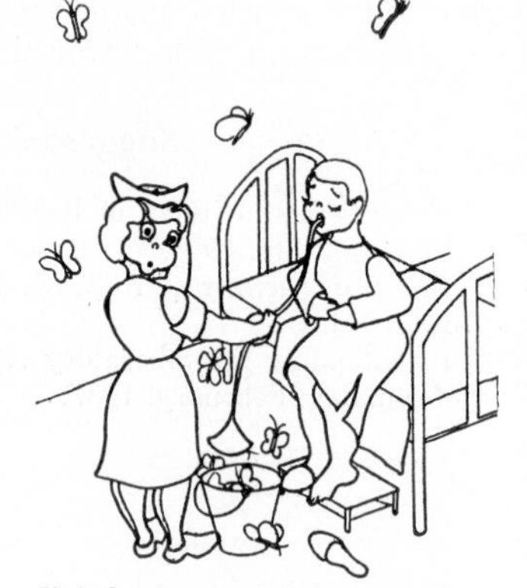

He's been complaining for a long time that he had butterflies in his stomach!

Diagnostic tests include various examinations made in the laboratory to aid the physician in making an accurate diagnosis so that effectual treatment may be prescribed for the patient. These examinations include scientific tests made on body discharges, secretions, and excretions, and tests performed with special equipment to determine specific factors related to the functioning of an organ or part. Numerous laboratory tests made as an aid to diagnosis are discussed under the various headings of this chapter, giving first the name and purpose of the test, a brief description of the procedure, the normal values, and the possible significance of the results.

DUTIES OF THE NURSE

In assisting with diagnostic tests the nurse performs one of the most exacting duties of her profession. On her accurate and skillful handling of specimens and preparation of equipment may depend the entire

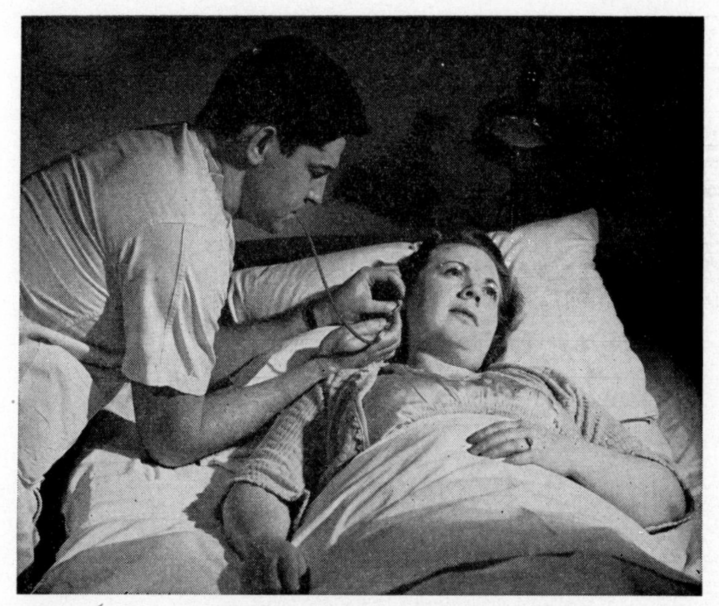

Fig. 129. A small cut made in the ear lobe provides blood required to test bleeding time. (Presbyterian Hospital, Chicago, Illinois.)

findings and subsequent prescribed treatment. A thorough understanding of the testing routine is essential if she is to carry out the procedure intelligently and efficiently.

The responsibility of the nurse is not the same for all tests, although usually she is expected to explain the procedure to the patient and to prepare him for the test.

Preparation of equipment to be used in obtaining the specimen or to be used by the doctor in performing the actual testing procedure is left almost entirely to the nurse.

Labeling of specimen containers, delivering them to the proper laboratory, and, at times, seeing that they are stored at correct temperature until ready for use are other responsibilities assumed by the nurse who assists with diagnostic procedures.

TESTS OF BODY FLUIDS, SECRETIONS, OR EXCRETIONS

Blood Tests. Blood tests mentioned here include determination of bleeding and clotting time, red and white cell counts, hemoglobin, sedimentation rate, and prothrombin time. Also included are Wassermann or Kahn test, blood chemistry, blood culture, and blood typing.

Bleeding Time. To determine the amount of time it takes for a cut to stop bleeding. A small cut or skin puncture is made, usually in the

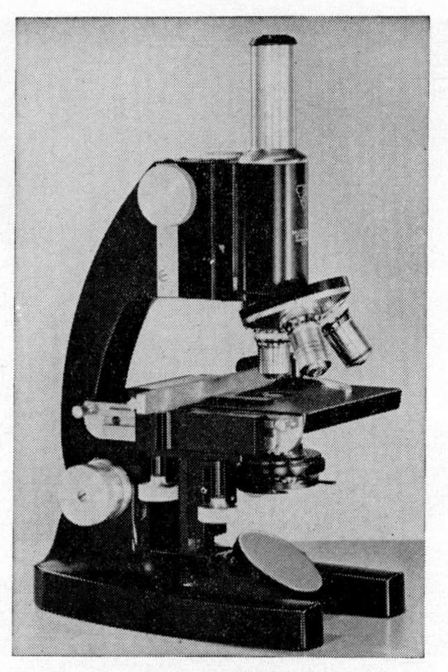

Fig. 130. The microscope—one of the most effective and valuable diagnostic aids available. (Bausch and Lomb Optical Co., Rochester. New York.)

ear lobe, and the time required for it to stop bleeding is observed. Normal value—two or three minutes. Significance—prolonged bleeding time may be a contraindication for some surgical procedures.

Coagulation Time. To determine time required for blood to clot after it leaves the blood vessel. A drop of blood is withdrawn from skin puncture of finger end, and time it takes for clot to form is timed. Normal value—three to five minutes. Significance—if coagulation time exceeds five minutes, surgical operations may be hazardous for the patient, as continuous oozing from severed blood vessels may occur.

Red Cell Count. To determine deviation from count of healthy individual. Through a small skin puncture (end of finger), a small amount of blood is withdrawn by means of a pipette, placed in a counting chamber, and examined under the microscope. The number of red cells per cu. mm. of blood can thus be determined. Normal value—4,500,000 to 5,000,000 per cu. mm. of blood. Significance—the red cell count is usually decreased in the anemias and in leukemia.

White Cell Count. To determine deviation in count from that of a healthy individual. The procedure is the same as for the red cell count. Normal values—5,000 to 10,000 per cu. mm. of blood. Significance—an increase in white cells may indicate the presence of infection or of leukemia; a decrease in the white cell count may indicate decreased resistance on the part of the patient.

Differential Cell Count. To determine the percentage of different kinds of white cells as a further aid to diagnosis. By the use of stains the white cells may readily be differentiated. Normal values—polymorphonuclears, 60–70 per cent; small mononuclears, 20–30 per cent; large mononuclears, 4–8 per cent; basophils, 1 per cent; eosinophils, 0.5 per cent. Significance—the various kinds of white cells vary in number in certain diseases and known variations are considered a part of the syndrome of a particular disease.

Hemoglobin. To determine the quantity of hemoglobin present in the red cells. Blood may be obtained for the test through a skin puncture or by venipuncture. The quantity may be estimated in various ways, the most common is that of comparing blood from the patient with a color chart showing known percentages of hemoglobin content. Normal values—14 grams per 100 cc. of blood, or 95–100 per cent. Significance—a marked decrease in hemoglobin may denote anemia, leukemia, hemorrhage, or the presence of a malignant disease.

Sedimentation Rate. To determine time required for red cells to settle to bottom of the container in which blood is allowed to stand. Blood is collected (in test tube) and allowed to stand. The rate at which the cells settle to the bottom is measured. Normal values—10–15 millimeters in an hour. Significance—the test is used to indicate the activity of the disease process, the rate of sedimentation being higher in the active stage of the disease.

Prothrombin Time. To determine prothrombin activity as a means of studying the disturbances in the clotting properties of blood in certain diseases. Blood is withdrawn by venipuncture. In the laboratory the plasma is separated out and a measured amount added to a measured amount of solution of calcium chloride and thromboplastin. The time elapsing between the addition of the plasma and the formation of a clot is the prothrombin time. Normal values—14–15 seconds. Significance—an increase in prothrombin time will be noted when there is a deficiency of vitamin K and in patients receiving anticoagulant drugs, as Dicumarol and heparin. A decreased prothrombin time may be noted in thrombosis. The test is used frequently as a guide in the management of anticoagulant drug therapy.

Wassermann or Kahn Test. To determine the presence of *Spirochaeta pallida,* the causative organism of syphilis. Blood is withdrawn by venipuncture (5–10 cc.). Normal values—negative. Significance—a positive result of the test indicates presence of the disease.

Blood Chemistry. To determine the content of various substances in the blood, one of the most common tests is that for blood sugar. A specimen of blood (5–10 cc.) is withdrawn by venipuncture after the patient has fasted approximately 12 hours. Normal values—80–120 mg. per 100 cc. of blood. Significance—increased sugar content of the blood may indicate the presence of diabetes mellitus.

Other important tests for chemicals in the blood (with normal values given per 100 cc. of blood*) include:

nonprotein nitrogen	25–35 mg.
calcium	9–11 mg.
cholesterol	150–230 mg.
creatinine	3–7 mg.
phosphorus	3–5 mg.
uric acid	1–3 mg.
chlorides (NaCl)	570–630 mg.
urea nitrogen	10–15 mg.

Blood Cultures. To determine the presence or absence of specific organisms. The blood is withdrawn by venipuncture, added to culture media and placed in an incubator at a temperature to encourage growth of the microorganism. Normal values—organisms not found in the culture. Significance—finding of the specific organism verifies diagnosis of the disease, as in typhoid fever.

Other tests on blood which are important therapeutically if blood transfusions are to be given are blood typing and crossmatching.

*Blood Typing.** To determine blood type pertaining to blood types O, A, B, and AB and to the Rh factor. Blood is withdrawn by venipuncture and typing is done by specially trained laboratory technicians. Significance—in general, when transfusions are to be given, the patient should be given blood of the type (O, A, B, AB) which is exactly the same as his or her own. All women under 50 years of age should be given blood of Rh factor (negative or positive) which is the same as their own.

Crossmatching. To determine the compatibility of two bloods (patient and donor) before transfusion is given. Blood groups are O, A, B, AB. Significance—undesirable reactions and, at times, death may result if incompatible blood is given by transfusion.

Urine Tests. Urine tests are made to aid in diagnosis, to determine constituents of urine, and to discover abnormalities of kidney function.

Routine Urinalysis. To determine various factors, such as reaction, constituents, and comparative weight of urine. A voided specimen is obtained or, if a sterile specimen is needed, the patient is catheterized. Normal values—reaction, slightly acid; specific gravity, 1.015–1.025; albumin, negative; sugar, negative; acetone, negative; microscopic examination for bacteria, pus, blood, negative. Significance—in disease conditions specific gravity may be lower or higher, indicating less or more waste solids in the urine. An increase in the number of cells, especially white cells, may indicate disease of the organs of the urinary system. Albumin in the urine results from inflammation of some part of the urinary tract; marked increase indicates the presence of nephritis. Sugar in the urine may be indicative of diabetes mellitus.

* From "Clinical Laboratory Diagnosis" by Levinson and MacFate, Lea & Febiger, Philadelphia, 1951.

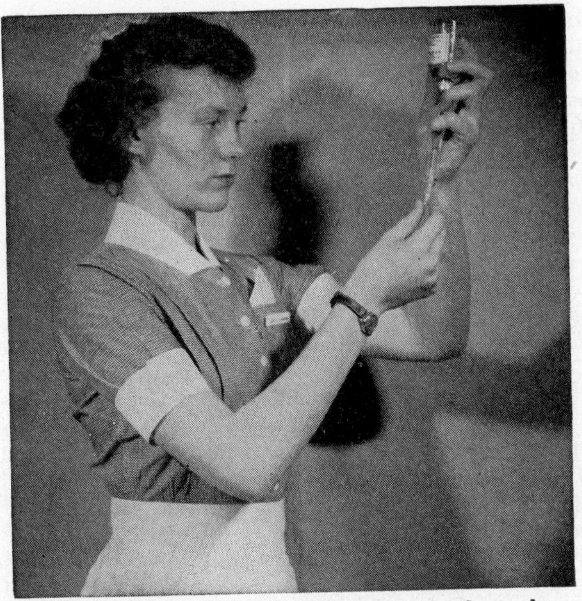

Fig. 131. Although the doctor usually administers the dye to be used for the P.S.P. test, the nurse may prepare the dye for injection. (Massachusetts General Hospital School of Nursing, Boston, Massachusetts.)

Twenty-four Hour Urine Test. To make a quantitative analysis of urine. All urine voided in a 24 hour period is saved and a small portion of it, or the entire amount, is sent to the laboratory so that the quantities, as well as qualities, of constituents can be measured. Normal values—same as for routine urinalysis. Significance—the total quantities of various waste products found in urine are indicative of the metabolism of the body and the proper functioning of the various organs. Through such findings proper diet may be prescribed and medical treatment outlined.

P.S.P. (Phenolsulphonephthalein) Test. To determine the functioning of the kidneys. Phenolsulphonephthalein, a dye that is excreted only by the kidneys, is injected intravenously or intramuscularly and urine is collected at stated intervals (see Chapter 19). The colorimeter is used to determine the amount of dye excreted in each specimen of urine. Normal values—60–80 per cent of dye has been eliminated at completion of the test. Significance—variation from normal values indicates impaired kidney function and aids in the diagnosis of nephritis.

Dilution and Concentration Tests. Tests to determine kidney function.

Dilution Test. The dilution test measures power of kidney to dilute urine. The patient is given no breakfast, fluids are increased (1500 cc. water), urine specimens are collected frequently. Specific gravity and amount of each voiding is recorded. Normal values—specific gravity of at least one specimen should be 1.003.

Concentration Test. The concentration test measures power of kidney to concentrate urine. The patient is given a carefully planned diet and no fluids. Specimens are collected at intervals during the day. The amount voided and specific gravity of each collection is recorded. Normal values—at least one specimen should show specific gravity of 1.025–1.030.

The dilution and concentration tests may indicate presence of disease when other tests have failed to do so.

Tests for Sugar (Benedict's and Fehling's Tests). To determine the presence and comparative amount of sugar in the urine. The tests are made with a single specimen of urine, and can be done by the nurse. Patients, instructed by the nurse, can soon do the tests for themselves.

Fehling Test. About 3 cc. of urine is put in a test tube and 5 cc. of boiling Fehling's solution is added. The mixture is boiled and the tube is placed in the rack. Formation of a typical red or golden yellow precipitate indicates the presence of sugar.

Benedict's Test. Five cc. of the reagent and 8 drops of urine are placed in a test tube, which is immersed in a water bath of boiling water for exactly five minutes. The tube is removed and allowed to cool. If the fluid becomes opaque, it indicates that sugar is present. If no sugar is present, the fluid remains clear, or only a faint turbidity results.

Normal values—negative.

The tests may be done often at home and serve as a guide to indicate accuracy of medical treatment and the amount of foodstuffs to include in the diet so that urine remains sugar free and diabetes is controlled.

Aschheim-Zondek Test. To determine if the patient is pregnant. An early morning specimen of urine is collected from the patient, and a small quantity is injected into the experimental animal (rabbit, mouse, or frog). If the patient is pregnant, ovaries of the animal will show hemorrhagic follicles in 24–48 hours.

Urine Culture. To detect presence of a specific organism. The patient is catheterized to prevent contamination of the specimen. Normal values—negative. Significance—presence of the specific organism indicates presence of the disease.

Sputum Tests. Sputum may be collected to determine its amount, color, and consistency, and to detect the presence of certain specific bacteria.

Specimens are obtained by having the patient expectorate into a waxed sputum cup. Early morning specimens are preferable, and the patient should be instructed to "cough up" or raise the material from

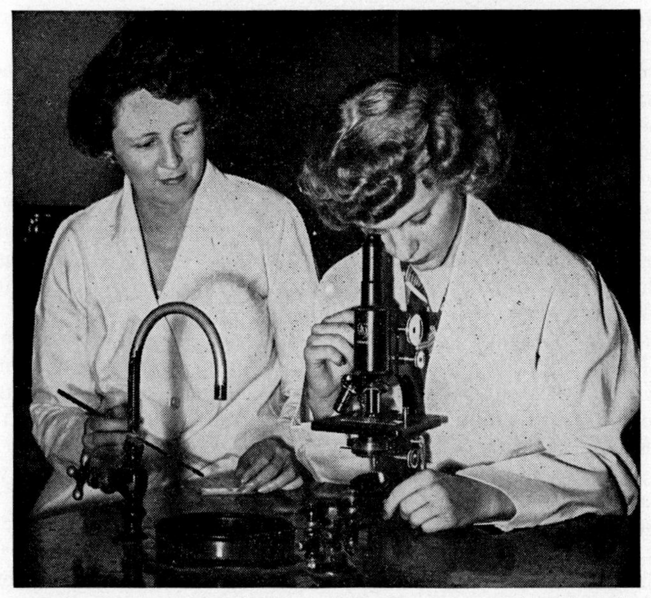

Fig. 132. Sputum is examined microscopically for the presence of specific bacilli. (Presbyterian Hospital School of Nursing, Pittsburgh, Pennsylvania.)

the lungs rather than merely expectorate saliva or other discharge from the mouth or nose. Normal values—no sputum is expectorated in a normal healthy condition. Significance—in disease in which sputum is produced the amount may vary from very little to extensive. Blood may be observed through color. Bright blood indicates bleeding at the present time; dark blood indicates the bleeding occurred several hours previously. The odor may vary from none at all to very offensive, as in lung abscess. Consistency of sputum may vary from a thin watery fluid to a thick purulent material. Microscopic examination may reveal specific bacilli; the presence of tubercle bacilli verifies the diagnosis of tuberculosis.

Tests Related to the Gastrointestinal Tract. Disease conditions affecting the gastrointestinal tract may be detected through various tests.

Examination of Feces. To determine the presence of parasites or of blood. Microscopic examination is for bacteria, ameba, and tiny worms. Chemical examination is usually for the presence of blood or bile. The stool specimen is collected in a bedpan and transferred by means of a wooden spatula to a waxed container. All stool specimens should be sent to the laboratory immediately after collection. When the examination is for ameba the specimen must be kept warm so the amebae will be active and their presence can be noted. Nomal values

—negative. Significance—the presence of parasites in the intestinal tract may be demonstrated. Traces of blood in feces may lead to diagnosis of gastric ulcer or of carcinoma in the upper intestinal tract.

Gastric Analysis. To determine presence of such conditions as gastric ulcer, carcinoma, anemia, and pulmonary tuberculosis. All food and fluids are restricted for several hours, and histamine solution is given to stimulate gastric secretion. A Levin tube is passed into the stomach, a syringe is attached, and stomach contents are aspirated. Normal values—0.1–0.2 per cent acidity. Significance—marked increase in the amount of hydrochloric acid may indicate presence of gastric ulcer. Absence of hydrochloric acid may denote pernicious anemia, gastritis, or advanced carcinoma.

Biliary Drainage Test. To determine volume and constituents of bile. The Levin tube is passed through the stomach into the duodenum. A weak solution of magnesium sulfate is introduced to stimulate the flow of bile, and contents of the duodenum are allowed to drain into bottles. Significance—absence of bile indicates obstruction to bile ducts; appreciable amounts of bile pigments and cholesterol crystals indicate the presence of stones in the gallbladder.

Tests of Discharges from Wounds or Body Cavities. It is necessary at times to examine discharges from wounds or from body cavities to determine the causative agent of a disease condition and the proper treatment.

Smears or Cultures. To determine the presence of bacteria. An applicator is touched to the affected area or to the discharge, the material is then spread on a slide for the smear or put in culture media and incubated for growing a culture. Normal values—negative. Significance—the presence of specific organisms helps to determine the treatment to be used, especially facilitating the choice among the various antibiotics available. Antibiotic tablets are sometimes placed immediately on the culture, to determine which one more effectively inhibits growth.

Tests Related to Fluids Obtained by Puncture. Examination of fluids normally or abnormally present within the body is sometimes important diagnostically.

Cerebrospinal Fluid (Lumbar Puncture). To determine pressure, cell count, specific gravity, color, reaction, and presence of bacteria. With the patient in proper position, the doctor inserts a special needle into the subarachnoid space between the third and fourth lumbar vertebrae to allow the spinal fluid to drop into sterile test tubes. The procedure is done with sterile equipment and with sterile technique. Normal values—pressure, 7.5–15 mm. Hg; cell count, 0–5; specific gravity, 1.001–1.010; color, clear; reaction, alkaline; bacteria, negative. Significance—increased pressure may indicate presence of a tumor of the brain or inflammation of the meninges. A cloudy or yellow color, marked increase in cell count, and presence of causative organisms indicate an acute infection. Blood may be indicative of in-

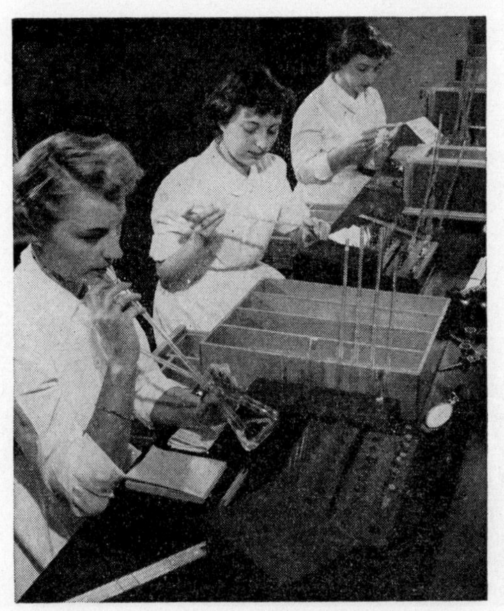

Fig. 133. Trained technicians carry out laboratory procedures in testing body fluids. (Presbyterian Hospital, Chicago, Illinois.)

jury to the spinal cord above the site of puncture. Cell count may be increased in poliomyelitis, encephalitis, and meningitis.

Pleural Fluid (Thoracentesis). To examine for pressure and for presence of bacteria. The procedure is done by a doctor, using aseptic technique. A long needle is inserted into the chest cavity, and fluid is withdrawn by means of a syringe. Normal values—negative for bacteria; pressure, 4 to 5 cm. of water. Significance—increased pressure may denote a condition of pleural effusion. Finding of a specific microorganism establishes the presence of the disease, as in tuberculosis.

Ascitic Fluid (Abdominal Paracentesis). To examine for the presence of bacteria. Aspiration (sterile technique and equipment) is done by the physician. A cannula with trocar is inserted in the midline of the abdomen two to four inches below the umbilicus. When the trocar is removed, fluid drains from the cannula. Normal values—negative. Significance—detection of the causative organism verifies diagnosis of the disease.

Pericardial Fluid (Aspiration of the Pericardium). To examine for presence of bacteria. A sterile needle and syringe is used by the physician to aspirate fluid from the sac enveloping the heart. Normal values—negative. Significance—presence of the organism may confirm diagnosis of tuberculous or purulent pericarditis.

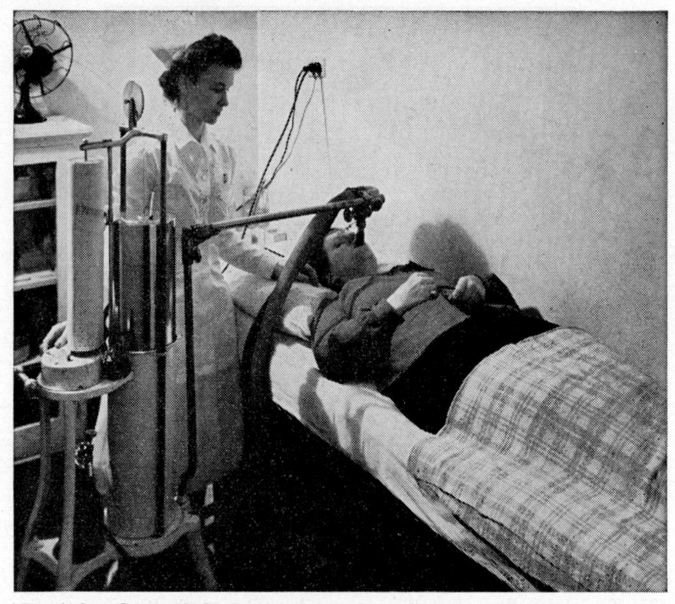

Fig. 134. A basal metabolism test determines the amount of oxygen consumed in a given time. (Presbyterian Hospital, Chicago, Illinois.)

Joint Fluid (Aspiration of a Joint). To examine for bacteria. A sterile needle and syringe is used by the physician to aspirate fluid from a joint cavity. Normal values—negative. Significance—presence of the organism confirms diagnosis.

BASAL METABOLISM

A basal metabolism test is made to determine the amount of oxygen consumed in a given time and thus measure heat production and heat loss or the rate at which chemical changes (metabolism) takes place in the body.

The test is performed by a trained technician, using special apparatus. The test should be taken after the patient has slept overnight and has been without food during that time. The patient should be at complete rest and thoroughly relaxed while he breathes oxygen from the machine and the graphic recording is made.

The normal value is −10 to +10. The normal basal metabolic rate is 38–40 calories per square meter of body surface per hour. A rate of −10 means 10 per cent below the normal level. A rate below −10 may be present in hypothyroidism; and a rate above +10 may be present in hyperthyroidism.

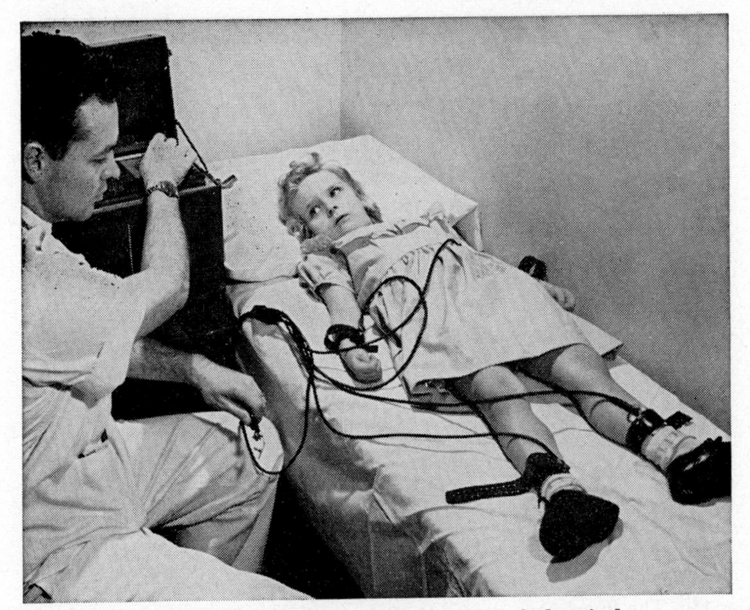

Fig. 135. The electrocardiogram is a graphic report of electrical currents produced by activity of the heart muscle. (Presbyterian Hospital, Chicago, Illinois).

TESTS RELATED TO ELECTRIC IMPULSES

Electric impulses are generated in the normal activity of various organs of the body, such as the heart, brain, or voluntary muscles. These may be amplified and recorded, by use of various devices, to permit detection of any variation from what has been established as a normal pattern.

Electrocardiography. To present graphically the electric impulses produced by activity of the heart muscle. A special apparatus, known as the electrocardiograph, is used, with connecting wires (leads) which are fastened to the patient's body, permitting transmitted electric impulses to be recorded on a graph (electrocardiogram). Study of this graph makes possible a more accurate diagnosis of the particular type of heart disease present.

Electroencephalography. To present graphically the electric impulses produced by activity of the brain. Electrodes are fastened to the head, and impulses are transmitted to a special instrument which records them in graphic form. Study of the graph aids in differential diagnosis of various conditions producing impairment of brain activity.

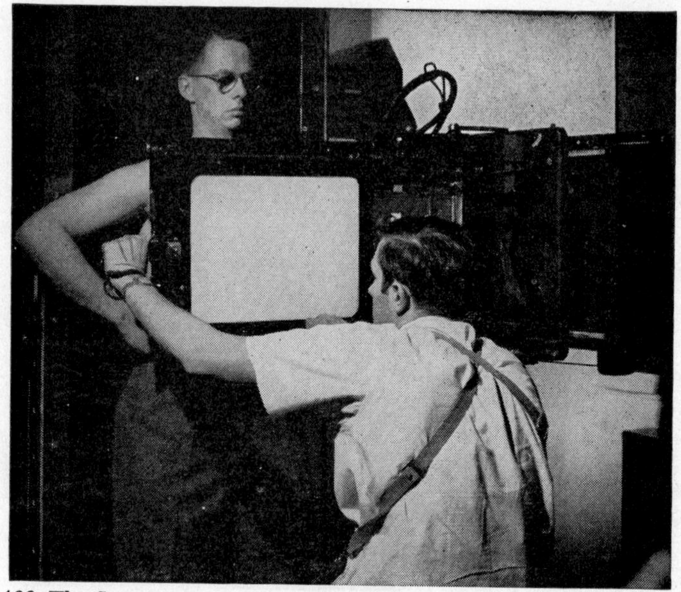

Fig. 136. The fluoroscope is used to study position, contour, and activity of the gastrointestinal tract. (Presbyterian Hospital, Chicago, Illinois.)

TESTS RELATED TO X-RAY

The condition and functional activity of various internal organs of the body may be observed directly or recorded on film by use of x-rays, or roentgen rays, which are capable of penetrating the body.

Gastrointestinal Series. To examine position, contour, structure, and activity of the gastrointestinal tract by means of a series of x-ray films or by fluoroscopy.

Barium sulfate is administered by mouth or by rectum. The barium has greater density than the soft tissues of the body and causes greater contrast on the x-ray film, outlining the part of the intestinal tract to be studied.

Normal values—normal outline of the organ; a schedule near the average normal for the course of a barium meal through the gastrointestinal tract: Reaching stomach a few seconds after being swallowed, stomach should be empty of barium in about 6 hours, barium should reach the cecum in about 5 hours, the ileum should be empty of barium in about 9 hours, and barium should be present in the colon after 24 hours.

Gallbladder Series. To determine time required for the gallbladder to fill and empty, the presence of gallstones, and to study the size and contour of the organ. A white, odorless powder which acts as a dye is

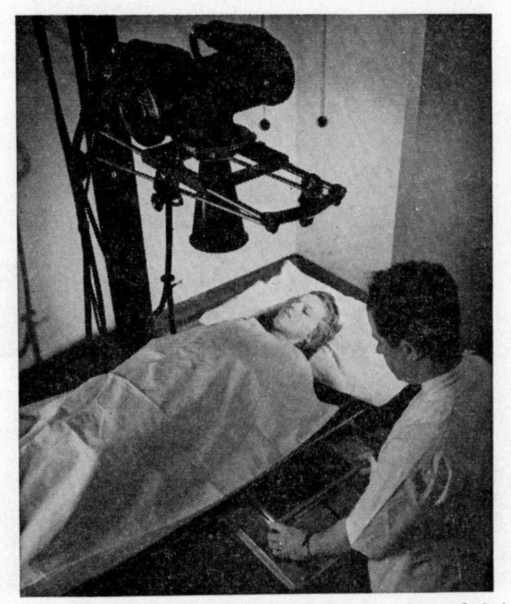

Fig. 137. X-ray is used to determine structural damage through injury or disease. (Presbyterian Hospital, Chicago, Illinois.)

administered orally or by intravenous injection. Several hours after the dye is given an x-ray picture is taken. A special diet high in fat content is then given, and another x-ray picture taken. Normal values —the gallbladder should be clearly visible in the first picture and not visible in the picture taken after the fatty meal.

Chest X-Ray. For study of the lungs. The patient stands against the x-ray machine and holds his breath while the picture is being taken. Normal values—lungs should be clear of shadow. Significance—structural damage through injury or disease is apparent if the x-ray film is not clear. Diagnosis of active pulmonary tuberculosis may be confirmed by x-ray of the chest.

X-Ray of Bones. To determine outline of bony part being studied. The part to be studied is placed in proper position and an x-ray picture is taken. The procedure is done by a trained x-ray technician. Normal values—normal outline of the structure. Significance—an abnormal outline, or a break in the continuity of the outline will indicate abnormality of the bone. The extent and kind of fracture of a bone can be determined by x-ray. Satisfactory progress in the healing of a fractured bone may also be checked by x-ray examination at stated intervals.

Other Tests. Other laboratory tests are performed as a means of helping to diagnose a condition accurately. Many factors must be

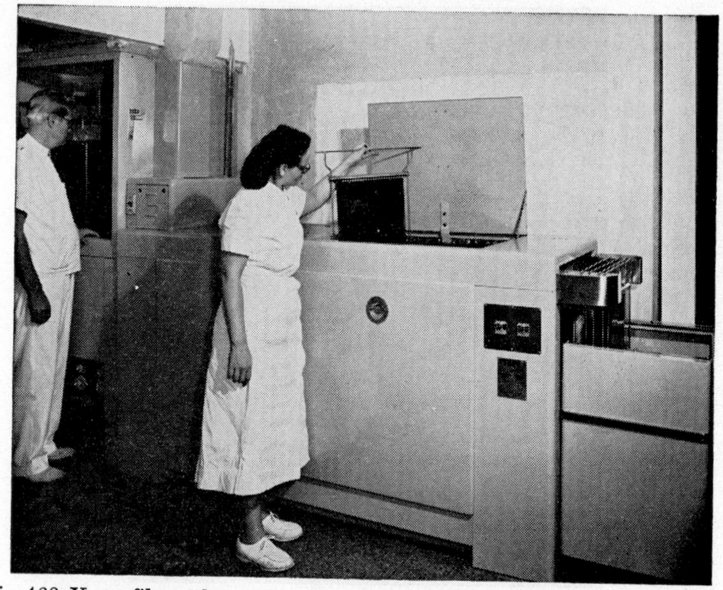

Fig. 138. X-ray films taken at stated intervals will show progress in the healing of a fracture or of a disease condition. (Presbyterian Hospital, Chicago, Illinois.)

considered in evaluating laboratory findings, and each hospital usually provides its own laboratory manual so that testing procedures will be carried out with some degree of uniformity.

The nurse who plans to work in departments where testing procedures are an important part of the daily routine should be well versed in all such procedures and should have greater knowledge of diagnostic tests than can be imparted in this brief résumé of the most common tests now in use.

Care of Equipment after Use

Containers used for specimens which are sent to the laboratory are cared for in the laboratory after the contents have been tested.

Trays used for collecting specimens related to puncture fluids should be thoroughly cleaned and returned to Central Supply where they can be made ready for use again.

Summary of Important Factors

Diagnostic tests are used not only to aid in making a diagnosis but also to confirm a diagnosis already made.

To be helpful in various laboratory procedures the nurse should

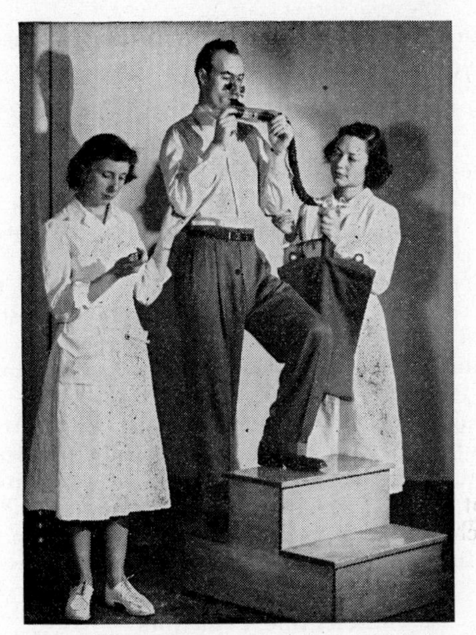

Fig. 139. A common laboratory procedure is to test before, during, and after exercise so results can be studied on a comparative basis. (Presbyterian Hospital, Chicago, Illinois.)

know the purpose of the test, the method of collecting specimens, and her responsibilities in helping perform the testing procedure.

Tests for bleeding time and coagulation time should be done before a patient undergoes surgery.

To understand and correctly interpret laboratory reports the nurse must know normal values for diagnostic tests which are commonly used in most hospitals.

Sedimentation rate indicates activity of the disease process.

Prothrombin time is an essential factor in anticoagulant drug therapy.

Before transfusion is done blood typing and crossmatching must be carried out if danger to the patient is to be avoided.

Routine urinalysis is an important part of the admission procedure for the patient being hospitalized.

All specimens should be placed in suitable containers, properly labeled, and kept at proper temperature (refrigerated, if necessary) until time for testing.

Stool specimen for ameba must be kept warm so the amebae will remain active and can be seen by the laboratory technician.

If meals are omitted as part of the testing procedure, the nurse should make sure that food is served the patient immediately after the tests are completed.

Factors To Teach the Patient

General purpose of the test to insure his cooperation.

Method of obtaining the kind of specimen needed for the test and the importance of using a proper container, if the patient is to be responsible for collecting the specimen.

Diabetic patients should be taught the procedure of testing urine for sugar. The relationship of diet, insulin, and the testing of urine for sugar should be clearly understood by the patient.

Sputum specimens should consist of sputum "coughed up" from the lungs.

That the accuracy of the basal metabolism (B.M.R.) test depends on cooperation of the patient, who must be relaxed physically and free from strain mentally during the test; that all activity requiring energy from the patient, even lifting an arm, affects the test findings.

Tests in which apparatus is used for electric impulse recording or for x-ray visualization are not painful and need not be feared.

Scientific Principles

Anatomy and Physiology. Body secretions and excretions, by containing abnormal constituents, furnish evidence of certain disease conditions. Diagnostic tests are based on deviations from normal in content, outline, or functioning of the fluid, organ, or part being studied.

Examination of urine and of blood may reveal the presence of bacteria or other characteristic evidence of disease.

Examination of stomach contents or of feces may reveal abnormal functioning of the digestive system.

Sputum examination may show the presence of bacteria in the respiratory system.

Special tests, as electrocardiography and basal metabolism tests, may be of value in diagnosing disease.

Chemistry. The body secretions and excretions normally contain various chemical substances. Deviations from normal content of these chemical substances aid in diagnosis of disease.

Sugar is not normally present in the urine.

Chemical tests are used to detect occult blood in the stool.

Microbiology. Tests to determine the presence of causative microorganisms are done as sterile procedures, and sterile equipment is needed. For a catheterized specimen of urine the container must be sterile. Most specimens should be kept in the refrigerator until ready for testing, as cold inhibits the growth of bacteria.

Because bacteria are found on the skin, when a needle is introduced through the skin to obtain a specimen of body fluid the skin should first be cleansed with an antiseptic solution.

Pharmacology. Drugs are used extensively in diagnostic procedures, to react with a secretion or excretion, to serve as a dye to outline a body cavity, and to stimulate activity so a specimen may be obtained: Phenolsulphonephthalein is a dye used to test kidney function. Glucose is used to test tolerance for sugar. Sodium benzoate is used to test liver function. A laxative may be used to stimulate evacuation and obtain a stool specimen. Barium sulfate is used in x-ray examination. Iodized oils and air are other mediums used in x-ray examination of various organs.

Physics. Withdrawal of fluids from the body is dependent on differences in pressure, all confined body fluids being under a pressure which is greater than the atmospheric pressure. Body fluids flow to the area of less pressure when a needle or cannula is inserted.

Pressures within a cavity may be measured in centimeters of water or millimeters of mercury. Mercury has a weight thirteen times that of water.

A smooth, slick surface of a tube or catheter makes insertion into a body cavity easier because of reduced friction. Stomach tubes are immersed in ice water, catheters are lubricated before use.

Electric impulses produced by activity of the brain and heart may be recorded graphically, for better examination of the two organs.

Because the penetration of body tissue by x-rays varies with the density of the tissue, x-rays may be used as a diagnostic aid.

Psychology. Patients may be apprehensive and nervous regarding laboratory tests, fearing the procedure itself as well as the outcome of the test. To overcome such fear, the nurse will need to give a careful explanation of the test.

Most tests may be conducted more effectively if the patient is relaxed and unafraid.

When food is withheld because of a laboratory test that fact should be explained to the patient and food should be served immediately on completion of the test.

Privacy should be given the patient for tests involving passage of a tube or catheter.

When x-ray or electrical equipment is used in testing, the patient should be reassured and informed that the equipment will not cause pain when in use.

Sociology. Cooperation of nurse, doctor, technician, and patient is needed for best results of diagnostic procedures.

The patient's stay in the hospital should not be prolonged because of carelessness in scheduling or performing various diagnostic tests.

Specimens may be sent by mail to state or local health departments.

Some laboratory tests are done without charge at free clinics.

Diagnostic tests may be done in a doctor's office, in special laboratories, in clinics, and in the hospital.

Situation Type Problem

1. A patient scheduled for a basal metabolism test did not have the procedure properly explained to him and understood only that he was to remain quietly in bed until time for the test. He was somewhat disturbed to find that he was not permitted to eat breakfast when he asked the nurse why his breakfast tray had not been served. After the nurse left the room he raised the window shade, which she had lowered, telephoned downstairs for the morning paper and a package of cigarettes. The nurse who was to take him for the test found him sitting up in bed, reading the paper, and smoking his third cigarette. He mentioned to her that he had been refused a breakfast tray, but hadn't fared too badly since a basket of fruit had been delivered the previous day and he had eaten several apples and a banana. What would you have done?

Suggested Reference Reading

"Interpreting laboratory reports," Deborah M. Jensen; American Journal of Nursing, July, 1950.

"Renal function tests for the clinician," Gregory S. Slater; American Practitioner, November, 1952.

"Diagnostic tests for Nancy," Helen S. Kaelin; American Journal of Nursing, November, 1952.

"If you see blood," Louis Schneider; American Journal of Nursing, February, 1953.

"What to expect of x-rays," Philip Lewin; Today's Health, October, 1952.

CHAPTER 21

Temperature—Pulse—Respiration

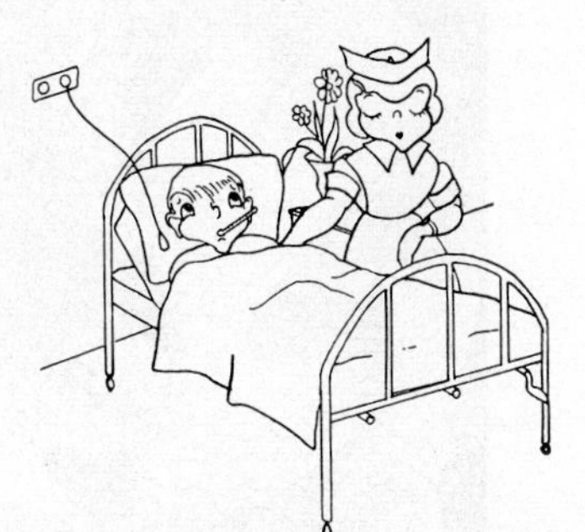

He lets go of the conversation at least twice each day—at 8 A.M. and 4 P.M.

TOPICAL OUTLINE

Temperature

HEAT PRODUCTION
HEAT LOSS
HEAT REGULATION
VARIATIONS OF TEMPERATURE
FEVER
NURSING CARE OF FEVER PATIENTS
THE CLINICAL THERMOMETER
METHODS OF TAKING TEMPERATURE
FREQUENCY OF TAKING TEMPERATURE

Pulse

THE NORMAL PULSE
VARIATIONS IN PULSE
CHARACTERISTICS OF PULSE
SITES FOR TAKING PULSE
METHOD OF TAKING PULSE
APICAL—RADIAL PULSE
FREQUENCY OF TAKING PULSE
TYPES OF PULSE

Respiration

ORGANS OF RESPIRATION
MECHANICS OF RESPIRATION
REGULATION OF RESPIRATION
NORMAL RESPIRATION
VARIATIONS IN RESPIRATION
METHOD OF COUNTING RESPIRATION
CONDITIONS RELATED TO RESPIRATION
TYPES OF RESPIRATION

In health, temperature, pulse, and respiration remain nearly constant and are at, or very near, the "normal" values which have been set at 98.6° F., 72, and 18, respectively. Any change in body functioning will produce a change in these values; any deviation from normal is symptomatic of disease and the degree of change may indicate certain stages of the disease process.

Because temperature, pulse, and respiration, by variation, may show any abnormal condition affecting the body, they are of major importance in the observation of a patient and furnish an accurate indication of his state of health. For this reason these important symptoms are termed "cardinal symptoms" or "vital signs." Even when the

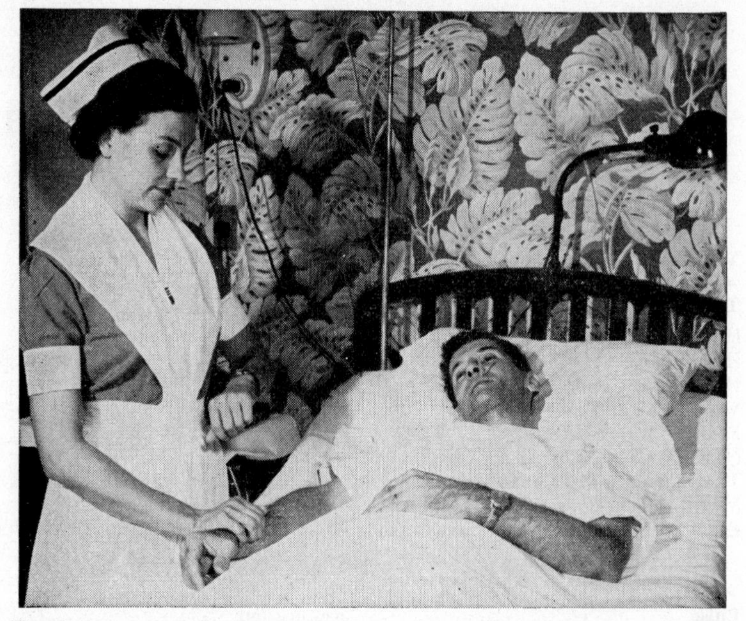

Fig. 140. Temperature, pulse, and respiration should be taken for each patient at least twice daily. (Saginaw General Hospital School of Nursing, Saginaw, Michigan.)

record shows very little variation from normal, the nurse should continue to observe and record their measurement at least twice each day. Any variation from normal in temperature, pulse rate, and respiration rate requires that more frequent observations and recordings be made.

Because of the importance of each of the cardinal symptoms the nurse must be very accurate in the recording and must check the result if there is any doubt as to the accuracy of the original findings. Graphic charts are made to show not only variations from normal for each of the three "signs," but also the relation of each to the other two.

Temperature

Body temperature is defined as the degree of heat maintained by the body; it is the balance maintained between the heat produced, as the result of the oxidation of food, and heat lost through perspiration, respiration, conduction, convection, radiation, and excretion.

So that food taken into the body can be burned to produce heat the respiratory tract supplies needed oxygen. In breathing, oxygen is inhaled, and excess heat, carbon dioxide, and other waste products are eliminated from the body with the exhaled air. The amount of oxygen inhaled determines to some extent the amount of heat produced in the body. In this manner a close relationship exists between body temperature and respiration.

HEAT PRODUCTION

Heat is produced mostly in the muscles and glands of the body. Factors causing an increase in the amount of heat produced are:

1. Exercise—the work of the muscles will increase heat production and cause a feeling of warmth throughout the body.
2. Shivering—another form of muscular activity which produces heat.
3. Ingestion of food—by increasing the fuel supply body heat is increased.
4. Strong emotions—excitement, anxiety, nervousness, and similar emotions cause increased activity of secreting glands to increase heat production in the body.
5. Increased temperature of environment—high room temperature or a hot water bath may increase body temperature.
6. Brief exposure to cold—stimulates the body to increased heat production, to compensate for heat lost by radiation and conduction. Prolonged exposure to cold will reduce the temperature of the body.
7. Very high external temperature—may upset the balance of heat regulation and produce high body temperature, as in sunstroke.

Factors causing decreased heat production include:

1. Illness—muscular activity is curtailed and less heat is produced.
2. Fasting—an inadequate supply of food or fuel leads to decreased heat production.
3. Lowered vitality—in conditions of illness or injury in which resistance is lowered body functions are slowed and muscular activity diminished so heat production is decreased.
4. Sleep—during sleep, when the body is less active, less heat is produced and body temperature is lowered.
5. Depression of the nervous system—mental depression, unconsciousness, the use of narcotic drugs, all act to lessen body activity and thus decrease heat production.

If a temperature balance is to be maintained in the body, heat must be lost as well as produced. Heat is lost by several means, including:

1. Perspiration—as the secretion from the sweat glands evaporates heat is lost from the body, the amount of loss depending on the amount of perspiration secreted.
2. Respiration—expired air is warmer than that inspired and carries

a large content of water vapor. Through expiration heat is lost from the body.

3. Excretion—the excretion of urine, feces, and saliva, at body temperature at the time of elimination, provides for some heat loss from the body.

4. Conduction—heat is lost by radiation of heat from the skin to cooler surroundings.

The total amount of heat loss varies with climate and with conditions affecting the immedite surroundings of the body.

HEAT REGULATION

Man belongs to the class of so-called warm-blooded animals whose body temperature is maintained at a certain level, regardless of the variations of temperature in different climates and in different seasons of the year. Body temperature normally remains constant because of the control over heat production and heat loss which the heat-regulating mechanism exerts.

Centers in the nervous system that control the circulation of blood through the skin and the secretion of perspiration also control, to a great extent, the amount of heat lost through the skin. The many minute capillaries of the skin bring to the body surface a large volume of blood which gives off its heat to the cooler atmosphere before returning to the larger blood vessels deep within the body.

In the winter, when the surrounding atmosphere is very cold, the vasomotor nerve centers that control the size of the blood vessels cause them to contract, so that less heat is lost from the body. The secretion of perspiration may be decreased by nerve center action, so that less heat will be lost by evaporation. An extremely cold atmosphere may cause the nerve endings in the skin to stimulate nerve centers that are active in producing heat. Shivering may occur, with muscular activity generating heat, and the appetite may be stimulated so that additional food (or fuel) is taken into the body.

In summer, when the atmosphere is warmer, blood vessels in the skin dilate, a greater volume of blood flows through them, and more heat is lost from the body. The appetite and muscular activity may be markedly decreased, and excessive perspiration helps to dissipate body heat.

Because the heat-regulating mechanism of the nervous system is not fully developed in infants and young children, their body function is more easily disturbed, causing variation in temperature, pulse, and respiration. They are also more apt to be influenced by temperature of the atmosphere.

VARIATIONS IN DEGREE OF TEMPERATURE

With a basic understanding of the heat-regulating mechanism which keeps body temperature at the standard "normal" level, the

Table 5. COMPARISON OF CENTIGRADE AND FAHRENHEIT THERMOMETRIC SCALES

*Centigrade**	*Fahrenheit*†
100°	212° (Boiling point of water)
90°	194°
80°	176°
70°	158°
60°	140°
50°	122°
40°	104°
39°	102.2°
38°	100.4°
37°	98.6° (Normal body temperature)
36°	96.8°
35°	95°
30°	86°
20°	68°
10°	50°
0°	32° (Freezing point of water)
10°	14°
20°	4°

* To convert Centigrade to Fahrenheit—multiply by 9/5 and add 32
† To convert Fahrenheit to Centigrade—subtract 32 and multiply by 5/9

nurse may soon learn to recognize the significance of any variations.

By close observation she may even detect changes in temperature of the patient before the change is measured on the clinical thermometer. Any change in appearance or manner indicating a variation in temperature requires that the temperature be taken and recorded. Symptoms of rising body temperature include flushed face, dry, hot skin, dry, parched, and tremulous lips, restless hands, and rapid, shallow respirations.

Normal body temperature taken orally has been standardized at 98.6° F. (37° C.), since that is the average temperature for persons in good health.

Numerous factors influence body temperature and cause deviation from normal. When the deviation is slight and remains constant, the variation may be considered "normal."

Temperature of the internal areas of the body is higher than that of body surface. Temperature of the blood is normally 102° F., that of the skin 90–92° F. Skin temperature varies, too, since temperature is increased at the surface if an underlying muscle is activated.

Recorded temperature may also vary slightly according to the blood supply to the part of the body where temperature is being taken. Findings vary consistently, depending on the method of taking temperature. Taken orally (by mouth), normal body temperature is 98.6° F., taken by axillary method (at the armpit) it is 97.6° to 98° F., and taken rectally it is 99.6° F.

Normal body temperature may be influenced by the amount and kind of food eaten, type of work being done, and by age and temperament. A person living very quietly and engaged in a sedentary occupation may have a lower "normal" temperature than the person engaged in strenuous outdoor activity. Normal temperature of a child may be about one degree higher than that of an adult. The very old person, like the very young, may have a slightly higher "normal" temperature.

Normal body temperature will vary during the day, being lowest in the very early morning hours and highest in the late afternoon and early evening. The increase in temperature each day is caused by food and exercise, so the person who sleeps during the day and works at night will have the lowest rate in late afternoon and highest in the early morning hours. Because of this daily variation in "normal" temperature, patients should have their temperature taken at the same time each day so the day by day measurement represented on the graphic sheet of the chart will provide accurate comparison. These slight daily variations of temperature (ranging from 97–99° F.) are not considered abnormal and are compatible with health.

SIGNIFICANT VARIATIONS FROM NORMAL TEMPERATURE

Slight variations above or below normal temperature, especially those which occur because of factors mentioned above, are not significant. Variations of a greater degree, or unexplained by such factors as age, exercise, and time of day, *are* significant since they indicate a disturbance of function in some organ or part of the body.

The degree of elevation of temperature above normal does not always indicate the seriousness of the disease or the condition that may be causing a rise in temperature. Acute infections which may prove fatal sometimes produce only mild elevation of temperature. A continuous high temperature is always an alarming symptom and is indicative of serious illness.

Temperatures are commonly classified according to differences in degree as: very high, 105° F. and over; high, 102°–105° F.; moderately high, 100°–102° F.; slightly elevated, 99°–100° F.; normal, 98°–99° F.; subnormal, 96°–98° F.; collapsing, below 96° F.

For variations of temperature requiring corrective measures the nurse is expected to carry out certain routine nursing procedures without waiting for them to be ordered by the doctor.

Elevated Body Temperature. When body temperature is above normal the nurse should make certain that the temperature of the room or unit is not above 72° F. Surrounding air that is too warm will tend to make the patient's temperature rise. The kind and amount of top covers being used for the patient should be checked. They should afford enough warmth but should not be heavy, thus causing too much additional warmth to the body.

All unnecessary noise or excitement should be prevented and activity of the patient should be restricted. Exercise or exertion on the part of the patient, sitting up in bed, carrying on animated conversation with visitors, turning, lifting, or moving himself, or straining to use bedpan or urinal, may cause a rise in temperature. The nurse may restrict or forbid the above activities if she feels it is wise to do so.

Other measures to prevent temperature elevation may be prescribed by the doctor and include: freedom from worry or mental unrest; increase in amount of fluids taken into the body; local application of cold, as by ice cap; sponge bath (ordered usually if temperature reaches 102° F.); and a special diet low in fats and carbohydrates, the foodstuffs that yield more heat and energy.

Subnormal Body Temperature. When the temperature is below normal, measures are required to increase heat production in the body and to prevent heat loss. Room temperature may be increased above 72° F., and hot water bottles or other means of applying external heat, such as hot blankets, may be used.

Hot drinks, unless contraindicated, may be given. The doctor may prescribe a hot foot bath, friction applied to the body surface, or a hot enema. In marked subnormal temperature the patient is in a state of shock and emergency shock treatment must be instituted without delay.

FEVER

Fever is defined as "the elevation of body temperature above normal." The technical term for fever is *pyrexia.* Many diseases are given a name which includes the word "fever" and the name of the causative agent of the disease, as "malarial fever." Some diseases are given a name that describes the characteristic graphic record of the fever, as "relapsing fever," an infectious disease marked by alternating periods of fever and of absence of fever. Other diseases are named to describe a characteristic symptom of the disease, as "scarlet fever," a disease characterized by inflammation of the throat and a scarlet rash on the skin.

Causes of Fever. The immediate cause of fever is a disturbance of the heat-regulating mechanism. Heat production is increased, without corresponding increase in heat loss. If the heat-regulating center is so disturbed that it fails to return to normal functioning within a short time the condition of the patient will become serious. With the onset of a disease causing fever the heat-regulating mechanism may be set at a higher level so the body temperature will rise to the point where better protection against the invading microorganism is achieved. Fever is a symptom invariably present in most disease conditions, and the treatment depends on the various causative factors.

In sunstroke, fever as high as 108–110° F. may be present as the result of the extreme external heat. The temperature may remain high for a long period, and every available means of reducing it must be employed if the patient is to survive. The extremely high body temperature in sunstroke causes chemical changes in body tissues which will result in death if not soon controlled.

Other causes of fever include acute infectious diseases, acute inflammatory conditions, acute and prolonged pain, extreme nervousness, emotional stress, hysteria, and trauma or injury to body tissue Fever may be induced artificially to aid in treatment of certain diseases. Dehydration or injudicious use of drugs may also cause increased body temperature.

In conditions of inflammation and infection the elevation of body temperature is a desirable defensive reaction which helps to destroy the bacteria or microorganisms causing the disturbance and helps to combat the toxins absorbed into the blood stream from the bacteria. The body seems better able to defend itself against disease-producing microorganisms when the temperature is elevated.

Symptoms of Fever. Although fever is in itself considered a symptom, various signs or symptoms are indicative of a rise in body temperature. The characteristic symptoms which cause the observant nurse to take the patient's temperature to determine the degree of variation present may include any of the following:

Flushed face with skin dry and hot. By placing the hand at the back of the patient's neck and noting that the skin feels very hot the nurse may detect rising temperature.

Eyes bright and somewhat anxious in expression are an indication of fever.

Rapid, shallow breathing and increased pulse rate may indicate increased body temperature.

Unusual thirst, loss of appetite, headache, and complaints of nausea may be noted in temperature elevation.

If the temperature increase is extreme the symptoms may become more severe. Urine may be scant and concentrated, and there may be diarrhea or constipation, and delirium.

Course of Fever. Regardless of the type of fever the patient may have or the length of time it persists, the course of fever will be the same. The graphic representation on the temperature chart shows the course of the fever and in some instances is typical of that seen in certain diseases so that diagnosis may be made merely by observation of the temperature graph.

The period of *onset* or *invasion* of fever, when the body temperature is rising, is usually characterized by a feeling of chilliness and general discomfort. The onset of fever may be sudden, or it may be a very gradual process, depending on the disease or condition causing it.

The *fastigium,* or *stadium,* of fever is the period when body temperature has reached its maximum and remains fairly constant and at

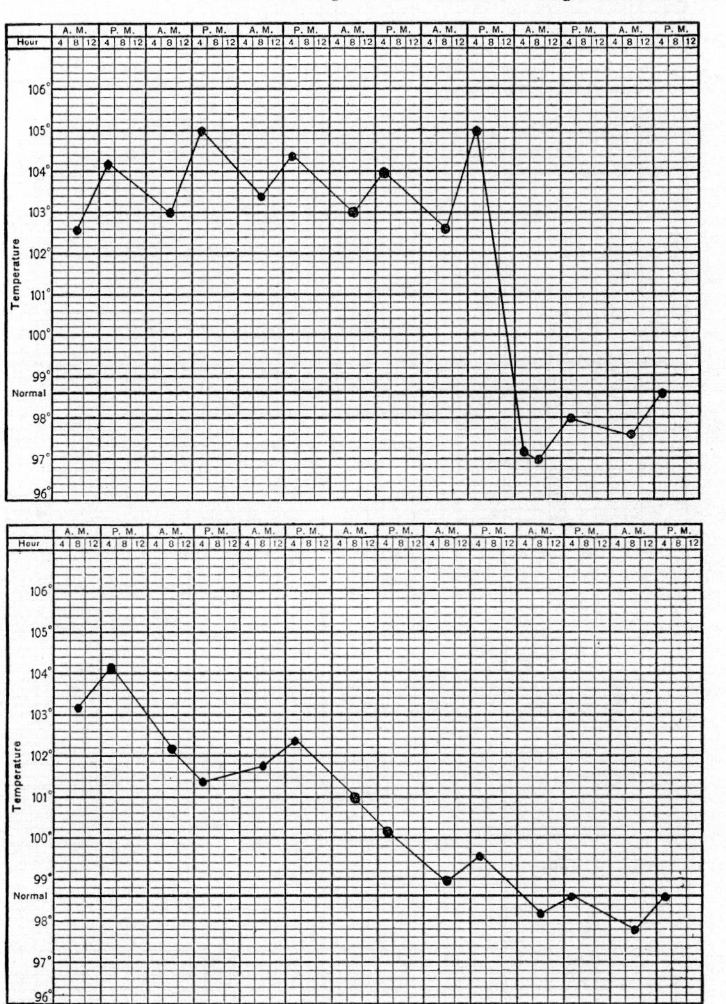

Fig. 141. Fever may decline by crisis (sudden drop) or by lysis (gradual return to normal).

a high level. This period may last from a few days to a few weeks.

The *defervescence*, or *decline* in fever, is the period when the elevated temperature returns to normal. If the temperature drops suddenly, returning to normal or below in a few hours, it is said to have dropped by *crisis.* If temperature returns to normal gradually, and over a period of several days, subsiding slightly more each day,

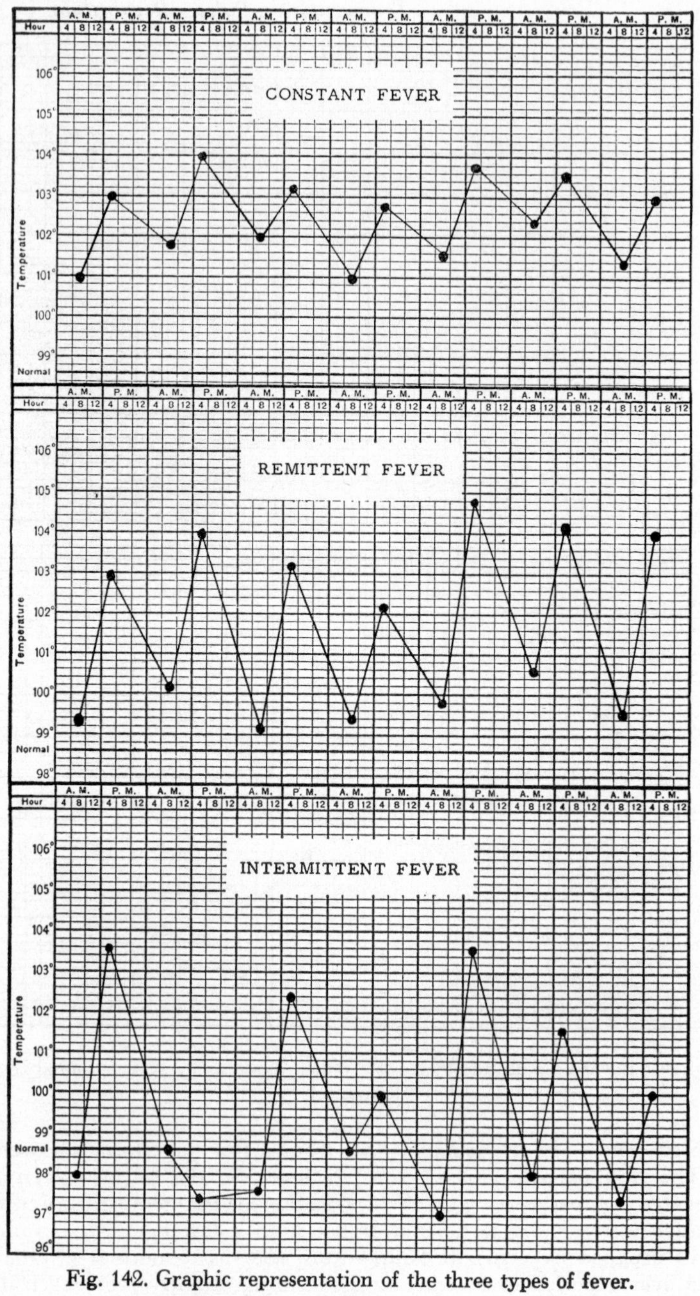

Fig. 142. Graphic representation of the three types of fever.

it is said to have dropped by *lysis*. When temperature falls by crisis the patient needs to be closely watched. If other symptoms are lessened and improvement in condition is noted, the period of crisis may indicate the beginning of recovery for the patient. If the temperature drops suddenly, but other severe symptoms persist or are noted, as increased pulse rate, rapid, shallow respirations, and increasing weakness, a complication, such as internal hemorrhage or perforation, may be present, and the patient's condition may rapidly become critical.

A rapid drop in fever may be brought about by chemotherapy, shortening the usual course of fever and the period of *fastigium*.

Since both pulse and respiration rate increase naturally as body temperature is increased, decrease in temperature should be accompanied by a corresponding decrease in pulse and respiration. Any change in temperature not followed by similar change in pulse and respiration may be considered undesirable and will require the attention of the physician.

Types of Fever. Fever may be classified as one of three types, based on the extent of daily variation, although its over-all course may follow the same general pattern.

Constant fever, sometimes termed *continuous* fever, is one in which the temperature remains constantly high throughout the day. It may vary slightly in degree (one or two degrees Fahrenheit), but does not fall below the moderately high level.

Remittent fever, a type of fever which may vary as much as two or three degrees Fahrenheit during the day but never quite returns to normal level.

Intermittent fever, a type of fever in which there are wide variations (of several degrees) during the day. The fever may rise suddenly or may drop with equal suddenness to normal or slightly below. This particular type of fever is characteristic of severe infectious diseases.

NURSING CARE OF FEVER PATIENTS

Although care of the patient depends largely on the disease causing the fever and on specific orders of the doctor, there are a few procedures in nursing which are always needed in giving care to the patient with fever.

In addition to accurate taking and recording of temperature at regular intervals, the nurse will be called on to use such measures as alcohol back rub, frequent bathing of face and hands, change of position, and special attention to bed linens to keep the patient comfortable.

Sufficient fluids must be given and food which is served the patient must be made as attractive as possible. Lack of appetite which may be present in fever patients quite often becomes a challenging problem to the nurse. Food will need to be made palatable and desirable, so that a proper diet will be eaten.

Special care of the mouth is necessary when the body temperature remains elevated. Lips are apt to become dry and cracked, the tongue may be swollen, and sordes may be present, requiring continuous attention and treatment. If blisters appear about the mouth or lips (herpes simplex), treatment for that condition must be instituted and made part of daily nursing care.

THE CLINICAL THERMOMETER

The self-registering clinical thermometer, used for measuring body temperature, is available in both Fahrenheit and Centigrade scales. The highest degree of temperature indicated on the scale is 110° F. (43.4° C.) and the lowest is 94° F. (34.5° C.)

The thermometer, made of glass, consists of an end bulb containing mercury and a stem in which the column of mercury may rise. The graduated scale, representing degrees of temperature (and marked in subdivisions of two tenths of one degree), is clearly visible along the stem of the thermometer. The back of the stem of the thermometer is flat to facilitate reading of the scale and to lessen the danger of breakage since the flat plane prevents the thermometer from rolling if it is placed on table top or other smooth surface.

Thermometers are made with end bulbs of different sizes and shapes. The long slender bulb is indicative of the *oral* thermometer; thermometers with short rounded, pear-shaped, or colored bulbs are used in taking temperature *rectally*. Difference in thermometers should be distinct so that thermometers used for each of the two methods will not be confused.

The principle on which the thermometer is constructed is the expansion of mercury when subjected to heat. The height to which the column of mercury rises in the stem of the thermometer depends on the degree of heat to which the bulb is subjected and thus accurately indicates the degree of body temperature. The column of mercury remains at the height to which it rises until it is shaken down. A constriction slightly above the point where the bulb and stem of the thermometer are joined prevents the mercury from receding back into the bulb. A quick snapping wrist movement, while holding the thermometer, will force the mercury downward into the bulb. A thermometer in which the mercury drops without being shaken down is no longer dependable and should be discarded.

Handling the Thermometers. Clinical thermometers are easily broken and should be handled with care. Each time, before use, the column of mercury should be shaken down to a point just below the 94° F. reading on the scale.

To hold the thermometer correctly, the upper part of the stem should be grasped firmly between thumb and fingers. To shake the column of mercury down, with the bulb end of the thermometer held downward, the hand should be brought up sharply and then with a snap of the wrist extended suddenly downward again. Devices are available which shake down a dozen or so thermometers at one time. The mechanical shaker prevents breakage and allows thermometers to be shaken down in greater numbers and in less time.

When at the bedside of the patient the nurse should stand away from bed or bedside table while shaking the thermometer, taking care not to strike it against anything on the downward movement which could cause it to be broken.

A clinical thermometer should never be rinsed in hot water because a temperature above 110° F. with cause the mercury to expand beyond the stem's capacity and the thermometer will be broken. The thermometer should never be held at the bulb end; warmth from the hands will cause further expansion of the mercury and produce an inaccurate reading, and microorganisms from the patient's mouth will be transferred to the hands of the nurse if she handles the bulb end of the thermometer immediately after it is removed for reading.

Reading the Thermometer. To read the thermometer the nurse should hold it at the upper end of the stem with one hand. Standing with her back toward light from window or lamp, she should hold the thermometer in a horizontal position at eye level.

By rotating the thermometer slightly back and forth the markings on the graduated scale can be clearly seen. The reader should follow with her eyes the column of mercury as it extends upward in the stem from the bulb of the thermometer. At the point on the scale where the column of mercury ends the reading should be taken. The long lines on the scale represent degrees of temperature; each of the shorter lines represents two-tenths of one degree.

After reading the thermometer the temperature should be recorded so there will be no question as to its accuracy. If there is reason to doubt the accuracy of the measurement recorded on the thermometer, the temperature should be taken again with a different thermometer.

The patient should not be permitted to handle the thermometer since there is danger of its being broken and since it is not advisable for him to know the degree of temperature being recorded.

Care of the Thermometer. Individual thermometers should be provided for all hospital patients and should be kept clean by washing in soap and water and rinsing with cool water.

When not in use the thermometer should be kept in a covered jar or other container so that it is immersed in an antiseptic solution, such as bichloride of mercury (1:1000 solution). A small cotton pledget should be placed at the bottom of the jar to protect the end of the thermometer. When removed from its container the thermometer should be passed through a folded cotton pledget to remove excess solution. After the temperature is taken the thermometer should again be passed through a folded cotton pledget to remove any secretion or discharge which may adhere to it. After the reading has been made the thermometer should be washed, rinsed, and returned to its container.

A thermometer used for an isolated patient must be kept in the isolated unit and clearly labeled so it will not be mistakenly used for another patient. When the period of isolation is over the thermometer must be completely disinfected before being put into general use again.

METHODS OF TAKING TEMPERATURE

To determine the accurate degree of body temperature the thermometer must be placed where it will be in contact with body tissues that are amply supplied with heat from nearby blood vessels. The temperature of the interior of the body may be taken by placing the thermometer in the mouth, the axilla, the groin, the rectum, or the vagina. The most commonly used sites for taking temperature are the mouth, rectum, and axilla.

Taking the temperature orally is the simplest, most convenient, and most comfortable method. Rectal temperature, considered the most accurate of the three commonly used methods, is one degree higher than oral temperature. Use of the axillary method is not desirable, since it is considered very likely to result in an inaccurate reading. The axillary temperature is one degree lower than temperature taken orally.

Taking the Temperature Orally. In taking temperature orally the thermometer should be placed so that the bulb containing the mercury is directly beneath the tongue. The lips should be closed firmly around the stem of the thermometer while the patient breathes through the nose only. The thermometer should be left in place for three minutes. If hot or cold fluids or food has been taken into the mouth, oral temperature should not be taken for at least 10 minutes.

If oral temperature (normally 98.6° F.) seems unusually low or is elevated more than a few tenths of a degree, it should be taken again with another thermometer or taken rectally.

Contraindications. The oral method should not be used for very young children or uncooperative older children. The thermometer may be broken by the child, and glass particles or fragments of mercury may be swallowed.

Adult patients who have a head cold or are breathing with difficulty should not have the temperature taken orally since it will be impossible for them to hold the mouth closed for the desired three minutes.

A patient with persistent and frequent coughing attacks should not have the temperature taken orally.

In cases of extreme weakness when the mouth is apt to fall open during the time the thermometer must remain in position, oral temperature is contraindicated.

Patients who are extremely nervous, delirious, unconscious, hysterical, or mentally confused should not have their temperature taken orally because the thermometer may be broken and there is small likelihood of an accurate measurement of body temperature being obtained.

After surgical operations on the mouth or nose, and during acute oral infections, temperature should not be taken by mouth.

Taking the Temperature Rectally. Since the rectal temperature is the most accurate, that method is used for the very ill patient, for infants and very young children, and for irrational or uncooperative patients.

The rectal thermometer should be well lubricated to prevent injury to the wall of the rectum and minimize stimulation of rectal muscles. It should be inserted into the rectum to a distance of 1½ inches. The nurse should hold the thermometer in place for three to five minutes, since that length of time is required to insure accurate measurement.

In patients with temperature above 102° F. temperature should be taken rectally, since their condition requires that the recorded temperature be as accurate as possible.

Contraindications. The temperature cannot be taken rectally following surgical procedures involving the rectum and perineal region, when the rectum is inflamed or diseased, or when it is distended with fecal material.

Taking the Temperature by the Axillary Method. The axillary method of taking temperature should be avoided if it is possible to use the oral or rectal method. If the temperature is to be taken at the axilla, the oral thermometer may be used. The axilla should be dry. The bulb end of the thermometer should be placed in the center of the axilla and the arm brought down across it to hold it in place. A period of ten minutes is required for the thermometer to register.

In some vascular diseases skin temperature may be required as a diagnostic measure. Special equipment is needed and the procedure is performed by the physician.

Taking the Temperature at Other Sites. Temperature taken "per groin" or " per vagina" is one degree lower than that taken by mouth, and the thermometer should be left in place for at least five minutes.

FREQUENCY OF TAKING TEMPERATURE

The frequency with which temperature is taken and recorded depends on the condition of the patient and the orders of the doctor. In most hospitals temperatures are taken twice daily on all patients, usually about 8:00 A.M. and 4:00 P.M.

Patients with an elevated temperature and all postoperative patients (for 48 hours) should have their temperature taken every four hours. For the patient with a very high fever, the interval may be two hours or even less.

When it is necessary for the nurse to report to the doctor on the condition of a patient it is good practice for her to take the patient's temperature, pulse, and respiration first, so these important signs may be reported, too. Most doctors will want to know the latest recorded temperature, pulse, and respiration for a patient on whom they have requested a report.

Although temperature is a very important symptom and often furnishes an index to the patient's condition, the nurse should not waken a patient at night to take the temperature unless specifically ordered to do so by the doctor.

If the temperature is elevated at 8:00 P.M., the night nurse should take the temperature again whenever the patient may waken during the night.

Pulse

The rhythmic expansion of an artery produced by increased volume of blood forced into it by contraction of the left ventricle at each heart beat is termed "pulse."

Each time the ventricle contracts it forces about 70 cc. of blood into the already filled aorta, causing increased pressure within the "closed tube" arterial system. Since the walls of the arteries are elastic they stretch or expand as the increased amount of blood passes through them. The intermittent pressure and expansion of the artery causes the blood to move along in a wavelike motion, toward the capillaries. The top of the wave is felt when the artery expands to accommodate the increased volume of blood. The lower curve of the wave is felt when the artery contracts to push the blood along its way. The upward curve of the pulse wave corresponds to the systole, or working period of the heart; the downward curve corresponds to the diastole, or resting period of the heart.

Any change in the volume of blood pumped through the heart, any interference with the functioning of the heart, any variation in the rate of heart beat, and any change in elasticity of the arterial wall will cause a change in the pulse. Hence, taking the pulse is a quick and simple method of determining the condition of the heart, blood vessels, and circulation.

Since the heart and blood vessels are controlled or regulated by the nervous system, a change in pulse may be brought about by interference with normal functioning of the nervous system.

An abnormal condition of the body will bring about a change in the heart and blood vessels and will be noted by a change in pulse. The pulse is often an important factor in diagnosis and treatment of disease and may serve to indicate the possible prognosis for a particular patient.

The nurse should learn to quickly recognize changes in the rate and quality of the pulse since symptoms that indicate failure of heart action are always serious in nature. By observing details about the pulse she will have more knowledge of the patient's general condition.

Although instruments such as the electrocardiograph record more accurately certain characteristics of heart activity, the taking of the pulse at frequent intervals is still an important part of routine nursing care for each patient.

THE NORMAL PULSE

Normal pulse rate for the healthy adult is 72–80 beats per minute. Pulse rate for the infant varies from 130–140 beats per minute. During the first few years of life the normal pulse rate decreases to approximately 110–120 beats per minute. In old age the normal rate is decreased to 60–70 beats per minute. The pulse rate for women is usually slightly more rapid than that for men. The normal pulse rates (average, per minute), at different ages, are: before birth, 140–150; at birth, 130–140; first year, 115–130; second year, 100–115; third year, 90–100; fourth to eighth year, 86–90; eighth to fifteenth year, 80–86; adult, 72–80; old age, 60–70.

FACTORS CAUSING VARIATION IN PULSE

Factors that may cause slight or marked variation in pulse rate or in other characteristic qualities of the pulse include:

Age—the very young have a rapid pulse rate; the adult has a normal range in rate of 72–80 beats per minute; the very old have a relatively slow pulse rate.

Sex—the female has a slightly more rapid pulse than does the male.

Physique—the short person with small body build has a slightly more rapid pulse than does the tall, heavy individual.

Exercise—increased muscular activity will increase the pulse rate temporarily. Because of this most doctors will take pulse rate before and after exercise as part of the procedure of physical examination. The time required for the rate to return to normal after exercise is also significant.

Food—ingestion of food causes a slight increase in pulse rate for several hours.

Posture—the pulse rate is higher with the body in standing position than when in a sitting or reclining position.

Mental or Emotional Disturbance—such disturbances will temporarily increase pulse rate.

Increased Body Temperature—when the body temperature is elevated pulse rate tends to rise about ten beats per minute for each degree of temperature elevation.

Disease Conditions—heart disease, thyroid disturbance, infections, and various other disease processes have a marked effect on pulse rate.

Drugs—stimulant drugs will increase pulse rate; depressant drugs will decrease pulse rate.

Blood Pressure—when blood pressure is low the pulse rate is increased in an attempt to increase the flow of blood and thus increase the pressure; in high blood pressure the pulse rate is decreased.

VARIOUS CHARACTERISTICS OF THE PULSE

Rhythm. The pulse is usually *regular* in rhythm, that is, the beats are of uniform force and separated by equal intervals of time. A disturbance in rhythm of the pulse may relate the force of the beat or the interval between beats. If the intervals of time between beats, are unequal, the pulse is termed *irregular* or *intermittent.* In an intermittent pulse a beat may be missed at regular intervals (every two, three, or four beats) or at irregular intervals.

Volume. The volume of blood in the vessels of the circulatory system is fairly constant. If the volume of blood is normal the pulse will be *full* or *large.* If the volume is decreased, as by hemorrhage, the pulse will be *small, feeble, weak, thready,* or *flickering.* The volume is determined by the size of the pulse wave against the fingers being used to take the pulse, which depends also on the force of the heart beat and on the condition of the arterial walls. If the pulse is large or full and also rapid in rate it may be described as *bounding.*

Tension. As the individual grows older arteries tend to lose some of their elasticity and to become hardened. Such arteries are less easily obliterated by pressure of the fingers in taking the pulse. The amount of pressure required to obliterate the pulse will depend on the pressure being exerted by the force of the blood and the resistance offered it by the arterial wall. Tension of pulse is usually described as high or low. A pulse of high tension is hard to the touch, and the artery is difficult to compress. A pulse of low tension is soft to the touch, and the artery is easily compressed.

Changes in pulse tension are indicative of changes in blood pressure, and the nurse should be able to recognize changes in the pulse that are caused by abnormal blood pressure.

The normal or average pulse for the adult may be described as one with a rate of 72–80 beats per minute, a regular rhythm and full volume. The artery should be clearly defined and compressed without difficulty by pressure of the fingers.

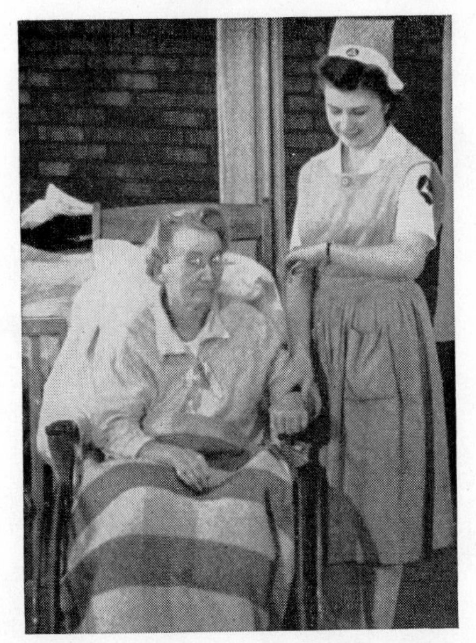

Fig. 143. Pulse may be taken at various sites, the one most commonly used being at the wrist, over the radial artery. (Ravenswood Hospital School of Nursing, Chicago, Illinois.)

SITES WHERE PULSE MAY BE TAKEN

Pulse may be taken at any place on the body where an artery near the skin or body surface can be compressed against a firm (bony) background. Sites most commonly chosen for taking pulse are: radial artery (at the thumb side of the wrist just above the radial artery), temporal artery (just above and to the outer side of the outer canthus of the eye), mandibular notch (at the outer angle of the lower jaw just above the facial artery), dorsalis pedis artery (on the instep of the foot), carotid artery (on either side of the neck, directly in front of the ear lobe), femoral artery (in the groin, between the anterior superior spine of the ilium and the symphysis pubis, just below the inguinal ligament).

The pulse is usually taken at the radial artery in the wrist, because this site is easily accessible and convenient for both nurse and patient.

METHOD OF TAKING PULSE

Before taking pulse the nurse should see that the patient is comfortably sitting or reclining, and that the arm or part being used is at rest and well supported.

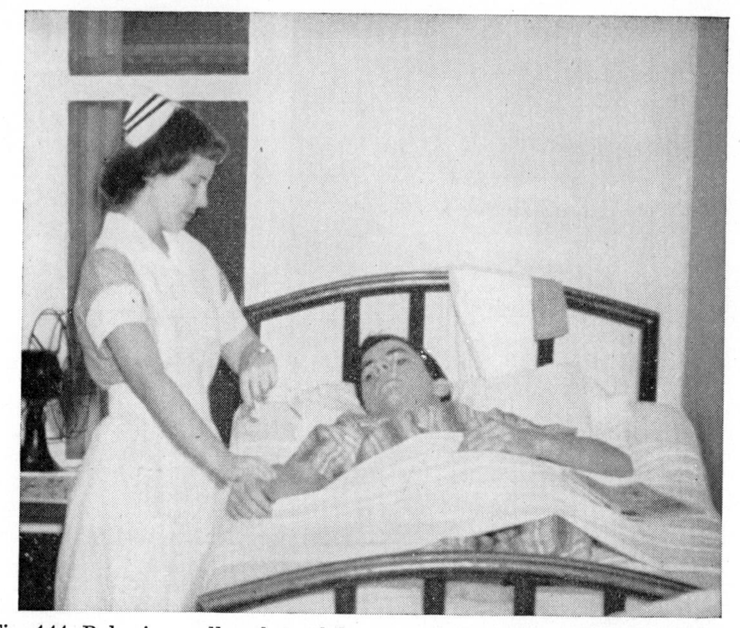

Fig. 144. Pulse is usually taken while temperature is being taken. (Mississippi Baptist Hospital School of Nursing, Jackson, Mississippi.)

Pulse is usually taken while temperature is being taken. If for any reason the patient is nervous, excitable, or extremely self conscious, the nurse should make an effort to induce him to be calm and relaxed before attempting to take the pulse.

In taking pulse the nurse should use the first three fingers of her right hand to compress the artery, using just enough pressure to make the pulse beat quite distinct and not enough to completely obliterate the pulse wave. She should never attempt to take pulse by placing her thumb above the artery where pulse beats are to be felt. Pulsations from a superficial artery in her own thumb may be confused with pulsations in the radial artery of the patient.

The pulse should be counted for one full minute by the student nurse who is not thoroughly familiar with the procedure. When she has become adept at counting pulse it may then be counted for one-half minute and multiplied by two to give an accurate count for one full minute.

The rate, regularity, force, and tension of the pulse should be noted so that a meaningful report may be given to the doctor.

Pulse should not be taken for routine daily counts immediately after physical exertion on the part of the patient or when the patient has just undergone a trying physical or mental exper-

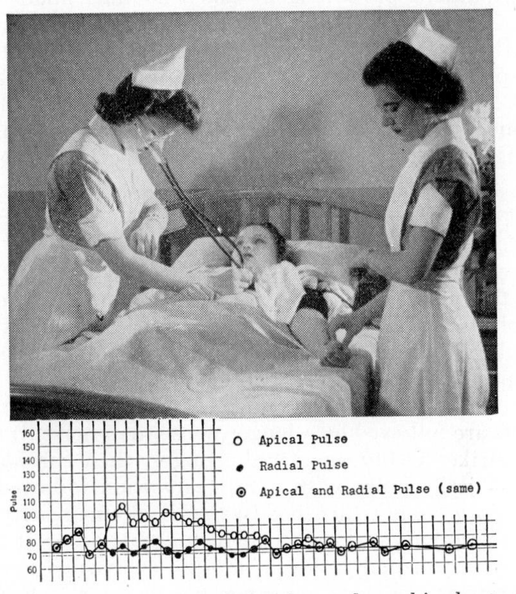

Fig. 145. Method of taking apical-radial pulse, and graphic chart of the results. (State University of Iowa College of Nursing, Iowa City, Iowa.)

ience which may greatly affect the pulse rate for a short period of time.

APICAL-RADIAL PULSE

In some instances the doctor will request that the radial pulse be counted at the same time a count is made of the apex beats of the heart. A difference between the two counts, termed *pulse deficit,* indicates that not all apex beats are being transmitted to or felt at the radial artery. The degree of difference in the apical-radial pulse may help to determine medication and treatment for the patient.

In taking apical-radial pulse one nurse must count the beats at the radial artery at the same time another nurse is counting the heart beats at the apex by means of a stethoscope. Both nurses must count during the same exact period of time, and the count should be for one minute.

FREQUENCY OF TAKING PULSE

Pulse is counted as a routine measure at least twice each day for hospitalized patients, at the time temperature and rate of respiration are being determined.

For some patients pulse may be taken at much more frequent intervals, depending on the doctor's orders and condition of the patient. The critically ill patient may have pulse taken very frequently, since change of pulse may be one of the first indications of a change in condition.

Postoperative patients, as well as those undergoing special treatments, experiencing severe symptoms, as pain, and receiving special nursing care may require frequent taking of pulse.

TYPES OF PULSE

Because the pulse is of such great importance in indicating the condition of the patient many different and characteristic types of pulse have been defined. A few of the most commonly used descriptive terms pertaining to types of pulse include: *apical*—counted with stethoscope at the apex of the heart; *bigeminal*—one in which two regular beats are followed by a longer pause than normal; *collapsing*—one which strikes feebly against the finger, then subsides abruptly; *Corrigan's*—a jerky pulse with a full expansion followed by sudden collapse; *dicrotic*—one which has two marked expansions in one beat of the artery; *irregular*—one in which the beats occur at irregular intervals or are of unequal strength; *labile*—one which is normal with the patient resting but increases when he sits up, stands, or exercises; *regular*—one in which the length of beat, the number of beats per minute, and the strength remain uniform; *running*—one with small, weak, irregular beats; *soft*—one of low tension; *tremulous*—one with small, weak, irregular beats; *water-hammer*—one with a short, powerful, jerky beat, followed by sudden collapse; *wiry*—a small, tense pulse that feels like a cord or wire.

Because taking the pulse is a nursing procedure that is used often for many patients, the nurse has ample opportunity to study and learn the characteristics of the normal pulse, to compare those characteristics with similar ones of the abnormal pulse, and to recognize abnormalities of pulse as being characteristic of certain specific disease conditions.

Respiration

Respiration may be defined simply as the act of breathing. It is the continual process of drawing in, then expelling air from the lungs; the taking in of oxygen and the elimination of carbon dioxide, water, and other products of oxidation.

Applied to all living matter, respiration is the exchange of gases between an organism and its environment. A common characteristic of all living things, it is essential for the chemical changes of metabolism which must take place if life is to be maintained.

THE ORGANS OF RESPIRATION

The organs which make up the respiratory system of the human body include the *lungs* and all those parts that serve to conduct air to the lungs: the *nose*—the external organ through which air is inhaled and exhaled; it serves the purpose of warming and moistening the air and of filtering it of impurities or foreign bodies before it enters the respiratory tract; *the pharynx*—the muscular, membranous tube between the mouth and the larynx; *the larynx*—a structure of muscle and cartilage, lined with mucous membrane and located at the top of the trachea, just below the root of the tongue; the organ of voice; *the trachea*—the cylindrical, cartilaginous tube extending from the larynx to the bronchi; the windpipe; *the bronchi*—the two main branches of the trachea which extend into the lungs.

The *bronchioles* are the finer branches or subdivisions of the bronchial tree within the lungs, leading to the *alveoli*, which are the functional units of respiration, since through them the exchange of gases occurs. The *paranasal sinuses*, within the bones of the skull, are accessory structures of the respiratory tract.

MECHANICS OF RESPIRATION

Each cell in the body requires oxygen and food for maintenance of life and for normal functioning. The chemical processes of metabolism take place within the cells so food and oxygen must be supplied to all body cells. The universal waste product of metabolism, carbon dioxide, must be eliminated not only from the cells but from the body itself. This exchange of gases is provided for in man by the combined action of the respiratory and circulatory systems.

The exchange of gases between the blood and the air in the lungs is termed *external respiration*. Through external respiration oxygen is taken into the body and carbon dioxide and other wastes are given off. The exchange of gases between the blood and the tissue cells is termed *internal respiration*. Through internal respiration the oxygen which has been absorbed by the blood in the lungs and transported to the tissues is absorbed by tissue cells. Carbon dioxide, and other wastes given off by tissue cells, is transported by the blood back to the lungs, where it is eliminated from the body.

External respiration depends on changes in capacity of the chest cavity produced by contraction of muscles and movements of the ribs and sternum. When the thorax enlarges in all directions the lungs tend to follow the movements of the chest wall, and air flows into the lungs until the pressure there is the same as atmospheric pressure. This stage of respiration is termed "inspiration," or the inspiring of air into the lungs.

With relaxation of the diaphragm and the external intercostal muscles, the chest cavity is decreased in size and air is forced from the lungs until the pressure within the lungs is again equivalent to atmospheric pressure. This stage of respiration is termed "expiration," or the expulsion of air from the lungs.

THE REGULATION OF RESPIRATION

To a limited extent regulation of respiration is under voluntary control. For short periods of time respiration may be regulated so that various other activities may be carried out. In swallowing food or fluids it is necessary to exercise some control over respiration since the entrance for the respiratory tract and for the digestive tract is a common part of the throat. In speaking, singing, or laughing, respiration is subject to control and plays an important part in each of those activities. Coughing and sneezing may alter the rate and character of respiration for short periods of time.

Breath may be held voluntarily, stopping respiration for a limited period, although when the limit of time has been reached, involuntary control will bring about contraction of the chest muscles and inspiration will occur.

The respiratory center in the brain, the nerve fibers of the autonomic nervous system, and the chemical composition of the blood are factors that help to regulate respiration. The respiratory center, located in the medulla, automatically sends out motor nerve impulses to cause the contraction of the chest muscles which is necessary for respiration. Sensory impulses travel to the respiratory center through the vagus from the lungs and larynx and directly from the cerebrum. Stimulation of any sensory nerve in the body may stimulate the respiration center reflexly and alter the rate and character of respiration.

Under normal conditions the control of respiration is, in the main, involuntary in action.

Since it is possible to revive a patient who has stopped breathing, if the respiratory center is not paralyzed, by artificial respiration (alternate forcible expansion and contraction of the lungs), it is thought that sensory fibers of the vagus from the lungs and larynx regulate the rhythmic movements of respiration.

The chemical composition of the blood regulates rate and depth of respiration. Activity of the respiratory center is increased in direct relationship to increase or decrease in the amount of carbon dioxide in the blood.

If the blood contains a small amount of carbon dioxide and a greater amount of oxygen, respirations will be weak and slower in rate.

NORMAL RESPIRATION

The rate of respiration for healthy adults ranges from 16–20 per minute. The usual ratio of respiration rate and pulse rate is approximately one to four. If the pulse rate is increased, respiration rate will usually show a corresponding increase. The rhythm of normal respiration is even and regular. The rise and fall of chest and abdominal walls is uniform, so that respirations are of the same depth.

The normal rates of respiration (average, per minute), at different ages, are: at birth, 30–40; first year, 26–30; second year, 20–26; adolescence, 20; adult, 16–20; middle age, 16; old age, 14–16.

FACTORS CAUSING VARIATION IN RESPIRATION

Many factors influence the rate and character of respiration. Those most commonly observed include:

Age—in the newborn respiration is much more rapid and in the adult 16–20 per minute. In old age the rate tends to be decreased slightly.

Sex—the female tends to have a slightly more rapid rate of respiration than the male.

Rate—increased respiration rate causes the breathing to become shallow. If the respiration rate is decreased the depth of respiration becomes greater.

Exercise—muscular activity causes a temporary increase in respiration rate.

During digestion—respiration may be somewhat increased in rate during the digestion of food.

Emotion—strong emotion, such as fear, may markedly influence respiration, usually causing an increased rate.

Disease Conditions—the rate of respiration may be increased or decreased by disease, depending on the disease and its effect on the body.

Drugs—depressant drugs, such as morphine or general anesthetics, will cause respiration to become slower and deeper. Caffeine and atropine stimulate respiration, increasing the rate and causing shallow breathing. Carbon dioxide, a stimulant to the respiratory center, is often used after administration of a general anesthetic to help overcome the depressant action of the anesthetic drug.

Application of Cold—by stimulating nerve endings in the skin the breathing may be made fuller and deeper.

Application of Heat—as in hot water bath, may increase respiration temporarily and cause more shallow breathing.

Pain—severe pain or pain having an effect on vital processes tends to increase rate of respiration.

Toxins—present in the body as a result of acute infections toxins stimulate the respiratory center and cause increased respiration.

Fever—related to pulse and respiration, usually causes an increase in rate of both.

Hemorrhage—the lessened volume of blood, with subsequent decrease in oxygen content supplied to tissue cells, will cause increased respiration.

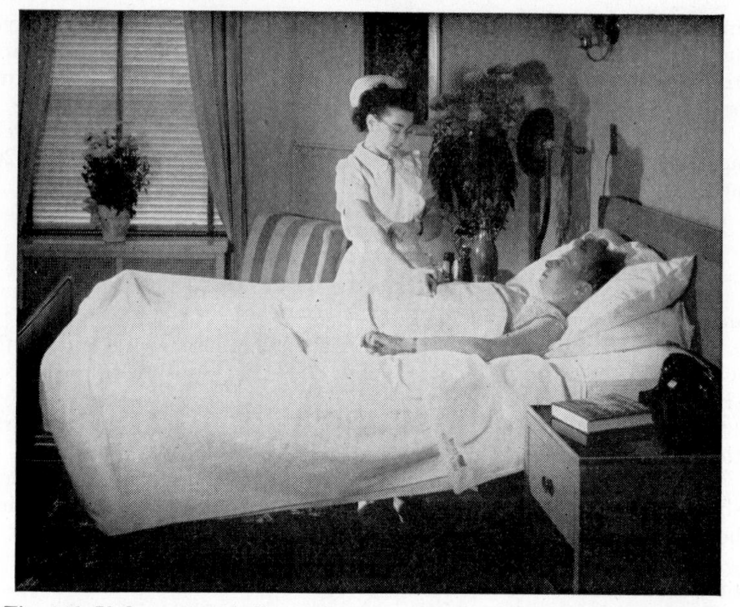

Fig. 146. If the patient believes the pulse is being counted the nurse may obtain a more accurate count of the respiration rate. (Presbyterian Hospital, Chicago, Illinois.)

Shock—with the congestion of blood in large abdominal veins, will cause increased respiration.

Change in Atmospheric Pressure—in high altitudes, as in the mountains or in an airplane, the atmospheric pressure is quite low and insufficient oxygen is available for external respiration. The respiration rate will increase in an attempt to supply more oxygen to the tissue cells. The normal amount of oxygen in the air is approximately 20 per cent, which is ample to meet the needs of the cells of the body. In high altitudes the amount of oxygen is decreased and the margin of safety, from the standpoint of body needs, is greatly reduced.

If the ascent to high altitudes is gradual, the body makes adjustments in the respiratory mechanism so that the oxygen supply remains fairly constant. In modern air travel pressurized cabins supply air with normal oxygen content for the crew and passengers in the plane.

METHOD OF COUNTING RESPIRATION

The patient should be relaxed and in a comfortable position before respirations are counted. Since respiration is, to some extent, under voluntary control, it should be counted, if possible, without awareness on the part of the patient.

In counting respiration the nurse needs to note, for one minute, the number of times the chest rises and falls.

If the patient's arm is placed across his chest and the nurse maintains finger pressure on the wrist, as in taking pulse, she may readily feel, as well as see, the movement of the chest wall. If she regulates her own respiration rate to correspond to that of the patient it will facilitate the counting of his respiration.

While counting respiration to determine rate the nurse should also be aware of the depth of respiration and other characteristics which may be of interest to the doctor and indicative of the patient's general condition.

CONDITIONS RELATED TO RESPIRATION

The rate and character of respiration is of significance in determining the patient's general condition. Other factors, too, which are related to respiration may be even more indicative of the patient's condition or of a change in condition. Conditions related to respiration include *apnea*—a temporary period of time when there is cessation of breathing; *dyspnea*—difficult or painful breathing; *hyperpnea*—increased respiration—both rate and depth may be increased; *orthopnea*—inability to breathe when in a horizontal position; *cyanosis*—blueness or discoloration of the skin and mucous membrane caused by lack of oxygen in the blood; *air hunger*—a characteristic symptom indicative of lack of sufficient oxygen for proper functioning of tissue cells.

TYPES OF RESPIRATION

Certain variations in rate and character of respiration have been given descriptive names. Some types are associated with specific disease conditions and have become characteristic symptoms or manifestations of the disease. The descriptive terms most commonly used in medical and nursing records include: *abdominal respiration*—accomplished chiefly by the muscles of the abdomen and the diaphragm; *absent respiration*—in which respiratory sounds are suppressed; *amphoric respiration*—accompanied by a sound similar to that produced by blowing over the opening of an empty jar; *cavernous respiration*—marked by a peculiar, prolonged hollow sound, usually caused by presence of a cavity in the lung; *Cheyne-Stokes respiration*—marked by variation in intensity, with successive cycles of gradually increasing depth of respiration until a stage of dyspnea is reached, then depth of respiration gradually decreasing until breathing ceases altogether for a short period; *costal respiration*—accomplished chiefly by the rib muscles; *diaphragmatic respiration*—accomplished chiefly by the diaphragm; *irregular respiration*—varying in depth and in rate of the rise and fall of the chest wall; *Kussmaul respiration*—performed with difficulty, occurring in paroxysms, and often preceding diabetic coma; *labored respiration*—performed with difficulty; *shallow respiration*—breathing only in the upper part of the lungs; *stertorous respiration*—accompanied by abnormal sounds resembling snores; *vicarious respiration*—increased activity in one lung when that in the other lung is decreased.

Care of Equipment after Use

The thermometer should be washed in soap and water and rinsed in cool water.

Individual oral thermometers used on clinical service departments should be immersed in an antiseptic solution.

The antiseptic solution should be changed every few days in the thermometer container.

Rectal thermometers should be washed and rinsed and submerged in an antiseptic solution for several hours, then returned to the rectal thermometer tray.

Summary of Important Factors

TEMPERATURE

Normal body temperature range 98.6–99° F.

Stages of fever: *onset*—period when temperature is rising; *stadium*—period when temperature remains elevated; *decline*—period when temperature returns to normal.

Types of fever: *constant*—varies less than 2 degrees, always above normal; *intermittent*—varies greatly, ranging above and below normal; *remittent*—varies greatly, remains above normal.

Methods of taking temperature: *orally*—by mouth, for 3 minutes; *axillary*—at axilla, for 10 minutes; *rectally*—by rectum, for 3–5 minutes.

Conditions when oral temperature is contraindicated: When patient is under five, uncooperative, unconscious, delirious, mentally ill, dyspneic, or has had oral surgery.

Rectal method is most accurate.

Rectal temperature 1° higher than oral; axillary temperature 1° lower than oral.

Shake mercury to below 94° F. before taking temperature.

Do not rinse thermometers in hot water.

The patient should not be told the exact reading of the thermometer, especially if his temperature is highly elevated.

PULSE

Normal range (adult) 72–80 beats per minute.

Variations: in rate, rapid—slow; in rhythm, regular—irregular; in volume, weak—full—bounding.

Pulse deficit: Difference between number of heart beats and number of pulsations counted at the wrist.

Common sites for taking pulse: radial artery—wrist; temporal artery—temple; internal carotid—beneath and to front of jaw bone.

Method: lightly compress artery with three fingers; count for one-half minute and multiply by two.

Always record pulse rate in even numbers.

RESPIRATION

Normal respiration rate (adult) 16–20 per minute.

Count respiration without patient being aware that you are doing it.

Patient should be in reclining or sitting position for temperature, pulse, and respiration, arm at rest.

Factors To Teach the Patient

TEMPERATURE

To keep lips closed on oral thermometer and to refrain from conversation while temperature is being taken.

To wait five minutes after taking hot or cold food or liquids before taking temperature orally.

Not to turn or change position suddenly while temperature is being taken rectally.

The thermometer must be left in place longer for taking axillary temperature.

Proper method of cleaning and disinfecting the thermometer.

PULSE

Muscular activity increases pulse rate.

If pulse is to be taken frequently an explanation should be made to the patient to prevent anxiety as to his condition.

RESPIRATION

Since respiration is, to some extent, under the control of the will, the patient's cooperation is necessary if respiration count is to be accurate.

Ascent to high altitudes should be made gradually so that oxygen supply will remain fairly constant.

Scientific Principles

Anatomy and Physiology. The center for heat regulation is in the hypothalamus, frontal portion of the brain.

Receptors for sensation of heat or cold are just below the surface of the skin.

Vasoconstriction and vasodilation affect loss of heat by radiation and influence moistness of the skin.

Heat elimination must be directly related to heat production or body temperature will be elevated.

Heat is produced by oxidation of food and by muscular exertion.

Heat loss occurs chiefly through the skin and lungs.

Temperature taken rectally is the most nearly accurate.

Pulse is observed in all arteries but can be readily counted in the radial, carotid, temporal, and femoral arteries.

Under normal conditions of rest the heart pumps approximately 4 liters of blood per minute.

The respiratory tract is lined with ciliary mucous membrane. The exchange of oxygen and carbon dioxide takes place in the alveoli of the lungs.

Red blood cells carry oxygen from the alveoli to the body tissues.

Internal respiration is a chemical reaction occurring within body cells; external respiration, or breathing, is a physical and mechanical process.

Inhaling and exhaling is accomplished through the action of the ribs, diaphragm, and muscles concerned with respiration.

Chemistry. Heat is produced in the body by oxidation of food.

Internal respiration is a chemical process whereby gases are exchanged.

Most biochemical reactions are brought about by the action of enzymes which are sensitive to temperature changes.

Force and rate of heart beat are determined by the presence of calcium, sodium, and potassium ions in the blood.

Inspired air contains about 78 per cent of nitrogen. In certain respiratory conditions fatigue and dyspnea may be relieved by giving the patient helium and oxygen with a molecular weight much less than that of nitrogen.

Microbiology. Moderate fever hastens destruction of bacteria by increasing phagocytosis.

The nurse will need to protect herself when caring for patients with diseases of the respiratory tract.

Increase in pulse and respiration rates may be caused by disease organisms in the blood stream.

Thermometers should be kept thoroughly clean by use of disinfectant solutions; 70 per cent alcohol or bichloride of mercury 1:1000 is usually used for this purpose. Solutions in these strengths are able to penetrate organic matter and destroy bacteria.

Pharmacology. Drug stimulants increase the pulse rate; drug depressants decrease the pulse rate.

The usual flow of oxygen for an adult patient varies from 6 to 14 liters per minute. Drugs used to increase body temperature are called pyretics; those used to decrease body temperature are termed antipyretics.

By preventing or inhibiting the action of bacteria, antibiotic drugs tend to lower body temperature.

The action of the respiratory system may be stimulated or depressed by drugs.

Physics. The clinical thermometer is so shaped that the front acts as a lens to magnify the fine bore in which mercury rises when expanded by heat from the body of the patient.

Radiation is the transfer of heat from the body to another object without any change in the temperature of the air. Loss of heat from the body by radiation constitutes 60–65 per cent of the total loss of heat.

The diffusion of oxygen into the blood stream and the diffusion of carbon dioxide from the blood stream into alveoli depend on a difference in pressure of these gases. When respirators are used the chest wall expands as air pressure in the chamber is reduced; when normal air pressure is restored in the respirator, air in the lungs is forced out by natural elasticity of the chest walls.

Psychology. The patient should be calm before pulse is taken.

The findings on temperature, pulse, respiration, and blood pressure are usually not told to the patient.

For taking rectal temperature the patient should be screened and properly draped to avoid embarrassment.

Many respiratory diseases require that the patient be isolated and guarded against loneliness since visitors to isolated patients are restricted.

Sociology. Oxygen may be supplied to patients at home, if necessary, through the home service departments of oxygen supply companies, who will arrange to meet requests for home service made by the attending physician.

Visiting restrictions for the isolated patient should be carefully explained to his family and friends.

The public health nurse may be required to take temperature, pulse, respiration, and blood pressure as part of her routine nursing duties.

Situation Type Problem

1. A preclinical student nurse was asked to chart temperature, pulse, and respiration for a graduate nurse who had taken and recorded in a notebook T.P.R. for all patients on the department. In charting for one particular patient the student noticed that the pulse rate recorded in the notebook was much faster than that recorded on the graphic sheet for the past several days. She mentioned the great difference in rates to the head nurse, who asked her to check the patient's pulse rate by counting it at that time. The patient asked why she was counting her pulse and not those of the other three patients in the

room. The student told her that she was checking to see if she got the same count as that obtained by Miss Smith, the graduate nurse. The patient said, "Miss Smith didn't count my pulse, she only took my temperature. In fact, she hasn't counted my pulse for the past week when she has taken temperature." What would you have done?

Suggested Reference Reading

"Postural changes in respiration," E. B. Franseen and F. A. Hellebrandt; American Journal of Physiology, January, 1943.

"Basal pressure and pulse rate in adolescents," N. W. Shock; American Journal of Diseases of Children, July, 1944.

"Effect of emotions on patients' temperature," L. Slatin; Modern Hospital, September, 1944.

"Changes in oral temperature," K. Brim and B. A. Chandler; American Journal of Nursing, December, 1948.

"It must be the heat," James A. Brussel; Hygeia, July, 1949.

"Control of body temperature," Modern Hospital, February, 1950.

"Disinfecting mouth thermometers," American Journal of Nursing, October, 1952.

"Water mattress and elevated temperatures," Frances Gibson; American Journal of Nursing, May, 1953.

CHAPTER 22

Blood Pressure

TOPICAL OUTLINE

DEFINITION OF TERMS
ARTERIAL AND VENOUS BLOOD PRESSURE
NORMAL BLOOD PRESSURE
FACTORS CAUSING VARIATION IN BLOOD PRESSURE
APPARATUS USED IN TAKING BLOOD PRESSURE
METHOD OF TAKING BLOOD PRESSURE

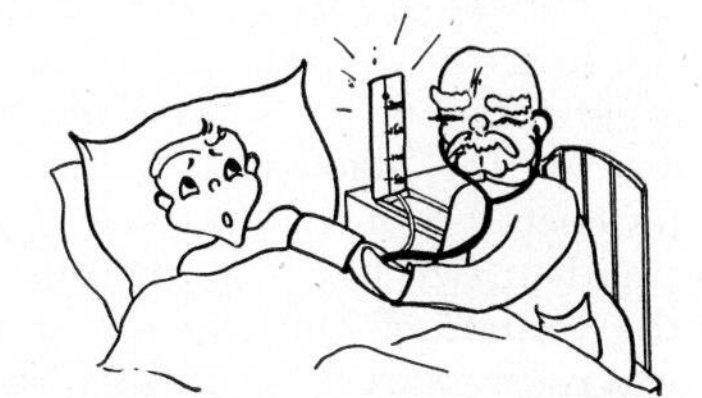

"Your blood pressure is normal, but for these times that's not so good!"

The circulatory system, made up of heart, arteries, veins, and capillaries, is a closed system or passageway for the circulation of blood throughout the body. Because the system is closed, blood flows through it under pressure.

DEFINITION OF TERMS

Blood pressure is "the force exerted by the blood against the walls of the blood vessels as it flows through them."

Systolic pressure is the highest degree of pressure exerted by the blood against the artery walls as the left ventricle contracts and forces the blood from it into the aorta.

Diastolic pressure is the lowest degree of pressure, or the point of lessened pressure when the heart is in its resting period just before contraction of the left ventricle.

Pulse pressure is the difference between systolic and diastolic pressure, and represents volume output of the left ventricle. Pulse pressure is indicative of the tone of the arterial walls and is important in diagnosis and treatment.

Hypertension is a condition of abnormally high blood pressure; *hypotension* is a condition of abnormally low blood pressure. Blood pressure will vary at different times during the day; since blood pressure readings are usually taken for the purpose of comparison with previous readings they should be taken at the same time each day.

ARTERIAL AND VENOUS BLOOD PRESSURE

Under normal conditions the degree of pressure is determined by the force of the contraction of the heart and the elasticity of the artery walls. The large arteries with elastic, muscular walls exert pressure and resistance to the blood flowing through them.

The blood circulates through the body with different degrees of pressure in different parts of the circulatory system. The blood leaves the heart at the left ventricle and is sent into the large arteries with great force. In these arteries the pressure is highest. From the large arteries the blood is sent into smaller arteries, where the pressure is lessened. From small arteries blood flows into arterioles which are very small in size but so numerous that there is ample accommodation for the volume of blood. From arterioles blood flows into the capillaries, where pressure is so greatly reduced that the blood flows in a steady, constant stream and the force of the heart beat is imperceptible.

Returning to the heart by way of the veins the pressure is still diminished since the veins are large vessels and pressure is lower because of ample room provided for the return flow.

Because of the differing blood pressure in the circulatory system, blood may be lost in a characteristic manner, depending on the kind of blood vessel cut or injured. If a large artery is cut blood will spurt out in jerks and with great force. If a small artery is cut the blood may still spurt out, but with much less force. From a severed capillary blood will slowly ooze out from the tissues, and from a vein blood will flow in a steady, continuous stream.

In addition to force of the heart beat and elasticity of the vessel walls, several other factors influence blood pressure to some extent, including the amount of peripheral resistance, the quantity of blood in the circulatory system, and the viscosity of the blood.

The pressure of the blood within the vessels may be determined in a number of accessible parts, but is usually measured at the inner bend of the arm, where the brachial artery nears the surface.

NORMAL BLOOD PRESSURE

Blood pressure readings are recorded as a definite number of millimeters of mercury (mm. Hg). A manometer is used to measure blood pressure. It is a device which bears a graduated scale beside a hollow tube in which a column of mercury can ascend to a certain height according to the pressure exerted against the vessel wall. Readings are taken at the point where the mercury stands at certain designated periods during the heart beat cycle. The average blood pressure for the healthy adult is usually about 120/80 (systolic pressure 120 mm. Hg and diastolic pressure 80 mm. Hg, with pulse pressure—the difference between them—40 mm. Hg). Normal blood pressure may gradually increase with age until at age 60 it may be approximately 140/90.

Normal venous pressure may range from 40 to 110 mm. of water.

FACTORS CAUSING VARIATION IN BLOOD PRESSURE

Factors which cause variation in blood pressure and which must be taken into consideration in determining whether blood pressure is normal or abnormal include:

Age—blood pressure is much lower in children than in adults. The young adult will have a blood pressure of approximately 120/80; in an older adult a blood pressure of 140/90 may be considered "normal."

Sex—the average blood pressure for men is slightly higher than that for women of a comparable age, although the difference is not considered significant.

Body build—the individual who tends to be obese will probably show higher than average blood pressure.

Exercise—muscular exertion will increase blood pressure, although the return to normal will occur very shortly after exercise is discontinued.

Pain—severe pain may cause a temporary and marked increase in blood pressure.

Emotion—fear, worry, excitement, and other emotions will cause blood pressure to rise sharply. The nurse should relieve emotional strain for the patient before attempting to take blood pressure. A reading taken at the time the patient is emotionally disturbed will be inaccurate.

Disease—diseases affecting the circulatory system, as sclerosis, those producing bacterial toxins, and disease affecting the kidneys may increase blood pressure. Diseases that weaken the heart action may lower blood pressure.

Hemorrhage—by decreasing the volume of blood in the vessels, hemorrhage causes lowered blood pressure. When internal hemorrhage is suspected the doctor may order blood pressure to be taken every few minutes, as a change in blood pressure may be the first definite indication of such hemorrhage.

Intracranial pressure—brain injuries or surgical treatment involving the brain indicate need for frequent taking of blood pressure. Pressure within the cranium will usually produce a rise in blood pressure.

Shock—lowered blood pressure is a characteristic symptom of shock and indicates the need for emergency treatment if the patient's life is to be saved.

APPARATUS USED IN TAKING BLOOD PRESSURE

In measuring arterial blood pressure, usually implied by the term "blood pressure," the sphygmomanometer and stethoscope are used. The manometer may have a dial, on which blood pressure is indicated by a pointer attached to a spring mechanism, or a graduated scale on which the height of a column of mercury is indicated.

For measuring venous pressure a water manometer is used. To

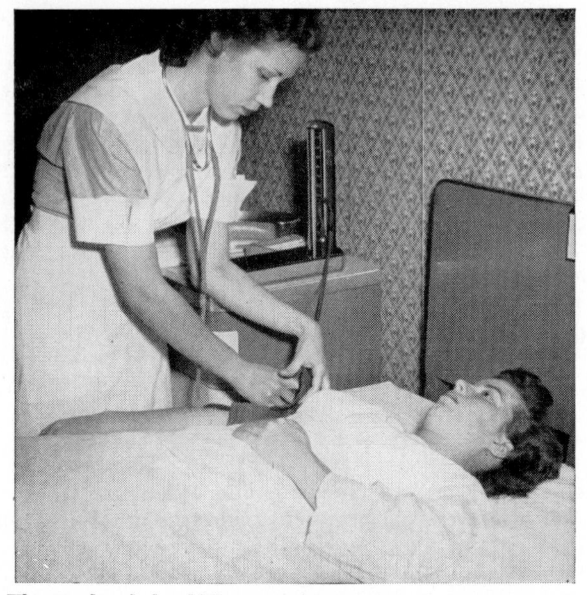

Fig. 147. The armband should be wound around the arm as a circular bandage would be applied. (Baylor University School of Nursing, Waco, Texas.)

measure such pressure directly, a needle connected with the manometer is inserted into a vein. Pressure within the vein causes the blood to rise in a connecting tube. Venous pressure is much lower than arterial pressure and cannot be accurately measured with a mercury manometer. Mercury is a heavy liquid and venous pressure may not be sufficient to make notable changes in the level of a column of mercury.

METHOD OF TAKING BLOOD PRESSURE

Before attempting to take blood pressure the nurse should explain the procedure to the patient. If he is assured that the examination is relatively simple, and not at all painful, he will be less apt to become nervous or to show concern, either of which reactions may cause the blood pressure to rise. For the patient who has not had a previous experience of having blood pressure taken it may be necessary to repeat the procedure to get an accurate reading.

The left arm should be used for taking blood pressure unless for some reason this is contraindicated. Although there is usually little difference in the blood pressure readings in the two arms, the left is used in almost all instances for uniformity and for an accurate comparison of different readings.

The patient should be reclining or sitting, with the left arm relaxed

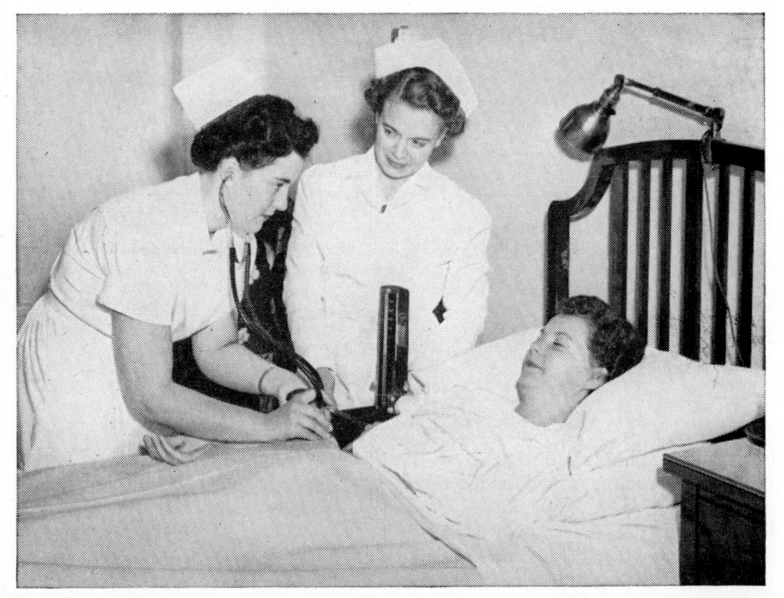

Fig. 148. Skill in the taking of blood pressure comes with practice. (Reading Hospital School of Nursing, Reading, Pennsylvania.)

and supported on the bed or a low table. He should be instructed not to close the hand into a tight fist or bear his weight on the left arm during the procedure.

The sphygmomanometer should be placed on a nearby table so that the measuring scale is turned away from the patient's line of vision. The box type device should be placed so the scale is at eye level for the person taking the reading. If the aneroid or spring type manometer is used the dial should be attached to the cuff by the hooks provided for that purpose.

The soft cuff is generally used and consists of a compression bag and cloth armband. The compression bag should be placed over the brachial artery on the inner surface of the upper arm at a level with the heart, and the armband wound around the arm as a circular bandage would be applied. The band, if wound too tightly, will bind the arm and be uncomfortable for the patient. If wound too loosely the sounds will be deadened by the cushion of air required to tighten the band sufficiently to compress the brachial artery.

The rubber tubes attached to the compression bag should not be crossed or allowed to come in contact with each other, as the sounds produced will interfere with sounds which determine the blood pressure reading.

Before inflating the cuff the pulsation of the brachial artery should

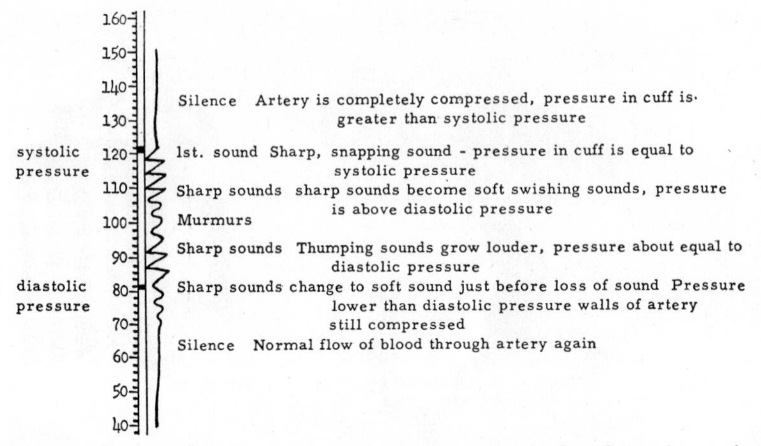

Fig. 149. Graphic illustration showing change of sounds that determines point at which reading is made when taking blood pressure: this reading, 122/82.

be felt lightly with three fingers to determine the point where the pulsation is strongest. The end of the stethoscope should be placed at this point, directly above the artery.

With the stethoscope in position, the cuff is inflated by means of the rubber bulb. The cuff should be inflated until the pulsation of the artery, originally heard clearly through the stethoscope, is no longer audible. Then air should be allowed to escape very gradually from the cuff, until once more the sound is heard. At this point on the manometer where the sound is first heard as the cuff is being slowly deflated the systolic reading should be taken.

The cuff should then be further deflated, with close attention to the change in sounds occurring as the air is gradually released from the confining armband. The first sound heard becomes a definite loud thumping, which changes to a soft thumping sound. Then once again the sounds become sharper in intensity then change to a muffled, soft thumping and gradually disappear entirely. At the point where the sharp thumping sound changes to a softer sound just prior to becoming inaudible, the diastolic reading should be taken. As soon as both readings have been made the air should be entirely released from the cuff and the cuff should be removed from the patient's arm.

Students who are just learning the procedure of taking blood pressure should practice it for a number of times on a healthy person (another student nurse) so they become adept at handling the apparatus, at winding the cuff, and at taking an accurate reading of blood pressure, before they attempt to do the procedure for patients in the hospital. A student who is unsure of her findings should ask a nurse more experienced in the procedure to check the reading and thus determine its accuracy.

Figure 149 should be helpful to the beginner who must learn to recognize the change in sounds which are important in determining blood pressure readings.

Care of Equipment after Use

The Sphygmomanometer. When removed from the patient's arm, all air should be released from the cuff, which should be folded and replaced in the box. The box containing the device should be returned to its usual storage place.

The Stethoscope. A cotton pledget saturated with alcohol should be used to sponge off the ear pieces and the bell of the stethoscope. The instrument should then be returned to its usual storage place.

Summary of Important Factors

Blood pressure is the force exerted against the vessel walls by the blood.

Systolic pressure is the highest degree of blood pressure; diastolic pressure is the lowest degree of blood pressure. Pulse pressure is the difference between systolic and diastolic pressures.

Normal blood pressure is approximately 120/80 mm. Hg. As age increases blood pressure becomes higher.

In shock and hemorrhage blood pressure will be lowered. Exercise, emotion, and some diseases increase blood pressure.

The left arm should be used, when possible, for taking blood pressure.

The systolic reading should be taken when the sound first becomes audible as the cuff is deflated. The diastolic reading is taken when the sound changes from sharp to soft just before it disappears.

Factors To Teach the Patient

That the taking of blood pressure is not painful and need not be feared.

If blood pressure is to be taken a second time for accuracy it need not indicate that the pressure may be abnormal.

If the doctor thinks the patient should know what his blood pressure is, he will tell him, so there should be no need to question the nurse in regard to the matter.

Scientific Principles

Anatomy and Physiology. Pressure of the blood in the arteries depends on the force of the contraction of the left ventricle, the amount of blood forced into the aorta, and the resistance offered by the smaller vessels. The force and rate of the heart beat influence the arterial pressure.

An increased volume of blood, as in transfusion, increases blood pressure. A decreased volume of blood, as in hemorrhage, decreases blood pressure.

The term "blood pressure" refers to arterial pressure usually.

Blood pressure is affected by emotion, exercise, age, pain, and conditions of hemorrhage or shock.

Chemistry. Mercury is used in the sphygmomanometer because it reacts quickly to slight variations of pressure. Mercury is 13.5 times as heavy as water.

Microbiology. Toxins from bacteria may constrict blood vessels and cause increased blood pressure.

The sphygmomanometer and stethoscope should be kept clean at all times. The sphygmomanometer and stethoscope used in taking blood pressure for a patient in isolation require special care.

Pharmacology. Vasodilators are used to decrease blood pressure; vasoconstrictors are used to increase blood pressure.

Carbon dioxide stimulates the respiratory center by increasing the hydrogen ion concentration of the cells in that center.

Sedatives may lower blood pressure by relaxing the muscles.

Physics. Transmission of sound through a stethoscope is possible because sound waves pass through glass, liquids, and solids.

Gravity affects blood pressure; pressure in arteries below the heart are greater when the person is in a standing position.

The instrument used in taking blood pressure accurately measures pressure within the blood vessels, the pressure being transmitted to a column of mercury on which its effect can be measured.

Psychology. Many patients are fearful of having blood pressure taken for the first time. Their emotional reaction to the procedure may increase the pressure so that an accurate reading cannot be obtained. An explanation of the procedure with demonstration will reassure the patient, and an accurate reading may be obtained when the procedure is done the second time.

Sociology. Heredity may be a factor in the cause of high blood pressure.

Patients being cared for in their own homes may have blood pressure taken by a nurse from the Visiting Nurse Association.

Situation Type Problem

1. A preclinical student nurse was asked to take blood pressure for a patient who had just been returned to the clinical service department from the postoperative recovery room. The student had had a difficult time in practicing the procedure in the classroom a few days before and felt that she was not really qualified to do the procedure ac-

curately. She expressed her doubts to the head nurse, who told her that the only way she could learn was to do it.

After taking the blood pressure reading the student still felt unsure about it and asked a senior student to check it for her. The senior student was called away to assist with a surgical dressing for another patient. A young intern came in to see the patient whose blood pressure had just been taken and the student asked him to check the reading of the blood pressure. The intern took the patient's blood pressure and his reading was the same as that obtained by the student a short time before.

After the intern had left the room the patient asked why her blood pressure was being taken so many times. The student was reluctant about admitting that she felt unsure of her ability to do the procedure accurately so explained to the patient that it was regular practice for the blood pressure to be taken by several different persons. The patient had been in the hospital a number of times and knew that it was not "regular practice." She became unduly alarmed about her physical condition and asked to see the head nurse. The head nurse was delayed for several minutes, so that by the time she did appear the patient was emotionally upset. The head nurse tried to explain that there was no cause for alarm and, when the patient asked that her doctor be called, tactfully suggested that he would be in before long to make his routine daily call.

As soon as the head nurse left the room the patient asked the student nurse to telephone the doctor and ask him to come to the hospital right away. What would you have done?

Suggested Reference Reading

"Technic of taking blood pressure," Veronica F. Murray; American Journal of Nursing, November, 1934.

"Nursing the patient with sympathectomy for hypertension," T. Feddar; American Journal of Nursing, October, 1948.

"The personality of high blood pressure," Grey Collins; Your Health, Spring Quarter, 1949.

"Blood pressure," Jennie Q. Adatto; Hygeia, July, 1949.

"Hypertension, arteriosclerosis and diet," Andrew W. Contratto; American Journal of Nursing, October, 1952.

CHAPTER 23

Dismissal of the Patient

TOPICAL OUTLINE

ORDER FOR DISMISSAL
NOTIFICATION OF PATIENT DISMISSAL
ATTENTION TO PATIENT'S PERSONAL PROPERTY
INSTRUCTIONS REGARDING SUBSEQUENT CARE
THE PATIENT'S DEPARTURE
CARE OF THE HOSPITAL RECORD
TRANSFER OF THE PATIENT

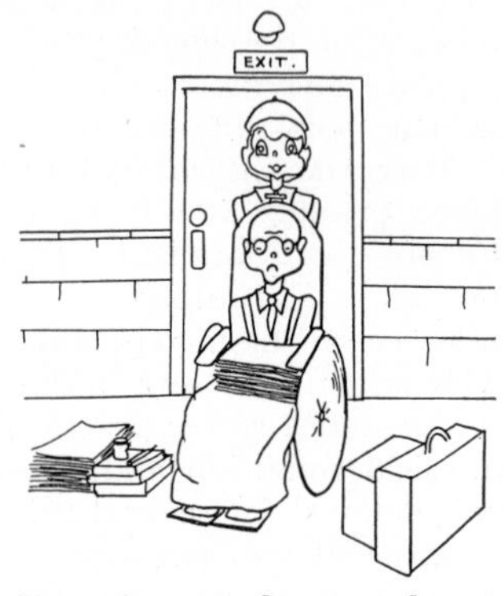

If you're too busy to laugh, you're too busy!

The experience of hospitalization, whether for a brief or prolonged period, is one that makes a lasting impression on the patient. Just as the events and procedures involving admission remain vividly in the mind, so will various factors pertaining to dismissal be important in the patient's remembrance of the total experience. If admission and dismissal are accomplished without misunderstanding or mishap, small inconveniences he may have encountered while in the hospital will soon be forgotten. Unpleasantness or disagreeable experiences related to dismissal will remain in the patient's mind and bear marked influence upon his reaction to need for hospitalization in the future and to remarks he will make to family, friends, and acquaintances about the hospital and the service it renders to the community.

The nurse should exercise the same care and understanding in establishment of good public relations for the procedure of dismissal that she employs in helping establish good relations with the patient during the admission procedure. Attention given the patient on the day of departure should be as considerate and as extensive as that accorded him on admission and during the period of his stay in the hospital.

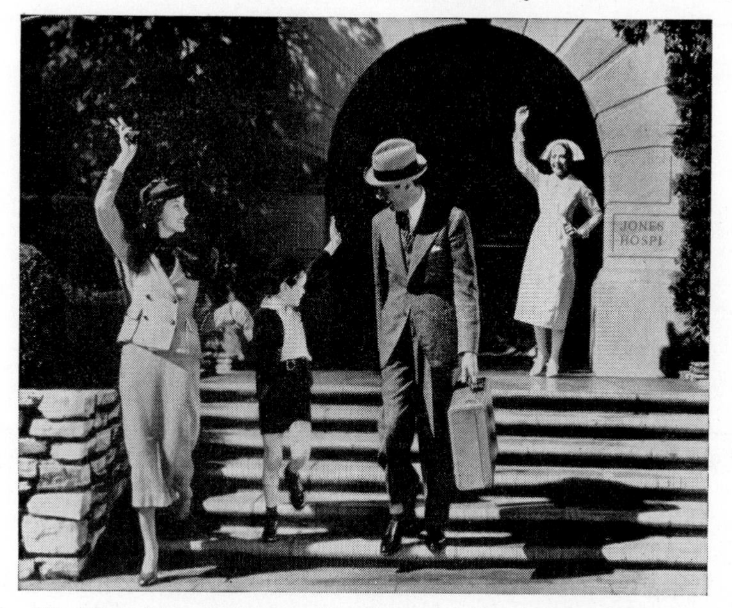

Fig. 150. When Johnny goes marching home, he leaves new friends behind in the hospital. (Parke, Davis & Co., Detroit, Michigan.)

ORDER FOR DISMISSAL

Because of legal implications involved in the dismissal of a patient from the hospital, the attending physician is required to give a written order for dismissal and to sign the patient's chart or hospital record. By writing the order for dismissal the doctor assumes full responsibility for continued improvement and well-being of the patient outside the hospital. If the doctor is not satisfied that the patient is able to leave the hospital, he may insure continued hospitalization by failing to write the dismissal order.

If a patient decides to leave the hospital against the advice of his doctor and without a written order for dismissal he must do so at his own risk. In such cases the hospital will require that the patient sign a "Release" form. Such a form (Fig. 151) states that the patient is leaving against the advice of the doctor in charge of the case and that neither the doctor or the hospital can be held responsible for any ill effect which may result to the patient because he is no longer receiving treatment.

The nurse is expected to assume the responsibility of obtaining the patient's signature on the release form if he is leaving the hospital without a written order of dismissal from the doctor.

RELEASE FORM

Discharge against advice Date____________

I, the undersigned, hereby leave the____________

hospital against the advice of Dr.____________. I release

the hospital and the doctor from all further responsibility.

Signed____________

Witness____________

Fig. 151. Typical release form to be signed by patient on leaving hospital against physician's advice.

NOTIFICATION OF PATIENT DISMISSAL

When the doctor has written the order for a patient's dismissal the nurse will need to institute plans so that the dismissal will be accomplished at the date and time designated by the physician.

Several days may be needed to complete arrangements for dismissal for some patients, and for that reason orders are usually written in advance of the actual date dismissal is to occur.

The family of the patient will need to be notified so arrangements can be made for caring for the patient at home. It is necessary for them to arrange for a member of the family to accompany the patient from the hospital.

The financial office at the hospital will need to be notified so the statement of expenses may be complete and ready for the patient at the time of dismissal. If the hospital bill is not paid in full at the time of dismissal, arrangements should be made by the patient or a member of his family for subsequent payments.

The clothes room will need to be notified so clothing that has been stored for the patient can be checked and returned to him on the dismissal date.

If the patient is on a special diet or needs to be instructed in regard to diet, the dietitian will need to be notified of his dismissal. Diets may be planned for use by the patient while he is being cared for at home.

If the patient or a member of his family must be taught certain procedures necessary for continued treatment and care after dismissal the nurse is responsible for teaching the procedure to the person who will be asked to do it as a part of the home care given the patient.

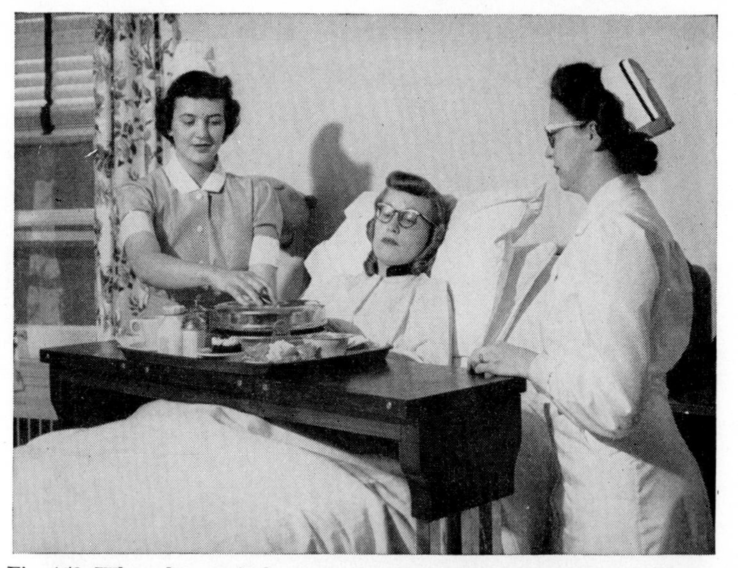

Fig. 152. When the surgical patient is given a general diet she is usually sufficiently recovered to ask about being dismissed. (St. Luke's Hospital School of Nursing, Denver, Colorado.)

The drug room should be notified and orders for medication which is to be taken home by the patient should be placed so that on the day of dismissal the medication is available. All drugs sent home with patients should be clearly labeled, with specific directions as to correct dosage, and frequency and method of administration. If unusual symptoms or undesirable reactions may result from use of the drug, the patient or a responsible member of his family should be warned and given instruction on remedial measures that might be required. If the drug is to be used over a long period of time, the pharmacist should tell the patient where and how to obtain additional quantities of it.

The social service department should be notified if its services may be required, as when a patient will be unable to return to his former type of employment or to lead a normally active life.

The admissions clerk will need to be notified as to exact date and probable time of dismissal, so she will know when the room may be available for another patient.

The receiving desk will need to be notified of the patient's dismissal and his home address should be left, so that mail received for him after dismissal may be forwarded to his home.

If the patient has been receiving the daily newspaper, notice should be sent to the dealer or newsboy so that its delivery can be discontinued.

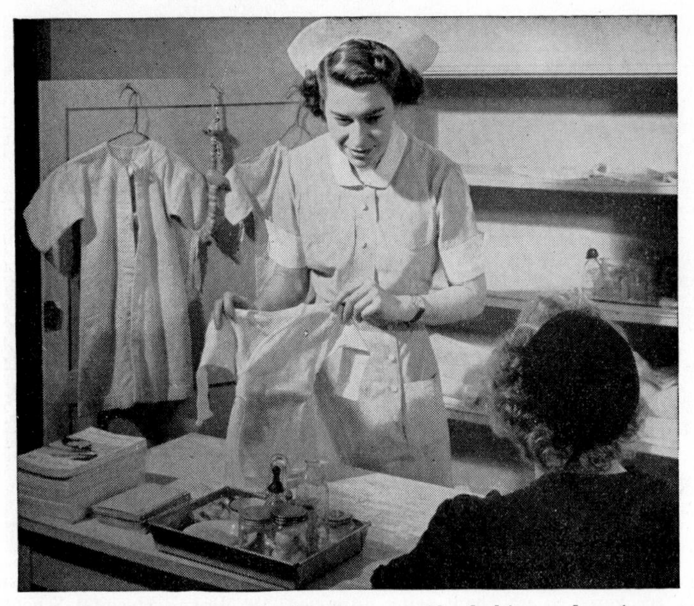

Fig. 153. It is necessary for the family to provide clothing and equipment that will be needed for home care of the patient at time of dismissal. (Johns Hopkins Hospital School of Nursing, Baltimore, Maryland.)

ATTENTION TO PATIENT'S PERSONAL PROPERTY

The care and attention given to personal possessions of the patient are important in the procedure of dismissal.

Clothing and valuables that have been sent from the patient's unit for proper care and safe keeping will need to be returned on the date of dismissal. If the patient has been hospitalized for a long period of time it may be necessary for the family to bring different clothes, suitable to the weather, for him to wear when leaving the hospital. A heavy suit or overcoat worn to the hospital in January would be most inappropriate for the patient leaving the institution in July, and lightweight articles of summer clothing would be inadequate for the patient dismissed from the hospital during a heavy snowstorm. Since the nurse in charge of the patient knows of his dismissal several days in advance of the actual date of departure, she has ample time to see that clothing he will wear is suitable, clean, and in good condition.

On the date of dismissal the list of clothing made at the time of admission should be carefully checked, and the patient should sign that all articles of clothing are accounted for and being taken with him from the hospital.

Money and other valuables, such as jewelry, should be returned to the patient, and again he should sign the form on which they have been listed, indicating that they are once more in his possession.

Several hours before time for the patient to leave the nurse should pack or help him pack all the belongings that may have accumulated during his stay in the hospital. She should ascertain his wishes in regard to the disposal of magazines, newspapers, cut flowers, plants, and other articles which he may have acquired and may not wish to take away with him. Many patients at the time of departure will gratefully accept the suggestion of the nurse that magazines, plants, and similar belongings be given to patients remaining in the department.

Shortly before time for the patient to leave the nurse should carefully check the clothes closet, dresser, and bedside table, and make sure that all personal belongings, such as radio, clock, electric fan, or other appliances, are packed and ready to be taken with the patient.

Since patients often return to the hospital after dismissal to inquire about personal belongings they failed to take with them on leaving, hospital administrators have sought various means of emphasizing to personnel the importance of careful handling of property belonging to patients. In one institution the nurse responsible for the dismissal of a patient is held responsible if belongings of the patient are overlooked at the time of departure. All items of wearing apparel and articles belonging to the patient which are inadvertently left behind when the patient is dismissed must be taken or sent to him by the nurse at her own expense. Nurses at that hospital, recognizing that their carelessness may inconvenience the patient, are willing to accept the responsibility of delivering to him any article left behind at the time of his dismissal.

INSTRUCTIONS REGARDING SUBSEQUENT CARE

The head nurse in charge of the department from which a patient is dismissed is responsible for giving instructions to the patient, or to a member of his family, about further care and treatment which may be required.

If diet has been an important factor in treatment, the dietitian will need to confer with the patient and his family. Special diets may be planned for a period of time in the future, and the dietitian will wish to be sure that the patient understands the kind of diet he is to have and why he must adhere to it if he wishes to regain health and return to normal activities. It may be necessary to teach the diabetic patient how to weigh his food and how to plan the diet so it includes the proper percentage of each of the foodstuffs.

Before the day of dismissal the doctor will confer with the patient and leave definite orders in regard to treatment, medication, and care after he has left the hospital. Since the nurse will need to interpret and explain in detail all such orders, she should be present at the conference between doctor and patient. She should write out all instruc-

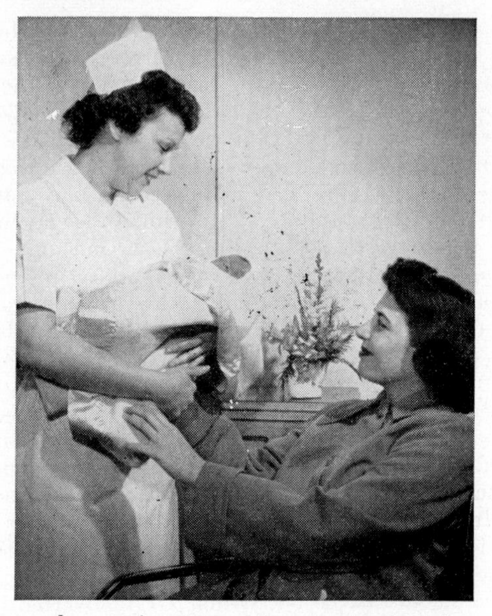

Fig. 154. The mother receives instructions to take the baby at regular intervals to the pediatrician for check-up. (Mercy Hospital School of Nursing, Des Moines, Iowa.)

tions which the patient is to follow and should carefully explain each one. In writing instructions for the patient, she should avoid medical terminology which may not be meaningful to the patient. If an order pertaining to medicine should read "Give drams 2 H.S." she would explain to the patient and rewrite the directions to read "Give 2 teaspoonfuls at bedtime."

If dressings or special supplies will be needed at home, the nurse should arrange for the patient to take a supply with him from the hospital or should tell him where the needed articles can be purchased.

She should remind him of the date, time, and place he is to see the doctor again, and should emphasize the importance of keeping any appointment for a check-up.

She should include in the instructions the doctor's suggestion in regard to rest periods during the day and to limited activity during waking hours. She should caution the patient against returning to work too soon and, if necessary, should refer him to the social service department or local rehabilitation office for help in planning for the future.

When instructions are given to the patient, plans for "follow-up" should also be made, with a definite appointment for his return to

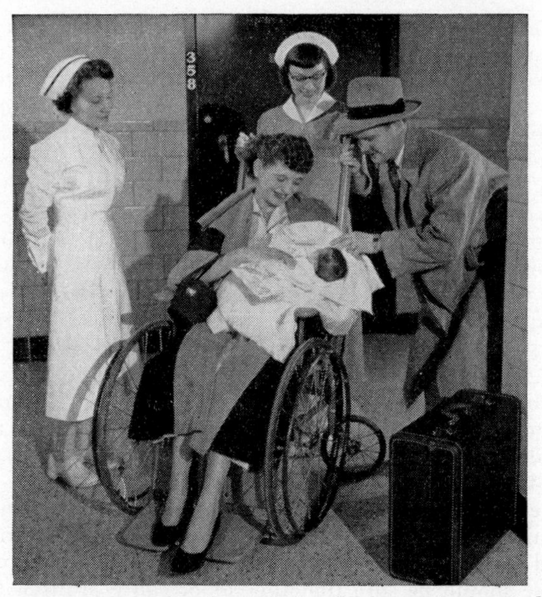

Fig. 155. Persons accompanying the patient as he leaves the hospital are usually members of his family. (Wesley Hospital School of Nursing, Wichita, Kansas.)

the out-patient department or to his own physician's office. Appointments for such follow-up visits should be made in writing, to avoid misunderstandings.

THE PATIENT'S DEPARTURE

Details of the actual departure of the patient from the hospital should be arranged several hours before the time set for dismissal so haste will not be necessary. Most patients feel some apprehension and excitement over departure and are thus more readily fatigued by the physical exertion of being dressed and of making the trip from the hospital to their home. In making arrangements for dismissal, factors to be considered will include time of dismissal, who is to accompany the patient, and mode of transportation.

The time of dismissal should be set so that it meets with hospital regulations, in regard to giving up the room or unit which he has occupied. Dismissal time should also be convenient for the patient, his family, and especially the person who will accompany him from the hospital. The person accompanying the patient, usually a member of the family, must be someone who is capable of looking after him, should need arise, during the trip from the hospital to the home.

Mode of transportation will depend on the condition of the patient, the distance he will need to travel, and the transportation facilities which are available. In a city, if the distance is relatively short and the patient is able to sit up without strain or fatigue, a taxicab or the family car may be the most suitable means of transportation. Patients who must remain in a horizontal position should be moved by ambulance. Whatever mode of transportation is decided on, arrangements should be made well in advance, so the patient does not worry or feel uncertainty as to proper dismissal procedure.

The nurse responsible for dismissing a patient should understand the mixed emotions which the patient will experience. He will derive satisfaction from having recovered sufficiently to be permitted to leave the hospital; he will be pleased at the thought of returning to his family; he will be greatly appreciative to hospital personnel who contributed to his care; and he will, at the same time, be somewhat reluctant to assume responsibilities which he had relinquished on admission to the institution. He may be greatly concerned about the effect on his physical condition which leaving the hospital may have, and for that reason he may seem reluctant to depart.

The patient will need to be reassured again and again, and he will overcome his misgivings if he is given reassurance by the nurse who has assisted in caring for him and in whom he has great confidence.

The nurse should be sure that the car or cab is waiting to receive the patient, then she should accompany him to the appropriate hospital exit. The patient should be taken to the exit in a wheelchair. Even if he is ambulatory, the wheelchair should be provided. Then if there is unexpected delay in his departure, the patient will not be unduly fatigued by being forced to stand for a prolonged period.

If the patient is being moved by ambulance, the stretcher will be brought to the hospital room. The nurse should accompany the patient to the hospital exit where the ambulance is waiting to receive him.

CARE OF THE HOSPITAL RECORD

After the patient has been dismissed and that procedure correctly recorded, the chart should be completed and made ready for permanent filing. Charts for patients are kept on file in the hospital and provide an accurate medical history should the patient be readmitted to the hospital later. Many hospitals keep the charts permanently; others may keep them for 25 or 30 years.

The nurse who dismissed the patient is responsible for checking the chart to see that it is complete. All chart headings should be accurately filled out, graphic sheets should be complete and up to date, and the final procedure, that of dismissal, must be accurately recorded. Hospitals vary in the arrangement of the contents of the chart for permanent filing, but instructions will be available so that the nurse can ascertain the correct order of the chart if she is not already familiar with it.

If the routine of dismissal requires that discharge slips be completed and sent to various departments in the hospital, the nurse will need to attend to that matter.

The completed chart should be taken to the record room, where it will be properly labeled and filed for future reference.

Transfer of the Patient

Because hospitals are sometimes unable to place patients immediately in the type of accommodations they prefer, it is often necessary to admit a patient to one room and later transfer him to another. At the time of transfer a procedure similar to that of dismissal is followed. The admitting office, financial office, receiving desk, diet kitchen, drug room, and nursing office should be notified that the transfer is being made.

If the patient is to be transferred to a different department, that department should be notified in advance so the room to which he is assigned will be ready to receive him.

Clothes and other belongings should be carefully checked and a record kept so that at the time of dismissal there will be no question as to whereabouts of articles of clothing.

The patient's chart should be complete and up to date, and all treatment and medicine cards should be sent with the chart to the nurse in charge of the department receiving the patient.

The patient, with his immediate belongings or personal possessions, should be transferred by stretcher or wheelchair, depending on his condition. He should be introduced to the head nurse of the department to which he is being sent, and she should see that the medical staff, the person in charge of visitors permits, and all departments concerned with treatment and care of the patient are notified as to the change in room number for the patient.

Summary of Important Factors

The patient is experiencing a certain amount of emotional stress, since he is pleased and excited at going home yet may be fearful and anxious about being removed from security and safety as represented by the hospital.

All arrangements should be made well in advance of actual departure time.

The doctor must write and sign the order for dismissal.

The nurse is responsible for correct interpretation of doctor's orders in instructing patient or family in regard to care after dismissal.

Clothes and valuables should be carefully checked at the time of dismissal and a signed receipt obtained from the patient.

Plans for "follow-up" should be made at the time instructions are being given the patient in regard to subsequent care.

A patient leaving the hospital without an order of dismissal from the doctor should sign a "Release" form.

The patient should be accompanied to the proper exit by a nurse who leaves him in the care of a responsible relative or friend.

Mode of transportation from the hospital should be determined by the patient's physical condition, distance he must travel, and facilities available.

The nurse who carries out the dismissal procedure should correctly record that procedure and properly care for the hospital record.

Transfer of a patient is a procedure very similar to the dismissal procedure. Care should be taken that all personal belongings and all hospital records pertaining to the patient are transferred with him.

Factors To Teach the Patient

The personal risk involved if he plans to leave the hospital without a written order for dismissal from the attending physician.

Importance of diet, and how to plan and prepare it at home, especially if a special diet has been ordered.

Nursing procedures necessary for his care at home. If the patient is to perform the procedure he should be taught the proper method. If it is to be performed by a member of the family, that person will need to be taught.

Detailed instructions as to continued medication and treatment and return visits to doctor or hospital.

Suggestions that will help the patient in adjusting to a life of restricted activity if such restriction is indicated. Such factors might include: slow and gradual return to work, change of work, daily rest periods, provision for longer hours of sleep and rest at night, change of recreational activities to conform with physical condition, and development of new interests in keeping with restricted activity.

Various social and health facilities available in his community should the patient need assistance that can be rendered by such organizations.

Scientific Principles

Anatomy and Physiology. After prolonged illness muscles are weak, vitality is low, and exertion in any form may be tiring to the patient. He is apt to be nervous and irritable, demanding more care and attention than is really necessitated by his physical condition.

Return to normal, physically and mentally, may be slow and at times the patient may be discouraged.

Microbiology. The patient should be clean and be dressed in clean clothes for departure from the hospital.

Care of the room or unit after dismissal should insure cleanliness and order for the next occupant.

Pharmacology. The nurse will need to interpret orders regarding medicine, giving directions in general terms that the patient can understand.

The patient should be told where to obtain needed pharmaceutical preparations.

Symptoms that indicate medicine now being given is having a questionable effect upon the patient should be reported to the attending physician.

Psychology. Impressions made at the time of dismissal are as lasting as those made on admission.

Farewell from the nurse should be that of a hostess for a departing guest.

The nurse should encourage the patient, who has become dependent on her and the hospital routine, to become self sufficient and return to active participation in home life.

If the patient has a chronic illness he should be fully informed as to limitations imposed by his physical condition and how to live happily and successfully within them.

Sociology. Social and health facilities for the patient after hospitalization should be made known to him.

Plan of subsequent care for the patient should be worked out by the family doctor, the family, and, if necessary, a social service worker.

Relatives of the patient should be told of his physical condition and suggestions made on how they may adjust to his changed condition and attitude.

If special equipment is needed for home care of the patient, the nurse should inform family members where it may be obtained.

Provision for return to work or for diversion if he is unable to work should be made at the time the patient leaves the hospital.

Situation Type Problem

1. A patient who had been in the hospital only two days and was being prepared for a surgical operation on the third day informed the student nurse that he had decided to leave the hospital. He refused to sign a release form and demanded that his clothes be brought to him. He had been permitted ambulatory privileges so had his clothing in his room, except for coat, hat, and shoes. The head nurse told the student she should refuse to take the articles of clothing to the patient. She also commented that the patient was "bluffing" in his stated intent to leave the hospital.

The student explained to the patient that it would be impossible to give him the clothing he had requested. The patient seemed to accept the explanation and made no further demands.

About 45 minutes later the student nurse glanced from a window in the nurse's station and saw the patient standing on the corner at the bus stop. It was snowing lightly and the patient was without hat or top coat and was wearing the light canvas "hospital slippers" which he had worn after being admitted. As the student watched, a bus came to the corner and stopped, the patient entered the bus and it moved away from the curb and into the line of traffic. What would you have done?

Suggested Reference Reading

"Teaching patients is easy," Charlotte Kerr; American Journal of Nursing, March, 1951.

"Protecting the patient's property," Hospital Management, February, 1952.

"Teaching patients to take care of themselves," Prudence I. Priest; American Journal of Nursing, December, 1952.

"Teaching social factors in illness," Sidney Liswood; Hospital Management, December, 1952.

PART IV

Procedures for Advanced Preclinical Study

CHAPTER 24

Counterirritants

TOPICAL OUTLINE

How Physical Reaction Is Achieved
Purpose of a Counterirritant
Effects of a Counterirritant
Classification of Counterirritants
Methods of Application
- Local Application
- Inunction
- Poultices and Plasters

Chemical Counterirritants

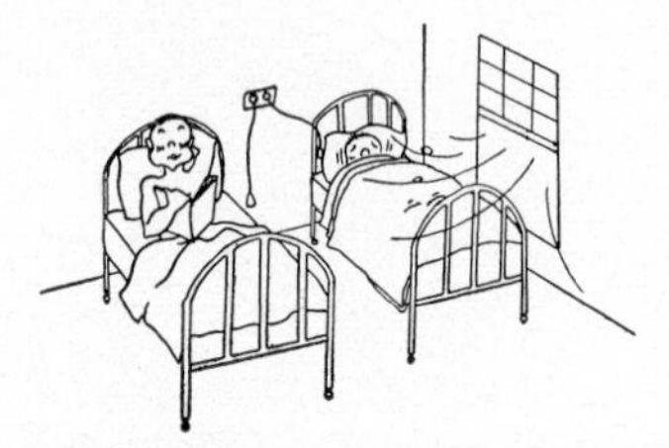

Some like it cold, some like it hot;
Some freeze while others smother,
And by some fiendish, fatal plot,
They share a room, and battle one another!

A counterirritant is an agent applied to the skin to produce an inflammatory reaction there, thus relieving congestion in an underlying organ or part.

HOW PHYSICAL REACTION IS ACHIEVED

Physical reaction which takes place when a counterirritant is applied to the skin is achieved by an impulse generated within the nervous system which produces changes in the congested or diseased part. In the deeper organ or part the inflammatory process has caused hyperemia and a transudation of blood serum and cells. When an irritant is applied to the skin the superficial vessels there are dilated and blood is drawn to the surface of the body from the deeper vessels thus relieving congestion in the affected area.

PURPOSE OF A COUNTERIRRITANT

The primary purpose of a counterirritant is to relieve congestion and inflammation through improved circulation in the affected area. The counterirritant also acts to promote absorption and gradual removal of deposits left by the inflammatory process. Pain in the organ or part is relieved when pressure on nerve endings is decreased as the swelling and congestion subsides.

EFFECTS OF A COUNTERIRRITANT

Counterirritants produce a local effect when applied to the body surface. The capillaries in the skin become dilated, increasing the flow of blood to the area and drawing it away from the deeper vessels, thus decreasing internal congestion.

The application of a counterirritant to the skin may affect organs or parts of the body far removed from the site of application. The stimulus felt in the nerve endings of the skin is transmitted to associated nerve endings in the underlying organs, improving circulation and relieving congestion caused by the inflammatory process. As swelling is reduced and the debris of blood cells and blood serum is removed the normal physical state and normal functioning of the affected part is restored.

CLASSIFICATION OF COUNTERIRRITANTS

Each agent, physical or chemical, which is applied to the skin for irritation produces the same effect but in different degrees of intensity, depending on the strength and amount of agent used.

Counterirritants are classified according to their effect or the degree of irritation produced, as follows:

Rubefacients. This is the most simple form of counterirritant. It merely reddens the skin, a reaction produced by dilatation of the capillaries and the subsequent increase in the supply of blood to the part.

A rubefacient is effective immediately on application. The effect lasts only a short time, with the skin rapidly returning to normal color and condition when the irritant is removed. A rubefacient allowed to remain on the surface of the body for a prolonged period may cause blister formation and injury to the skin.

Agents used as rubefacients are: mustard, turpentine, flaxseed, liniments, and arnica.

Vesicants. This particular form of counterirritant is used to produce blister formation on the skin. Such an agent acts to draw fluids from deeper tissues to the body surface, where blisters are formed. A counterirritant of this type may be used effectively for treatment of inflammatory processes affecting joints, the fluid being aspirated under aseptic conditions so an autogenous vaccine may be prepared and used in treatment. The formation of a blister for any other purpose is dangerous, since it may cause infection in the area being treated.

Agents used as vesicants include cantharides and iodine.

Escharotics. Escharotics are agents which destroy tissue and cause it to slough away. Such substances, termed caustics, are used effectively in the treatment of skin diseases. When it is necessary to destroy tissue which has become infected, an escharotic agent is employed. This type of counterirritant is used, too, in counteracting the poisonous effect of bites from insects or animals.

Examples of escharotic agents include caustic soda, silver nitrate, and lunar caustic.

Pustulants. Pustulants are irritant agents which produce a severe irritation and cause the formation of pustules on the skin.

Examples of pustulants include croton oil and antimony, agents which are rarely used now in medicine.

Agents not included in this classification of counterirritants, yet commonly used for counterirritant effect, include applications of heat and cold (hot water bottle, ice cap, or ice collar), cold compresses, fomentations, stupes, hot compresses, electric pads, and footbaths. Detailed discussion of these agents, included in other chapters, may be readily found by consulting the index.

METHODS OF APPLICATION

Local Application. In applying medicine to the skin, a cotton applicator or atomizer may be used for liquids; ointments may be applied with a tongue blade or spoon handle, and a powder may be dusted on. Ethyl chloride, applied to produce local anesthesia, is sprayed on the skin from a glass container.

Inunction. Inunction is defined as "the act of applying an ointment or medicine to a part or area by rubbing it into the skin." In this procedure the nurse should wear a rubber glove so that the ointment is absorbed through the skin of the patient rather than that of her hand. The part to which inunction is given should be held steady, while the gloved hand exerts light pressure and rubs the part with a continuous circular motion. A period of 20–30 minutes may be required to rub the ointment into the skin. Liniments may be applied in the same manner; those which will not produce an undesirable effect on the nurse may be applied with her bare hand, and the area or skin surface to which they are applied may be briskly rubbed.

Poultices and Plasters. Although not used as extensively as in previous years, because heat applied in various other ways is easier, produces the same results, and is less likely to cause burns, poultices and plasters are still used occasionally for their counterirritant effect. Commercial plasters, available in all drug stores, are easy to apply and produce the same effect as the plaster made by the nurse or other member of the nursing service staff.

Poultices. A poultice (cataplasm) is a hot, moist mass contained between two layers of muslin or similar material and applied to the skin as a counterirritant. It may be used to promote a suppurative process (by hastening the localization of infection), to relieve pain

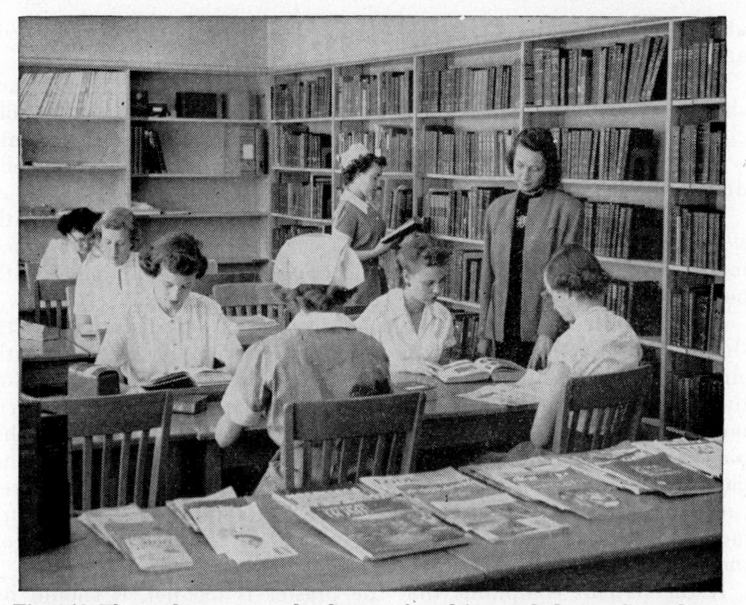

Fig. 156. The student nurse today learns of poultices and plasters from the textbook or from reference reading, rather than from experience with them. (University of Denver Basic Nursing Program, Denver, Colorado.)

and congestion, and to reduce distention. To be effective, the poultice should be large enough to cover the area to which it is applied, light in weight yet thick enough to retain heat, and smooth in consistency.

As soon as the poultice has been made it should be placed against the nurse's cheek to be tested for accurate temperature and should then be immediately applied to the patient.

Ingredients most frequently used in making poultices include: flaxseed, mustard, bread, hops, digitalis, soap, and various volatile oils.

If the poultice is to be applied frequently or if the skin is tender, oil should be applied before the poultice is placed in position. In applying a poultice it should be placed gently on the skin, the corners being raised and lowered until it can be left in place without discomfort to the patient. If applied to the back, the patient should rest on one side since lying flat on the poultice would decrease radiation and make the heat more intense. Under such conditions there is danger of the patient being burned. The poultice should be removed before it becomes cold.

If a second poultice is to be applied it should be ready and at the bedside before the first one is removed. A newly prepared poultice should be carried to the bedside of the patient on a hot water bottle. A poultice, properly applied, will remain warm and comfortable for about an hour. After that time, if the treatment is to be continued, another poultice should be prepared.

After a poultice has been removed the skin of the affected part should appear pink and healthy. It should be patted dry with a soft cloth, dusted lightly with powder, and be covered for a short time with a cotton pad and binder to prevent chilling and subsequent discomfort to the patient.

Plasters. A plaster (sinapism) is a cloth foundation spread with a medicated substance to be used as a counterirritant. The substance most commonly used is mustard, although plasters are made with belladona (to check secretions), capsicum, and cantharides.

For an adult the plaster should be made of one part mustard with three parts flour. For a child the usual ratio is one part mustard with eight parts flour. Enough water should be used to make a paste of the right consistency to spread evenly. Heat tends to destroy the irritant action of the mustard, so hot water should not be used. The plaster should be placed on a hot water bottle to be taken to the patient's bedside. It should be applied with the same care and precautions as outlined for a poultice. Oil is not applied to the skin surface before placing the plaster in position, as the irritant action of the mustard will not penetrate the oil.

If the patient complains that the plaster is too hot, it should be removed immediately; otherwise it may be left in place 15–20 minutes. At frequent intervals the nurse should lift one corner of the plaster to observe the condition of the skin beneath it; if the skin becomes reddened, the plaster should be removed.

After the plaster has been removed oil should be applied to the affected skin area and a lightweight pad or binder placed over it.

CHEMICAL COUNTERIRRITANTS

Chemical counterirritants are used in the same manner and have the same effect as hot applications. They reduce the amount of blood in a deep seated and congested region by drawing blood to the superficial tissues. Such irritants have been used in treatment of headache, pneumonia, bronchitis, pleurisy, lumbago, abdominal distention caused by flatulence, and other conditions.

Chemical counterirritants still used occasionally include *acetic acid* (used most commonly as an astringent and styptic to check the flow of blood as an emergency measure); *ammonia* (used as an irritant ingredient in various liniments); *silver nitrate* (used locally as an astringent and germicide in conditions affecting mucous membrane; in contact with living tissue it causes formation of a dense film of coagulated albumin, the affected area being white and then becoming black after a short time, the tissue is destroyed and sloughing follows). Cantharides, croton oil, iodine, mustard, and myrrh are still used in various forms as chemical counterirritants. Besides these, many varieties of counterirritant ointments are on the market. These preparations contain mustard, menthol, eucalyptus, and other similar drugs and their use should be governed by directions on the package in which they are purchased.

Care of Equipment after Use

Bottle caps and ointment jar lids should be closed tightly after liniment or ointment has been used from bottles or jars.

Tongue blades used in applying ointment should be discarded.

Poultices and plasters removed from the patient should be discarded.

Containers used in making mustard plaster should be washed in warm soapy water, rinsed, and returned to the proper place.

Containers of mustard, flour, and other ingredients should be closed tightly and returned to the proper storage place.

Summary of Important Factors

A counterirritant is an agent applied to the skin to relieve congestion in an underlying organ or part.

The relief of congestion and inflammation is brought about by improved circulation in the affected area.

Pain is relieved when pressure on nerve endings is decreased.

Counterirritants are classified according to the degree of irritation produced: rubefacients—redden the skin; vesicants—produce blister formation; escharotics—destroy tissue; pustulants—cause formation of pus.

Medication may be applied to the skin by inunction (rubbing into the skin). The person giving an inunction should wear rubber gloves.

A poultice is a hot moist mass contained within layers of cloth, applied to the skin as a counterirritant.

Oil applied to the skin will serve as protection if the skin is tender or frequent applications of the poultice are to be made.

A plaster is a cloth foundation spread with a medicated substance and used as a counterirritant.

Oil should not be used on the skin before applying a mustard plaster as the irritant action of the mustard will not penetrate the oil.

Chemical counterirritants are used for the same effect as that produced by hot applications.

Factors To Teach the Patient

When an irritant is applied to the skin the superficial vessels dilate and blood is drawn to the surface, relieving congestion elsewhere in the body.

Counterirritants applied for mild effect (to redden the skin) usually become effective immediately and the effect lasts only a short time.

Counterirritants applied for mild effect may cause blisters or damage the skin if allowed to remain in place for a prolonged period.

Strong counterirritants should be used only under a doctor's supervision.

A poultice should always be removed before it becomes cold.

Care should be taken so that a poultice is not allowed to remain in place too long.

A mustard plaster usually may be left in place 15 to 20 minutes, but should be lifted at the corner at frequent intervals to see if the skin is becoming reddened.

The ratio of flour and mustard to be used in making a mustard plaster is much greater for the child than for the adult patient. There should be no undissolved lumps of mustard when the paste is prepared. Hot water should not be used in making the mustard paste, since heat destroys the irritant action of the mustard.

Scientific Principles

Anatomy and Physiology. Numerous capillaries in the skin, when dilated by action of counterirritants, can hold a large supply of blood. Blood may be thus drawn from a deep-seated congested area to the skin or surface area. The increased supply of blood to the area where a counterirritant is applied causes the skin to become reddened.

The effect of a counterirritant on deep-seated areas of congestion is made possible through nerve reflexes. Sensory nerves convey the sensation of heat to the spinal cord, and impulses are transmitted through the sympathetic ganglia and by means of the sympathetic nerves to the affected internal organ.

Chemistry. Heat increases the speed of a chemical reaction and speeds metabolism.

The chemical reaction occurring between the mustard and warm water in a mustard plaster produces a volatile oil which causes the production of heat that makes the plaster effective.

Flaxseed contains oil which makes it a useful ingredient in hot moist poultices or applications.

Microbiology. To avoid unnecessary contamination, the nurse should wash her hands before carrying out a procedure involving the use of counterirritants.

The skin surface to which a counterirritant is applied should be clean and unbroken.

Plasters or poultices which are not sterile cannot be used as counterirritants on an area where a sterile procedure is required.

Pharmacology. Turpentine and mustard are commonly used irritant drugs. Turpentine is usually used in conjunction with oil. Mustard is applied in plaster form or used as a medicated bath.

The active ingredient in mustard is destroyed by hot water, so water used in making a mustard plaster should be lukewarm.

Irritant drugs may cause blisters or injury to the skin if left on too long. When a counterirritant is applied, the affected skin area should be observed frequently; the application should not be left in place after the skin shows definite redness.

Physics. Heat may be transferred by conduction when a counterirritant such as a poultice or plaster is applied to the skin. The heat retained in the softened mass of a poultice or the active ingredient of a mustard plaster makes such applications an effective means of producing counterirritation.

A layer of oil on the skin will prevent evaporation and conduction of heat and so will prevent burns that might be produced by a counterirritant.

Friction produces heat and aids the counterirritant effect of liniments and lotions.

Psychology. Because of danger from burns, the patient may be apprehensive. The treatments should be explained, and application of the counterirritant should be made slowly, with frequent examination of the site of application. The patient should be watched carefully during the treatment. The nurse can reassure the patient and relieve anxiety as to harmful effects of the treatment if she visits the patient often while the counterirritant remains in place.

Sociology. The nurse has a legal responsibility to the hospital in the procedure of applying a counterirritant to a patient; carelessness or negligence may cause the patient to be burned and furnish the basis for possible litigation.

Situation Type Problem

1. A graduate nurse applied a counterirritant, in the form of a commercial preparation made up as an ointment, to the chest of a patient being treated for an inflammatory condition.

The patient expressed some concern about the treatment, explaining to the nurse that her skin was "tender" and that she had to be extremely cautious because she was easily burned. When hospitalized previously she had been severely burned by a hot water bottle which would not have been too hot for the average patient.

The nurse assurred the patient that the ointment was mild and would not burn, then she placed a large piece of flannel over the chest and fastened it securely in place with a snug breast binder.

Five minutes after the graduate nurse left the room the patient asked a student nurse to remove the binder and to look for reddening of the skin which might indicate that the ointment was too strong for her use.

As the student was unfastening the binder the graduate nurse returned to the room. She sharply reprimanded the student, refastened the binder without looking at the skin surface beneath the flannel covering, and once more left the room. What would you have done?

Suggested Reference Reading

"A home-made counterirritant," Freddie O. Jones; American Journal of Nursing, February, 1936.

CHAPTER 25

Compresses—Fomentations—Stupes —Packs

TOPICAL OUTLINE

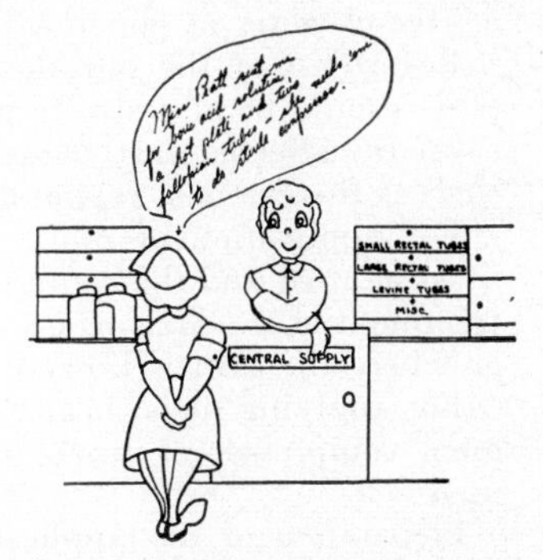

Some people are like blotters—they soak it all in, but get it all backwards!

THE APPLICATION OF MOIST HEAT

When given the responsibility of carrying out nursing measures which include the application of moist heat, the nurse should thoroughly understand the effect of such measures on the patient. She must bear in mind that each application will increase original tolerance to heat, and that after repeated applications the patient is unable to judge accurately whether the compress is hot enough to burn, so the nurse must be extremely careful if undesirable effects are to be avoided.

The average patient who has not yet developed increased tolerance for the heat of moist applications may be asked whether the application is too hot as it is applied, but the nurse should not depend on the judgment of a diabetic or edematous patient or one with circulatory impairment. The very young, the very old, and the critically ill patient are particularly susceptible to heat and are more likely to be burned by hot moist applications.

Purpose of the Application. The application of moist heat serves essentially the same purpose as application of dry heat, being used to warm the skin or surface area, to produce hyperemia, to relieve pain and muscle spasm, and to aid the process of suppuration.

Because water conducts heat much better than air, hot wet applications are a more effective means of conducting heat to the skin or body surface than the various forms of dry heat. To prevent possible burning of the patient's skin all hot wet applications must be wrung as free of water as possible.

Regardless of the purpose for which the heat is applied, the compress should be of a size to permit easy handling and still adequately cover the affected part. Gauze compresses are required for small areas, such as the eye or a region of the head or face.

For application of moist heat to a part where aseptic technique must be used and the compress or dressing must be sterile, such as for treatment of the area where a recent surgical incision has been made, or where the skin is broken, gauze compresses should be used.

For applying moist heat to relatively large areas, such as the abdomen, compresses of linen, flannel, or woolen material are usually used.

Preparation of the Application. In preparing hot wet applications the material used, such as toweling, linen, or flannel, should be boiled for at least five minutes so that heat will be retained for a longer period when the application is made to the body surface. The material should be wrung from the hot solution as dry as possible. Moisture retained in the application is in the form of live steam and may readily cause a burn when the application is covered by oiled silk, waxed paper, or cellophane. To retain heat an additional covering of turkish toweling, flannel blanket, or binder is provided, the latter being used to hold the entire application in place.

Methods of Making the Application. Moist heat is applied to the body in a number of different ways, depending on the condition requiring such treatment and the amount of body surface to be covered.

A hot water bottle or heating pad placed over the application inside the binder will help maintain the desired temperature. If the hot application is placed beneath the patient (weight of the patient causing pressure on the application) the electric pad should not be used to help retain the heat; the pressure of the patient's body causes a deeper penetration of heat and increases the danger of burns.

All hot moist applications should be made gradually, with the nurse retaining her hold on the material and lifting it from time to time until the skin surface of the affected area becomes accustomed to the increased temperature and the application can be tolerated without pain or discomfort.

When hot moist applications are first begun the patient may be able to determine accurately whether the application is too hot. Any complaint of discomfort should be accepted by the nurse as a warning that a burn may result.

Hot wet applications are usually continued for 20 to 30 minutes and application is made every 2 to 4 hours. Prolonged application of moist heat has an undesirable effect on the skin, tending to soften and weaken the tissues.

Solutions most commonly used for application of moist heat are tap water, normal saline, and a weak boric acid solution. Temperature of the solution will need to be maintained well above the desired temperature of the application, since the process of wringing and applying the compress permits it to cool and much of the original heat is lost.

COMPRESSES

The Hot Wet Compress (Unsterile). Gauze or linen is used as a compress for hot moist applications applied to the patient's face or to a small surface area.

If the compress is to be applied to the face, a linen towel wrung from hot water may be folded lengthwise, tested and applied, the length of the towel encircling the nose and entirely covering the rest of the face.

Two towels will be needed so that one can be used while the other is being prepared. Frequent changing of the towels ensures continuous hot application. The pillow under the patient's head should be protected with a rubber cover and utility towel. Such applications are effective in relieving pain caused by sinusitis or neuralgia.

For the application of hot wet compresses to the eye, see Chapter 30.

The Hot Wet Compress (Sterile). When hot compresses are to be applied to the area of a surgical incision, to broken skin, or to a wound, all supplies and equipment should be sterile and aseptic technique should be observed.

For an abdominal incision the 4 x 4 gauze yard roll is required and the compress is handled with a pair of sterile hemostats. The sterile compress should extend beyond the area of incision in all directions and should be covered with oiled silk and other dressings as indicated. An abdominal binder, pinned securely, is usually applied for the purpose of holding the compress and dressings in place.

For the back of the neck several sterile 4 inch gauze squares may be placed on the area to be treated and moistened with warm, sterile solution from an Asepto syringe. The compress is then covered with oiled silk and an ice collar half filled with water heated to a temperature of 125° F. may be applied directly over the compress. A towel or suitable covering may then be pinned around the throat to hold the compress and collar in place.

Compresses may be applied to arms, legs, or other parts of the body as outlined above, with the final covering wrapped and pinned so that it fits the part and holds the hot wet application in place.

Hot sterile compresses that are to remain on the affected part for longer than one hour should be moistened with the sterile solution at

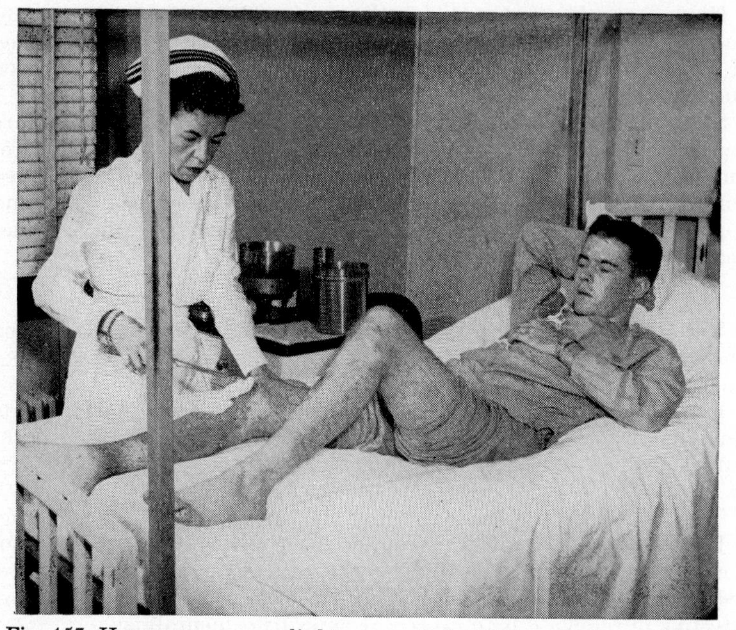

Fig. 157. Hot compresses applied to a surgical incision require sterile equipment and use of sterile technique. (Bureau of Medicine and Surgery, Navy Dept., Washington, D.C.)

intervals and the hot water bottle should be reheated when necessary to maintain correct temperature. At the end of two hours, if the treatment is to be continued for a longer period, the compresses should be removed and fresh ones applied.

Sterile compresses applied to the face or head may be kept warm by use of the infant size hot water bottle, which can be held in place by a suitable bandage.

When sterile compresses are removed, a dry, sterile dressing should be applied to the affected area. The dry dressing may be held in place by a bandage or by adhesive tape.

The Cold Wet Compress. Cold compresses are used frequently on the forehead to relieve simple headache or on parts of the face to relieve pain and congestion. A wash cloth, small linen towel, or several gauze squares may be used, depending on the part to be treated. Four by four gauze squares are used for the eyelids.

A moderately large piece of ice placed in a basin lined with gauze (the gauze lining prevents the ice from rattling or striking against the sides of the basin) will be needed, in addition to the other essential equipment. If the gauze squares are moistened with cold water before being placed on the ice they will cool more rapidly. Each

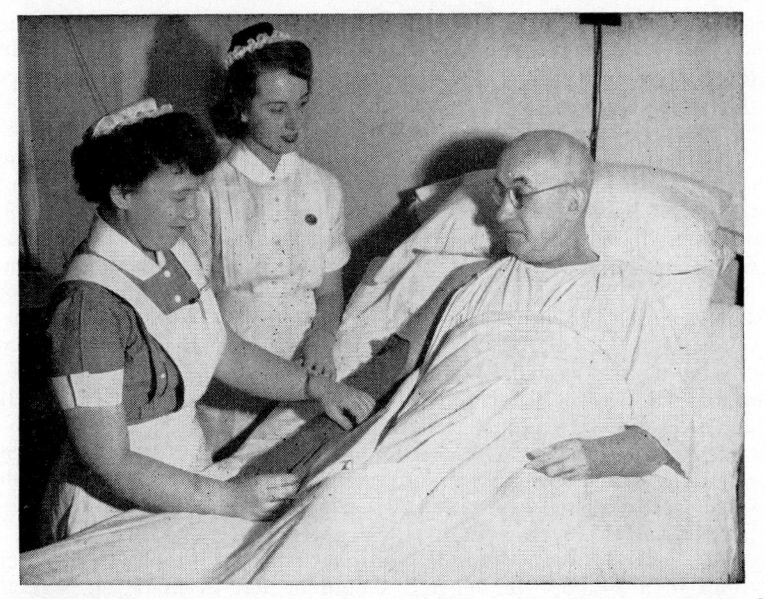

Fig. 158. Fomentations are a means of applying moist heat in the form of unsterile hot packs. (Massachusetts General Hospital School of Nursing, Boston, Massachusetts.)

compress should be wrung dry before being gently applied to the eyelid. At no time during the treatment should pressure be exerted on the eyeball. As one compress is placed on the eyelid another is put on the ice so it will be ready to apply within a few minutes. Compresses soiled by discharge or secretion from the affected eye should be discarded when removed after their first application.

Moist cold compresses are usually applied for 15 to 20 minutes.

Cold compresses are used to relieve swelling and discomfort caused by bruises. Before applying the compress the bruised area should be gently cleansed with warm water and soap, using sterile gauze or sterile cotton applicators for the cleansing procedure.

If the skin is broken at the site of a bruise the choice of antiseptic to be applied should be made by the attending physician.

FOMENTATIONS

The term fomentation is defined as "a hot, wet application used in treatment of pain and inflammation" yet, through common practice, is used chiefly to designate the application of moist heat in the form of an unsterile hot pack. Wool or flannel packs are usually used when a large area or surface of the body is to be treated.

The patient should be draped so that only the area to be treated is exposed. The hot pack should be removed from the pack machine or the basin containing the heated solution and should be wrung thoroughly dry. The pack should be tested by touching the back of the hand, to make certain it is not too hot, then should be placed gradually on the part to be treated. When the pack is placed in position one corner should be placed first against the skin surface and the rest of the pack then slowly lowered into place, the nurse continuing to hold at least one corner which may be lifted to permit the escape of steam. It may be necessary to lift this last corner of the fomentation several times before it is placed permanently in position. The wet pack is covered with a dry pack or towel and left in place for several minutes, while a second pack is immersed in the heated solution and then made ready for application. The second pack, when wrung dry and tested, is placed in position as the first pack is removed, care being taken to keep the skin surface covered so it will not be cooled by exposure to currents of air.

When the procedure has been completed the skin surface treated should be patted dry, the patient placed in a comfortable position with sufficient covers to ensure warmth, and all equipment should be removed from the room or unit.

Hot packs to relieve muscle pain or spasm may be applied several times in a 24 hour period and should be left in place for several hours at a time. Such packs should be cut to fit the part of the body to which they are applied. After the original pack has been put in place it is covered with oiled silk or some other water-resistant material, the part is wrapped in a blanket or other covering, and a hot water bottle or electric pad is applied to help maintain the desired temperature of the application.

Since fomentations are usually prepared at the patient's bedside and he can see that the solution is heated to a high degree of temperature, it is necessary to assure him that proper precautions will be taken to prevent possibility of a burn. The apprehensive patient, fearful of being scalded or burned, will usually relax and readily accept the treatment if he understands that the pack will be tested before it is applied and that it will be immediately lifted from place if it is too hot to be borne without causing discomfort.

If the electric pack heater or other special device designed for the preparation of hot wet packs is not available, the pack may be placed in a pack wringer immersed in a basin of solution which is heated by means of an electric plate. Wringer sticks will be needed to wring the fomentation dry, since the nurse will be unable to handle the pack wringer with her bare hands.

STUPES

The term "stupe" has been defined as "a cloth or sponge wrung out of hot water and applied, usually with a counterirritant, to the surface of the body as a means of treatment." Except for the counterirritant effect, the procedures of applying stupes and fomentations are identical. Through common practice, however, the term stupe is used when the procedure is done for the counterirritant effect.

Turpentine is used to increase the irritating effect of the heat produced by the stupes. One part turpentine to three parts oil is the mixture usually used or ordered by the physician. A heavy oil, such as cottonseed or mineral oil, is preferable. The turpentine and oil mixture should be spread thinly (with a cotton applicator) over the skin area before the hot wet pack is placed in position. After the counterirritant has once been painted on the affected area, the next two or three hot wet applications should be made without additional use of the counterirritant. With use of the counterirritant each time the irritating effect of the stupes might be increased to the point where it would cause damage to the skin surface being treated.

BODY PACKS

Hot Wet Pack. The purpose of the hot wet pack is to increase perspiration, and in doing so to aid elimination, to relax the muscles in spasmodic conditions where general relaxation is desired, to reduce blood pressure, and to quiet the patient who is extremely restless or in a condition of emotional excitement or delirium. Because of the danger involved such treatment is, as a rule, used only for conditions that are in themselves extreme, such as uremia, eclampsia, and acute nephritis.

The hot pack has a systemic effect since it covers the entire body. In general, the treatment stimulates sweat glands, and through increased perspiration furthers the elimination of nitrogenous waste products and the removal of toxins from the tissues. It soothes the nerves, relaxes the muscles, dulls sensation, and increases body temperature by checking the evaporation of body heat.

The patient's temperature, pulse, and respiration should be checked and recorded before the procedure is begun and, if he is able to understand, an explanation of what is to be done should be made. Patients to whom the procedure has not been explained are apt to be frightened because of the restraint to movement imposed by the pack.

The bed should first be protected by a rubber sheet, which is used to enfold the patient after the hot moist blankets have been properly applied, and which serves to retain the heat of the pack.

Bath blankets are immersed in water of 180° F., wrung dry, and placed snugly around the entire body surface of the patient, except for the head.

Two nurses are needed for administering a body pack, since the application must be made quickly to prevent chilling of the patient. Special care should be observed in wrapping the blankets snugly, so that large air pockets are not formed, increasing the danger of burning. Too tight wrapping is to be avoided, as it would tend to cause discomfort to the patient. Covered hot water bottles should be placed at the feet and sides of the patient, and an ice cap placed on the patient's head.

The pulse (at the temporal artery) should be counted frequently during the procedure, which usually requires 30 to 40 minutes.

Perspiration appearing on the patient's face is an indication that perspiration is occurring over the entire body. To further promote perspiration during the treatment the patient should be encouraged to drink freely of hot fluids which are made available to him frequently.

During the application of a hot wet pack, complaints of nausea and vertigo or symptoms such as extreme pallor, cyanosis, or shallow and irregular respiration should indicate to the nurse that it is necessary to discontinue the treatment at once.

While the treatment is in progress the patient should not be left alone. When removed from the pack he should be left for an hour or so between dry blankets, until perspiration has ceased. After that time he should be given a complete alcohol rub, and gown and bed linens should be changed so that he is dry and comfortable. Temperature, pulse, and respiration should be taken and recorded one hour after the treatment has been discontinued.

Because of lowered blood pressure and general weakness resulting from the treatment the patient should remain in bed for several hours.

Cold Wet Pack. The cold wet body pack, which acts as a sedative, is used extensively for treatment of psychiatric patients. It is used to quiet restlessness and to overcome insomnia.

Before the pack is applied the room should be made quiet and shades should be partially drawn. This treatment, like the hot wet pack, increases urinary output, so the patient should be encouraged to void just before the pack is applied.

With the bed made ready as in the hot wet pack, the patient is wrapped in cold, wet sheets (wrung from water that is 60–70° F. in temperature). The first effect, caused by contraction of cutaneous blood vessels, is undue chilliness, and the patient may exhibit pronounced shivering. In 5 to 15 minutes this initial reaction subsides and as the blood vessels dilate a peripheral hyperemia occurs and the skin becomes comfortably warm. Heat given off by the body surface is held within the wrapped blankets and the patient is surrounded by a layer of moist warm air which induces quiet and relaxation. It is not unusual for the patient to fall asleep during the treatment.

The pack may be left in place for 60 to 90 minutes. For greater comfort, an ice cap may be placed at the patient's head and a hot water bottle at the feet. If the patient desires, water may be given by mouth while the pack is in place.

The patient should not be left alone during the treatment, and he

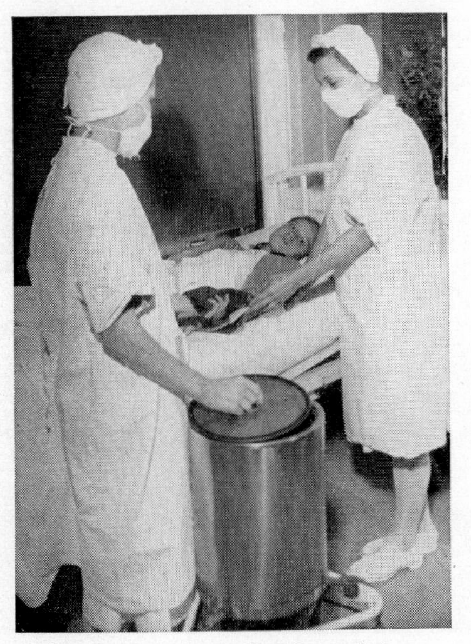

Fig. 159. Packs used in the treatment of poliomyelitis are made of flannel and cut to fit the part to which they are applied. (Mercy Hospital School of Nursing, Hamilton, Ohio.)

should be closely observed. If the pulse decreases in rate and becomes weak, if the face becomes markedly flushed, or if the patient, after 30 minutes, is still restless, the pack should be discontinued.

After the pack is removed the patient should be given a brisk alcohol rub and be placed between dry, clean sheets, made comfortably warm, and allowed to rest for as long as he wishes.

For the elderly patient or one with cardiac involvement cold wet packs are contraindicated.

Kenny Pack. Packs adapted for use in the treatment of poliomyelitis, termed "Kenny" packs in recognition of the Australian nurse, Sister Kenny, are modifications of the hot wet packs first used by her in the treatment of muscles weakened or paralyzed as a result of that disease.

The material used is flannel (chosen for its heat-retaining qualities), and pieces are cut to fit the part to which they are to be applied.

The flannel pieces are taken from the pack heater with lifter forceps and are tested by the nurse (by placing against the inside of her wrist) before being applied to the area to be covered. Parts are covered adequately with the moist hot pieces of flannel, with joints being left free so they are movable. The packs should be applied

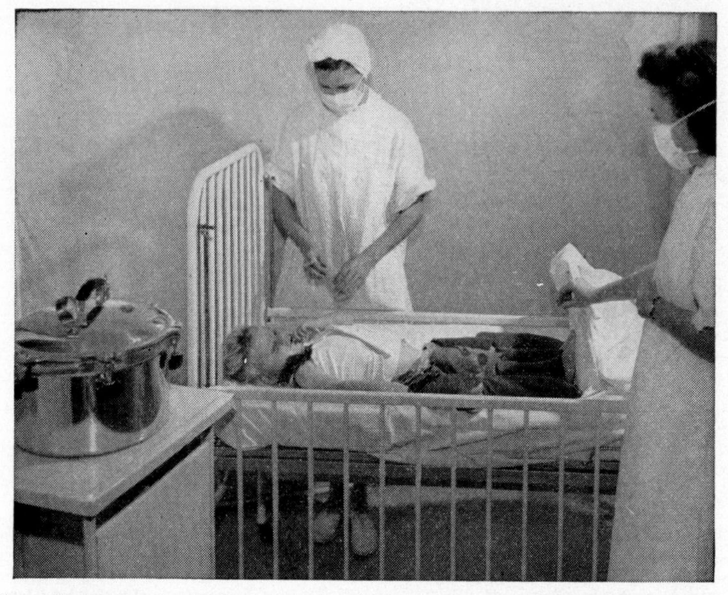

Fig. 160. Packs should be applied quickly and covered; they are changed as ordered by physician. (Mercy Hospital School of Nursing, Hamilton, Ohio.)

quickly, covered with Koroseal or Cellophane, and changed as frequently as ordered by the physician.

Care of Equipment after Use

Material used for hot wet applications and hot or cold packs should be sent to the laundry and thoroughly washed before being used for another patient.

Gauze compresses should be discarded after use. Gauze rolls used for stupes may be sent to the laundry and then made ready for use again.

Cellophane or oiled silk should be cleaned and returned to central supply.

Basins used for hot or cold compresses should be cleaned and returned to central supply. If used for sterile compresses they will be sterilized and made ready for use again.

Hot water bottles and ice caps used for pack treatments should be cared for after use as described in Chapter 8, "Local Applications of Heat and Cold."

Summary of Important Factors

Boiling the material used for hot wet applications increases its ability to retain heat.

Applications not wrung dry contain live steam and are more apt to burn the patient.

Moist heat applications are used to produce hyperemia, relieve pain and muscle spasm, and promote the process of suppuration.

If infection is present, hot compresses should be used only once, then discarded.

Sterile compresses should be handled with sterile forceps and the procedure carried out with aseptic technique.

A bruised area should be cleansed with soap and water before the application of cold compresses.

The term "fomentation" has come to mean, through common usage, the application of moist heat in the form of an unsterile hot pack. The term "stupe" is usually applied to fomentation used with a counterirritant drug.

The procedure should be explained to the patient so that his cooperation will be obtained.

In using turpentine or other forms of counterirritant, the treated area should be closely observed for signs of injury from increased irritant effect.

Factors To Teach the Patient

If the treatment is to be done by the patient at home, the method of procedure should be demonstrated and, if necessary, improvised equipment suggested.

Factors that increase the danger of burns from hot moist applications.

The danger of applying heat to the abdomen unless such treatment is recommended by a physician.

The effects desired and the symptoms that indicate an undesirable reaction, in order to prevent burns.

Scientific Principles

Anatomy and Physiology. The effect of moist heat or cold is more marked than that of dry.

Live steam of moist heat increases danger from burns.

Moderate heat increases perspiration.

Hot or cold wet body packs help to relax muscle tissue and are soothing to nerves.

Chemistry. Heat will increase the speed of a chemical reaction, thus speeding up body metabolism.

Oil, as an inert substance, is used to proctect the skin from excessive heat in applying hot compresses; in the application of a stupes it may be mixed with the counterirritant, such as turpentine.

Microbiology. All supplies and equipment used for unsterile fomentations or compresses should be clean.

Soap is mildly antiseptic and can be used to cleanse a bruised area to which compresses are to be applied.

Application of heat or cold to open wounds requires sterile supplies and equipment and must be done under sterile technique. A sterile thermometer should be used in taking temperature of solutions to be used for sterile compresses.

Pharmacology. An irritant drug reinforces the effect of a hot wet application.

Drugs used for hot moist compresses have a mild antiseptic action. Drugs most commonly used in solution for hot compresses are boric acid and sodium chloride.

Physics. Water is a conductor of heat, and danger of burns is increased if heat is applied as a wet application. For this reason wet applications should be wrung as dry as possible before being applied. Pressure on a hot application increases the danger of burns by reducing air layers within the application.

Psychology. Explanation of the procedure reassures the patient and lessens his fear of being burned or injured by the application of moist heat.

If the patient complains that the moist application is too hot it should be removed and gradually reapplied.

To prepare the patient for a marked difference in temperature of hot or cold applications the nurse should explain the purpose of the treatment.

Sociology. The patient should be informed as to services which are available to him through the Visiting Nurse Association.

Legal suits against a hospital are not unusual and often result from carelessness or negligence on the part of the nurse in applying heat or cold, especially when moist heat is being applied and there is danger of burning or scalding the patient.

Careful instruction of the patient is necessary if he is to perform the procedure of applying hot or cold wet applications for himself.

Situation Type Problem

1. A nurse had applied hot compresses, which were to remain in place for 30 minutes, on a patient's legs. After the application had been made the patient stated that she wished to walk to the adjoining bathroom. She had bathroom privileges and refused to use the bedpan.

The compresses, which were rolled strips covered with Koroseal, would not stay on the legs if the patient stood. It had taken the nurse 15 minutes to prepare the application, and she had to be in class before she would have time to reapply compresses for the patient. What would you have done?

Suggested Reference Reading

"The evolution of a stupe kettle," Pauline Carlson; American Journal of Nursing, June, 1937.
"Improvising a hot pack," Sister M. Humilitas; American Journal of Nursing, June, 1937.
"The nurse in physical medicine," George Morris Piersol; American Journal of Nursing, July, 1945.
"Deep freeze unit for ice bags," Fred G. Carter; American Journal of Nursing, March, 1948.
"Keeping hot packs hot," American Journal of Nursing, July, 1952.

CHAPTER 26

Preoperative Care

TOPICAL OUTLINE

Physical Preparation
Mental Preparation
Spiritual Preparation
Immediate Preoperative Nursing Care
Duties of Nurse while Patient Is in Surgery

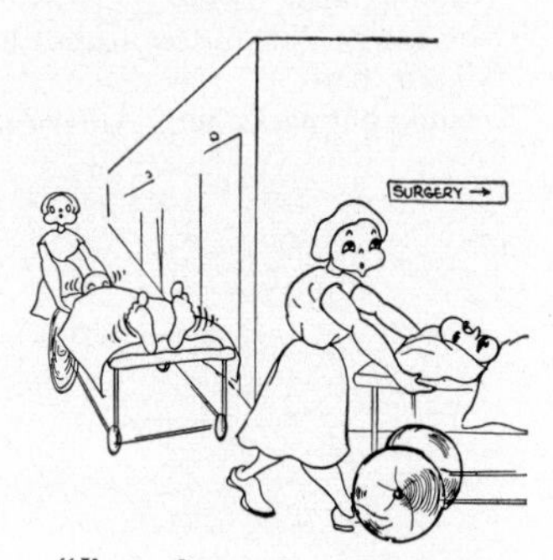

"I've changed my mind!"

Many patients enter a hospital with dread and apprehension, and quite often the patient being admitted for surgical treatment experiences fright that is nearly akin to terror. An understanding and sympathetic nurse can help to overcome this extreme fear by supporting the confidence the patient has in his doctor and by building up confidence in the medical and nursing staff at the hospital. Whatever sympathy she may feel for the patient should not be expressed in words or actions since it might serve only to increase his fear and anxiety regarding the proposed surgical procedure.

Regardless of the kind of surgery planned, the patient requires special physical, mental, and spiritual preparation which calls for skillful and thoughtful care on the part of the nursing personnel.

PHYSICAL PREPARATION

Physical preparation of the patient for surgery is still an important part of preoperative care, although it no longer is the only form of preparation with which doctors and nurses are concerned. The most important factor of total physical preparation of the patient is the complete physical examination, which determines largely whether or not surgical treatment should be undertaken.

Physical Examination. The surgeon in charge of the operation, or a doctor designated to act for him, should perform the following preoperative procedure: carefully examine the patient to determine if surgical risk is too great, recognize any indication for postponement of surgery, decide what diagnostic laboratory procedures are indicated, and decide on the type of anesthesia which should be administered.

Personal History. In addition to the physical examination, a complete personal history should be taken and properly recorded. Such a history includes family history as well as past and present medical history of the patient. It includes, too, information on childhood diseases, previous operations, and serious illnesses or injuries which the patient may have had in recent years. The report should include an explanation as to the onset of the present complaint and a detailed description of symptoms.

Laboratory Tests. All surgical patients are subjected to routine laboratory tests which include complete blood count (red cell count, white cell count, hemoglobin content), differential count of white cells, coagulation time, urinalysis, and Wassermann reaction (to determine presence of syphilis). Other laboratory tests may be indicated for patients with complicating conditions, such as diabetes mellitus or cardiac or renal disease.

The patient's blood pressure should be taken and recorded at the time of the physical examination, to provide a reading for comparison with those which will be made during and after the operation.

Food and Fluids. Food is given the patient the day preceding surgery, but should consist of so-called "light" foods which are nourishing yet easily digested. Additional carbohydrate (sugar in the form of orange juice or other sweetened fruit juce) should be taken to provide more energy to heart muscles and to prevent acidosis following the operation.

Fluids are given freely to the patient for a few days before operation and water may be given to within four hours of the time scheduled for the operative procedure. In some cases water is given to within two hours or less of the designated time for the operation. One of the greatest reasons for discomfort immediately after surgery is thirst, and the surgeon who permits water to be given until within a few hours of the operation does so in an effort to alleviate postoperative thirst of the patient. Such excessive thirst is caused not only by loss of blood during the operation but by profuse perspiration immediately after surgery, by emesis, in which more body fluids may be lost, and by the restriction of fluids postoperatively. Intravenous fluids help prevent postoperative shock, as does the administration of blood or blood plasma.

Enema. A cleansing enema of soapsuds or saline is usually given a few hours before the operation. This prevents involuntary defecation during surgery when the sphincter muscle of the rectum is relaxed from anesthesia. A cleansing enema also tends to reduce nausea and

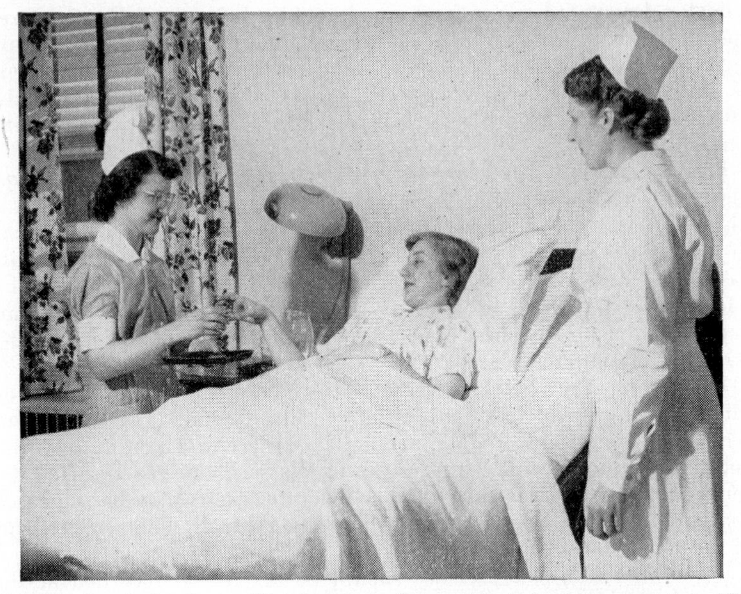

Fig. 161. A sedative is usually administered the night before the operation. (St. Luke's Hospital School of Nursing, Denver, Colorado.)

vomiting after surgery and lessens the formation of gas in the intestines which causes distention and the discomfort commonly referred to as "gas pains."

Skin Preparation. Shaving and cleansing of the skin of the operative field, a very important factor in the physical preparation for surgery, is usually done the evening before the operation is scheduled to take place. The area to be shaved and cleaned and the way in which this is done varies in different hospitals and with different surgeons. All phases of the skin preparation procedure should be done by nurses specially trained in operating room technique, so no detailed instructions are included here. The nurse giving general preoperative care need only make certain that the area involved is clean and ready for the special skin preparation procedures that will be used to render the operative field as nearly sterile as possible.

Sedation. The night before surgery, the patient is usually given a sedative which insures sleep and thus lessens anxiety and fear in regard to the impending operation. If the sedative medication is not ordered in sufficient amount to cause the patient to sleep and he is still awake and restless after a few hours, the nurse should report to the attending physician or resident doctor so a second dose of the drug may be administered if indicated.

Care of Dentures, Other Prostheses, and Valuables. Unless the anesthetist specifies otherwise, dentures should be removed, wrapped in a piece of gauze and submerged in a glass (or other suitable container) of water. The receptacle in which the dentures are placed should be properly labeled to prevent breakage of teeth or their removal from the room and subsequent loss.

Some artificial teeth are not removable and the anesthetist should be notified that such is the case so he will not break a very expensive denture in a futile attempt to remove it from the patient's mouth.

Artificial eyes or other prostheses should be removed and carefully labeled and put away for safekeeping while the patient is in the operating room and until such time as he has sufficiently recovered so that he may require their use again.

Large sums of money, expensive jewelry, and other articles of value which the patient may possess should be given to the closest relative for safekeeping while the patient is in the operating room and during the first few postoperative days.

If valuables are not given to a relative they should be placed in a special envelope provided by the hospital, with each article listed on the outside. The envelope should be sealed in the presence of the patient and a responsible witness and then placed in the hospital safe until the patient has recovered sufficiently to be responsible for the articles.

If the patient is wearing a wedding ring and dislikes having it removed, it should be securely tied to her wrist by means of 1-inch bandage or fastened to her finger with strips of adhesive tape so there will be no danger of its accidental loss in the operating room.

MENTAL PREPARATION

Doctors and nurses now recognize the close relationship existing between the physical and mental condition of a patient and know the important part mental attitude plays in achieving physical recovery. To successfully prepare the patient for the procedure of surgical operation attention must be directed toward mental characteristics which will markedly influence physical reaction.

Fear of the Operation. A surgical operation may assume major proportions for the person concerned, and regardless of whether the operation is *major* or *minor* the mental stress and strain may cause more harm to the patient than the physical condition for which surgery is being done.

Even patients who are suffering physical pain or disability and are convinced that relief can be obtained only by surgical treatment may have definite feelings of doubt and anxiety. The nurse should encourage the patient to talk about a forthcoming operation and to express his fear and concern. By a few well chosen remarks in regard to the rapid recovery made by other patients who submitted to the same operation she may reassure the patient and relieve tension caused by worry. An explanation of the necessity for the operation, mentioning factors already brought to the attention of the patient by his doctor, will tend to quiet the patient who may be inclined to feel that he should have refused surgery or at least postponed it for a time.

His fear may be chiefly concerned with the mysteries of anesthesia, and a brief explanation by the nurse as to modern means of producing satisfactory anesthesia may suffice to overcome fear and dread.

Whatever the cause of mental unrest, the nurse should do her utmost to dispel unnecessary fear and worry. Her obvious familiarity with hospital routine and her apparent assumption that the surgical procedure is merely a temporary interruption of nursing care given the patient on the clinical department makes it easier for the patient to accept surgical treatment.

Economic Problems. In addition to anxiety regarding the operation, the patient may be mentally disturbed because he is the sole support for his family. His concern for their welfare may be an even greater cause for worry than is his own physical condition. If his family will be unprovided for during his stay in the hospital and he is greatly worried by this fact, the nurse should suggest that the family seek help from community agencies which are established for just such needs. The patient who can be reassured by an understanding nurse, that his period of convalescence need not be prolonged and that his return to work and to the status of a wage-earner can be accomplished in a comparatively short time, will be mentally relieved and better able to adjust to the experience of undergoing surgical treatment.

Confidence in Doctors and Nurses. The nurse should let the patient know that she believes he has chosen wisely in selecting the doctor who is to perform the necessary surgical operation. Even though the patient may have complete confidence in the ability and skill of his doctor he will like to have that confidence confirmed by a nurse who works with the doctor and is in an excellent position to evaluate his qualifications for doing the operative procedure. If the surgeon is not one the nurse would have chosen were she herself to undergo surgical treatment, she should still bolster the patient's confidence and trust in the doctor by indicating that she has the utmost confidence in his ability. The confidence the patient has in his doctor plays an important part in his reaction to surgical treatment, and the nurse should never, by statement or by implication, cause doubt in the mind of the patient regarding the skill or ability of his attending physician or surgeon.

By performing nursing duties efficiently and quietly, and by being skillful in her own work, the nurse may gain the confidence of the patient who can then mentally relax, certain that he has placed his physical well-being in the hands of competent medical and nursing personnel.

Permit for Surgery. A written permit must be signed before surgery can be performed. If the patient is of legal age, he must be thoroughly informed as to the meaning of the permit before he is asked to sign it. If he is under legal age or is unable to sign, the permit must be signed by a close relative who is considered legally responsible for the patient. The signed permit is a protection for the doctor and for the hospital, and the nurse should accept the responsibility for making sure that the patient's signature is obtained well in advance of the time surgery is scheduled. No court would accept the signature of a patient who had been wakened from a preoperative narcotic or sedative and forced to sign the permit which the nurse had carelessly forgotten and which must be properly executed before the operation can take place.

Notification to the Family. The family of the patient should be notified in advance as to the date and exact time the operation is to be performed. If possible, members of the family should be present at the hospital during the operation, although they should not expect to accompany the patient to surgery or to be permitted to attend the operation. In some instances the patient will request that his family not be notified. If such a patient is under age, the request will have to be ignored, since a member of the family must legally be responsible for signing the permit. If the patient is of age and has signed the permit, the request may be honored, although some provision should be made to notify a close friend or other person who could be at the hospital during the operation.

SPIRITUAL PREPARATION

Associated with fear and mental anxiety so often felt by the preoperative patient is the need and desire for spiritual aid resulting from worry over the outcome of the operation.

Request Must Come from the Patient. No nurse should ever suggest to a patient that he ought to seek religious guidance before he submits to a surgical operation. To do so is to imply that the operation may not be successful and that recovery is, at best, very doubtful. Such an implication would cause the most quiet and resigned patient to become emotionally upset and seriously concerned as to his prognosis.

The request for spiritual help must originate with the patient, but once such a request is made the nurse is obligated to comply, whether it is to call a minister, priest, or rabbi, or to read from the Bible whatever verses the patient would like to hear.

When a patient has requested spiritual aid and the clergyman arrives in answer to that request, the nurse should see that absolute privacy is provided. The spiritual adviser, through his training and experience, is best fitted to help the patient and they should be left alone so both may talk freely without thought of another person being within hearing distance. Benefits to be derived from the presence of the clergyman will more than justify any effort which may be involved in making arrangements for his visit.

Special services of a religious nature which may be required for patients of certain faiths are discussed in Chapter 37, "Spiritual Needs of the Patient."

IMMEDIATE PREOPERATIVE NURSING CARE

Nursing care given just before surgery has been clearly defined and is basically the same in hospitals throughout the country. The nurse assigned to preparation of the patient for surgery is expected to perform the following nursing procedures: taking temperature, pulse, respiration, and blood pressure; observation for symptoms of cold; bath; care of mouth; care of hair; attention to voiding; correct apparel for the operating room; administration of preoperative medication; explanation and instruction to visitors; and transfer of the patient to surgery.

Temperature, Pulse, Respiration and Blood Pressure. The nurse responsible for the immediate preoperative care of the patient should take and record temperature, pulse, and respiration. If the temperature is elevated, that fact should be reported to the nurse in charge who will inform the surgeon. Blood pressure should be taken and recorded at the same time the temperature is taken.

Observation for Symptoms of Common Cold. While taking the temperature the nurse should be observant for signs of head cold, sore throat, or interference with normal respiration; any one of these symptoms may be sufficient cause for postponement of the operation. Any signs which indicate that the patient has a cold should be reported to the nurse in charge, who will report to the attending physician. The abnormality in respiration caused by manifestations of the common cold may have an important effect on the patient's tolerance for general anesthesia.

Bath. A bath should be given the patient unless a tub bath was taken previous to admission and the patient is to go to the operating room soon after being admitted.

Care of Mouth. The mouth should be thoroughly cleansed and teeth brushed to insure mouth cleanliness during and immediately after the operation.

Care of Hair. Hair should be neatly combed. If the patient has long hair, all hairpins should be removed and the hair braided loosely into two braids; if it is tightly braided it may be very uncomfortable for the patient. The braids should be securely fastened at the ends with rubber bands or a piece of 1-inch bandage.

Attention to Voiding. Before being transferred to the operating room the patient should be placed on a bed pan or given a urinal and encouraged to empty the bladder. This prevents involuntary urination on the operating table and may prevent accidental injury to the bladder during the operation.

If the patient is unable to void the operating room nurse and the

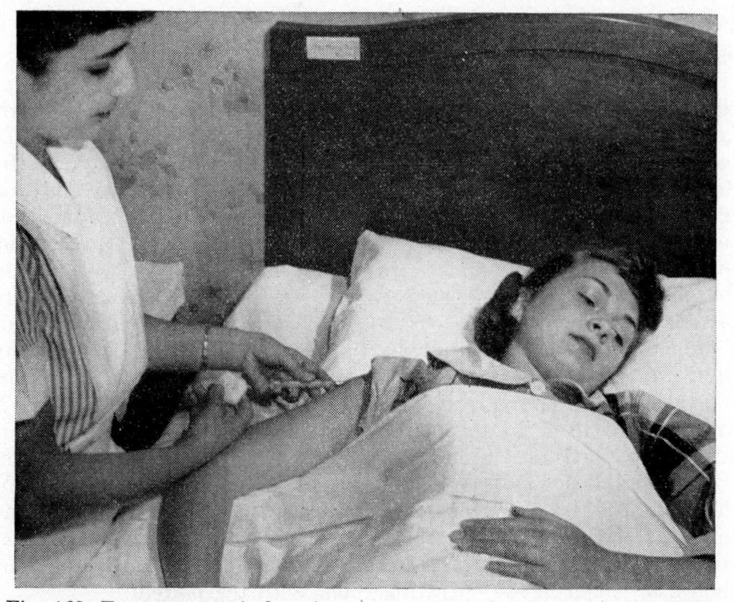

Fig. 162. For some surgical patients preparation for surgery begins several days before the scheduled operation. (Delaware Hospital School of Nursing, Wilmington, Delaware.)

surgeon should be notified and the failure to void should be recorded on the chart. Some surgeons ask that the patient be catheterized in the operating room, to make certain that the bladder is empty. Such precautions are necessary in abdominal surgery, and are especially important in surgery of the pelvic region.

Correct Apparel for the Surgical Patient. The usual attire for the patient being prepared for surgery consists of a cap, which may be of stockinette material and made in rounded shape, or of cotton material cut in triangular shape, worn to keep the patient's hair confined and to prevent chilliness.

The standard hospital gown which reaches only to the patient's thigh and is fastened in the back is required for wear by all patients being received in the operating room.

Surgical stockings or leggings are provided as part of the suitable operating room dress to partially clothe the patient and help keep him warm during and immediately after surgery.

Administration of Preoperative Medication. The drug used as preliminary medication for surgery is selected in accordance with the wishes of the surgeon, and doctors differ in their choice.

It is almost standard practice to give morphine, which makes the patient drowsy and relaxed, and atropine, which decreases the secretion of saliva and mucus in the mouth and thus facilitates the giving of inhalation anesthesia. Preoperative medication is usually administered by the nurse about 30 minutes before the operation.

Explanation and Instruction to Visitors. After the preoperative narcotic has been given the nurse should explain to members of the family, or to friends who are present, that it is necessary for the patient to refrain from talking and to have the room quiet and restful. Relatives and others should be asked to leave the room and wait in a nearby waiting room or lounge. If the patient wishes one close relative to remain in his room such a request should be granted, but the relative should be instructed not to carry on conversation with the patient and to remain absolutely quiet so the patient may receive benefit from the preoperative drug that was given. Window shades should be drawn or blinds partially closed and all unnecessary lights should be turned off to promote an atmosphere of quiet and relaxation. All nursing duties should have been performed prior to or immediately after the medication was given, and the patient should not be disturbed until time for him to be taken to the operating room.

Transfer of the Patient to Surgery. The nurse should accompany the patient to the operating room, walking at the head of the stretcher so that the patient is reassured by her presence. The chart, complete with all necessary notations relative to preoperative nursing care, should be taken to the operating room with the patient.

When the stretcher is brought to the room for the patient the nurse and orderly should assist the patient in getting on the stretcher, and care should be taken not to jerk or jar the patient during transfer to the surgical department. The elevator floor should be at exact floor level when the stretcher is wheeled into the elevator, and it should be operated smoothly with no sudden stops or starts to jostle or disturb the patient.

In surgery, if the patient is required to wait for a few minutes, the stretcher should be wheeled into a comfortable and quiet waiting room provided for that purpose. There is little use to provide excellent care and conditions for the preoperative patient on the clinical division of the hospital and bring him to the surgical department with only a minimum of nervousness or apprehension, and then subject him to the terrifying experience of waiting for a long period of time in a brightly lighted, well traveled corridor where all his fears and anxieties return in greater degree than before. Under such conditions, when he is finally wheeled into the operating room, he may well be so tense and fearful that the problem of administering a successful anesthetic is greater than it would otherwise have been.

DUTIES OF NURSE WHILE PATIENT IS IN SURGERY

When the nurse has accompanied the patient to the operating room and leaves the chart in the proper hands, her immediate duties to the patient end and she is expected to return to the clinical department to continue her duties there.

Preparation of Room for Patient's Return. The nurse will need to prepare the room for the return of the patient from surgery if there is no postoperative recovery room in that department. The standard anesthetic bed, as described in Chapter 7, should be made up in the patient's room.

Articles which may be needed in caring for the postoperative patient should be provided, including two emesis basins, a package of Celluwipes or paper handkerchiefs, padded tongue depressors, paper scratch pad and pencil for noting blood pressure, pulse, respiration, and other data pertinent to the immediate postoperative condition of the patient. A paper bag should be pinned to the side of the mattress near the head of the bed. The sphygmomanometer, if not in use on the department, and a stethoscope may be placed in the room to be available when needed. If the nature of the operation is such that special equipment, such as shock blocks, hot water bottles, oxygen tent or equipment for nasal administration of oxygen, electric suction machine, or special drainage bottles, may be needed, the equipment should be obtained and placed where it can be reached conveniently.

The room should be cleaned and aired, and blinds should be opened to permit sunshine to enter. All old magazines, newspapers, etc., should be discarded. Furnishings and equipment should be arranged in an orderly fashion. The temperature of the room should be correctly adjusted to the needs of the returning patient and care must be taken to prevent drafts.

Reassurance of the Family. During the operation the period of waiting is a time of extreme anxiety for the patient's family. An understanding nurse will go to the operating rooms once or twice (if the patient is subjected to prolonged surgery) to learn the condition of the patient. Anxious relatives and friends should be given, if possible, an estimate of the time which will elapse before the patient can be returned to the room.

The nurse should not give the relatives information regarding the findings of the surgeon. Information of this nature will be given the family by the surgeon who visits the patient soon after the operation is completed and then reports to the family on the results of surgical treatment and the physical condition of the patient.

Care of Equipment after Use

Equipment used in giving care to the preoperative patient depends on the kind of surgical treatment to be performed. The care of equipment has been discussed in previous chapters in which the various routine nursing procedures have been described.

Summary of Important Factors

Preoperative care involves preparation of the patient for surgery from the physical, mental, and spiritual standpoint.

Physical examination and personal history may reveal factors that must be carefully considered in preparing the patient for surgery.

Temperature, pulse, respiration, and blood pressure should be taken before surgery for comparison with those taken during and after surgery.

Light, easily digested food should be served the preoperative patient the day before surgery. Fluids may be given up to a few hours before surgery, depending on the doctor's orders.

Thirst, following a surgical procedure, may be caused by loss of blood during operation, perspiration, restriction of fluids, and emesis.

A cleansing enema, before surgery, will tend to prevent distention and reduce postoperative nausea and vomiting.

Skin preparation is usually the responsibility of operating room personnel.

Sedation is usually ordered the night before operation to insure rest and sleep for the patient.

Dentures and other prosthetic appliances should be removed before the patient is taken to the operating room.

Valuables should be cared for by a relative or placed in the hospital safe.

Fear and worry should be relieved by the nurse through explanation of benefits to be derived from surgery, expression of confidence in the doctor, and suggestions for solving economic or social problems.

A written permit for surgery must be signed, by the patient if he is of age; if he is under age a responsible relative should sign for him.

The family should be notified of the date and exact time of operation, and a member of the family should be at the hospital during the operation.

Spiritual aid should be at the patient's request, not suggested by the nurse.

Symptoms of a common cold may indicate need to postpone the operation.

Shortly before going to surgery the patient should void; if unable to void, he may need to be catheterized.

After the preoperative narcotic has been given the patient should not be disturbed by relatives or friends.

The nurse who gives preoperative care to a patient should accompany him to the operating room.

The return of the patient from surgery requires special preparation of the bed and of equipment for the bedside table.

Reassurance of the family during the operation is a responsibility of the nurse.

Information to the family as to the extent of surgery and probable outcome should be given by the doctor.

Factors To Teach the Patient

Complete cooperation in giving medical history will aid the doctor in making diagnosis and determining the extent of surgery required.

Preparation for surgery, adequately done, will lessen discomfort during the immediate postoperative period.

Valuables should be entrusted to a relative or placed in the hospital safe until the patient can again assume responsibility for their care.

Modern methods of operating room procedure reduce danger to the patient.

Social agencies that are interested in helping solve his economic or social problems.

The meaning of the surgical permit and why he is asked to sign it.

That a member of his family or a very close friend should be at the hospital during the operation. Decisions affecting his physical condition may need to be made when he is unable to make them for himself.

The desire for spiritual aid and encouragement is experienced by most preoperative patients.

The purpose of the preoperative narcotic and need for quiet and rest after it has been given.

That personnel in the operating room are just as interested in his welfare as those with whom he has become acquainted in the clinical department.

Scientific Principles

Anatomy and Physiology. A preoperative bath should be given to free the skin of perspiration, dirt, and waste before an operation is performed.

In all operations in which an incision must be made through the skin the area must be shaved and made as clean as possible. In orthopedic surgery special skin preparation (treatment with alcohol or other strong antiseptic and protection with sterile towel covering) is required to help prevent infection.

Fluids are limited for several hours preceding surgery to avoid nausea and vomiting as postoperative complications.

Diet is restricted to facilitate the giving of an anesthetic and to reduce the possibility of gastric complications.

Dentures and other prostheses should not be worn to the operating room.

A complete physical examination is required for the preoperative patient except in cases of an emergency nature.

All vital centers are depressed by the action of a general anesthetic.

Chemistry. Diagnosis of various conditions requiring surgical treatment may be made through chemical tests used to detect occult blood in the stool.

Chemical elements of the blood may be affected by the administration of an anesthetic, with acidosis resulting.

Pharmacology. A sedative is given to insure rest and sleep the night before operation.

A preoperative medication may be given hypodermically to prevent excessive secretion from the respiratory tract, to promote relaxation, and to help prevent shock.

Each anesthetic drug produces a characteristic reaction in the body.

Physics. The patient should be protected from drafts and the possibility of taking cold.

Coagulation time must be determined preoperatively.

Nail polish and cosmetics should be removed so the patient may be closely observed for change of color by the anesthetist.

Ether and chloroform are volatile and diffuse rapidly through the air.

Psychology. The patient may desire spiritual help and be reluctant to request it—the nurse may mention religious services which are available without seeming to suggest that there is *need* for spiritual aid.

A patient who dreads or fears surgery may benefit by talking with other patients who have had the same experience.

The patient who fears pain and discomfort following operation should be reassured by the nurse with an explanation of the use of narcotics as needed to relieve pain. She should also explain that doses of narcotics are gradually reduced in size and frequency, so there is no danger of resultant addiction.

The presence of the nurse is comforting to the patient, and she should accompany him to the operating room.

Sociology. Relatives should be advised not to worry or distress the patient by discussion of family or financial problems, and should be instructed not to attempt to carry on conversation with him after the preoperative narcotic has been given.

The relatives should be informed of the approximate time that will be required for the operation. During the operation they should receive a report at intervals to reassure them as to the condition of the patient.

Foreign-born patients may need to be given instructions or an explanation of various procedures in their own language. Procedures should be explained in simple terms to the patient with limited educational background.

Religious and social welfare organizations may need to be informed of needs of the patient.

Overanxious relatives convey anxiety to the patient and may cause mental strain or apprehension.

For a child or mentally incompetent adult the operative permit must be signed by a person responsible for his welfare.

Situation Type Problems

1. A student nurse, assigned to give preoperative care to a patient who was scheduled to have major surgery done, had completed all

the necessary procedures and administered the preoperative narcotic when the patient's wife came into the room. She ignored the presence of the nurse and began an animated conversation with the patient, as follows, "I'd have been here sooner, but the car just doesn't work right. I told you, John, a week ago you should have it in for check up. You look ghastly, didn't you sleep last night? Oh, well, you'll be here long enough, you'll get a good rest. You know Mr. Hart had much the same kind of operation four months ago and he said he still doesn't dare do much. He came over to borrow the lawn mower, said he'd just keep it until you get home again. Well, I did tell him that you'd just had it sharpened. I couldn't very well refuse to loan it to him, could I?"

The nurse signaled the patient's wife to come out into the hall and once out of hearing of the patient she explained to her that the patient had had a hypodermic injection which would make him very drowsy and that he should not attempt to converse with her. She asked the wife to refrain from talking to the patient, but to sit quietly in the room until the stretcher came to take him to the operating room.

A few minutes later the nurse entered the room again to find the wife of the patient reprimanding him for not paying attention to what she was trying to say when it was of vital importance to both of them. She explained to the nurse that she had just remembered to ask the patient about payments of his life insurance. "He is so forgetful I have to constantly check on such things, and certainly this is no time to get careless with his insurance."

The nurse again beckoned the wife to withdraw from the room and when they were in the corridor she suggested that it would be preferable for her to wait in a lounge at the end of the corridor. The wife resented being asked to wait elsewhere than in the patient's room and informed the nurse that so long as she was paying for the hospital room she felt she had every right to be in it whenever she chose. What would you have done?

Suggested Reference Reading

"Knowing about operations helps," Dorothy E. Curtis; American Journal of Nursing, January, 1943.

"Nursing care as related to anesthesia," T. H. Seldon, J. S. Lundy, and R. C. Adams; American Journal of Nursing, August, 1944.

"Nurse—listen please," Elizabeth Fink; American Journal of Nursing, January, 1951.

"I'm going to have an operation," May Richstone; Today's Health, July, 1952.

"Anxiety—a factor in nursing care," Dorothy E. Gregg; American Journal of Nursing, November, 1952.

CHAPTER 27

Postoperative Care

TOPICAL OUTLINE

IMMEDIATE POSTOPERATIVE CARE
GENERAL POSTOPERATIVE CARE
POSTOPERATIVE COMPLICATIONS
  Hiccup—Shock—Hemorrhage—Distention
  Pulmonary Complications
  Cardiovascular Complications
  Renal Complications
  Wound Infections
EARLY AMBULATION

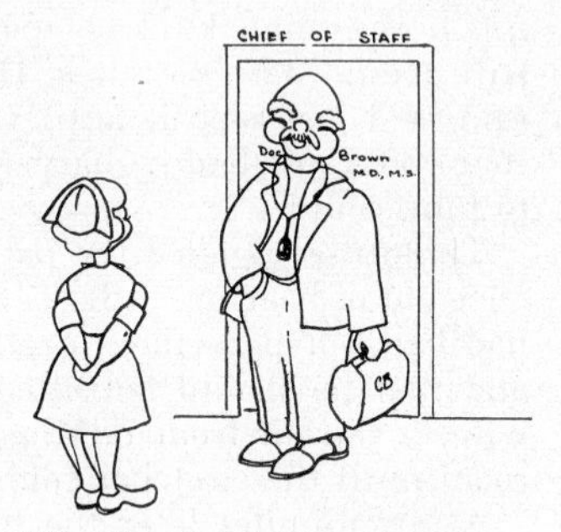

"You have to do your own growing—no matter how tall your grandfather is!"

The nurse in charge of a patient who has just returned from the operating room will need to practice a goodly number of skills she has attained and put into use the knowledge that is hers. She will need to be keenly observant of the patient's general condition, to recognize early symptoms of a change in condition, and to be capable of performing the required nursing procedures in a calm and efficient manner. The safety of the patient may depend on her degree of nursing skill and her ability to properly evaluate his needs.

IMMEDIATE POSTOPERATIVE CARE

Receiving Patient in the Recovery Room. In many hospitals the newly operated patient is transferred from the operating room to a recovery room where he remains several hours after operation. Care should be taken to avoid jarring the patient, he must be lifted with great care, especially if he is unconscious from anesthesia and is thus completely relaxed. He should be well covered with blankets to prevent chilling as he is transported by stretcher from one room to another. In the recovery room the patient should be placed in the bed

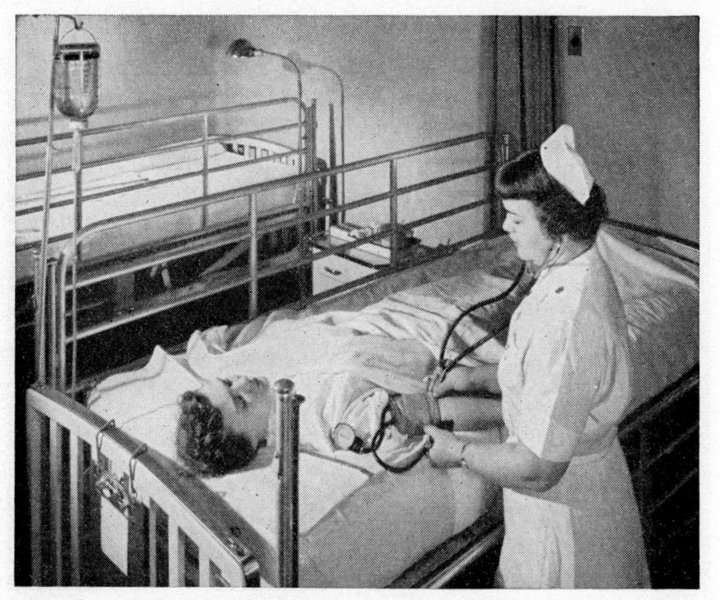

Fig. 163. The anesthetic bed is needed for the postoperative patient. (Presbyterian Hospital School of Nursing, Chicago, Illinois.)

which has been brought there from the room he occupies on the clinical division of the hospital.

In lifting the patient from the stretcher to the bed his body should be well supported and kept in a straight line position. Sudden, jerky movements, as well as strain on the operative area, should be carefully avoided. If the head of the stretcher is placed at right angles to the foot of the bed three persons, the anesthetist, orderly, and nurse, standing side by side in the order named, with the anesthetist at the patient's shoulders, may lift the patient and, supporting his weight against their chests, walk together toward the head of the bed and deposit him safely and gently on the bed. Care should be taken to avoid exposing the patient unnecessarily as the transfer is being made.

When the patient has been placed in bed he should be turned to one side, unless that position is contraindicated. With the head turned to one side respiration is facilitated and the danger of aspiration is lessened. The arms should be flexed in front of the body, the lower leg extended until it is almost straight, and the upper leg flexed. A pillow may be placed between the legs and another at the back, with a small pillow against the abdomen to relieve strain on that part of the body.

The patient should quickly be placed in the position described above and the top covers should immediately be brought into position over him to keep him warm. Care must be taken that he isn't made

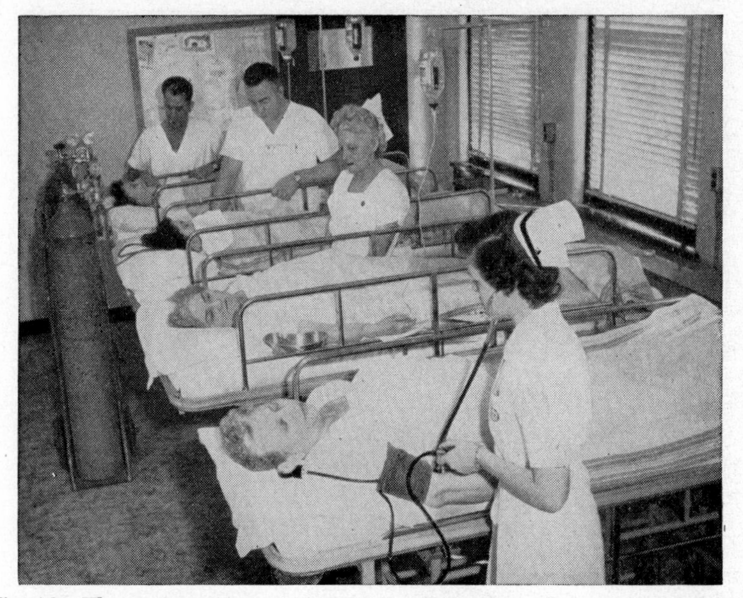

Fig. 164. The postoperative patient may be retained in the recovery room for several hours. (Ravenswood Hospital School of Nursing, Chicago, Illinois.)

so warm that profuse perspiration occurs, with resultant excessive loss of body fluids.

The cap and leggings worn during the operation may be removed soon after the patient is placed in bed.

Observing the Patient. The newly operated patient should not be left alone until he has reacted from the anesthetic and is fully aware of his surroundings. The nurse should observe and record the time the patient is brought from the operating room, the pulse and respiration rate, and the color and condition of his skin, which should be warm and moist. Immediately after surgery the patient's pulse may be rapid; however, it should soon return to its normal rate. Pulse rate should be taken every few minutes and recorded every 5 to 10 minutes until the patient regains consciousness. Blood pressure should be taken several times postoperatively at intervals of about 15 minutes.

Minor movements of the patient should not be restrained, since restraint would increase restlessness. If necessary to prevent injury to himself or others, a very restless patient may be properly restrained.

Close observation of the dressing over the wound should be part of the immediate postoperative care, to detect early symptoms of excessive drainage or of hemorrhage.

Respiration. Immediately after surgery respirations should be regular and fairly deep. Any sudden change should be noted as it may be

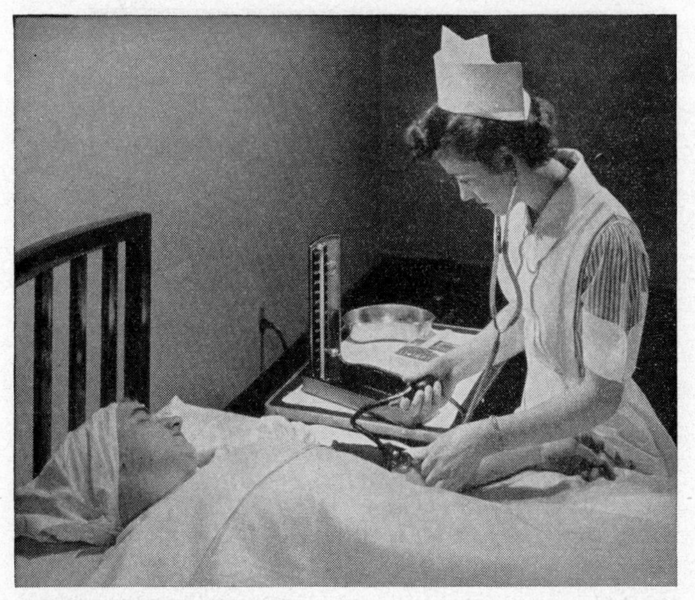

Fig. 165. Blood pressure should be taken at frequent intervals postoperatively. (St. Luke's Methodist Hospital School of Nursing, Cedar Rapids, Iowa.)

caused by an obstruction in the throat, especially if it is accompanied by cyanosis or change of color in the skin. If the obstruction is caused by retraction of the tongue, this condition may be relieved by exerting pressure on the angle of the lower jaw, pushing it forward while keeping the mouth open. If necessary, an airway may be inserted to insure proper passage of air into the lungs.

Pain. As the patient reacts from anesthesia he is apt to become increasingly uncomfortable because of pain at the site of operation. To prevent the pain and other unpleasant effects many surgeons order morphine to be given soon after the operation has been completed. For major surgery, morphine, or some other drug ordered for relief of pain, is usually given every 4 hours for several doses. Since morphine is a respiratory depressant the rate of respiration should be carefully watched. If it is decreased to 14 or less per minute the interval between doses of morphine will need to be lengthened. Since morphine is habit forming its continued use is undesirable and another drug may be substituted if the need for such relief is prolonged.

If pain is due to pressure from safety pins, rubber drains, or a too tight dressing or binder, the nurse should be aware of the fact and, if possible, alter the condition to give relief to the patient.

Complaints of muscle stiffness or of an ill-defined muscular ache in back or limbs may be caused by a restricted or unnatural position.

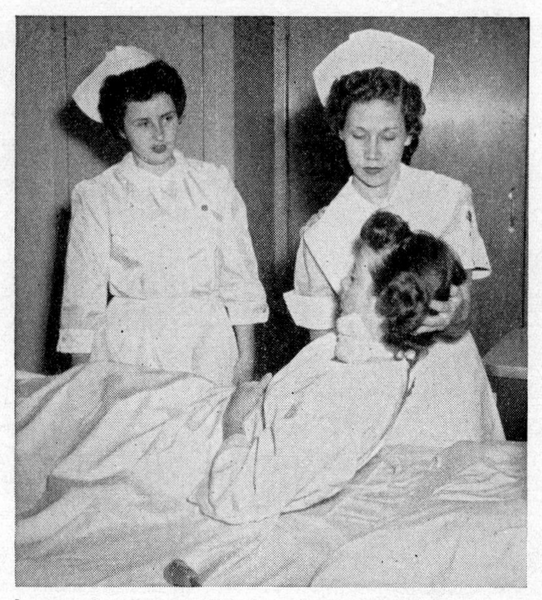

Fig. 166. A change of position will help relieve the patient of muscular discomfort. (Baylor University School of Nursing, Waco, Texas.)

Such discomfort will usually be relieved by change of position, by gentle massage, or by rearrangement of supporting pillows. Reassurance to the patient as to satisfactory progress toward recovery should frequently be given.

Severe headache may be caused by effects of the anesthetic, by nervousness, or by an overheated room. Absolute quiet, fresh air, and an ice cap to the head will usually afford relief. Visitors should be excluded, and the nurse should be extremely quiet in all her movements about the room.

Prolonged and persistent pain and discomfort should be brought to the attention of the surgeon.

Thirst. Excessive thirst after surgery is caused by loss of fluid from body tissues. The blood lost from the circulatory system at the time of operation is partially compensated for by withdrawal of fluid from the tissues, and profuse perspiration causes an additional loss of fluid.

As soon as nausea and vomiting have ceased the patient may be given water in very small amounts. Some surgeons insist that only hot water be given, others permit the patient to have small amounts of cool water or chips of ice. All agree that ice water should be withheld since it is thought to cause abdominal distention.

If sufficient fluid cannot be given by mouth it may be administered by various other means, such as intravenous or subcutaneous injection.

The postoperative patient will be more comfortable if a mouth wash is used to keep his mouth fresh and moist, and if his lips are kept moistened to prevent the parched sensation usually caused by excessive dryness.

Nausea and Vomiting. After administration of a general anesthetic the patient usually experiences a period of nausea and vomiting. With modern methods of anesthesia the duration of nausea has been markedly decreased, lasting less than an hour or so after the patient has regained consciousness. In cases of persistent nausea and vomiting Wangensteen suction may be employed to bring relief.

Vomiting, if continued, may cause dehydration, and it is well to give fluids to replace those lost. If the patient is unable to take fluids by mouth it may be necessary to give the needed fluids intravenously. Nausea may be somewhat controlled by judicious use of morphine to induce rest. Some postoperative patients will be relieved of nausea and vomiting by drinking water. Water taken by mouth may temporarily increase nausea for a very short time and then serve to control completely postoperative nausea and vomiting.

Apprehension. When the postoperative patient begins to react from anesthesia he may be exceedingly apprehensive; he is fearful of experiencing pain, worried about the results of the operation, and afraid of being nauseated and of being left alone. During the initial period of returning consciousness the patient needs to be assured that he is back in his bed, that the operation is over, that he is in good condition, and that now rest and quiet will effect complete recovery.

At this time the nurse should be constantly at the bedside, since the patient wakens at frequent intervals and needs the feeling of security and comfort which her presence will give him. Relieved of anxiety and sure that he is being cared for by a competent nurse, the patient will often relax and sleep quietly for several hours.

Restlessness and Sleeplessness. As rest is an essential factor in the recovery of the postoperative patient, the nurse must provide conditions conducive to rest and sleep. In addition to the narcotic ordered for relief of pain, usually a mild hypnotic or sedative should be used to insure adequate rest. Restlessness and sleeplessness can be prevented if the nurse will thoughtfully keep room temperature properly regulated, prevent unnecessary noise, and keep the patient comfortable by the use of pillows and change of position when indicated.

GENERAL POSTOPERATIVE CARE

Whether the first few days after surgery are to be days of never-ending discomfort and fatigue or a rather hazy, not unpleasant time of only partial awareness of immediate surroundings depends on the ability and skillfulness of the nurse. If she understands the needs of the patient and acts to provide them she will contribute much to his comfort and welfare. She will understand that she should not "fuss over" him or tire him out by too much attention to details involved in nursing care. For the first day or two after surgery she should be as inconspicuous as possible—performing procedures that are necessary but adjusting them to fit the needs of the patient. She must protect him from anxious relatives and friends and help him conserve energy and gain strength.

General care of the postoperative patient usually requires that a daily bath be given and linen changed. An alcohol back rub after the bath will refresh the patient and keep the skin in good condition. The mouth should be given special care to keep it clean and fresh. A mouthwash may be used soon after the patient has reacted from the anesthetic. No attempt should be made to brush the teeth soon after surgery, since the procedure is very tiring and might tend to increase postoperative nausea.

Hair should be kept neatly combed. If the patient has long hair, it should be parted in the center and braided into two braids which are allowed to hang down the back.

During the first few days after surgery the physical needs of the patient are of paramount importance. As his physical condition improves and the operative wound heals, psychological needs begin to take precedence and the nurse must accept responsibility for keeping him comfortable and contented. Visitors may be permitted, at this time, in greater numbers, and should be encouraged to stay for a longer period of time. Occupational therapy should be provided to help strengthen weakened muscles and to promote a desirable mental attitude. The nurse should encourage the patient to begin to do things for himself, and by gradually withdrawing her aid to him she can facilitate his return to health and to a resumption of normal activities.

Diet. After surgery the diet, which is ordered by the doctor, varies according to the kind of surgical treatment that was done and the condition of the patient.

As soon as water can be tolerated it is given in small amounts, then in gradually increasing amounts until the patient may have all he wishes. The first diet given the patient usually consists of clear liquids only (broth, tea, and fruit juice). Milk is not included with a clear liquid diet. By the third day after operation the patient is usually given soft foods, such as eggs, cereals, and custards. Solid foods are gradually added to the diet until by the time the patient is able to be up and about he is allowed a fairly normal diet.

If the site of operation was not the abdomen or gastrointestinal tract, the patient may be given a general or normal diet very early in the postoperative period.

Elimination. Normally the postoperative patient should void within 8 to 10 hours after the operation, although a patient who is nervous or apprehensive may be unable to void for a much longer period. Doctors differ in their opinion on the length of time that should elapse before the patient is catheterized. The nurse does not catheterize a patient without an order from the doctor, but it is her responsibility to inform the surgeon if the patient has not voided after 10 to 12 hours. If failure to void causes abdominal distention or discomfort and all nursing measures to induce voiding have been employed without success, the doctor should be notified.

Since preoperative care included a cleansing enema and the postoperative diet is limited to liquids for the first 24 to 48 hours defecation is not expected until about the third postoperative day.

A mild laxative or low enema will probably be ordered when the patient begins to eat solid foods, or if he complains of abdominal distention. As the patient's physical condition improves and he is gradually able to take a normal diet and return to normal activities, a re-establishment of healthful evacuation habits should be encouraged by the nurse.

POSTOPERATIVE COMPLICATIONS

Although with modern methods of surgery the operative risk for the patient and the incidence of postoperative complications have been reduced, complications still occur and must still be given consideration by surgeon and nurse.

Very often the nurse, taught to be especially observant, is the first to detect early symptoms of the development of postoperative complications. Her management of the situation in a calm and efficient manner will prevent undue alarm on the part of the patient. A report of her observation of undesirable symptoms should be made immediately to the attending surgeon.

Hiccup. Hiccup is brought about by spasmodic contraction of the diaphragm and the sudden closing of the glottis. The cause is unknown, and the attack may vary from a mild episode lasting only a few minutes to a severe attack which may continue for such a long time that it becomes a serious complication.

The most commonly used treatment for hiccup is inhalation of a mixture of oxygen and carbon dioxide.

Shock. Shock is a condition of marked depression of practically all bodily functions, varying from a feeling of slight weakness to complete failure of vital organs to continue functioning.

The most important symptoms are a feeble, rapid, and irregular pulse, decreased blood pressure, and cyanosis or an ashen gray color of the skin. The patient is usually very apprehensive and wears a pinched and anxious expression. The skins feels cold and clammy, and the face is usually covered with perspiration. Extreme pain may be a contributing factor, as are strong emotions, such as grief and fear. In severe cases the patient may lose consciousness, and if the condition is not immediately and successfully treated death may ensue.

Treatment of shock includes administration of fluids (preferably whole blood or plasma) to restore blood volume, elevation of the foot of the bed to help supply blood to vital centers, application of external heat to help increase body temperature, and treatment to keep the patient free from pain.

Hemorrhage. Hemorrhage is sudden and excessive bleeding which may be clearly visible (*external*) or of an insidious nature (*internal*).

Hemorrhage may occur from an artery, with spurts of bright red blood, from a vein, marked by a steady flow of dark red blood, or from capillaries, with merely an oozing of blood.

The symptoms of hemorrhage may be very slight at first and go unnoticed unless the nurse is alert and watchful. The patient may complain of thirst or of some slight difficulty in breathing. As the hemorrhage is prolonged or increased in extent, symptoms become more pronounced. The patient may experience a ringing in the ears, with some dimness of vision and a definite feeling of apprehension. Pulse and respiration rate will be increased, the skin may be dry and warm, the face is flushed and wears a look of anxiety. The patient may become quite restless and show symptoms of marked air hunger as a result of the limited amount of oxygen being supplied the body.

When hemorrhage occurs its immediate control is of primary importance to doctor and nurse. Both should work quietly and without evident haste or concern.

The head of the bed should be lowered; if the bleeding is from an extremity, the part should be elevated and a tourniquet applied. The patient should be kept quiet, morphine being administered if necessary. Warm blankets should be used to supply additional warmth, and the patient will need to be protected from drafts.

If the hemorrhage is difficult to control, emergency treatment may need to be supplemented in the operating room by reopening of the wound and ligation of the bleeding vessels.

After the hemorrhage has been controlled a transfusion should be given to replace the blood lost. The patient should be left in the position described above. Fluids may be given by mouth, extra warmth should continue to be provided, and pulse and respiration as well as blood pressure should be checked at frequent intervals. Morphine or a similar drug may be given to keep the patient quiet, to relieve apprehension, and to insure rest.

Distention. After abdominal surgery patients usually have some degree of discomfort caused by distention. Distention is due to an accumulation of gas in the intestines, and "gas pains" are caused by muscular contractions occurring in an attempt to expel the gas.

Symptoms of distention are: complaints of cramplike pains from the patient, a characteristically tense and firmly rounded abdomen, and the presence of slight or excessive nausea.

Treatment consists of measures prescribed by the doctor, which may include application of heat to the abdomen, insertion of a colon tube into the rectum to facilitate expulsion of gas, an enema, and, if indicated, intubation with a Miller-Abbott tube.

Pulmonary Complications. Complications affecting the lungs have decreased in direct relationship to improvement in methods of administering anesthetic agents. However, some postoperative patients are still subject to pulmonary complications, the most common is that of *atelectasis* or partial lung collapse.

Symptoms are rapid, shallow breathing, cyanosis, and a sharp rise in temperature. This complication results when a mucus plug obstructs a large bronchus. If coughing fails to dislodge the plug, mechanical suction may need to be used.

Atelectasis may be prevented by altering the position of the patient frequently, and by having him perform deep breathing exercises and occasional coughing.

If atelectasis is not successfully treated, a more serious complication, postoperative pneumonia, may result. Symptoms are persistent coughing, rust-colored sputum, increased pulse and respiration rate, and a rapid increase in body temperature.

At the present time postoperative pneumonia does not occur as frequently as in the past. The complication is controlled largely through improved administration of anesthetics and the use of antibiotic drugs.

Cardiovascular Complications. Postoperative complications affecting the circulatory system usually are not apparent until the patient has reached the stage of convalescence. The most common is thought to result from inflammation of a vein (phlebitis). Inflammation leads to formation of a blood clot which adheres to the wall of the vein (thrombosis). If a portion of the clot breaks away and is free to move with the circulating blood, it becomes an embolus, which may lodge in a large pulmonary vessel, causing almost instant death. If a smaller vessel is occluded, the patient may complain of severe chest pain and difficult respiration. He may expectorate blood-tinged sputum. Usual treatment is absolute quiet and rest.

Surgeons who favor early ambulation for postoperative patients believe that such treatment is effective in decreasing the number of cardiovascular complications. Part of their postoperative treatment is encouragement of frequent turning of the patient, leg exercises for the bed patient, and anticoagulant therapy.

Surgical removal of an embolus is possible and may provide the patient a greater chance for recovery.

Renal Complications. Several factors may combine to cause urinary retention as a postoperative complication. The enforced horizontal position in bed, prolonged anesthesia, and nervousness on the part of the patient may cause inability to void.

Several measures the nurse may institute to induce urination are: providing the patient with absolute privacy, allowing him to sit or stand in an upright position while attempting to void, allowing him to hear the sound of running water, and pouring warm water over the external genitalia. If, after the above measures, the patient is still unable to void, the surgeon should be notified. Catheterization should be done before the bladder becomes overdistended, as marked distention decreases bladder tone and lessens resistance to infection which may be produced by bacteria normally present in the bladder.

A more serious renal complication is suppression of urine, in which the kidney fails to secrete urine. This complication may be caused by inflammation produced by the irritating effect of the anesthetic agent. Symptoms are scanty urine of low specific gravity, headache, dizziness, nausea and vomiting, puffiness of the eyes, and restlessness.

Measures which may be ordered for effecting improvement or recovery include forcing the patient to drink a large amount of fluids, giving hot enemas, and using hot packs to increase elimination of fluid through the skin. The doctor may order diuretic medication to be given orally or subcutaneously.

Wound Infection. Wound infections are usually caused by a break in aseptic technique by surgeon or nurse just before or during the operation. Such complications include stitch abscess, cellulitis, and wound disruption.

Stitch Abscess. Stitch abscess, which is one of the most common of wound infections, is recognized by symptoms which include tenderness, redness, and the appearance of pus around a suture. Temperature may increase suddenly or may be elevated for a longer period than is normally expected.

Treatment consists of drainage of the infected area and application of hot wet dressings until the wound has healed.

Cellulitis. Cellulitis is a generalized infection of the entire operative site, characterized by a higher and more prolonged temperature elevation than usual and by local symptoms of heat, redness, swelling, throbbing pain, and loss of function. Treatment requires removal of sutures and insertion of a drain to help the escape of pus. Large hot packs and irrigation of the area may be ordered.

The infection is usually treated systemically by means of chemical agents, this treatment also helps to prevent the infection from spreading to some other part of the body and becoming localized there.

Wound Disruption. Wound disruption, although relatively rare, occurs often enough to warrant mention here. Predisposing factors include extensive postoperative nausea and vomiting, coughing, and distention.

The patient usually complains that he "felt something give way beneath the dressing." A profuse amount of serosanguinous discharge may be found on the dressing, and inspection will reveal that the incision edges have separated and parts of the abdominal viscera are protruding from the opening. The patient should be assured that what has occurred may be quickly remedied by surgical treatment.

A sterile towel should be placed over the wound and the surgeon notified immediately. The patient should be watched carefully for symptoms of shock.

If the patient's condition permits, he is returned to the operating room for resuturing of the wound. If this is not feasible, the wound is strapped with adhesive tape, the edges approximating as closely as possible, and supportive treatment and care is given.

EARLY AMBULATION

Early Ambulation Explained. The term, "early ambulation" denotes a method of management of surgical patients which differs greatly from the generally accepted method that had been used for many years.

The outstanding feature of this method is that of getting the patient out of bed very soon after surgery. As soon as the patient has reacted from the anesthesia he is allowed or encouraged to get up. During the first 24 hours after surgery he is out of bed several times. After the initial out-of-bed experience, which lasts only a very short time, the periods of activity out of bed are gradually increased, until by the third day the patient is up frequently and for as long as he desires.

The chief benefits derived from early ambulation are: (1) to clear the lungs of mucus (by induced coughing); (2) to restore normal functions of the body as soon as possible; (3) to control or prevent postoperative complications; and (4) to facilitate or stimulate rapid recovery of the patient.

Uninformed persons who believe that it is "cruel" to get patients out of bed soon after operation fail to understand the benefits of such treatment. If getting out of bed at the earliest possible moment prevents postoperative complications, adds to the patient's comfort, and shortens the period required for recovery, then the most cruel practice possible would be that of forcing the patient to remain immobile in bed with threats of what might happen should he be active.

Brief History of Early Ambulation. The idea of early ambulation is not new, Emil Ries having first reported this method of management of surgical patients in 1899. Although it is now rather generally accepted as standard treatment, in many localities it is still not known or practiced.

Many surgeons who profess to practice early ambulation keep their patients in bed until the fourth or fifth postoperative day. Others consider it "early rising" if patients are out of bed on their second or third postoperative day, while still others claim that the true practice of early ambulation requires that the patient be out of bed as soon as he has reacted from anesthesia. When local anesthesia is used, the patient walks back to his room from the operating theater.

Dr. D. J. Leithauser, chief of surgery at St. Joseph's Mercy Hospital in Detroit, Michigan, who reported work in early ambulation in 1946, became interested in the procedure in 1938 when an uncooperative patient forced him to give the problem his attention and consideration.

The patient, a man 38 years old, after appendectomy refused to follow instructions of the doctor and nurses. He was out of bed a few hours after the operation and, even though warned by the doctor of the danger involved, left the hospital on his second postoperative day and drove 30 miles to Detroit, spending some time on errands in the downtown business district. He worked in his garden at home on the third and fourth postoperative days, and on the fifth day drove 40 miles for his first medical inspection after leaving the hospital. Examination showed him to be in excellent physical condition. The doctor was deeply interested in the unusually rapid recovery of the patient and began to practice "early rising" methods on all appendectomy cases. The beneficial effects were so marked that soon he treated all of his young adult surgical patients in the same way.

Other surgeons have used this particular form of treatment during the past few decades, and it has been practiced extensively by surgeons in the armed forces.

Improvement in administration of anesthesia and progress in surgery are largely responsible for the success of this different method of postoperative treatment and care.

Preoperative Care in Early Ambulation. The standard procedures for preoperative care of the surgical patient are employed usually for patients to be treated by early ambulation after surgery, although the routine enema the night before is considered unnecessary.

The patient is given a hypnotic the night before to insure a good night's sleep, and another dose of the hypnotic drug may be given the next morning about 6 o'clock.

Surgical Technique in Early Ambulation. The surgeon who seeks the beneficial effects of early ambulation is aware that the manner in which the operative procedure is performed may largely determine the success of the postoperative treatment.

The technical factors essential for safe and comfortable early ambulatory activity by the postoperative patient include: (1) the making of incisions for furthering security and comfort in early ambulation, that is, transverse, midline, or muscle-splitting incisions; (2) a minimum amount of tissue trauma during the operation; (3) the proper choice and use of suture material; and (4) a minimal use of drains.

Postoperative Care in Early Ambulation. To secure the best results through early ambulation it is essential that the patient understand the dangers of being confined to bed and that he be informed in regard to the practice of "early rising," so he will have no fear of getting out of bed soon after the operation.

There is usually no objection on the part of the patient; in fact, most of them are anxious to have early ambulation when they realize that the treatment causes no undue pain or discomfort and makes the convalescent period much more comfortable and much shorter.

The surgeon who practices the technique of early ambulation should be thoroughly versed in the procedure, and should get numerous patients up for the first time himself rather than delegate that responsibility to nurses who may be unfamiliar with the method and unconvinced as to its effectiveness.

Contraindications for Early Ambulation. In conditions of profound shock and of uncontrolled internal hemorrhage early ambulation is contraindicated, as it is in cases (such as advanced cancer) where the condition is hopeless and death seems imminent.

If the surgical procedure involved use of the mid-rectus incision and of absorbable or insecure sutures, activity and ambulation should be restricted during the immediate postoperative period.

Advantages of Early Ambulation. Since early ambulation shortens the period of postoperative recovery there is little need for continued use of sedatives or narcotics, although no patient should have narcotic drugs withheld if they are needed for relief of pain and discomfort.

When the patient is ambulant soon after surgery the need for enemas in the postoperative period is largely eliminated. The patient who is no longer subjected to the indignity of using the bedpan has little difficulty in establishing normal bowel evacuations.

Food is given to early ambulant patients as they desire, and appetite is recognized as the best guide as to when solid food should be given.

Most ambulatory patients are able to urinate, and catheterization is seldom necessary. Even if the patient cannot void and must be catheterized, repeated catheterization is usually not required.

Immediate Postoperative Management. For the average surgical patient under early ambulation treatment the routine includes:

(1) Position of lying flat on the bed to permit freedom of movement —pillows should not be used under the knees since they cause pressure on the veins of the legs, inhibit circulation, and may be a causative factor in postoperative thrombosis;

(2) Morphine or other narcotic to be used only for relief of pain;

(3) Water in small quantities, regulated by thirst;

(4) Patient to wiggle his toes frequently and to flex and extend ankles and knees four times every hour;

(5) Patient to be out of bed in 3 to 4 hours for deep breathing and coughing, and to begin walking about.

First Out-of-Bed Period. When the patient has recovered from anesthesia he is asked to turn to his side with feet extended over the edge of the bed. Through his own effort or with the assistance of the nurse, he assumes a sitting position, and then stands beside the bed.

He is then instructed to take two or three deep breaths, after which he is asked to cough. While the patient is coughing (two or three coughs) the nurse should place her hand on his back to determine the presence of rales. If rales are present, the patient is asked to continue coughing until the mucus is expectorated and the rales disappear.

No abdominal support is used or needed.

After clearing the lungs by coughing, the patient walks around the bed or across the room.

He returns to bed by stepping on the footstool, then sitting on the side of the bed, then supporting himself with both hands as he gradually assumes the recumbent position.

After the first out-of-bed period the patient is usually able to get up without assistance and may indulge in any activity he wishes. If he is fearful of getting out of bed or if he experiences faintness or weakness, he should be asked to bend over and try to touch the floor. Such exercise gives the patient confidence in the procedure and quickly dispels any fear he may have regarding his ability to get up and become active.

Hospital Dismissal. Under the early ambulation régime patients are usually permitted to go home when they wish if their condition is satisfactory and most patients who have had a simple appendectomy leave the hospital the day after operation. Some patients elect to stay until the second or third postoperative day.

All such patients are encouraged to resume normal activity, such as riding in a car, and returning to work (unless they perform heavy manual labor) within a few days.

Care of Equipment after Use

Surgical cap and leggings should be discarded, along with additional linen used in making the anesthetic bed, down the laundry chute.

The additional rubber sheets and rubber-covered pillows should be returned to their storage place in the clinical department.

The stethoscope and sphygmomanometer should be returned to their place of storage.

Used mouthwipes, tongue depressor, and paper bag should be discarded into the incinerator.

The emesis basins should be cleaned, one should be returned to the bedside table, the other to storage.

Notations made on the scratch pad should be transferred to the patient's chart.

Summary of Important Factors

In the recovery room a properly made anesthetic bed and fully equipped bedside table should await the patient.

Care should be taken in moving or lifting an anesthetized patient.

The patient should be placed in the proper position in bed.

Immediate postoperative care includes: frequent determination of pulse and respiration rate; determination of blood pressure every 15 minutes; frequent examination of the dressing for bleeding; minor movements not to be restrained; narcotic as ordered for relief of pain; frequent change of position; restriction of visitors; giving of fluids when indicated; and, reassurance of the patient to relieve mental anxiety.

General postoperative care includes: daily bath and routine nursing procedures; care of mouth; proper diet; attention to psychological needs; proper elimination; record of intake and output; and, careful watch for symptoms of complications.

Postoperative complications include: *hiccup*—cause unknown, if prolonged may become serious; *shock*, evidenced by feeble, rapid irregular pulse, decreased blood pressure, cyanosis, cold clammy skin, and apprehension—treatment includes: elevation of foot of bed, application of external heat, drug to relieve pain, and blood or blood plasma; *hemorrhage*—internal or external, evidenced by thirst, dyspnea, increased pulse and respiration rate, flushed face, pallor of lips, dimness of vision, and apprehension—treatment includes: immediate control, treatment for shock, and blood transfusion after control is established; *distention*—caused by accumulation of gas, treated by heat to abdomen, colon tube, or suction apparatus; *pulmonary complications*—atelectasis, postoperative pneumonia, combated by forcing fluids, chemotherapy, oxygen therapy; *cardiovascular complications*—phlebitis, embolism, treated by preventive measures, early ambulation; *renal complications*—retention of urine, suppression of urine, treated by catheterization, forcing fluids, diuretic medication for suppression; *wound infections*—stitch abscess, cellulitis, treated by specific therapy for the infective agent in both conditions; *wound disruption*—edges of incision separate, abdominal viscera protrude from the opening, treated by resuturing of the wound or close approximation of wound edges with adhesive tape.

In early ambulation, the first time the patient gets out of bed he should first turn to his side, then extend feet and legs over the edge of the bed, come to a sitting position, then step from the footstool to the floor in an upright position. Standing quietly, he should take two or three deep breaths and cough. Then he should walk a few steps, and return to bed by reversing the procedure by which he got up. He should get out of bed again during the day at intervals of a few hours.

Factors To Teach the Patient

That his room may be properly ventilated without danger of drafts.

Restriction of movement of a part may be necessary after surgery.

That movements of limbs, change of position, and early ambulation help to prevent postoperative complications.

That narcotic drugs are still effective in relieving pain, although they may be given in progressively decreased amounts and at less frequent intervals.

Intravenous therapy will relieve thirst by supplying needed body fluid.

Anxiety and apprehension may add to restlessness and discomfort; that he will be well cared for after surgery so he can relax and sleep or rest.

Recovery is facilitated when he begins to do things for himself instead of depending on the nurse for complete care.

His diet is planned to suit his own particular needs and he should adhere to it. Supplementing his diet with food brought from outside the hospital may cause gastric disturbances.

The nurse is alert for symptoms of postoperative complications; any subjective symptoms should be reported to her.

Early ambulation is the present accepted method of treatment for a great many postoperative patients.

Scientific Principles

Anatomy and Physiology. Trauma to internal organs during the operation may increase pain and discomfort later.

The head should be on the same plane with the rest of the body and turned to one side so there is less danger of aspiration of mucus or emesis.

Early ambulation helps to prevent complications caused by lack of movement or exercise and by shallow breathing.

Muscle tone is maintained by exercise so the patient is encouraged to move about.

Dressings are necessary for the protection of surgical wounds.

An accumulation of gas in the intestinal tract may cause the "gas pains" experienced after abdominal surgery.

If there is retention of urine the doctor should be notified before the patient becomes too uncomfortable.

Transfusion, by increasing the volume of blood, increases blood pressure.

Microbiology. The surgeons and nurses wear rubber gloves and use only sterile equipment as a safeguard for the patient.

Pharmacology. Narcotics are used to relieve pain and discomfort following surgery. Morphine decreases respiration which is already depressed by the anesthetic agent. Morphine should not be given unless the rate of respiration is 14 or more per minute.

Physics. The room should be comfortably warm, but not overheated—a surgical patient may be more susceptible to colds.

Pressure from a distended bladder may cause pain and discomfort.

Fowler's position aids drainage of the pelvic region.

More blood is sent to the heart to aid the patient in shock by elevation of the foot of the bed.

Psychology. Patients recovering from anesthesia are apt to react vigorously to restriction of movement.

The patient should be continually reassured that the operation is over and his physical condition is good during the time he is recovering from the anesthetic.

The attitude of the nurse in caring for the operated area may have a decided influence on the patient's mental outlook.

The patient should be constantly observed for symptoms of change in condition.

The patient should be familiar with the procedure of having blood pressure taken before surgery so he will not be alarmed when the procedure is done at intervals after surgery.

Sociology. The family of the patient should be informed as to how they may be most helpful in the immediate postoperative period. The nurse should insist that all members of the family who enter the room remain quiet so the patient will not be disturbed. Not more than two relatives should be in the patient's room at any one time.

Situation Type Problems

1. A student nurse assigned to care for a postoperative patient after he had been returned to his own room kept a careful record of all factors involved in postoperative care by making notations in a notebook which she carried for that purpose.

While the patient was resting quietly she brought his hospital chart to the room so she could transfer the notations to the chart and still be in the room to closely observe the patient.

The mother of the patient came into the room and asked to be permitted to read what the student was printing on the chart. She stated that she also wished to read the laboratory reports and operative record.

The student nurse attempted to explain that the chart was for the use of doctors and nurses only and that permission could not be granted for a lay person to read its contents.

The mother of the patient became very angry, charged the nurse and doctor with trying to conceal information from her, stated that she felt certain the operation had not really been necessary and that neither the doctor or the hospital would be paid until she had been allowed to read the chart. What would you have done?

2. The student nurse who was assigned to give postoperative care for a patient who had just been returned to his room on the clinical department had been informed by the nurse in charge as to results of the operation. The surgeon had found inoperable carcinoma of the abdomen and had not performed surgery. The doctor had specified that the patient was *not* to be told of his condition.

The patient had recovered from the anesthetic, had stated that he was not comfortable and was dozing when his older sister came into the room. The nurse indicated by gesture that the visitor should be seated. The patient appeared to be sleeping and the nurse continued with her work of completing notations on the chart.

The sister left the chair she had been sitting in, came to the bedside, and stood for a moment looking down at the patient. Then, without warning and before the nurse could intervene, she asked in a clear and distinct tone of voice, "Did *you* know, he's dying of cancer?" The nurse hurried the unthinking woman from the room after noting that the patient hadn't moved or reacted in any way to the blunt question. She explained, in a few words, to the startled woman that under no circumstances was she to say anything within the patient's hearing with reference to his physical condition.

The visitor went on her way and the nurse returned to the patient's bedside. He was lying quietly just as she had left him, but his eyes were wide open. She knew he must have heard the words his sister had spoken, so she was not totally unprepared when he asked, "Is what she said true? Am I dying of cancer?" What would you have done?

Suggested Reference Reading

"Early ambulation," Daniel J. Leithauser; American Journal of Nursing, April, 1950.

"Some recent advances in surgery," Louis T. Palumbo; American Journal of Nursing, October, 1950.

"What is shock?" Conrad R. Lam; American Journal of Nursing, February, 1951.

"Get out of bed and get well," Morton M. Hunt; Coronet, January, 1952.

"Post anesthetic and post operative recovery units," Sister Agnes Leon; American Journal of Nursing, April, 1952.

"I've just had an operation," May Richstone; Today's Health, August, 1952.

"Our recovery room experience," Marilyn Gassler; American Journal of Nursing, September, 1952.

CHAPTER 28

Surgical Dressings

TOPICAL OUTLINE

More than 50 per cent of all patients admitted to the hospital require some form of surgical treatment or emergency treatment of accidental injury. In either event, the patient suffers a mechanical injury to some part of the body and must be given treatment for the particular type of wound present.

Wounds may occur as the result of accidental injury or may be intentionally produced in surgical treatment.

In order to give intelligent care, for either type of inflicted wound, the nurse must possess a basic knowledge of the various types of wounds and understand the process by which wounds heal.

A wound may be defined as a break in the continuity of soft parts or tissues of the body, such as skin, mucous membrane, or muscle.

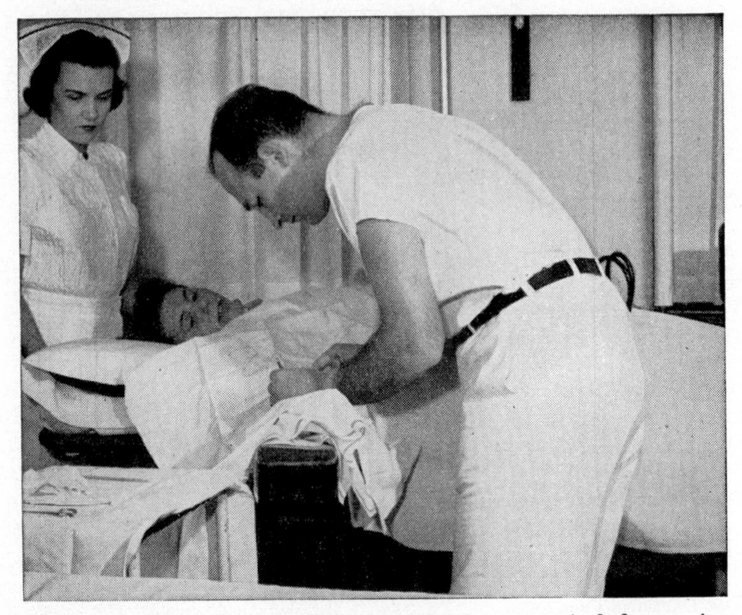

Fig. 167. Emergency treatment of accidental injury may include suturing a wound. (Mercy Hospital School of Nursing, Hamilton, Ohio.)

CLASSIFICATION OF WOUNDS

Wounds may be classified into two main groups according to the manner in which they are produced and according to their bacterial content.

According to Manner of Production. When classified according to the manner in which they are produced, wounds are described by the following terms:

Abraded Wound—One produced by friction which removes the superficial layers of the skin.

Incised Wound—One made by a sharp cutting instrument which produces a clean and simple separation of tissues.

Lacerated Wound—One in which the tissues are torn, the edges of the wound being jagged and irregular.

Penetrating Wound—One that passes through deep lying tissues to enter an important deep body cavity or organ.

Puncture Wound—One made with a sharp pointed narrow instrument piercing beyond surface depth, but making only a small opening on the body surface.

According to Bacterial Content. According to their bacterial content wounds are classified as follows:

Clean Wound—One in which no pathogenic organisms are present.

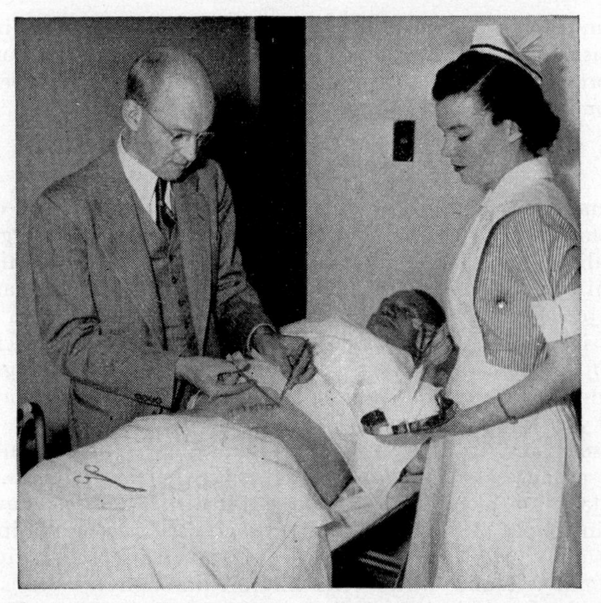

Fig. 168. The incision made in surgery usually heals as a "clean" wound. (Presbyterian Hospital School of Nursing, Charlotte, North Carolina.)

When an incision is made in surgery under aseptic conditions the wound should remain clean. It is impossible to produce a completely sterile wound since the patient's skin cannot be sterilized and there is no way of completely eliminating organisms that are air borne and continually present in the so-called "sterile field." Under desirable conditions, however, the few organisms introduced into the wound during the surgical procedure are usually rendered harmless by the defensive reaction exerted by the tissues. The wound or incision made in surgery usually heals without any apparent indication of the presence of an infection.

Contaminated Wound—One in which the number of organisms present is much greater than in a clean wound. All wounds acquired by accident are contaminated since no preventive measures, such as aseptic technique, can be applied. A surgical incision which must be made in a contaminated area is a contaminated wound. The wound resulting from hemorrhoidectomy is an example of such a wound. A contaminated wound, although liable to infection, may heal without clinical manifestation of infection.

Septic Wound—One infected with disease-producing microorganisms. Such a wound contains large numbers of organisms which have caused the destruction of tissue in the affected area. A clean or contaminated wound may become infected by the activity of organisms which multiply so rapidly that the defensive reaction of the involved tissues is ineffectual. A wound made at a site where infection is already present, such as an incision for drainage of an abscess, becomes a septic or infected wound immediately.

INFLAMMATION

Inflammation is the condition produced by the reaction of body tissues to injury or to invasion of disease-producing microorganisms. Many different types of inflammation have been defined, the most common being: *acute,* severe form with sudden onset, and marked by active processes of the defensive mechanism; *chronic,* a slowly progressive form that may result in the formation of connective tissue; *diffuse,* spreading over a large area; *serous,* producing a thin and watery exudate; and *specific,* caused by a specific microorganism.

Local Signs and Symptoms of Inflammation. Changes occurring in the tissues and in the vascular system during the inflammatory process produce the following signs and symptoms: *redness,* caused by dilatation of blood vessels at the affected site, with consequent increase in supply of blood to the part; *heat,* produced by the increased blood supply; *swelling,* caused by an exudative process in which serum and red and white cells migrate through the walls of the dilated blood vessels into the tissues; *pain,* caused by pressure on nerves and nerve endings as a result of the swelling produced by the inflammatory process, pain may also result from irritation produced by the toxins of bacteria and the decomposition of cells; *impairment of function,* as a result of the pain and swelling which characterize an inflammatory process. The action of white blood cells that ingest damaged tissue cells and pathogenic organisms and are themselves destroyed in the process is extremely important in the development and progress of inflammation.

INFECTION

Infection occurs when a part of the body is invaded by disease-producing microorganisms whose growth and proliferation results in the destruction of tissues in the affected area.

Signs and Symptoms of Local Infection. In addition to the characteristic signs and symptoms of local inflammation, a local infection will result in the formation of pus, a thick exudate made up of destroyed tissue cells, leukocytes, and dead or living microorganisms. An abscess is formed when the pus is successfully walled off from surrounding tissues by the defensive reaction of those tissues.

TREATMENT OF LOCAL INFLAMMATION AND INFECTION

Factors in the treatment of local inflammation and infection include the following: *rest of the part,* to overcome pain brought about by movement and to reduce the inflammatory process, thus lessening the absorption of toxic materials; *elevation of the part,* to relieve congestion and aid in removal of toxic products of the infection through blood and lymph vessels; *application of heat or cold,* to hasten the process of suppuration or to inhibit the inflammatory process; *incision and drainage,* when the suppurative process has resulted in abscess formation.

GENERAL SIGNS AND SYMPTOMS OF INFLAMMATION AND INFECTION

General signs and symptoms will be manifest when toxic substances from the inflamed or infected area are absorbed by the blood stream. Such signs and symptoms include: elevation of body temperature, increase in pulse and in respiration rate, a feeling of fatigue and weakness, loss of appetite, nausea and vomiting, headache.

If toxins are being rapidly absorbed into the blood stream, chills may occur. The number of leukocytes will be markedly increased as the cells and tissues of the body resist the inflammatory or infectious process.

GENERAL TREATMENT OF INFLAMMATION AND INFECTION

The primary purpose of giving general treatment to inflammation or infection is to increase the resistance of the patient and to overcome the microorganism causing the condition. Such treatment consists largely of *mental and physical rest,* with sufficient sleep to conserve the patient's strength and energy; *increased fluid intake,* to promote elimination, thus diluting toxins and removing them more rapidly from the body; *maintaining nutritional balance,* by means of a high-calorie, high-vitamin diet; *personal hygienic measures,* to insure cleanliness and comfort of the patient; *relief of pain,* by administration of drugs and careful attention to ordered treatments; *blood transfusions,* to help increase resistance to the infection and to combat anemia which may be a complication of the existing condition; *fresh air and sunshine,* to promote favorable mental attitude and help increase resistance to the disease condition; *chemotherapy,* with administration of antibiotic agents to effectively combat the causative organisms.

HEALING OF WOUNDS

Many wounds of a minor nature will heal without any special treatment or attention. Wounds heal according to the type of tissue involved. Wounds affecting tissue which cannot be replaced, such as that of brain, liver, kidney, and voluntary muscles, heal through the formation of connective tissue in the affected area. Wounds involving

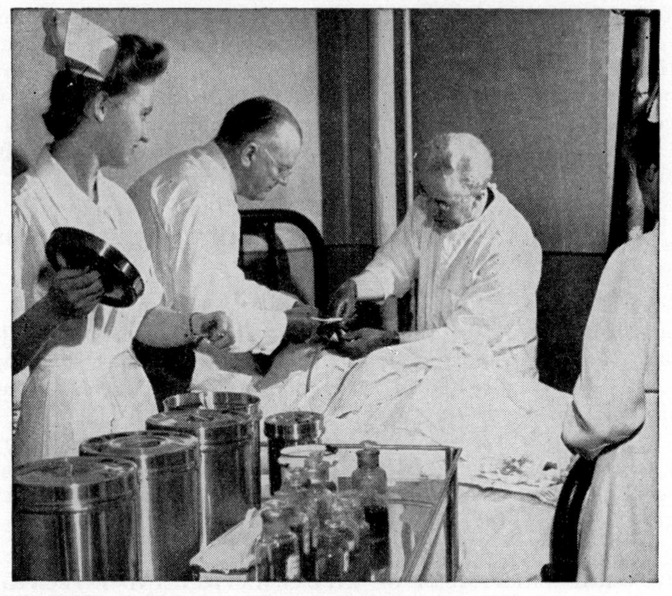

Fig. 169. Rubber tubes are used to conduct draining fluid from deep wounds. (Ravenswood Hospital School of Nursing, Chicago, Illinois.)

tendons, nerves, and bones heal through gradual growth and replacement of the injured tissue.

Primary healing. Healing by first intention occurs when the wound heals promptly. The wound edges are approximated so that contamination is slight, very little granulation tissue is required, and only a very small or narrow scar results.

Secondary Healing. Healing by second intention occurs when the wound edges are widely separated, a large amount of granulation tissue is required, infection commonly occurs, and a large scar or deformity results. Such wounds heal slowly because of the various interferences to the reparative process.

Wound Irrigation. When infection is present irrigation may be used as a means of cleansing the wound and removing waste products of the suppurative process. Such treatment helps to maintain free drainage from the wound and aids the healing process.

Drainage Tubes. Tubes used to conduct the exudate or draining fluid materials from deep wounds are made of rubber; a rubber dam or folded strip of gauze may also be used. The rubber drainage tube is prevented from slipping further into the wound by a safety pin fastened crosswise at the exposed end of the tube.

From time to time, as dressings are changed, the surgeon may

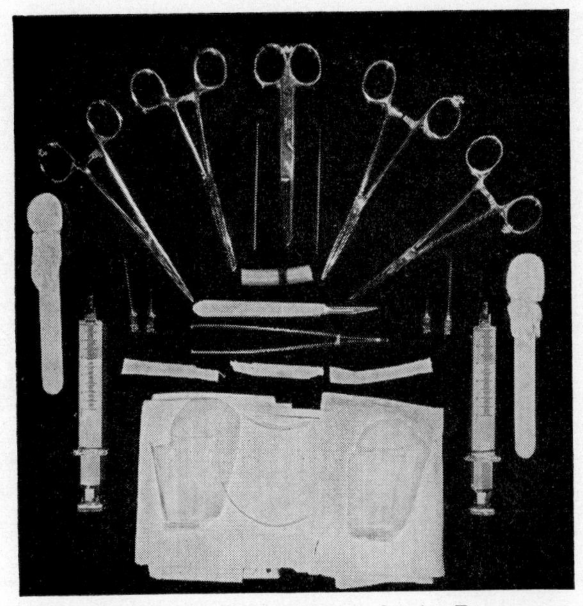

Fig. 170. Incision and drainage set. (Nursing Service Department, New England Center Hospital, Boston, Massachusetts.)

shorten the tube by cutting an inch or more from the end. Each time the tube is shortened a sterile safety pin is fastened in place with sterile forceps. The safety pin not only holds the tube in place but will serve as a marker to locate the tube by x-ray should it disappear into the depths of the wound. When drainage is profuse, the tube in the wound may be attached by a sterile glass connecting tube to a longer rubber tube which conducts the draining material to a collection bottle. Bottle holders that clamp to the bedside hold the collection bottle in place, and by judicious use of safety pins and rubber bands the drainage tube may be kept free from tension and danger of being pulled from the wound. Drainage material collected in the bottle should be measured and discarded at least once in each 24 hour period. When the drainage bottle and long tube are used the dressing will need to be changed less frequently.

If it is necessary to cleanse the glass connecting tube and the long rubber tube, aseptic technique should be used in the procedure. The nurse should wear rubber gloves and use sterile water or normal saline solution which is injected from an Asepto syringe to forcibly rinse the tubing. If drainage is continued for a long period the connecting tubes should be removed at regular intervals and replaced with sterile tubes of the same size and length.

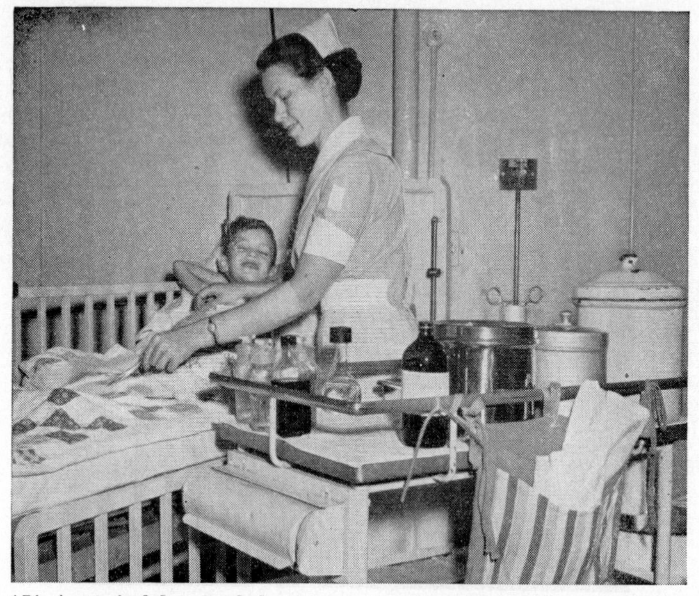

Fig. 171. A surgical dressing helps to prevent contamination of a wound. (Indiana University, Medical Center, School of Nursing, Indianapolis, Indiana.)

THE PURPOSE OF SURGICAL DRESSINGS

A surgical dressing is a protective sterile covering of gauze or other material applied to an operative wound to (1) protect the wound from injury; (2) prevent contamination of the wound, especially to protect it from pathogenic microorganisms; (3) keep the edges of the wound in close approximation by immobilizing the affected area; (4) provide for local application of drugs; (5) apply pressure to the area; (6) absorb material being discharged from the wound.

The procedure of removing a soiled or used dressing, treating the wound so that healing is promoted, and applying a new dressing is termed "dressing the wound." The way the term is used in a sentence will determine whether reference is made to the material applied over a wound or the actual process of caring for or treating the wound.

MATERIALS USED TO MAKE SURGICAL DRESSINGS

Dressings used to cover or protect surgical wounds are made of a variety of materials, depending on the purpose for which they are needed.

Gauze sponges are used extensively to swab or cleanse a wound and to apply antiseptic solutions when their use is indicated.

Gauze squares are used as compresses for a sterile covering applied directly over a surgical incision.

Cotton applicators are made in different sizes and have a variety of uses; the most common use is that of applying medicine to a wound or of cleansing with an antiseptic solution.

Absorbent cotton is used to supply bulk in surgical dressings. Its chief disadvantage lies in the fact that it adheres to the wound, so it must be enclosed in one or several layers of gauze when it is made into a dressing.

Cellucotton is a fluffy, absorbent material used for wounds in which there is profuse drainage or discharge. This material, too, must be enclosed in layers of gauze to prevent its disintegration when saturated with fluid drainage.

Pads for use as surgical dressings are made of absorbent cotton and Cellucotton, covered with layers of gauze to preserve their shape. Many such pads contain a top layer of non-absorbent cotton which is always placed on the outer side of the dressing to prevent seepage of drainage material through the dressing.

Rubber dams or rubber drains made from India rubber sheeting are used to keep drainage tracts in a wound open.

Gauze and silk drains or tampons are also used to help remove discharge or fluid drainage.

Ointment gauze, gauze strips impregnated with an ointment, is used to apply the ointment to the wound or to the skin surfaces around a wound.

Petrolatum gauze strips or drains may be removed from wounds with less pain and injury than are occasioned by use of plain gauze.

EQUIPMENT NEEDED FOR THE DRESSING PROCEDURE

Besides the materials used for drains or drainage tubes and dressings, many other articles, both sterile and nonsterile, are necessary for the application of surgical dressings.

Sterile Articles. Articles used in applying surgical dressings which must be sterile, include:

Sterile drugs or ointments commonly used with dressings;

Rubber catheters or rubber tubing used in irrigating wounds;

Rubber gloves which are essential for the performance of the procedure under aseptic conditions;

Glassware, such as glass syringes and the glass barrel of the Asepto syringe;

Enamelware or stainless steel basins and other utensils that might be needed;

Instruments used in handling the sterile dressings, including forceps, scissors, probe, and other equipment needed to handle sterile supplies;

Safety pins, rubber bands, wooden tongue depressors—all sterile and ready for use when needed.

Non-Sterile Articles. Non-sterile articles that may be required in dressing wounds include roller bandage, binders, adhesive tape, matches, alcohol lamp, and receptacles for soiled instruments and dressings.

Equipment needed for the dressing procedure should always be collected and made ready for use prior to the arrival of the doctor who is to change the dressing. All the equipment should be taken to the patient's room in the surgical dressing basket or the dressing cart.

PRECAUTIONS FOR APPLYING OR CHANGING A DRESSING

In applying or changing a dressing it is necessary to maintain strict surgical aseptic technique to prevent contamination or secondary infection of the wound. Attention should be given to the patient's comfort during the procedure, but the necessity for precaution against careless handling of supplies and equipment is of paramount importance. Precautions that are essential to prevention of contamination include the following suggested rules for nurses and doctors:

Careful washing of hands with soap and water before starting the procedure.

Freedom from respiratory or other infections for the person doing the dressing.

The wearing of a mask during the procedure.

Making certain that air in the room is quiescent and that doors and windows are closed to prevent drafts. This precaution lessens the possibility of contaminating the wound by air-borne microorganisms which would be present in increased numbers if air was in movement.

The wearing of sterile gloves if the wound requires manipulation by hand.

Careful handling of instruments and supplies to insure aseptic technique throughout the procedure.

Avoid reaching directly over the sterile field while doing the dressing.

Refrain from handling sterile supplies unnecessarily, as additional handling increases the danger of contamination.

When handling sterile instruments touch only the handles of the instruments. At all times during the procedure keep unsterile instrument handles outside the sterile surgical field.

Cleanse the lips of solution bottles by pouring a small amount from them before pouring the solution to be used in doing the dressing. Never allow the bottle opening to come in direct contact with the sterile sponge when pouring solution upon it.

If there is some delay in doing the procedure after the sterile field

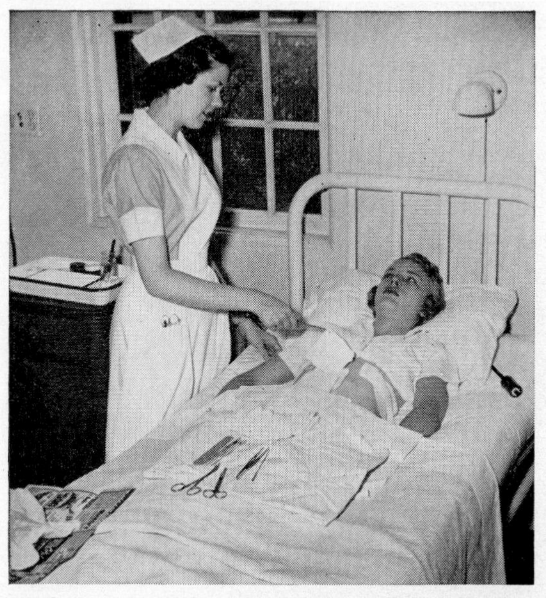

Fig. 172. Unsterile instrument handles should be kept outside the sterile field. (Good Samaritan Hospital School of Nursing, Phoenix, Arizona.)

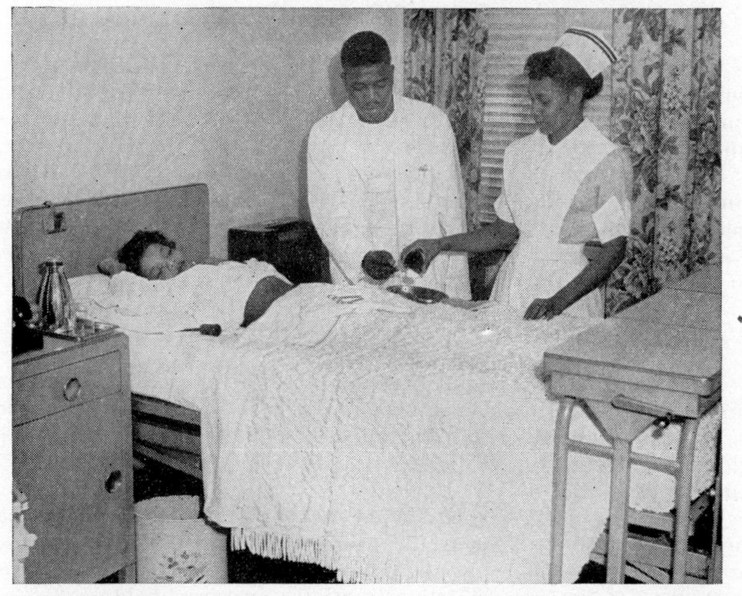

Fig. 173. The bottle should not come in contact with the sterile sponge when an antiseptic solution is being poured. (Provident Hospital School of Nursing, Chicago, Illinois.)

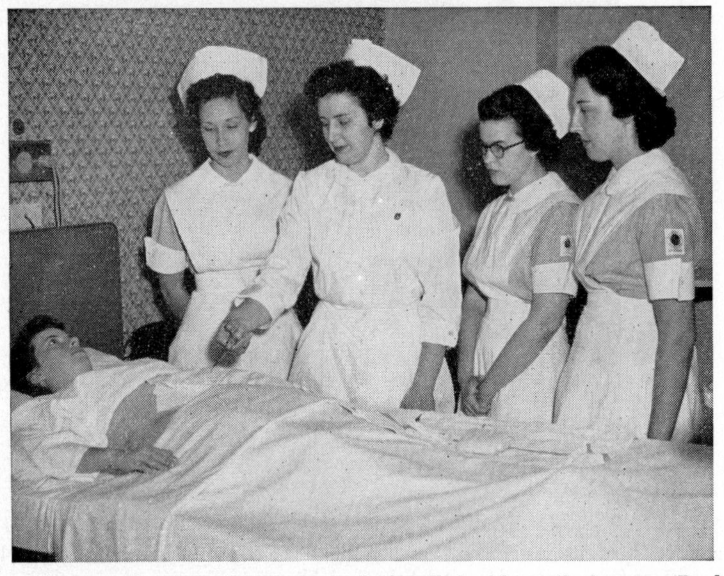

Fig. 174. Inner dressings should always be handled with sterile forceps. (Baylor University School of Nursing, Waco, Texas.)

is made ready, cover the area with a sterile towel. If there is a long delay, all instruments and supplies that have been exposed for that time should be replaced with other sterile instruments and supplies and a new sterile field should be set up.

Do not remove the inner dressing from a surgical incision before time for the dressing procedure to be performed. The doctor or other person doing the dressing must be in attendance and prepared to carry out his part of the procedure at the time the incision is exposed to view.

THE DRESSING PROCEDURE

Before starting the dressing procedure the patient should be screened, properly draped, and given an explanation as to just what is to be done.

Sufficient lighting should be provided so that the affected area is clearly visible. Artificial light is usually required in the form of a lamp or flashlight.

If there is a disagreeable odor to the soiled dressing or if the patient prefers not to witness the procedure a towel may be draped around the face just below the chin to serve as a screen which prevents the patient from directly viewing the operative field.

If there is a binder or bandage holding the dressing in place it should be unfastened or removed. The outer layers of the dressing should be removed and placed in the receptacle provided to receive soiled dressings.

Inner dressings are to be handled with sterile forceps, preferably by the doctor or person applying or changing the dressing.

When all dressings have been removed, the wound should be cleansed and treated as indicated by its appearance. Fresh dressings are then applied, being handled with sterile instruments and applied in such manner that they remain sterile during application.

Throughout the entire procedure everything that comes in contact with the wound, directly or indirectly, must be sterile.

The new dressing should be fastened securely in place by means of a binder or by use of bandage and adhesive tape.

TO ASSIST THE SURGEON IN DOING A DRESSING

The basic requirement for giving adequate assistance to the surgeon doing a dressing is ability to anticipate his wants and to have all necessary articles or supplies immediately available at the time he may need them. In assisting the doctor so that his work is neat and efficient the nurse needs to be well versed in the correct method of handling and presenting to him such articles as those listed here.

Sterile gauze squares should be placed, with a sterile forceps, directly on the sterile field or extended to him so that he may take them from the wrapper without danger of contaminating his sterile gloves.

Sterile safety pins, as well as rubber bands, should be placed on the sterile field and the doctor permitted to pick them up as he chooses.

Adhesive tape should be held at each end, with the length of tape pulled taut, and extended within easy reach of the doctor's hands.

Unsterile safety pins should be presented with the point downward and directed away from the doctor, so that when grasped by the doctor the pin is in proper position for use.

Roller bandage should be unwound about six inches, the free end held in one hand and the roll, on top of the bandage strip, with the other, and extended to the doctor.

Unsterile rubber bands should be placed over tips of fingers and thumb of the right hand and then transferred over the tips of fingers and thumb of the doctor's extended hand.

The nurse who handles articles with efficiency, works without detailed instructions from the surgeon, and refrains from unnecessary conversation during the procedure will be appreciated by the doctor who is able to do the dressing in a shorter period of time. She will also earn the gratitude of the patient, who experiences only a minimal amount of discomfort and apprehension during the dressing procedure.

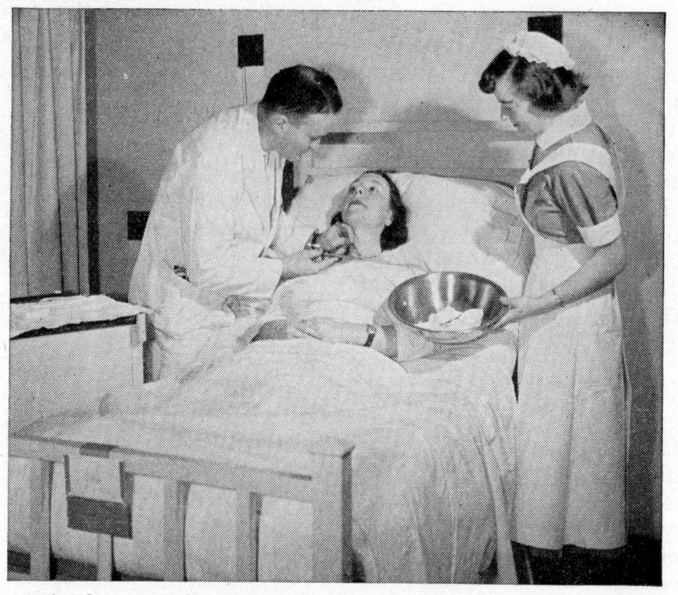

Fig. 175. The nurse should be able to assist the doctor without detailed instructions from him. (Massachusetts General Hospital School of Nursing, Boston, Massachusetts.)

Often the doctor will perform the procedure only to the point where fresh inner dressings have been applied and will then leave completion of the dressing to the nurse. In such event the nurse should continue to use aseptic technique and complete the procedure, making sure that the dressing is securely fastened or held in place by adhesive tape and bandages or a suitable binder.

TO HOLD DRESSINGS IN PLACE

Dressings are held in place chiefly through use of adhesive tape, which may be placed directly across the dressing, extending out over the skin surface, or may be made into tie straps and laced together with gauze bandage for use when the dressing must be changed frequently. If the patient is allergic to adhesive tape, scotch tape or some other means may be used to hold the dressing in place.

If adhesive tape is to be used to approximate and hold the edges of the wound together, it should be flamed so that it is relatively safe to be in close contact with the wound itself. To do this, the desired length of tape is passed back and forth, cloth side down, through the flame from an alcohol lamp. When the adhesive mass begins to blister the tape is ready for use. Time for the tape to cool sufficiently should be allowed so the skin surface will not be burned. Flaming of

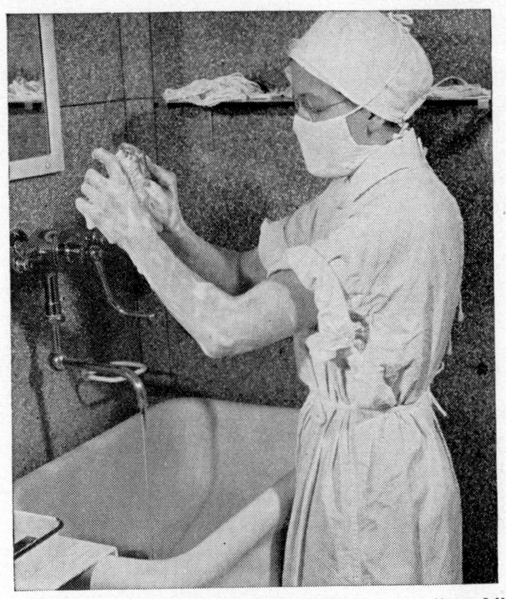

Fig. 176. It would be impractical to ask the nurse to "scrub" for dressings when sterile articles may be safely handled with forceps. (Presbyterian Hospital School of Nursing, Chicago, Illinois.)

adhesive tape increases its adhesive quality, so that it becomes more useful as well as more safe.

Tie straps of adhesive tape used to hold in place a dressing that will need to be changed frequently are made by unrolling tape of 1 or 2 inch width for about 15 inches. The tape is then folded back upon itself at one end, leaving about 6 inches of tape with adhesive side exposed. The adhesive side is applied to the skin, and the double thickness portion, with a small hole through it near the end, extends across the dressing. Two or three such straps are fastened in place on each side of the dressing, so that when brought across the dressing they may be tied together with small strips of gauze bandage passed through the holes.

Small dressings applied to the face may be held in place with liquid adhesive preparations which make the dressing much less conspicuous.

ASEPTIC TECHNIQUE IN OPENING STERILE SUPPLIES

Packages of sterile supplies consist of the outer wrapper, an inner wrapper and the folded drapes, towels, gowns, dressings, or other needed surgical supplies. All sterile packages are opened in such a way that only the outside portion of the outer wrapper is touched by the nurse. The contents and inner portion of the wrapper can be considered sterile only so long as they are handled by a "scrubbed" nurse wearing gloves or by sterile forceps, and so long as they are not contaminated by contact with articles or persons not "sterile."

To successfully open a sterile package the "unsterile" nurse holds it firmly in her left hand and opens the wrapper by grasping the top corner on the outer side, turning it back over her left hand and arm. Then in turn she grasps the corner of the right side, the left side, and the lower corner, turning each back to expose the contents of the package. The sterile nurse then grasps the gown, towel, or other sterile contents and places them where needed on the sterile table. Small packages may have only one wrapper.

ASEPTIC TECHNIQUE IN HANDLING STERILE SUPPLIES

Many sterile supplies or articles are handled so frequently by nurses engaged in general bedside nursing that it is impractical to require the nurse to "scrub" or to wear rubber gloves so the sterile articles will not be contaminated. Such articles or supplies, as sterile instruments, dressings, tongue blades, ointments, etc. may be removed from their sterile containers and handled safely by means of long-handled forceps or sponge sticks. These handling forceps are kept in containers of antiseptic solution and are used in such manner that they do not become contaminated and may therefore be replaced in the solution and used again when needed.

Forceps are always held with the ends pointed downward. Only the lower part of the forceps is sterile (that part immersed in the antiseptic solution). If the forceps should be held so that the ends point upward, the solution adhering to them when the instrument is removed from the container would travel across the unclean or contaminated region of the forceps. Then when the forceps is held point down this contaminated solution would, in turn, contaminate the ends of the forceps and make them unsuitable for handling sterile articles.

In removing the forceps from the container, great care must be taken not to touch the sides and top of the container. Touching the forceps to any unsterile surface makes them unsterile and renders them useless for safe handling of sterile supplies.

Sterile articles removed from their containers by handling forceps must be taken by other forceps, dropped on a sterile towel, or placed in a sterile container.

When using handling forceps the nurse must be exceedingly cautious, bearing constantly in mind that the ends of the forceps which are sterile must come in contact only with sterile articles or sterile surfaces. Any contact with an article or surface that is not sterile will contaminate the forceps.

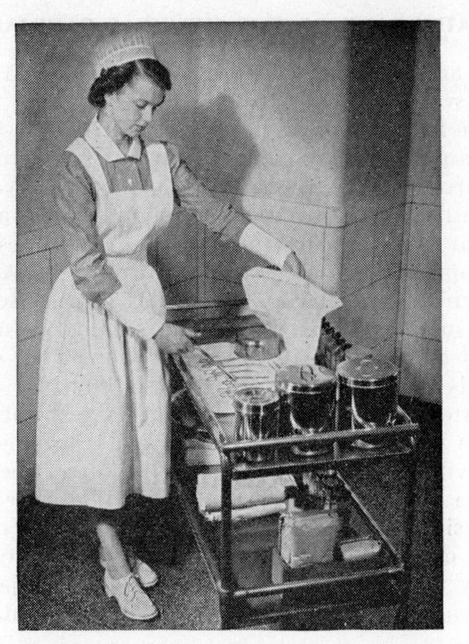

Fig. 177. Handling forceps should be used to place sterile instruments on a sterile field. (St. Luke's Hospital School of Nursing, Chicago, Illinois.)

Care of Equipment after Use

The dressing carriage or tray should be cleaned, all supplies should be replenished, and the equipment should be returned to its usual place.

Instruments used in doing the dressing should be washed and rinsed well before being sterilized and made ready for use again.

All enamel, stainless steel, and glass articles should be thoroughly cleaned and made ready for sterilization.

Rubber gloves should be rinsed under cold running water, both inside and out, then washed in warm soapy water, rinsed again, and placed on a glove drying rack. When the gloves are dry outside, they should be turned to permit drying of the inside.

All soiled dressings, bandages, used adhesive tape, etc. should be discarded into the incinerator.

Instruments should be rinsed in cold water, to remove blood, washed with soap and water, rinsed, and sterilized by boiling or autoclaving, then returned to instrument basin on the dressing carriage. When instruments have been contaminated by pus or feces, or when the doctor directs, they should be soaked in a strong germicidal solution for 30 minutes before being washed and rinsed.

DAILY CARE OF THE SURGICAL CARRIAGE

Remove all articles from the surgical carriage and wash carriage with soap and water.

Scrub sponge forceps and container and sterilize by boiling 10 minutes. Fill container with Lysol 1 per cent to 1 inch from the top.

Cleanse instruments by washing with soap and water, and rinse well. Wash instrument basin with soap and water and rinse well. Boil instrument basin and instruments for 10 minutes.

Replenish supplies on the carriage, returning to central supply all packages on which the expiration date has passed. Requisition daily from central supply all needed items, arranging sterile dressings in the order of dating, so that those with the earliest expiration date are most readily accessible and will be used first.

Pay close attention to articles with special expiration date. Iodoform wicks, in gauze-wrapped sterile metal container, are marked when opened with date four weeks from the date of opening. Iodoform gauze in sterile container with overlapping lid, secured by two strips of ½-inch adhesive tape, is marked when opened with date four weeks from date of opening. Ointments, contained in sterile glass jars, are sterile only until opened. After a single use, the jar should be returned to central supply even though it may still contain a supply of ointment.

WEEKLY CARE OF SURGICAL CARRIAGE

Wash containers thoroughly and boil 10 minutes then label and date one week from date of preparation. Fill containers with sterile supplies; cover those which should be in solution with aqueous Zephiran 1:1000.

Replace all supplies with recently sterilized supplies.

Label and date one week from date of weekly care.

Summary of Important Factors

To adequately care for surgical patients the nurse must have knowledge of wounds and wound healing.

Wounds are classified (according to manner produced) as abraded, incised, lacerated, penetrating, and punctured.

Wounds are classified (according to bacterial content) as clean, contaminated, and septic.

Inflammation is the reaction of body tissues to injury or pathogenic microorganisms. It may be acute, chronic, diffuse, serous, or specific.

Symptoms of inflammation include: redness, heat, swelling, pain, and loss of function.

Infection is the destruction of tissue by pathogenic microorganisms, the symptoms are the same as those of inflammation, with the addition of pus formation.

Local treatment consists of rest and elevation of part, application of heat or cold, and incision and drainage if pus formation is present.

General signs and symptoms of inflammation and infection include temperature elevation, increased pulse and respiration rate, fatigue, loss of appetite, headache, nausea, and vomiting.

General treatment of inflammation includes physical and mental rest, increased fluid intake, good personal hygiene, balanced diet, relief of pain, blood transfusion, fresh air and sunshine, and chemotherapy.

Wounds heal by first intention—prompt healing, with only slight contamination, and small scar formation; or second intention—slow healing, with infection present, and large scar formation.

The amount of drainage material on dressings should be specified, as scant, moderate, or excessive. Drainage that is collected should be measured.

Surgical dressings serve to protect the wound, prevent contamination, keep wound edges in close approximation, provide for local application of drugs, apply pressure, and absorb drainage from the wound.

Equipment needed for surgical dressings, which must be sterile, includes drugs, drainage tubes, rubber gloves, glassware, basins, and other articles, instruments, safety pins, tongue depressors, and dressings. Equipment which need not be sterile includes roller bandage, adhesive, binder and receptacle for soiled dressings.

All surgical dressings should be done with aseptic technique. For the dressing procedure, see that patient is screened and made comfortable, close windows and door to prevent movement of air in room, avoid reaching over the operative area, cleanse lips of all solution bottles used, keep sterile field covered with sterile towel if there is delay in doing the procedure, remove inner dressing only when ready to do procedure, anticipate needs of the surgeon. Dressings may be held in place by bands of adhesive tape, Montgomery strips, liquid adhesive, scotch tape, or binders.

Factors To Teach the Patient

That touching a clean wound with the hands may cause contamination or infection of the wound.

An inflamed part should be elevated and put at rest.

Treatment of wounds need not necessarily cause pain.

An accidental wound should be covered with a sterile or clean dressing.

All soiled dressings should be wrapped and burned.

The patient at home may obtain dressings from organizations that supply them and may arrange with the Visiting Nurse Association to have dressings changed.

There is little danger that surgical wounds will break open.

Scientific Principles

Anatomy and Physiology. Superficial wounds may affect only the skin surface. More severe wounds may affect connective tissue, fascia, and muscle, and may even involve blood vessels, nerves, and bones.

Because the skin contains nerve endings a superficial wound may be quite painful.

Wounds not infected will heal more rapidly than those where infection is present.

Factors which affect the rate of healing of a wound include age, physical condition, state of nutrition, and condition of circulation.

Lack of rest, hemorrhage, infection, and presence of a foreign body may interfere with healing of a wound.

A wound heals by primary intention when the edges are not widely separated, blood and lymph fill the narrow space, a clot forms to seal the wound, and the surface is covered with epithelial cells.

Wounds that are deep and wide or infected heal by secondary intention. The wound fills with buds or granulations of soft tissue, these enlarge to fill the space, the outer cells become elongated to form scar tissue, and the surface is gradually covered with epithelial cells.

Chemistry. Benzene is a solvent for adhesive and is used to remove the residue on the skin surface when adhesive tape is removed.

Urine held in a saturated dressing decomposes and is irritating to the skin surface.

Wounds need to be protected from strong chemicals.

Microbiology. All supplies and instruments used in surgical dressings should be sterile, and sterile technique should be used in applying or changing the dressing.

Because bacteria from the air can enter an exposed wound the door of the room should be closed and care should be taken not to handle bed linen so that air near the patient is agitated or set in motion when surgical dressings are being applied.

Soiled dressings should be wrapped in paper, then discarded into the incinerator.

Pharmacology. Alcohol 70 per cent is used for cleansing wounds. Alcohol coagulates the albumin of the bacterium and destroys the organism.

Iodine is used as a germicide for the skin. Because of its irritating effect on the skin its application is usually followed by the application of alcohol, which acts as a diluting agent.

Mercurochrome is used frequently as a skin antiseptic.

Zinc oxide ointment or powder helps prevent irritation of the skin by excessive drainage from a wound.

Penicillin is used in chemotherapy for open wounds.

Physics. When oil is removed from ordinary cotton it becomes more absorbent.

Gauze absorbs drainage, by capillary action, and by the same means conducts drainage from a wound. A rubber drain removes drainage from a wound by gravity.

Tension of sutures holds the edges of a wound together. As the strength of the sutures decreases, the support of the repaired wound is weakened and additional support of adhesive straps or a binder is needed.

Scissors and hemostats, levers of the first class, and tissue forceps, a lever of the third class, are instruments usually used in doing a surgical dressing.

Psychology. Accidental or surgical wounds have usually caused much pain to the patient, who fears and dreads treatment because of the possibility of more pain being caused.

The treatment should be explained to the patient before the dressing carriage is brought into the room.

When clips or stitches are to be removed, the patient should be informed that the procedure is not painful.

If the patient is informed that the method of suturing used in the operating room makes breaking open of the wound practically impossible, he will not needlessly worry about such a complication.

If the wound being dressed is such that an unpleasant odor is present, the nurse should not indicate by words or action that the duty of changing the dressing is distasteful to her.

Sociology. When operative patients return home a few days after undergoing surgery, dressings may often be changed in the home by a member of the Visiting Nurse Association.

Dressings are furnished by various societies and organizations to patients who cannot afford to buy them for home care.

Situation Type Problem

1. The Nursing Arts instructor had emphasized to a class of students the importance of keeping instruments and supplies sterile in assisting with surgical dressings. One of the students in the class was asked a few days later to assist one of the staff doctors in changing an abdominal dressing. She took the dressing carriage to the patient's bedside, carefully screened the patient from view, and had the outer dressing removed when the doctor came into the unit to change the dressing.

She was skillful and efficient in helping the doctor and everything went well until near the close of the procedure. The doctor had been using tissue forceps and scissors and in placing them on the prepared sterile field he placed the scissors too near the edge and they slid downward so that only the tip ends remained on the sterile towel. After a few minutes of examination the doctor seemed satisfied with the conditions of the wound and indicated he would need the sterile gauze square to be applied directly over the incision as the initial dressing. The gauze square given to him by sterile forceps in the hands of the nurse was evidently larger than he desired, so he picked up the scissors to cut it to desired size. The student promptly advised him that the scissors were contaminated and therefore the gauze dressing had been contaminated. She gave the doctor another sterile gauze square the same size as the one he had received before. He applied it to the incision, applied the necessary additional dressings, fastened them securely in place, assured the patient that the abdominal wound was in satisfactory condition, that he would see her again the following day, and left the room.

When the student nurse completed the procedure and brought the surgical carriage from the room the doctor was waiting for her in the corridor. He was finding it difficult to control his anger and he was most explicit in informing the student that under no circumstances was she ever again to make such a remark to him while assisting him with a treatment. What would you have done?

Suggested Reference Reading

"Care of surgical materials," Martin Frobisher, Jr.; American Journal of Nursing, April, 1941.

"A technique for dressing septic wounds," S. E. McAllister; American Journal of Nursing, June, 1947.

"Sterilizing surgical supplies," Phoebus Berman and John S. Beckett; American Journal of Nursing, October, 1952.

CHAPTER 29

Irrigations

TOPICAL OUTLINE

Purpose of an Irrigation
Equipment Needed
Gastric Lavage
Perineal Irrigation
Vaginal Irrigation
Wound Irrigation

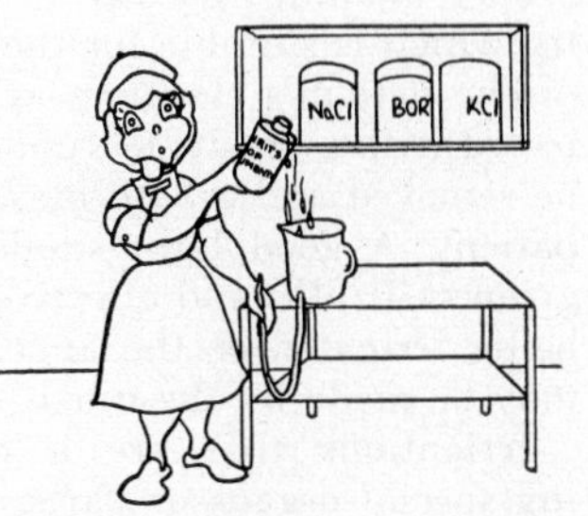

"*And I used to think that* irrigation *was a procedure related to agriculture!*"

An irrigation is defined as the washing out of a canal or cavity by the injection of a stream of water or medicated solution. The solution may be directed into the cavity in a fine spray or allowed to run freely in a stream that is kept at low pressure.

The procedure of irrigating a body cavity continues until the desired result has been obtained, or the amount of solution ordered has been used. Frequency of irrigations will depend on the physical condition of the patient, the organ or part being treated, and the orders of the attending physician. Symptoms indicating that the irrigation has an undesirable effect should be reported at once to the doctor, such symptoms require that the treatment be discontinued.

Areas and cavities of the body most frequently irrigated are the stomach, perineum, vagina, eye, ear, nose, and throat, and the lower colon.

PURPOSE OF AN IRRIGATION

In general, the purpose of an irrigation is to remove added secretions or excessive discharge from a mucous membrane, which is subject to attack by pathogenic microorganisms. Irrigations are given also to apply moist heat to a part, to apply an antiseptic or medicated solution, or to cleanse the area or cavity.

EQUIPMENT NEEDED FOR IRRIGATION

Equipment needed for the irrigation will vary somewhat, according to the kind of irrigation being given, but will be basically the same for most procedures. An irrigating can or container for the solution, a bedpan or other container for return flow of the solution, the proper amount and size of rubber tubing, and an irrigating tube or tip which is suitable for the part being irrigated.

The patient's clothing, as well as linens on the bed, should be protected with a plastic or rubberized cover. Top covers on the bed should be removed and a bath blanket should be used to cover and drape the patient. A good light should be provided so the treatment may be given skillfully and effectively and necessary observations, of the area being irrigated or the appearance of the return flow of the solution, may be made by the nurse.

Irrigations that are a part of the basic procedures for treating special organs or parts, such as the eye, ear, throat, and bladder, are discussed in detail in the chapters dealing with the particular organ or system. Those discussed below are largely related to organs or parts in which special nursing procedures are somewhat restricted.

GASTRIC LAVAGE

Lavage, defined as "an irrigation or washing out of a body cavity," through common usage has come to mean the washing out of the stomach. Written in correct terminology, washing of the stomach would be referred to as "gastric lavage."

Gastric lavage may be done to achieve any of the following purposes: to remove or wash from the stomach material, as poison, that will cause harm to the patient; to remove the stomach contents for diagnostic purposes; to relieve persistent nausea or distention caused by gas; or to wash out the stomach as a preoperative measure for gastric surgery.

The stomach tube is a flexible rubber tube about 5 feet in length. The end that is swallowed is rounded and has several small openings; the other end is shaped like a funnel. Some stomach tubes have a round bulb about midway on the tube. Pressure on the bulb will create suction, when needed, to start or maintain the flow of stomach contents.

The tube should be immersed in ice water for about one hour before the treatment to cool and stiffen it, making it easier for the patient to swallow. In an emergency, as in the case of poisoning, the tube may be lubricated with glycerin or oil to facilitate swallowing.

The physical process used in lavage is that of siphonage. The tube is introduced into the stomach and about 350 cc. of solution is poured into the funnel at the end of the tube. To establish siphonage, before all of the solution has passed through the tube into the stomach the free end of the tube (just below the funnel) is pinched tightly to prevent air from entering the tube. The funnel end of the tube is then lowered so that it is below the level of the patient's stomach. The solution in the tube will flow (because of force of gravity) in the downward direction, and siphonage will withdraw the stomach contents. When the flow ceases, the funnel end may be raised again and more solution poured through the tube into the stomach, and the siphonage is repeated. This process is continued until the ordered amount of solution has been given. In the tube with bulb attachment siphonage is established and controlled by compression and inflation of the bulb.

Solutions most commonly used are tap water, normal saline, sodium bicarbonate 5 per cent, boric acid 2 per cent, and magnesium sulfate. The temperature of the solution should be 100–105° F., and the quantity should be 2000–6000 cc.

The patient should be placed in a sitting position in the bed or, if permitted out of bed, in a straight chair. He should be well draped to keep him comfortably warm during the treatment and his clothing should be well protected.

Several layers of newspaper should be placed on the floor beneath the receptacle for return flow of the solution. Since the return flow may contain gases as well as fluids, it is returned at times with great force, so ample protection for doctor and nurse, as well as for the patient's clothing and bed linen, should be provided.

The procedure should be explained to the patient as equipment is brought into the room. When the tube is introduced he should be instructed as to what he is expected to do and encouraged to keep on swallowing as the tube is gently inserted through the esophagus into the stomach. If the patient wears dentures, they should be removed and stored safely away before he attempts to swallow the tube.

As the tube is inserted, care should be taken not to touch the back of the throat with the end of the tube. This will cause gagging and the tube may be coughed up; continued gagging will cause the patient to vomit, and the tube may be forcibly ejected.

If at any time during the procedure the patient begins to cough or becomes cyanotic, the tube should be withdrawn. If the patient shows signs of weakness or complains of severe pain, the procedure should be discontinued.

Stomach tubes are marked with a colored ring about 18 inches from the tip end. When the tube has been swallowed so that the ring is at the patient's front teeth, the end of the tube should be in the stomach. To make certain that the tube is in the stomach, instead of in some part of the respiratory tract, the funnel end should be inverted into a bowl of water. Bubbles arising from the bowl would indicate that the tube is *not* in the stomach. Crackling sounds within the tube will also indicate that the end of the tube is not in the stomach. If there is doubt as to the location of the end of the tube, a few drops of water allowed to run down the tube will cause the patient to cough if the tube is in the respiratory tract.

If a specimen has been ordered, it should be collected in a sterile container. A test tube quite often will hold the amount needed for performing the specified laboratory tests.

When the tube is withdrawn from the stomach, it should be tightly pinched to prevent aspiration of solution into the lungs. After the irrigation has been completed, the patient should be given a mouthwash to rinse and freshen his mouth and to remove any unpleasant taste of rubber caused by insertion of the tube.

PERINEAL IRRIGATION

Perineal irrigation is defined as "a periodic, aseptic, external irrigation of the vulva and the perineum." The perineum is the area of skin surface between the external genitalia and the anus.

The giving of perineal care periodically adds greatly to the comfort of the patient and helps prevent irritation to the vulva and perineal region from vaginal discharge. Infection may be prevented through the use of perineal irrigations after surgical treatment of the anus, urinary meatus, and perineum. The treatment is effective, too, for preventing discomfort and infection following childbirth and for cleansing the area after urination or defecation.

The patient should be screened to assure privacy and freedom from possible embarrassment. A good light should be provided and so placed that the external genitalia may be clearly viewed. Most patients for whom perineal irrigation is ordered will be wearing perineal pads. These should always be removed and discarded into a paper bag which is later placed in the waste disposal container or incinerator.

When removing a soiled perineal pad, the nurse should grasp the pad, on the outer side only, with thumb above and fingers below, folding the pad together with the soiled portion inside as she removes it from the patient. Top covers should be fan folded to the foot of the bed and the bath blanket used to drape the patient. When properly draped, one corner of the bath blanket extends over the pubic and perineal region and can be used to prevent exposing the patient unnecessarily. During the procedure the corner of the blanket should be folded upward over the patient's abdomen, exposing the perineal area to view.

The solution to be used will be designated by the attending surgeon or obstetrician and should be pleasantly warm (105° F.). In many instances, tap water is used instead of a sterile solution.

The amount of solution used must be known so that output of urine may be measured, if necessary. By using a pitcher with graduated markings for the procedure, the amount of solution used may be quickly and accurately determined.

In irrigating the perineum and vulva, the solution should be poured slowly and steadily from the pitcher, which is held only a few inches above the pubic area. In order not to startle the patient, the beginning stream of water should be directed to the outer part of the vulva or to the labia majora. When the patient is assured that the solution is of correct temperature, it may be directed toward the inner vulvar region. Perineal irrigation is in no way painful and should cause no discomfort to the patient.

If cleansing of the vulva or perineum is required, sterile cotton balls handled with forceps, or with the nurse's scrubbed hands, are used. In cleansing the vulva and meatus, each cotton sponge should be used to cleanse with one downward stroke, then the sponge discarded into the paper bag. After using sponges from the soap solution, sponges from clear water are to be used in the same manner, each sponge being discarded after one downward stroke.

If the cleansing takes place after defecation, the treatment should be given as above, then the bedpan removed and the patient turned to her side for cleansing and drying of the anal region and buttocks. In cleansing the anal region, the cotton balls should be used for only one stroke, the stroke beginning at the perineum and moving across or around the anus toward the lower back.

As soon as perineal care has been given a sterile pad should be placed over the perineum. The sterile pad should be touched only on the outer or topmost side, with the upper half grasped in the top center by the right hand and the lower half in the top center by the left hand, the pad is opened as it is put into position, the sterile side of the pad being placed against the perineum. A T-binder or sanitary belt should be used to hold the perineal pad securely in position.

Perineal care is usually given each time the patient uses the bedpan and should be given at least four or five times during the day, and at night about every four hours if the patient is awake.

Although the procedure just described is one of almost universal standard usage, a few recognized hospitals have adopted a more simple, although equally effective, method of perineal care: The parts are washed thoroughly with soap and water at the time the morning bath is given. A clean washcloth and towel are required, both being used for care of the perineum only.

Patients who require perineal irrigation should have the procedure explained and should be instructed to keep their hands away from the affected or operative area. They should also be cautioned against touching the perineal pads. Those who understand the necessity for handling the pads with aseptic technique are eager to cooperate and will usually respond readily to the suggestion that all stages of the procedure be carried out by the nurse.

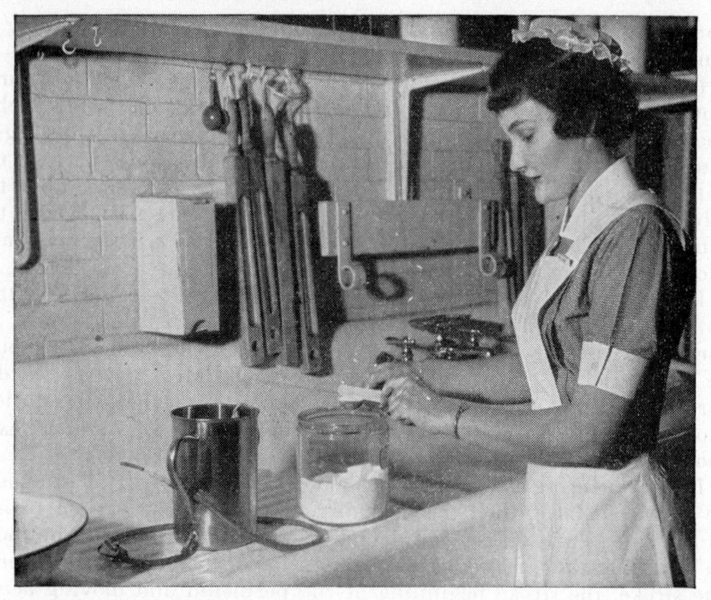

Fig. 178. The kind, amount, and strength of solution is important in any irrigation. (Massachusetts General Hospital School of Nursing, Boston, Massachusetts.)

VAGINAL IRRIGATION

Although the term "vaginal douche" is often used for this particular procedure, the correct term is vaginal irrigation. A douche, correctly defined, is a stream of water or medicinal fluid directed with force against a part. A vaginal irrigation, as carried out in the performance of nursing service, consists of introducing a solution *at low pressure* into the cavity of the vagina, the solution returning immediately.

Vaginal irrigations are prescribed as part of the patient's treatment, usually for one or more of the following reasons: to cleanse the vagina; to prevent infection by use of an antiseptic solution in irrigating the part; to destroy an offensive odor caused by vaginal discharge; or to lessen or overcome an irritating discharge from the vagina.

The procedure was used extensively in former years to apply heat in treating inflammation and to help control hemorrhage. It is now used much less frequently for those purposes, since mechanical devices now available for applying heat to the involved area are much more effective and more pleasant for the patient.

Vaginal irrigation is done only when ordered by the attending physician. Normally the mucous membrane lining the vaginal canal secretes a slightly acid substance which serves to protect the vagina against infection. Although a limited number of vaginal irrigations may help to prevent the growth of pathogenic microorganisms, frequent and excessive irrigation is likely to wash away the protective secretion and make the vagina even more susceptible to invasion by the causative agents of infection.

The most common use of the irrigation is for the purpose of cleansing the vagina, and this particular method of cleansing has been used to serve a variety of purposes. Cleansing the vagina following sexual intercourse has long been a part of many contraceptive measures; irrigation offers a means of reducing the amount of vaginal discharge produced by mechanical devices, such as pessaries, which are worn in the vagina to help support the uterus in proper position; the procedure is also used routinely to help overcome the offensive odor so often associated with gynecologic diseases, such as carcinoma of the cervix.

The kind, amount, and strength of solution used, as well as the temperature of the solution, are important in obtaining the desired results, and the doctor's order should be specific in regard to all four factors. For simple cleansing of the vagina, the solutions most commonly used are normal saline, 1 per cent, or plain tap water. The temperature of the solution should be 105° F. (40.5° C.). The amount of solution may vary, although usually about 2000 cc. (2 quarts) is required.

If the irrigation is for antiseptic purposes, to combat infection or offensive odor, potassium permanganate 1:2000, silver nitrate 1:10,000, or bichloride of mercury 1:10,000 may be prescribed.

For specific treatment, as in the application of heat, the temperature of the solution may be as high as 110–115° F. (43.3–46.1° C.) if it can be tolerated by the patient.

The length of the vagina is about 3 inches. It is lined with mucous membrane, which is continuous with the lining of the uterus and fallopian tubes and with the peritoneum. For this reason infection of the vagina may spread rapidly to the abdominal area, making it necessary to exercise care in irrigation of the vagina, so that solution will not be forced through the cervix into the uterus. The mucous membrane lining the vagina lies in convolutions or folds, called *rugae*, and a thorough cleansing of the organ is possible only when the numerous small sprays of solution coming from the douche nozzle are kept in constant motion with a rhythmic inward and outward manipulation of the nozzle which at the same time is slowly rotated in a half circle from right to left. The douche nozzle, 6 to 8 inches in length, is slightly curved to better follow the normal contour of the vagina. Glass tips or nozzles are easily cleaned and sterilized, but must be handled with extreme care to avoid being cracked or broken. The danger to the patient subjected to vaginal irrigation with a damaged glass nozzle is obvious.

In some conditions, such as presence of a particularly small vagina, of edema or swelling, or of an abnormality in structure or development, substitution of a soft rubber catheter for the douche tip may be necessary.

The choice as to use of a bedpan or douche pan for return flow of the irrigating solution will depend on the equipment available in the institution.

Since low pressure is indicated for the procedure, the lower end of the irrigating can should not be more than 18 inches above the level of the mattress. Pressure may be increased by raising the irrigating can and decreased by lowering it.

The procedure should be explained to the patient and if she has not had such treatment before it may be necessary to assure her that the treatment will not be painful nor will it cause damage to any part of the area involved. If temperature of the solution is above 105° F. the patient should be cautioned that the solution is quite warm but that it is not actually hot and there is no danger of her being burned.

The patient should be properly screened and draped and during the procedure should be exposed only as absolutely necessary. A suitable "treatment" sign should be placed on the door of the patient's room to prevent interruption by visitors or nurses and other employees of the hospital.

The top covers should be fan-folded to the foot of the bed and the patient should be draped with a treatment or bath blanket. If necessary, an additional blanket may be used so the patient will be comfortably warm.

All pillows, with the possible exception of one small one, should be removed from the bed, and the backrest should be lowered. The patient's hips should be elevated to a position slightly higher than her head and shoulders and this is accomplished by placement of the bedpan or douche pan.

If there is excessive vaginal discharge it may be necessary to thoroughly cleanse the part before beginning the irrigation.

When the irrigating can has been hung at the proper height the stopcock on the rubber tubing should be released enough to permit a small amount of solution to run through the douche tip so it will be warmed before it is inserted into the vagina. The douche tip should be inserted by being directed slightly upward, then backward to conform with the curve of the vagina.

Just before the last of the solution flows from the can, the tip should be withdrawn and the equipment replaced on the douche tray. The patient should remain on the bedpan and should be assisted to a sitting position to allow the remaining solution to drain from the vagina. The perineal region should be dried, the drapes removed and top covers replaced. After the patient has been made comfortable all equipment should be removed from the room, properly cleaned and returned to central supply or to its assigned location in the utility room on the clinical service department.

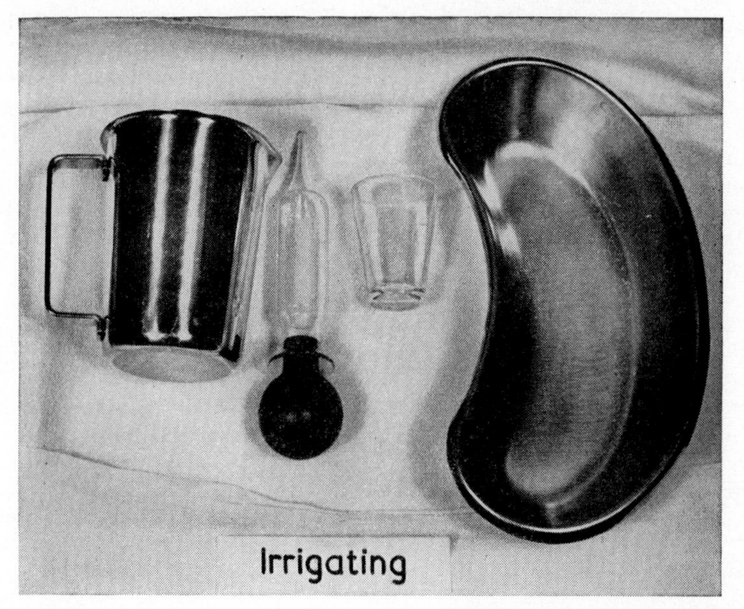

Fig. 179. A sterile tray for wound irrigation. (Central Supply, Hospital for Sick Children, Toronto, Canada.)

If vaginal irrigation is ordered for a patient just before or after menstruation or during the postpartum period, the danger of infection is increased because the cervical canal may be open, making the adjoining organs more susceptible. For vaginal irrigation under these rather unfavorable circumstances or following an operation on the generative organs, the solution must be sterile and aseptic technique must be strictly adhered to in carrying out the procedure.

If it is known that the patient is affected with gonorrhea, the nurse should wear rubber gloves and her eyes should be protected by goggles.

As the doctor often asks the patient to continue vaginal irrigations after she has left the hospital, the nurse should instruct the patient in the most effective and simplest manner of carrying out the procedure in her own home.

WOUND IRRIGATION

Irrigation of a surgical wound or of drainage tubes that have been placed in a wound may be ordered by the doctor.

Solutions usually used are normal saline, Dakin's solution, tyrothricin, and penicillin sodium.

An Asepto syringe with bulb is used for the irrigation, and a large curved basin is usually used for the return flow. All equipment should be sterile, and aseptic technique should be used. The irrigation should be continued until the solution returned is clear. When Dakin's solution is used, petrolatum gauze should be placed carefully over the edge of the wound to protect new granulation tissue.

If rubber drainage tubes are to be irrigated, it may be necessary for the nurse to hold the end of the tube with sterile forceps, or to wear a sterile rubber glove on her left hand so she may hold the end of the tube for insertion of the tip of the syringe. The drainage tube should be handled as little as possible during the procedure to avoid loosening or dislodging it from its place in the wound.

Care of Equipment after Use

GASTRIC LAVAGE

The stomach tube, including bulb and funnel, should be rinsed in cold water, washed in soap and water, rinsed again, and allowed to dry. It should be sterilized by being boiled or by being immersed in a strong disinfectant solution before it is used again.

Rubber aprons or protectors should be washed in soap and water.

All other equipment should be washed and returned to central supply.

PERINEAL IRRIGATION

A tray is set up for the use of each patient receiving perineal care. It should be kept continuously supplied with sterile cotton pledgets and sterile perineal pads. The small pitcher must be kept covered at all times and should be washed and resterilized at regular intervals.

VAGINAL IRRIGATION

All equipment used in vaginal irrigation should be sterilized by boiling or by being wrapped and autoclaved to prevent cross-infection.

WOUND IRRIGATION

The irrigating set should be washed and boiled for 10 minutes. The Asepto syringe should be boiled with bulb attached to the syringe. All other equipment used should be washed and boiled. All supplies used from the dressing cart should be replenished. All soiled dressings should be burned.

Summary of Important Factors

GASTRIC LAVAGE

The patient should be in sitting position during the procedure.

If the stomach tube is immersed for one hour in ice water it will be easier for the patient to swallow.

PERINEAL IRRIGATION

Proper draping of the patient will minimize embarrassment.

In pouring solution, the stream should be started slowly and gently so as not to startle the patient.

Correct handling of soiled perineal pads is essential for protection of the nurse.

VAGINAL IRRIGATION

Vaginal irrigation should be done only on order of the physician.

Pressure should never be used to insert the douche nozzle.

The irrigation should be discontinued during the patient's menstrual period.

Aseptic technique should usually be used.

The face (especially the eyes) should not be touched during or after the procedure, until hands have been thoroughly washed in soap and water.

Any drug used in making the solution should be thoroughly dissolved.

For patients known to have gonorrhea, the nurse should wear goggles and gloves to protect herself from possible contamination.

WOUND IRRIGATION

All equipment used should be sterile, and the procedure should be done with aseptic technique.

Drainage tubes should be handled in such a way that they are not loosened or dislodged from their original position.

Factors To Teach the Patient

GASTRIC LAVAGE

That the benefits of the treatment are well worth the unpleasantness or discomfort experienced in swallowing the stomach tube.

That swallowing the tube will be easier if he thinks in terms of swallowing a favorite food and, once started, keeps on swallowing until the tube is in the stomach.

PERINEAL IRRIGATION

The proper handling of a soiled perineal pad.

The perineum should be cleansed after urination and defecation from front to back so that contamination from the anal region is not carried toward the vagina.

The procedure is commonplace to the nurse and should cause no embarrassment.

VAGINAL IRRIGATION

Gonococcus which may affect the eyes is carried on the hands and may be transferred to the eyes unless hands are carefully washed.

That taking douches without the doctor's order may cause harm by washing away the protective secretions of the vagina.

How to prepare the solution and use equipment for taking the douche at home, if that is necessary.

WOUND IRRIGATION

To refrain from touching equipment or supplies, since all are sterile and aseptic technique is being used.

Scientific Principles

Anatomy and Physiology. The stomach is a hollow, muscular organ where much of the digestion of food takes place. The oral cavity and esophagus are lined with mucous membrane which secretes more mucus when irritated, as by introduction of the stomach tube. This facilitates swallowing of the tube, which is done primarily by muscular action. Gastric juice is secreted by glands in the walls of the stomach. Since little absorption takes place in the stomach, if poisons are removed before they enter the duodenum there is good possibility of saving the life of the patient.

External genitals of the female include labia majora, labia minora, clitoris, and vaginal orifice. The labia minora are located inside the labia majora. Both structures must be separated to permit introduction of the douche nozzle into the vaginal orifice. Bartholin's glands, secreting a lubricating fluid, are small glands on either side of the orifice. The vagina is a muscular, membranous canal about 3½ inches long. The direction of the vaginal tract is backward and slightly upward, a fact which should be borne in mind when the douche nozzle is being inserted.

Chemistry. Gastric juice is clear and acid in reaction. It is made up of approximately 98 per cent water and very small percentages of mucin, salts, pepsin, rennin, and gastric lipase, as well as hydrochloric acid.

Sodium bicarbonate is often used as an irrigating solution for the stomach, since it neutralizes stomach acidity.

A mild alkali is given for an acid poison.

A mild acid is given for an alkaline poison.

Normal reaction of the vaginal mucosa is acid and serves, therefore, as a protection against certain bacteria. Frequent vaginal irrigations will lower the acidity and lessen the effectiveness of the secretion.

Microbiology. All equipment used in lavage is kept clean, although it need not be sterile.

The tube used in stomach irrigations should be sterilized after use, by boiling or by being immersed in a bichloride of mercury solution.

Normal vaginal secretion is acid in reaction. Frequent irrigation of the vaginal tract removes protecting vaginal secretions and lessens resistance to pathogenic microorganisms.

Soiled perineal pads should be wrapped in paper and burned.

Organisms causing disease of the genitals are the gonococcus, *Streptococcus pyogenes*, staphylococcus, the colon bacillus, and tubercle bacillus.

Because the gonococcus attacks the conjunctiva of the eye and may cause blindness, the nurse should wear goggles when giving a vaginal irrigation to a patient with gonorrhea.

The colon bacillus may be found on the vulva and perineum, and care should be taken to prevent contamination of the vaginal canal.

Where stitches are present or there has been laceration of tissues, the vaginal irrigation should be done with aseptic technique. All equipment and the solution used should be sterile.

Pharmacology. Solutions used for gastric lavage are normal saline, sodium bicarbonate, or the specific antidote of a poison.

An antidote that mixes with the poison to prevent its absorption, as milk and egg whites with a metallic poison, is classified as a physical antidote. An antidote that reacts with the poison to neutralize it, as sodium bicarbonate for an acid poison, is termed a chemical antidote. An antidote that produces the opposite systemic effect, as caffeine for morphine poisoning, is a physiologic antidote.

Solutions used for vaginal irrigations are sodium chloride or sodium bicarbonate for cleansing, boric acid for antiseptic action, and potassium permanganate for deodorizing.

Physics. Gastric lavage is accomplished by siphonage, an action that results because of differences of pressure, and liquids exert pressure in relation to their weight. The irrigating solution flows into the stomach because of its weight. When the funnel is lowered below the stomach level, the fluid flows out, bringing the stomach contents with it.

Vaginal irrigations should be given under low pressure, so the irrigating can should never be elevated more than 18 inches or so above bed level. Since the mucous membrane of the vagina can tolerate a temperature of 110° F. or more it may be necessary to protect the skin around the orifice with a layer of oil. The skin may be burned if a solution of that temperature is used without such protection.

Gravity will aid the return flow of the irrigating solution if the patient is elevated by means of the backrest after the procedure is completed.

Psychology. Before introduction of the stomach tube, which is generally not a pleasant procedure for the patient, the benefits to be derived from the treatment should be explained. The patient needs encouragement and reassurance.

Many patients have vague ideas that disease involving the genital tract is disgraceful. Many are acutely uncomfortable and embarrassed at the necessity of exposing the genital area. The nurse should explain the procedure to the patient and by her own matter-of-fact attitude relieve the patient of embarrassment. If the patient has not had a vaginal irrigation previously, the nurse should inform her that the treatment is not at all painful and that the warmth of the solution is soothing and relaxing.

Sociology. In an emergency, as when poison has been taken, if a stomach tube is not available lavage may be accomplished by forcing the patient to drink large quantities of lukewarm salt solution. Sufficient solution will force the patient to vomit, thus emptying the stomach of much of the poison that was taken.

If vaginal irrigation is to be continued after the patient leaves the hospital, the nurse will need to teach the patient how to administer the douche for herself. It would be well to have her purchase the equipment she will use at home and learn to use it while she is still in the hospital and under the supervision of the nurse.

Situation Type Problems

1. A student nurse was assigned to care for a patient who had received vaginal irrigations each morning for several days. The procedure had been ordered to be given once daily. After setting up the tray and explaining to the patient that she was to give her the usual irrigation, the nurse draped the patient and placed her on the douche pan. As the treatment was about to be started a moderate amount of bloody discharge was noted at the opening of the vagina. During the previous days when the treatment was being given there had been no discharge and the return flow of the solution had been clear. What would you have done?

2. A patient for whom a wound irrigation had been ordered daily, refused to let the student nurse carry out the procedure. When questioned as to why she was refusing a treatment, which had been done for her several times before, the patient stated that the nurse who did the procedure on the previous day had been rough and careless and had made the treatment extremely painful. What would you have done?

3. In giving a perineal irrigation a student nurse accidentally touched the lip of the sterile pitcher over which the solution would be poured. She had washed her hands just before beginning the procedure. If she took time to return to Central Supply for another pitcher she would be late to class and the instructor had already told

her that if she was late to class again her grade in the course would be lowered. What would you have done?

Suggested Reference Reading

"Perineal care after delivery," Ann Kirchner and Elizabeth Peck; American Journal of Nursing, June, 1950.

CHAPTER 30

Eye, Ear, Nose, and Throat Procedures

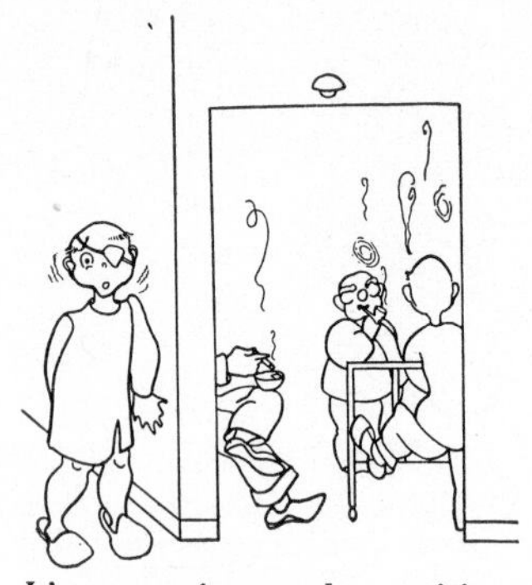

It's a comfort to have visitors occasionally—in fact, that's the best way!

The Eye

The eye is the special organ for the perception of visual images, commonly termed "the organ of sight." In giving nursing care or treatments involving the eye, the nurse should be very gentle, using the utmost caution to avoid pressure against the eyeball. The conjunctiva and cornea of the eye are extremely delicate in structure and form. The eye is considered one of the most sensitive organs of the body.

When entering a room the nurse should always announce her pres-

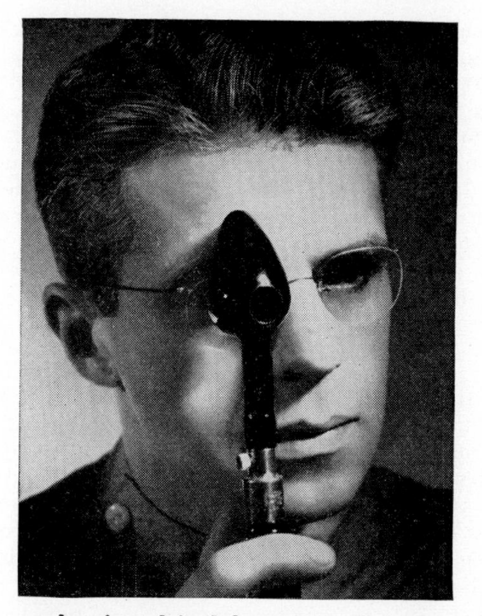

Fig. 180. If the procedure is explained the patient will not be needlessly frightened of an eye examination. (Bausch & Lomb Optical Co., Rochester, New York.)

ence to a patient who cannot see. She should avoid startling him by speaking suddenly or touching him when he is unaware that another person is in the room. In performing nursing service she should work smoothly and effortlessly, and all hand movements should be sure and skillful. The patient who cannot see develops confidence in the nurse in accordance with her ability to use her hands effectively, since he is unable to observe visually her method of performing nursing procedures.

The student who gives nursing service to a patient with eye involvement should keep her hands immaculately clean and fingernails fairly short and well rounded to facilitate the handling of eye dressings and to prevent possible injury, through scratching, to the region of the eyes.

Any procedure involving the eye should be carefully explained to the patient so he will know what is expected of him and cooperate in helping to obtain the best possible results.

LIGHTING, AS IT AFFECTS THE EYE

Daylight is preferable to any type of artificial light, but in rooms where close work is being done, artificial illumination may be needed to supply sufficient light on dark days. To further insure proper lighting it is necessary that walls and ceilings be kept clean. Dull-finished surfaces will minimize glare from lights. For handwork or for reading the light should come from over the left shoulder (right shoulder if the patient is left handed). This will prevent a hand shadow from falling across the work if handwork is being done.

In caring for the sick, all nurses should remember that light can be a source of much discomfort, chiefly because illness tends to increase light sensitivity. The bed in a hospital room should never be placed so the patient must face a window, and overhead lights should always have shields to direct the illumination away from the patient's eyes.

Reading and other close work should be limited to brief periods of time and should not be permitted at all if the patient is fatigued.

USE OF SUN GLASSES

Normally the eyes are able to adjust to ordinary daylight without discomfort, but when exposure to sunlight is prolonged the use of an eye shade or of sun glasses is indicated. Although the color of the lens in sun glasses is largely a matter of choice, it should be such that natural colors are not greatly altered when viewed through the lens.

Sun glasses should be worn only during periods of exposure to sunlight. To wear them indiscriminately may result in reduced tolerance to ordinary light.

SYMPTOMS OF EYE ABNORMALITIES

Symptoms that indicate the need for eye examination include: swollen, inflamed eyelids, or persistent crusting of lid margins; pain in the eyes, with redness and swelling; sudden change in vision, such as dimming sight or double vision; frequent formation of styes (hordeolum); discomfort, vertigo, headaches, and other signs of eyestrain; undue sensitivity to light; necessity of holding reading material very near or quite far from the eyes in order to see clearly; overuse of one eye; stumbling, misjudging height of steps, and other actions which indicate inability to see well.

EYE EXAMINATION

For examination of the eyes, the patient should be placed in a comfortable position. He may remain in bed with his head and shoulders elevated by means of the backrest or he may be placed in a sitting position in a chair near the source of light.

The doctor usually sits facing the patient. If a head mirror is worn by the doctor, the light should be back and to the right of the patient. Daylight is preferable to artificial light for general examination of the eyes.

To examine the interior of the eye, an ophthalmoscope, a lighted instrument designed for this particular purpose, is used, and the room should be darkened.

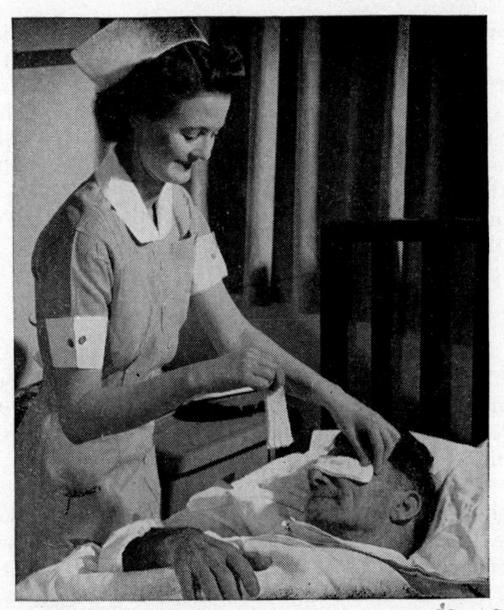

Fig. 181. Gauze compresses may be used to apply heat or cold to the eye. (Johns Hopkins Hospital School of Nursing, Baltimore, Maryland.)

If vision is to be tested, the familiar chart of various sized letters is used. If the largest letters on the chart are not visible to the patient, the examiner may hold the fingers of one hand before the patient's eyes and gradually move the hand away to determine the distance at which he is no longer able to distinguish separate fingers and therefore cannot accurately count those extended out from the hand.

TO APPLY MOIST HEAT TO THE EYES

A simple and effective method of applying moist heat to the eyes is to wring a large towel from boiling water, roll it in a dry towel and apply carefully to the eyes. The dry towel conserves the heat, and the application will remain hot for about 15 minutes. Heat applied in this manner is moist heat and therefore more desirable. Care should be taken not to burn the skin of the nose if a hot application is used for both eyes.

Hot compresses for use in treatment of various eye conditions are made of 4-inch squares of gauze. The squares are placed in a basin of solution heated to the desired temperature and maintained at that temperature throughout the procedure. Forceps must be used to wring hot water from the compress, which may then be tested and applied by hand.

Mineral oil applied to the eyelid before the treatment is begun will decrease the conduction of heat from the compress and there will be little danger of burning the area being treated.

If there is a discharge from the eye, each compress should be discarded after use. If both eyes are to be treated, separate equipment and supplies must be used for each eye, to prevent cross infection from one eye to the other.

If the patient is known to have gonorrheal infection of the eyes, the nurse should protect herself by wearing rubber gloves and goggles during the procedure.

EYE IRRIGATION

Irrigation of the eyes, usually with a solution of boric acid or normal saline, is done to apply heat to inflamed mucous membrane and thus relieve pain and congestion, to cleanse the eyelids of excess secretions, and to remove foreign bodies from the conjunctival sac.

Patients should be cautioned against rubbing an inflamed eye or touching the eyes with their fingers, which carry microorganisms.

For the irrigation, the patient should be turned to the side of the affected eye. The solution is expressed from a rubber bulb syringe and directed into the eye at the inner canthus. When correctly done, the solution runs across the eye and flows out the outer canthus into the emesis basin, which has been placed to receive it.

The temperature of the solution should be as ordered and just before doing the irrigation the nurse should test the solution by allowing a small amount to run across the inner surface of her wrist.

The patient's eye should be closed and a small stream of the solution allowed to run over the lid to reassure the patient that the solution is not too hot. The lid should then be cleansed with a cotton pladget, the eye opened, and the irrigation procedure begun. Care must be taken not to startle the patient by allowing the end of the irrigating syringe to come in contact with the eye or eyelid.

When both eyes are irrigated two sets of sterile equipment and two emesis basins must be used, and the patient is turned to the respective side as each eye is treated. These precautions are necessary to prevent cross-infection from one eye to the other.

EYE INSTILLATION

If the instillation of medicine in the eye is a new experience for the patient, it should be explained to him that his part in the procedure is to maintain a comfortable position, to look upward during the instillation, to refrain from jumping when the medicine is dropped on the lower lid, and to close his eyes gently instead of squeezing them tight together after the treatment. He should be told that the medicine may result in a change in vision or in the appearance of the eye for a short time.

The bottle containing the medicine should be open and ready for use before the eye is prepared to receive the medication. As the eye dropper containing the medication is removed from the bottle it should be held upright, with the medication remaining in the lower end. The dropper should not be inverted since the medicine should not be allowed to run into the rubber bulb end of the dropper. If the medicine dropper is in good condition, no medicine will drop from the open end when it is held downward unless pressure is exerted on the bulb.

In preparation for instilling medication into the eye a cotton ball or gauze square should be used to help draw the lower lid gently downward to prevent trauma and to insure a more steady hold on the eyelid.

The hand in which the dropper is held should be steadied by placing the little finger against the patient's forehead in the templar region. The patient should be instructed to look up, and the thumb of the other hand should be placed below the margin of the lower lid and gently pressed downward. The end of the dropper should be brought close to the outer corner of the lower lid and one drop of the medicine expressed. The dropper should be hastily removed from the vicinity of the eye as soon as the medicine has been instilled.

The drop of medicine, when well placed, will spread evenly across the lower lid and will not run over onto the patient's cheek. By placing the cotton ball or gauze with slight pressure against the junction of the inner canthus and nasal bone, excess medicine will be absorbed by the cotton and that instilled in the eye will not escape into the nasolacrimal duct.

Since it is necessary to touch the patient about the eyes, especially in drawing the lower lid into position, the thoughtful nurse will warm her hands, if necessary, before beginning the procedure.

APPLICATION OF EYE OINTMENTS

Eye ointments are used primarily: to treat infections of the eye; to dilate or contract the pupil; and to soothe or lubricate in burns of the conjunctiva.

Eye ointment is available in small collapsible tubes. A small amount should be expressed from the tube and discarded before the ointment is expressed in the eye.

The eyelids should be cleansed before ointment is applied. The lower lid should be gently pulled downward, with cotton ball or gauze square, and the patient should be instructed to direct his gaze upward. A thin line of ointment should be placed along the conjunctival surface

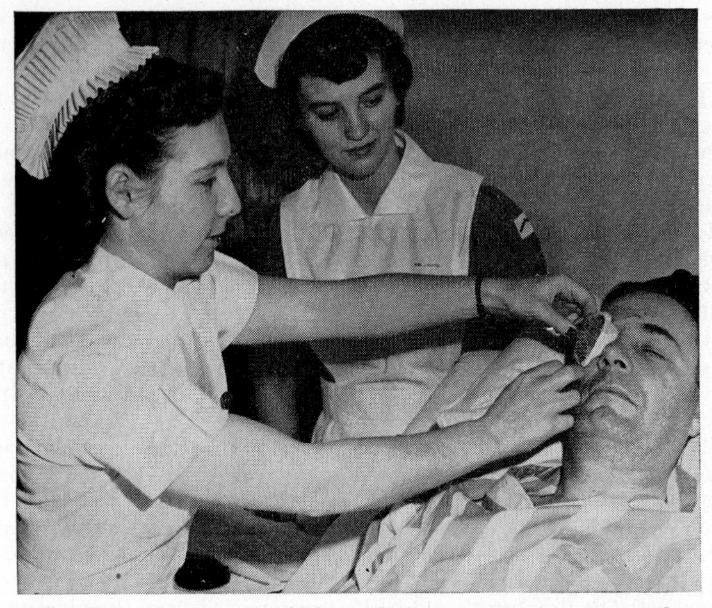

Fig. 182. All eye dressings should be applied so pressure is not exerted on the eyeball. (Miami Valley Hospital School of Nursing, Dayton, Ohio.)

of the retracted lower lid, extending from the outer to the inner canthus. Sufficient ointment should be used to lubricate the outer edge of both lids. When the patient closes his eye and rotates the eyeball from side to side the ointment will be dispersed over its entire anterior surface.

In applying ointment to the eye care must be taken not to touch the eyeball or the eyelid with the tip of the ointment tube.

EMERGENCIES INVOLVING THE EYE

Emergencies involving the eye, for which the nurse may be expected to know first aid treatment, include burns, incised wounds and lacerations, and foreign bodies.

Burns. Most burns affecting the eye are caused by acid or alkali. The solution or substance causing the burn should be washed out immediately at the scene of the accident. Ordinary tap water from a faucet or drinking fountain may be used, provided the flow of water is not strong enough to cause undue pressure on the eyeball. Irrigation of the eye should be continued until all irritating material has been removed from the eye and eyelids.

As soon as possible a doctor should be called to examine the eye and to order proper medical treatment.

Incised Wounds and Lacerations. Eye injuries of this nature usually require surgical treatment. The only immediate treatment which can be given is protection of the injured eye with a clean dry dressing. The dressing should be applied loosely, so that pressure is not exerted on the eye.

Foreign Bodies. Foreign bodies in the eye are very painful because of the extreme sensitiveness of the eyeball. Small particles, such as sand, coal, dust, cinders, and ashes, may cause minor abrasions of the eyeball. An object that has a sharp edge or enters the eye with great force may cause a more serious wound and become deeply embedded in the eyeball.

With the patient in a sitting position and face tilted slightly upward, the cornea and bulbar conjunctiva may be examined to locate the foreign body. If found on the cornea, the foreign body may be removed by gentle irrigation or by the corner of a clean handkerchief or gauze square.

If the foreign body is not found on the cornea, the conjunctiva of the lower lid should be inspected. If the foreign body is not found on the lower lid and the patient still complains of discomfort or pain in the eye the upper lid should be everted to permit inspection of that part of the eye.

To Evert the Upper Lid. For eversion of the upper lid the patient should be instructed to look down, and an applicator stick or toothpick should be placed horizontally across the eyelid, one-half inch from the margin. By grasping lashes firmly between thumb and index finger, the lid may be gently pulled down and forward, then up, folding it back over the applicator. The eyelid can then be held in position by pressing the lashes against the eyebrow with the thumb of the hand grasping the eyelid.

With the eyelid completely folded back on itself, the undersurface is exposed to view and a foreign body adhered to it may be quickly and easily removed. If the object cannot be removed without effort and in the first or second try, sterile olive oil or mineral oil should be put into the eye to help prevent further irritation and the patient should be seen by a doctor.

To return the eyelid to its normal position, the lashes should be grasped and the lid gently pulled forward and down, while the patient is instructed to look up.

All eye procedures should be done with the utmost care and gentleness, and the nurse's hands should be thoroughly washed before and after each procedure.

The Ear

The ear is the special organ of the sense of hearing. It is a receiving station for sound waves, and plays an important part in maintaining equilibrium or body balance.

DEAFNESS

The most common symptom related to hearing is deafness, which may range from complete loss of hearing to very slight impairment only.

Loss of hearing, to some degree, affects a large number of people and in many of these deafness could have been prevented. Programs for control of communicable diseases and for correction of remedial defects now help to check the growing number of persons with impairment of hearing.

Several factors are concerned in the underlying cause of deafness. Among the most common causes are: *physical injuries,* such as those caused by blows, cannon shots, dynamite, diving from great heights; *communicable diseases,* as scarlet fever, diphtheria, and measles; *the common cold; purulent infections of the middle ear; impacted cerumen* or *foreign bodies; drugs,* such as quinine, salicylates, nicotine, and morphine; *chemicals* encountered in industry, as lead or mercury; *deficiency in diet,* especially a lack of vitamins or of calcium; *noise* and other occupational hazards, as in boilermaking or riveting; *congenital defects* or malformation.

An effective program for the prevention of deafness depends largely on early discovery of the disease or defect which may produce loss of hearing.

Ear infections are often preceded by infection of the nose and throat. Adequate care of nose and throat conditions may help to prevent the more serious ear infections, as otitis media and mastoiditis.

EAR EXAMINATION

Examination of the ear usually includes a general hearing test, such as determination of the patient's ability to hear the ticking of a watch which is held at an increasingly greater distance from the ear, and observation of color, size, and shape of the ears. The presence of discharge from the ear should be noted, as should symptoms of inflammation or of tenderness on pressure in front or behind the ear.

An electrically lighted instrument, the otoscope, is used in examining the ear. A small rounded speculum attached to the otoscope fits into the auditory meatus, so that the examiner may clearly see the auditory canal inward as far as the tympanic membrane. The membrane itself should be examined for perforations or scars.

EAR WAX

A wax-like substance termed cerumen, secreted by the epithelial cells lining the external auditory canal, serves as a protection for the drum membrane since insects and other foreign bodies become imbedded in it and cannot enter the middle ear. When cerumen accumulates and hardens it forms a plug in the canal which may interfere with hearing. In some instances, irrigation of the ear or surgical treatment may be necessary for effective removal of the plug.

EARACHE

Infections or other disorders in any one of the three parts of the ear may cause earache which can be extremely painful.

Earache may occur as a referred pain caused by one of several disorders, such as facial neuralgia, dental caries or dental procedures, as tooth extraction, or the common cold, especially when pharyngitis occurs; earache may also be a postoperative complication of tonsillectomy.

EAR DROPS

Ear drops are usually ordered as a means of applying heat to the ear to relieve the pain of earache, to dry up a persistent discharge from the ear, or to soften a plug of cerumen so it can be removed by irrigation. Warm oil may be dropped in the ear for the purpose of killing an insect which has entered the auditory canal.

Ear drops may be of 2 per cent phenol and glycerin, olive oil, or a boric acid and alcohol solution, depending on the purpose for which they are used. The solution or medication should be warmed to 100° F. by placing the bottle or container into a basin of hot water for a few minutes.

With the patient in a dorsal recumbent position and the head turned to one side, the warm solution or oil should be dropped into the ear. Three or four drops is the amount usually instilled.

A small cotton pledget should be placed in the ear to prevent escape of the oil or medication from the auditory canal when the patient turns his head to a different position.

EAR IRRIGATION

Ear irrigation is the washing out of the external auditory canal with a prescribed solution, done usually to remove cerumen, a foreign body, or purulent discharge caused by infection.

A metal syringe or an irrigating can with the correct length of rubber tubing may be used for ear irrigation. The irrigating can should not be elevated to more than 6 inches above the level of the ear, and the irrigation should be given with only a minimum amount of pressure, since there is danger of involvement of the middle ear.

Solutions most commonly used are a 2–4 per cent boric acid solution, a weak sodium bicarbonate solution, and physiological saline solution. Temperature of the solution should be approximately 105° F. The amount of solution varies with the purpose for which the treatment is given. If the irrigation is done to supply heat to the affected area, 1000 cc. of solution is usually used.

The patient should be placed in a sitting position and instructed to hold the curved basin in which return flow of the solution is collected.

The external auditory canal should be straightened for the procedure. In the adult, the nurse may grasp the ear lobe and pull it gently upward and backward. In a child, the ear lobe should be grasped firmly and pulled downward and backward to straighten the canal.

The opening of the canal must not be blocked by the tip of the syringe or irrigating tube, since there must be ample room for return flow of the solution.

The stream of solution should be gentle and continuous and directed toward either side of the canal, rather than toward the ear drum.

During the procedure the patient should be watched for symptoms of pain or vertigo. Any signs of such unfavorable reaction to the procedure is an indication that the irrigation should be discontinued.

When the irrigation has been completed, the patient should be turned so that the affected ear is downward and drainage from the ear is facilitated. The opening of the canal should not be plugged with cotton after irrigation, as this tends to interfere with drainage from the middle to the outer ear.

EMERGENCIES INVOLVING THE EAR

Sharp or pointed objects used to remove wax from the ear may cause injury to the canal or to the ear drum. Patients should be warned against such practices as "cleaning" the ear with a hairpin, the head of a straight pin, or the pointed end of a fingernail.

Removal of foreign bodies is the most common emergency measure related to the ear. It is not unusual to find such objects as small rocks, cereal grains (corn, wheat, beans), and pieces of matches or other bits of material in the external auditory canal. For rocks and other hardened material, irrigation may be an effective means of removal. Irrigation cannot be used for removal of cereal grains, as the solution causes the grain to swell and may cause injury to the ear drum. Special instruments are needed for removal of such foreign bodies, and the procedure calls for the services of a specialist in the treatment of ear conditions.

When a live insect has entered the external auditory canal it should be killed immediately, to reduce the danger of further injury from bites or from damage caused by the insect's frantic efforts to escape. A few drops of oil or of alcohol instilled into the ear will kill the insect, which can then be washed from the canal by irrigation.

A swimmer may experience having water enter the ear and remain there instead of flowing out spontaneously. A sudden tap on the side

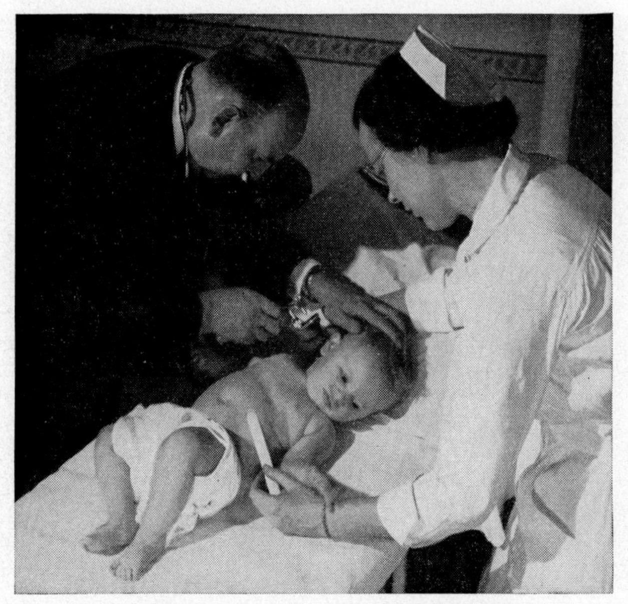

Fig. 183. Ear examination may reveal the presence of a foreign body in the ear. (Presbyterian Hospital, Chicago, Illinois.)

of the head just above the ear is usually sufficient to dislodge the accumulated water and cause it to flow outward through the auditory canal.

GENERAL CONSIDERATIONS

The nurse should know how to make the hard of hearing or the deaf patient comfortable. She should inspire confidence and cooperation which are essential if treatment and nursing care are to effect improvement of the ear condition. She should urge relatives and friends to treat the patient as they would any normal individual. She herself should always speak directly to him in a normal tone of voice, pronouncing each word distinctly.

If the patient is totally deaf it may be necessary for her to write notes to him, to make sure he understands the information she wishes to impart. To help the patient effectively, she should refer him to social agencies whose services are available and, if necessary, should inform him of the location of schools which are conducted for the hard of hearing and for the deaf.

The Nose

The nose is the special organ of the sense of smell. It serves as an air passageway and acts as an air conditioner for all inspired air. The

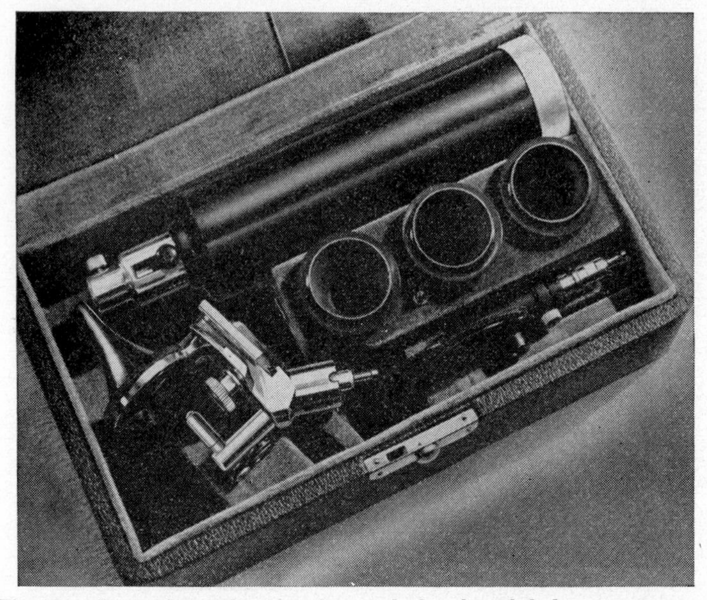

Fig. 184. The nasal speculum may be attached to the ophthalmoscope to convert it to an otoscope for examination of the nose. (Bausch & Lomb Optical Co., Rochester, New York.)

nose prepares inhaled air for entry into the lungs by warming it and by filtering out particles of dust, bacteria, and other irritating substances.

The nose acts as a resonance chamber to help produce a clear voice, and it aids in taste perception when food or drink is taken into the mouth.

EXAMINATION OF THE NOSE

The otoscope may be used for visual examination of each nostril, the nasal speculum being attached to the examining instrument.

For laboratory examination of nasal discharge, the nurse may be asked to obtain the material needed to make a nose culture. For this, test tubes containing the appropriate fresh medium slants will be needed, along with sterile cotton swabs. As a preliminary, the procedure should be explained to the patient. The swab should be passed directly back into one nostril without coming in contact with the outer surface of the nose. With the material adhering to the swab, it is carefully removed from the nostril and rolled over the slant surface of the culture medium. The tube should be accurately labeled and placed in the laboratory incubator as soon as possible. From the original cultures an

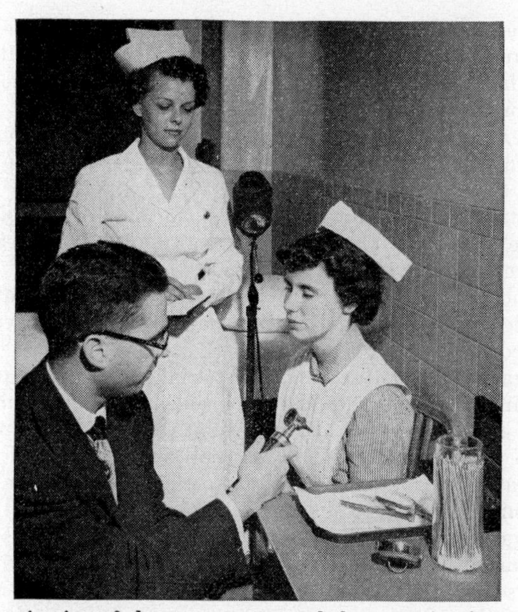

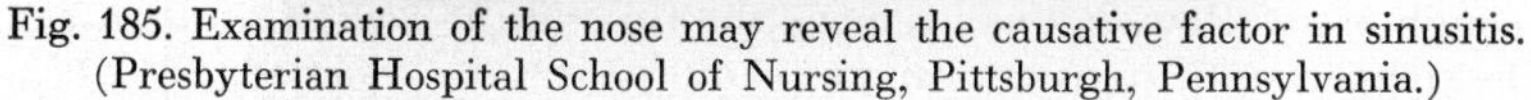

Fig. 185. Examination of the nose may reveal the causative factor in sinusitis. (Presbyterian Hospital School of Nursing, Pittsburgh, Pennsylvania.)

attempt is made to isolate pure cultures, with the inoculation of guinea pigs as a part of the diagnostic procedure.

NASAL SPRAY

The droplet dispersion of a liquid into the nasal passages by means of a jet of air is termed *nasal spray*. The spraying of a medicated substance in this manner is usually done with an atomizer. Sprays ordinarily are made up of aqueous or oily solutions and contain drugs such as ephedrine, menthol, camphor, eucalyptol, or methyl salicylate. The tip of the atomizer nozzle should be inserted well into the nostril and the solution directed upward in spraying. Enough force should be used that the spray reaches all parts of the nostril, but the force should not be great enough to force infection into the paranasal sinuses or eustachian tubes.

NASAL IRRIGATION

Nasal irrigation is the introduction of a solution into one nasal cavity so that return flow of the solution is from the other nasal cavity.

Nasal irrigation is usually used to cleanse the area, soften and remove dried secretions and crusts, remove purulent discharge, and relieve congestion, swelling, and pain.

The procedure should be explained to the patient so he will know the solution is injected into one nostril and returns through the other. He should be instructed to breathe through his mouth during the entire procedure.

The patient should be placed in a comfortable sitting position with head bent forward and slightly tilted to one side, to insure the flow of solution in the desired direction.

The solution most commonly used is normal saline solution, at a temperature of 105° F. The amount of solution used, which should be ordered specifically by the doctor, is 500–1000 cc.

Before the procedure is begun the patient's clothing and the bed must be adequately protected with a plastic or rubberized cape and other needed drapes.

The irrigating can is used with a special nasal tip attached to the rubber tubing. The can should not be elevated to more than four or five inches above the level of the patient's nose. Increasing the pressure or the force of the solution increases the danger of forcing infectious material from the nose into the sinuses. The stream of solution from the nasal tip should be that of a steady, gentle flow.

The irrigating tip should be inserted into one nostril just enough to prevent return flow of the solution through that nostril. If the patient is able to do so, he may hold the irrigating tip. If he feels impelled to cough or swallow, he may remove the tip and the flow of solution can be stopped until he is once more ready for it to be resumed.

Following the procedure, the patient should be instructed not to blow his nose for a short while, as to do so may force discharges into surrounding areas. He should not be permitted to go out into cold for an hour or so. The heat from the solution and increased blood supply in the mucous membrane of the nose makes the patient more susceptible to the common cold for a temporary period of time. If nasal irrigation follows a recent surgical procedure on the nose, the treatment will need to be given with sterile equipment and under aseptic conditions.

INSTILLATION OF NOSE DROPS

Nasal instillation is introduction of a liquid medication into the nostrils, drop by drop, so that it reaches the area to be treated without use of force, as in the nasal spray.

Nose drops are used usually to relieve inflammation and congestion of the nasal mucous membrane. They may be used to apply an antiseptic drug or a local anesthetic prior to surgical treatment of the nose.

The patient should be placed in the dorsal position, with head lower than the shoulders. If the pillow under the patient's head is moved downward so that it is well beneath the shoulders and the patient's head is allowed to tip backward on the mattress, the desired position will be obtained.

A medicine dropper is needed for instilling drops in the nose and the correct amount of solution can be regulated by drawing into the dropper the exact amount desired for instillation. The tip of the medicine dropper should not be inserted into the nostril more than about one-half inch.

Usually two or three drops of the solution is sufficient to reach all areas of the nasal cavity. After the drops have been instilled into both nostrils, the patient should be instructed to remain in the same position for at least five minutes, so the medication will spread throughout both nasal cavities.

Some of the solution is very apt to find its way into the mouth and, if it has a disagreeable taste, as is often the case, the patient should be supplied with paper handkerchiefs so the excess solution can be expectorated.

Although frequently employed in former years as a means of treating various nasal conditions, the use of nose drops is gradually giving way to more effective means of treatment, and the procedure should not be used unless prescribed by a physician.

EMERGENCIES INVOLVING THE NOSE

Epistaxis. Epistaxis, or the common emergency condition of nosebleed, may be caused by a sudden blow or injury, the presence of adenoids or of other small growths, or by spontaneous rupture of a blood vessel in conditions of hypertension.

Treatment of the condition depends on severity of the hemorrhage. For minor bleeding, ice compresses over the bridge of the nose or pressure exerted on the affected side may suffice to stop the bleeding.

For persistent or extensive bleeding it may be necessary to pack the nostril with a special pack made of gauze soaked in Adrenalin solution. For severe hemorrhage a hypodermic injection of a coagulant may be indicated.

Removal of Foreign Bodies. Children may put such objects as beans, nuts, beads, and marbles into the nostrils and push them upward with additional small objects so that their removal is not easily accomplished. If slight pressure exerted above and to the side of the foreign body does not dislodge it, the services of an eye, ear, nose, and throat surgeon may be required.

The Throat

The term "throat" usually refers to the cavity back of the mouth and in the neck, extending from the palatine arch to the opening of the esophagus.

EXAMINATION OF THE THROAT

Examination of the throat, which is an important part of the routine physical examination, is done usually after the head and face have

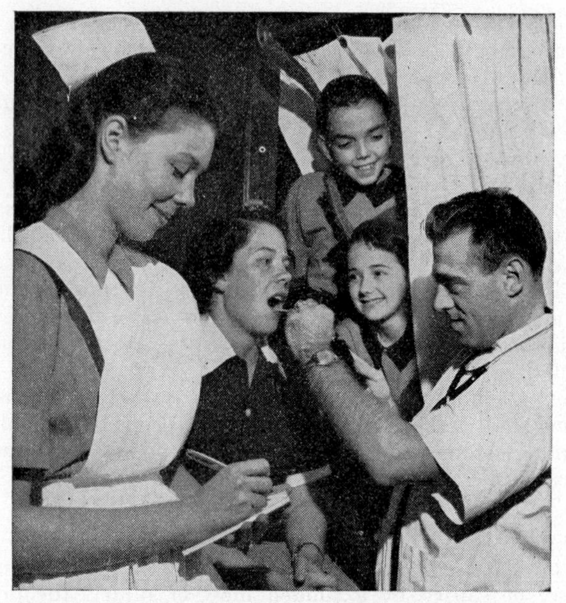

Fig. 186. Examination of school children affords an opportunity to swab or otherwise treat inflammation of the throat. (Presbyterian Hospital School of Nursing, Chicago, Illinois.)

been examined. Articles needed for the examination include tongue depressor and flashlight.

The nurse should hand the tongue depressor to the doctor in such a way that he will grasp the same part she has touched and the opposite end will not have been touched or contaminated. The uncontaminated portion of the tongue blade is put into the patient's mouth to hold the tongue down firmly so a clear view may be had of the throat.

TO SWAB THE THROAT

Swabbing the throat is the means used to apply medication directly to affected areas. In some localities "painting the throat" is the terminology used.

Articles needed to swab the throat include adequate light, head mirror, tongue depressor, cotton applicators, the prescribed medication, and a container for waste.

The patient should be placed in a comfortable sitting position with the light back of him so that reflection from the head mirror can be directed into the throat.

The procedure should be explained to the patient so that he will know how to cooperate to achieve best results of the treatment.

Just before the tongue depressor is brought into use, the cotton applicator should be made readily accessible and the top or cap should be removed from the bottle containing the medication.

With the tongue depressor extending slightly beyond the highest point in the arch of the tongue, gentle steady pressure should be exerted so the tongue is kept firmly in place and cannot obstruct view of the throat or interfere with application of the medication.

The applicator should then be dipped into the medication. While the patient says "AH," the applicator is moved quickly and smoothly in a half circle, swabbing one side of the throat. If the applicator is turned slightly during the movement, the medication will be applied evenly to all the affected surface area. The used applicator should be discarded and a fresh applicator used to apply the medication to the opposite side.

If care is taken not to use more solution than is needed, there will be no excess medication deposited in the mouth to create an unpleasant taste or cause gagging by flowing downward into the throat.

THROAT SPRAY

Sprays may be used to apply a soothing solution or a medication to the mucous membrane of the throat. An atomizer is used and the solution, in a stream of droplets, is directed into the throat. Temperature of the solution should be approximately 105° F.; and solutions used are specifically prescribed by the doctor. A solution that causes pain or discomfort to the patient may be too strong and the doctor should be notified so a further dilution of it can be made.

GARGLES

Gargling is sometimes used in conditions affecting the throat in which sprays or irrigations may be indicated.

Solutions used for gargling are normal saline, boric acid, and weak sodium bicarbonate. Temperature of the solution should be 115 to 120° F.

Although the patient should be instructed not to swallow the solution, no special ill effects result from swallowing a small amount.

Gargling is a tiring procedure for most patients, and many find it difficult to do. Because rigid control of the throat and of breathing is required, the treatment can be painful for those not adept in the procedure.

Physicians often disagree as to the effectiveness of this method of treatment and tend to prescribe sprays and irrigations as the preferred method of treating various throat disorders.

THROAT IRRIGATION

The introduction of a solution through the mouth, directed backward into the throat to cleanse or wash that area, is termed a throat irrigation.

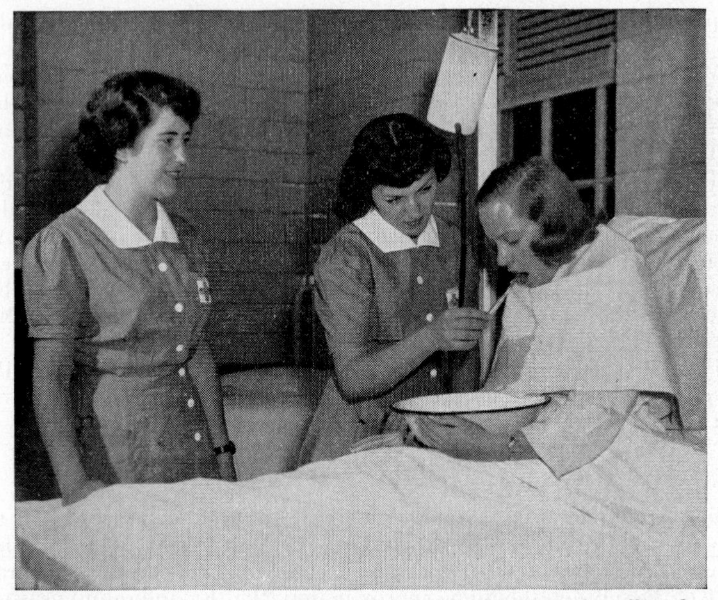

Fig. 187. Throat irrigation is a means of supplying heat to the affected area. (Bridgeport Hospital School of Nursing, Bridgeport, Connecticut.)

The treatment is used primarily to cleanse the area of exudate or of discharges. It may be prescribed for relief of pain caused by inflammation or infection of the tonsils or of the mucous membrane of the throat.

The chief value of the treatment lies in the application of heat to the affected area, and for that reason the solution should be quite hot (115 to 120° F.); 1000 cc. of a solution such as normal saline, sodium bicarbonate 2 per cent, or boric acid is usually used.

The irrigating can, with rubber tubing and a special curved irrigating tip, will be needed. The irrigating can should not be raised higher than 12 inches above the level of the patient's head.

The patient's clothing and the bed linen should be adequately protected with a plastic cape or with rubber protectors. Two large emesis basins will be needed for the return flow of the solution.

Before beginning the procedure, it should be explained to the patient, to insure his cooperation and achieve best results. In addition to understanding the beneficial effect of the treatment, the patient will need to know how he can help. If he is able to do so, he should be permitted to hold the irrigating tip so he can direct the flow of solution into the throat. By having control of the direction and flow of solution, the patient soon finds that the unpleasant experience of gagging can be avoided and normal breathing need not be curtailed during the treatment.

A sitting position is the most comfortable one for the procedure. If the patient is not permitted to sit up, he may be turned partly to one side, with his head slightly elevated. In either position, the head should be held forward over the emesis basin, so the return flow of solution is easily accomplished.

Whether the nurse or the patient controls the flow of solution, it should be directed toward the affected area; if the patient wishes, the flow should be discontinued once or twice during the treatment, so he can rest for a few minutes.

Care should be taken to prevent irritation of the mouth and chin from the hot solution used in throat irrigation. If the irrigation is repeated frequently, application of cold cream or olive oil will help keep the outer surfaces of the mouth and chin in good condition.

Care of Equipment after Use

Medication used for eye instillation should be kept in the dropper bottle tightly closed. The eye dropper tip should not be contaminated by contact with the patient's eye or the nurse's hands.

Compresses used in eye treatment should be discarded after use. Equipment used for eye irrigation should be thoroughly cleaned and sterilized. Equipment used in treatment of the ear, nose, or throat should be washed and dried and returned to central supply to be made ready for use again.

When the ophthalmoscope is used for examination of eye, ear, nose, or throat, the speculum should be cleaned with a cotton pledget which has been saturated with alcohol.

Summary of Important Factors

EYE

Illness increases light sensitivity.

Sun glasses should be worn only during exposure to bright sunlight.

Eye examination is indicated when symptoms of abnormality appear.

Never startle a patient who can't see by speaking to him or touching him without first announcing your presence.

Assure the patient that temperature of the irrigating solution is not too high by first allowing some of the solution to run over the closed eyelid.

Never touch the eyeball or eyelid with the medicine dropper or end of the irrigating syringe.

Avoid making pressure on the eyeball.

An eye specialist should be called for removal of a foreign body imbedded in the eye.

Separate equipment must be provided for each eye when both are to be irrigated.

In irrigating the eye the solution should flow from the inner to the outer canthus.

EAR

Common causes of impaired hearing include: injury, infection, cerumen, diet deficiency, occupational conditions, and congenital defects.

Earache may occur as referred pain.

Warm oil should be used as ear drops to kill an insect in the ear.

The ear should not be plugged with cotton following irrigation.

Cleaning the ear with a hairpin is a dangerous procedure.

The deaf patient should be treated as any normal individual.

NOSE

Treatment of nasal conditions is largely preventive.

The tip of the atomizer nozzle should be inserted well into the nostril for nasal spray.

The irrigating can should not be elevated more than a few inches above the nose.

The patient's head should be tilted backward for instillation of nose drops.

If slight pressure above a foreign body in the nose does not dislodge it, the doctor should be called.

THROAT

Tonsils are beneficial only so long as they function normally to help resist pathogenic microorganisms.

Sore throat, fever, cough, and loss of voice are common symptoms of throat disease.

Medication is applied directly to the throat by swabbing.

Throat treatments include sprays, gargles, and irrigations.

Cold cream or oil applied to the chin before throat irrigation will help to prevent irritation from the hot solution.

Factors To Teach the Patient

EYE

To place eye glasses on table so they rest on the frame and the lens will not be scratched.

Not to touch the eyes with the hands.

Sun glasses should not be worn except for exposure to sunlight.

Change in vision, headache, stumbling, and pain, redness, or swelling of the eyes indicate an eye examination is needed.

Not to jump or move suddenly when medicine is dropped on the lower lid.

An ophthalmologist treats eye diseases and eye defects.

An optometrist only examines the eyes.

An optician makes eye glasses and optical instruments.

EAR

Correction of remedial defects and cooperation in control of communicable diseases helps to prevent deafness.

Instillation of warm oil is an effective means of killing an insect in the ear.

Damage to the ear drum may result from cleaning the ear with a hairpin or other pointed instrument.

Deafness need not interfere with leading a normal life, although it will necessitate making adjustments.

NOSE

That cooperation is essential to success of nasal irrigation.

A doctor should be seen if a foreign body in the nose isn't easily removed by slight pressure from above it.

TONSILS

Tonsils should be removed when they are no longer able to help resist pathogenic microorganisms.

Gagging is less apt to occur in throat irrigation if the patient holds the irrigating tip and controls the flow of solution.

Scientific Principles

Anatomy and Physiology. Tears are constantly being formed and distributed over the eyeball by winking.

Stimulation of the cornea causes pain.

Eyestrain is caused by overuse of the eye or by improper lighting.

Vibrations of the eardrum produced by sound waves are transmitted through the middle ear to the inner ear, the stimuli being conducted from there by the eighth cranial nerve to the auditory center in the brain.

Acuity of hearing can be determined by use of the audiometer.

Inspired air is warmed and moistened as it passes over the nasal mucous membrane, and is filtered by cilia on the membrane lining the nasal passages.

The throat cavity communicates with the nose and mouth and is lined with mucous membrane.

Chemistry. Visual purple is a chemical substance that is altered by light.

Tears serve to keep the eyeball moistened. An increase in pH of tears produces a feeling of irritation, a decrease causes a feeling of dryness.

Microbiology. The eyes are protected from dust and impurities in the air by the eyelashes.

A protective chemical compound found in tears protects the eyes from infection.

Eye infections may lead to impaired vision.

Eye irrigations must be given so that cross-infection is prevented. Sterile equipment and sterile solutions are necessary for eye treatments.

Infection of the middle ear is termed otitis media.

Boils in the ear canal are very painful, since the canal is not yielding or flexible.

Cerumen helps protect the ear from infection.

Infection of the ear may be caused by diseased tonsils and adenoids. Blowing the nose may cause infection in the throat to be transmitted to the ear.

Many communicable diseases are first recognized by symptoms affecting the nose and throat.

Protection is needed from the spray of sneezing and coughing when the patient has a communicable disease.

The hydrochloric acid of the stomach helps to destroy bacteria that have been swallowed.

Pharmacology. A weak solution of boric acid or normal saline is commonly used for eye, ear, nose, and throat irrigations and for a gargle.

Argyrol and silver nitrate are used as antiseptics in treatment of the eye.

Atropine is used as a mydriatic to dilate the pupil for eye examination. Physostigmine is used to contract the pupil of the eye.

Vitamins A, B, C, and D have a marked effect on eye health.

Penicillin is used to treat eye infections.

Cocaine is used to anesthetize the eye.

Research is now being done in use of radiation (weak beta rays) for eye therapy.

Alcohol is used for ear irrigation if a foreign body has become lodged in the ear and can be shrunk by alcohol.

Hydrogen peroxide may be used to soften impacted ear wax.

Various antibiotic drugs are used to combat ear, nose, and throat infections.

Strong antiseptic drugs, as iodine or Mecurochrome, are used to paint the throat.

Physics. Light serves to stimulate the optic nerve. Increased light admitted into the eye will cause the pupil to contract.

Glare causes eye fatigue and eye strain.

The cornea and lens bend light rays so that images on the retina will be clear and distinct.

The eyeball is a closed cavity, therefore pressure on the surface will cause equal pressure on the retina and produce pain.

Tears prevent friction between eyelids and the eyeball.

The sensation of sound is produced as a result of vibration of air waves.

A decibel is the unit of measure for intensity of sound.

Hearing aids increase the intensity of sound and thus improve hearing.

Temperature changes affect the fluid of the inner ear. Irrigating fluid that is too hot or too cold may cause dizziness.

Pressure in throat irrigations may be controlled by changing the height of the irrigating can.

Gravity helps in instilling drops in the nose if the head is tipped backward.

Air reaches the upper part of the nasal cavity by diffusion. Sniffing or breathing forcibly hastens diffusion of air to the olfactory area.

Psychology. The eye is very sensitive and the patient may be fearful of eye treatment and of disfigurement or loss of vision.

When a patient who cannot see must be fed, his feeling of helplessness and dependence on others is increased. His mental state may depend a great deal on the tactfulness and gentleness of the nurse.

An artificial eye should be removed at intervals for care. The extreme sensitiveness of the patient who wears it should be recognized.

Patients wearing glasses or hearing aids may require help in adjusting to the condition necessitating such mechanical aid.

Persons who are totally or partially deaf may tend to withdraw from social contacts and will need help in overcoming the tendency to be suspicious or depressed. Persons with only a slight degree of auditory impairment resent being termed *deaf*.

In nose and throat treatments the patient should be permitted to help with the procedure (such as irrigation) if by doing so the pain and discomfort caused by the treatment may be reduced.

If isolation technique is required an explanation should be given the patient so he will know that friends and relatives cannot visit him and why care given him differs from that being given the average patient.

Sociology. After the age of 55 or 60 a very large percentage of persons have defective vision, impaired hearing, or both.

School children are examined regularly for visual or auditory defects and industrial programs are set up to help prevent those defects.

Blind persons are dependent on their families or on welfare organizations such as the National Society for the Blind, Prevention of Blindness, Vocational Rehabilitation, Foundation for the Blind, Braille

Institute and other local agencies. The nurse should know about such organizations and refer to them any patients needing help.

An agency that will help the deaf and hard of hearing is the American Society for the Hard of Hearing.

State schools are set up for the teaching of deaf children. The deaf tend to withdraw and need to be encouraged to learn lip reading, to wear hearing aids, and to adjust satisfactorily to their physical defect.

Serious diseases may begin with symptoms of a cold. Precautionary measures should be known and practiced by all persons. Each patient should be taught how to prevent exposing others to a nose or throat infection. The cause of the common cold is not yet known, but it is continuously pandemic and costs hundreds of millions of dollars each year in working days lost and in drugs and medical care given.

Situation Type Problem

1. The Director of Nurses had severely reprimanded a Senior student because she had accepted a $10.00 tip from a patient who was not always responsible for her actions. The student had defended her acceptance of the money on the basis that the code of ethics which prohibited it was out dated and was ignored by many other nurses. The Director of Nurses did not succeed in her attempt to justify the necessity for ethical standards in regard to the matter in question, but did succeed in making quite clear to the student the fact that she would be asked to withdraw from the school should she accept another such "tip."

A few months later the student, assisting a patient to make preparation for departure from the hospital, inadvertently came across a very expensive ophthalmoscope which the patient had packed with his belongings. The student recognized the instrument as the one which had been reported missing a week before and for which a diligent search had been made without results.

She suggested to the patient that she would be glad to take the piece of equipment to the administration officer and explain that she had found it elsewhere. The patient refused to accept her suggestion. She then informed the patient that she would have to report that the instrument was in his possession. Whereupon the patient became very angry. He reminded her of the many different "tips" which he had given to her and to her surprise and consternation showed her an account of the small tips she had accepted which represented a total sum of $35.00. The patient did not know that the student faced dismissal from the school if her acceptance of the tips was disclosed, but he threatened to claim that she had stolen the money and to report the "theft" if she mentioned to anyone that she had discovered the whereabouts of the missing ophthalmoscope. What would you have done?

Suggested Reference Reading

"Dropper instillation of eye medications," Eunice R. Parfitt; American Journal of Nursing, February, 1949.
"Glaucoma," Eugene M. Blake; American Journal of Nursing, April, 1952.
"Headaches caused by eye defects," Albert D. Ruedemann; American Journal of Nursing, September, 1952.
"Tracheotomy," John J. Conley; American Journal of Nursing, September, 1952.
"Otitis media," Harold Cutler; American Journal of Nursing, May, 1953.

PART V

Procedures for Clinical Study

CHAPTER 31

Catheterization

TOPICAL OUTLINE

NORMAL URINE
CATHETERS
PURPOSES OF CATHETERIZATION
TO STIMULATE NORMAL VOIDING
CATHETERIZATION OF THE FEMALE PATIENT
CATHETERIZATION OF THE MALE PATIENT
TO OBTAIN A STERILE URINE SPECIMEN
THE RETENTION CATHETER
IRRIGATION OF A RETENTION CATHETER
BLADDER IRRIGATION
BLADDER INSTILLATION
INSTILLATION INTO KIDNEY PELVES

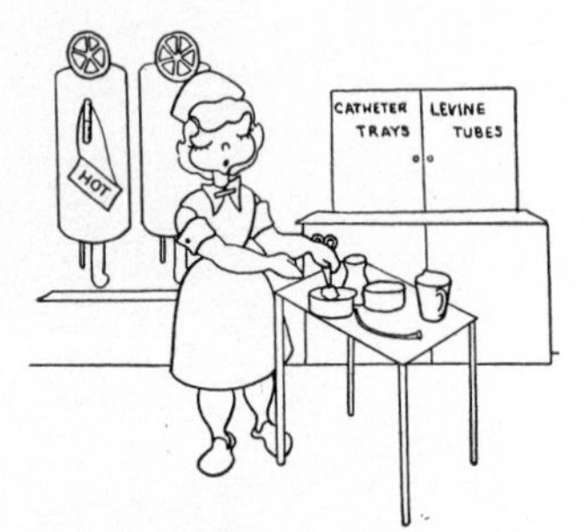

There's no future in any job— the future lies in the person who holds the job.

Catheterization is defined as "the removal of urine from the bladder by means of a catheter." A catheter is "a long narrow tube for withdrawing or injecting fluids through a natural body opening." To successfully perform catheterization the nurse must know the anatomy and physiology of the urinary system. This system is made up of the kidneys, ureters, bladder, and urethra. The kidneys secrete urine, which passes through the ureters to the collecting reservoir, or bladder.

When a few hundred cubic centimeters of urine has accumulated the patient experiences the desire to void and the urine is then expelled through the urethra, a narrow canal (about 1½ inches long in the female, 7 inches long in the male) extending from the bladder to the body surface. The external orifice of the urethra is termed the urinary meatus. Sphincter muscles closing the opening of the urethra are maintained in the contracted state, relaxing only to permit the voiding of urine.

The urinary bladder normally holds 300–500 cc. of urine, which is ejected in tiny spurts from the ureteral openings at intervals of only a few seconds. After several hours the accumulation of urine in the bladder causes stimulation of nerve endings in its wall, resulting in the desire to void.

Although normal capacity of the bladder is approximately 500 cc.

the walls of that organ are elastic and will stretch to accommodate a much greater volume of urine. It is not unusual to find a distended bladder containing 1000 cc. or an even greater amount of urine. When the urinary bladder is distended by more than a normal amount of accumulated urine the patient may experience discomfort caused by pressure against nerve endings and the other pelvic organs.

The procedure of catheterization should not be performed without a written order from the attending physician. In introducing a catheter into the bladder there is danger of introducing pathogenic microorganisms, too, even though sterile equipment is used and sterile technique is observed. Because of the danger involved, the nurse should not take the responsibility of resorting to catheterization unless it is specifically ordered by the doctor.

NORMAL URINE

Normal urine is yellow-amber in color and clear in consistency. Its odor is somewhat aromatic and not unpleasant, although it may change temporarily after ingestion of certain foods, beverages, or drugs. Coffee often acts as a diuretic, increasing the output of urine, and it is not unusual for the urine to have a distinctive coffee odor.

Normal urine is made up of approximately 95 per cent water and minute amounts of urea and bile salts, as well as such inorganic substances as sodium chloride, calcium, magnesium, potassium, and sulfates and phosphates. Normal urine is acid in reaction and has a specific gravity which may range from 1.015 to 1.025. The amount of urine voided in a 24-hour period may vary from 1500 to 2000 cc.

A definite increase in the usual amount of urine voided is termed *polyuria;* a decrease is termed *oliguria.* Failure to secrete urine is referred to as *anuria.* The secretion of urine containing abnormal constituents is named with the term designating the constituent, as: *pyuria* (pus in the urine), *glycosuria* (sugar in the urine), and *hematuria* (blood in the urine).

CATHETERS

A catheter is a long, slender tube, open at one end and having a rounded tip at the other extremity. The tip end of the catheter has one or several perforations, through which the urine may be drained from the bladder.

Catheters are made of various materials, such as rubber, glass, metal, woven silk, and other pliable materials, and are available in various sizes. The choice of size and length of catheter used depends on the size and sex of the patient to be catheterized. The rubber catheter is considered the most safe and is usually used for male patients, for young children, for restless or irrational patients, for pregnant women, for patients with a known structural defect (as stricture of the urethra) and for patients requiring vaginal packing.

Rubber catheters range in size from 10 to 22 French. A 14–18 French catheter is generally used for adults, and 8–10 French catheter is used for children.

If the catheter is pliable, rubber gloves should be used for handling it; for a stiff rubber catheter, forceps or sterile finger cots may be used. The finger cots are worn on thumb and index finger of the left hand, which is used to separate the labia in catheterization of the female. A normally stiffened catheter may be grasped far enough from the tip to be handled with the ungloved right hand of the nurse.

Woven silk catheters are pliable and can be handled easily, but they are destroyed by heat in sterilization and for that reason are not practical.

Metal catheters need to be very carefully inspected for roughened edges around the tip or the eyes, which could cause severe injury to the patient.

Glass catheters are easily cleaned and sterilized, but are hazardous for the patient. If they are cracked or broken during the process of sterilization, they may cut or injure the urethra or cause even greater damage by breaking off in the bladder.

Some doctors believe that glass or metal catheters may cause more trauma to the patient, while others maintain that the smooth, firm surface of the glass or metal catheter passes freely through the meatus and thus causes less trauma.

PURPOSES OF CATHETERIZATION

Catheterization may be ordered for a patient for a number of reasons, such as those discussed in the following paragraphs.

1. To relieve distention of the bladder, caused by retention of urine. Retention of urine occurs when there is interference with the normal process of emptying the bladder at intervals throughout the day. When the bladder is distended and the patient is unable to void, he may experience marked discomfort which increases in direct proportion to the increasing amount of urine retained in the bladder.

In most instances, retention of urine is a temporary condition and relief is afforded by catheterization. The condition may occur after a surgical procedure; it may be due to trauma, infection, or a mechanical obstruction, as the growth of a tumor or the insertion of packing into the vagina or rectum. Retention of urine may occur because of an emotional factor, such as extreme embarrassment at the necessity of having to use a bedpan.

In *complete retention* the patient is unable to void despite the distention. *Retention with overflow* is present when the patient voids a very small amount (approximately 50 cc.) and the bladder remains distended after the voiding. If a large amount is voided, yet the bladder is not completely emptied (approximately 50 cc. remaining after voiding), the amount retained in the bladder is termed *residual urine.*

2. To secure a sterile specimen of urine.
3. To determine whether inability to void is due to retention (the urine retained in the bladder) or to suppression (failure of the kidneys to secrete urine).
4. To prevent the patient from voiding, as after perineal surgery, and thus prevent infection.
5. As a diagnostic procedure. In conditions of suspected bladder infection, the causative organism may be found by examining a culture of the urine.
6. To keep incontinent patients dry.
7. To determine if residual urine is present in the bladder. Catheterization of the patient immediately after voiding will reveal the presence of any residual urine remaining in the bladder.
8. To obtain a clean specimen of urine, especially during the menstrual period of the female patient.
9. To make certain the bladder is empty before performance of a pelvic operation.
10. To empty the bladder before bladder irrigation or bladder instillation.

TO STIMULATE NORMAL VOIDING

Before resorting to catheterization to relieve bladder distention caused by retention of urine, the nurse should have employed all the measures to help the patient void which were discussed in Chapter 17. If catheterization is unavoidable, it should be done under aseptic conditions and with care and consideration.

EQUIPMENT NEEDED FOR CATHETERIZATION

Part of the equipment used for catheterization must be sterile and aseptic technique must be used.

Sterile Equipment. The sterile equipment necessary for the performance of catheterization includes a tray containing two towels, a sponge bowl, containing eight cotton sponges, a specimen bottle and labeled cap, an empty sponge bowl, a basin in which to collect the urine, two catheters, lubricating jelly, and two finger cots. Soap solution used must also be sterile.

Clean, Non-Sterile Equipment. The equipment necessary for catheterization which should be clean but need not be sterile includes: a drop light, paper bag, rubber square and utility towel.

CATHETERIZATION OF THE FEMALE PATIENT

To catheterize the female patient the factors to bear in mind relative to the procedure include: proper screening and draping of the patient and an explanation of the procedure. An understanding nurse

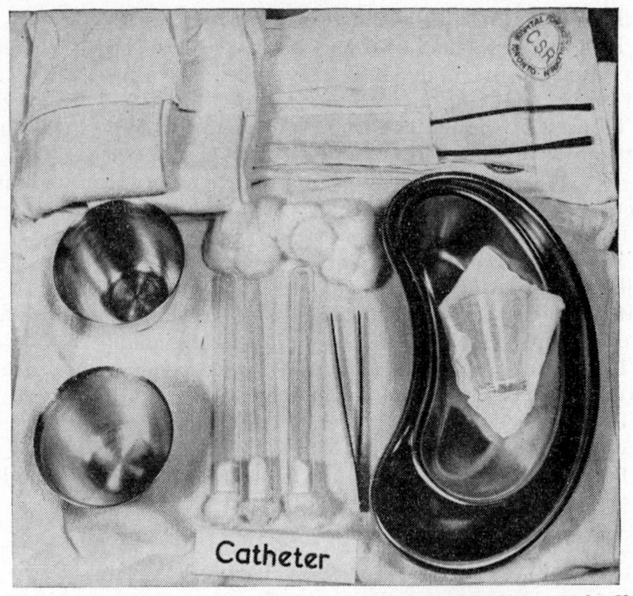

Fig. 188. Catheterization tray. (Central Supply, Hospital for Sick Children, Toronto, Canada.)

will realize that the patient may be unduly frightened or embarrassed by the necessity of catheterization, especially if she is reluctant to be exposed in the manner required.

Because catheterization may require 15 to 20 minutes, and the position which must be maintained by the patient may become uncomfortable, a pillow should be used to support one bended knee and the other should be allowed to rest against the nurse's chest, as she bends over the patient while urine is being withdrawn from the bladder.

For successful catheterization, a good light must be provided. A drop light or a special "caged" light which may rest on the bed is usually used. Ordinary lighting in the average hospital room is not adequate for this procedure. A good light is essential as the nurse must be able to see the urinary meatus before attempting to insert the catheter into the urethra.

Before beginning the procedure the nurse should carefully wash her hands in soap and water. The catheterization tray should be ready for use with solutions of proper temperature, amount, and strength being placed in the basins designated for them.

Catheterization is always performed as a sterile procedure. Sterile forceps should be used in setting up the tray. Aseptic technique should be used throughout the procedure, and great care must be taken to prevent contamination of the equipment and subsequent development of cystitis, which may result from a break in the technique.

The patient should be carefully draped so that she is exposed only during the actual performance of the treatment. Top covers should be fan-folded to the foot of the bed and the bath blanket should be used to drape the patient as for a gynecological examination. The patient unit should be screened to provide privacy. If the patient is in a private room a screen should be placed in front of the door.

Because of the nature of the procedure, catheterization may cause fear and emotional strain in the patient. Such emotional reactions may in turn cause constriction of the muscles of the urethra and contraction of the orifice, making introduction of the catheter exceedingly difficult. By assuring the patient of privacy, by careful draping, by explanation of the procedure, and the use of rubber gloves or finger cots for handling the genitalia, the nurse may help reduce embarrassment and relieve fear and tension.

The tray should be placed on the bed and sterile covers removed in such a way that equipment on the tray is not touched by contaminating hands or drapes.

Finger cots worn on the left thumb and index finger provide adequate covering for use in separating the labia.

Sterile cotton sponges, used to cleanse the vulvar area, are handled with forceps so the gloved fingers will be free of contamination when handling the catheter.

In cleansing the vulva and meatus, care should be taken not to cause pain or discomfort to the patient and not to contaminate the sterile equipment. Strokes made in cleansing the area are from above downward, and each cotton pledget is discarded after being used for one downward stroke. During the cleansing procedure the urinary meatus should be located, so the exact site of entry for the catheter is known.

Locating the orifice or opening of the urethra may be made difficult by abnormalities in structure of the urethra or the meatus. The meatus in the female is usually a very narrow slit or opening in the center of the papilla, just below the clitoris and just above the vaginal opening. If the vulvar area is inflamed or swollen or if the vagina has been packed following a surgical procedure, the meatus may not be readily located when catheterization is attempted.

When the location of the urinary meatus is known, the catheter should be picked up with right thumb and index finger, about four inches from the tip end, which must not come in contact with any of the equipment or with any part of the vulva. Skillful handling of the catheter is essential if the patient is to be catheterized without discomfort or injury. The catheter is under better control and can be handled with more sensitivity if it grasped by the fingers, rather than with forceps. Since a rubber catheter must be held within a few inches of the tip, rubber gloves should be worn by the nurse.

Lubricant used on the tip of the catheter may be mineral oil, a form of vegetable oil, or a lubricating jelly; enough should be used to facilitate entrance of the tip of the catheter into the urinary meatus.

After urine begins to flow from the open end of the catheter it is unnecessary to insert it further into the bladder. The catheter should not be inserted into the urethra beyond the point where the nurse has grasped it between thumb and finger of her right hand.

At no time should force be used in inserting the catheter. Whether a glass or rubber catheter is used, it should pass readily into the meatus and be easily pushed through the urethra until it reaches the bladder. If force is used in inserting the catheter and it is inserted farther than is needed, the bladder wall may be injured.

Urine should begin to flow from the catheter when it has been inserted approximately 1½ inches. If no urine is obtained when the catheter has been inserted, it should be removed and discarded. The urinary meatus must be located and a second catheter lubricated and inserted. The opening of the urethra appears only as a tiny slit in the folds of mucous membrane and it is not unusual to mistake a tiny fold or fissure for the meatus, in which event the catheter may pass directly into the vagina.

Resistance to passage of the catheter indicates presence of an obstruction or abnormality. In either case, the procedure should be discontinued and the doctor notified.

The basin for receiving urine and the specimen bottle, provided a specimen has been ordered, should be placed on the prepared sterile field within easy reach for use immediately after the catheter has been inserted.

While the urine is flowing from the bladder, the catheter should be held in place by the nurse. It should be maintained in a steady position, not being pushed farther into the bladder or pulled away so long as the urine is flowing.

If the bladder has been greatly overdistended by retention of 1500 or more cc. of urine, only about 1000 cc., should be removed at one time. There is danger of collapse of the bladder walls if an abnormally large amount of urine is suddenly withdrawn.

After urine has ceased to flow, the catheter should be pinched tightly between thumb and finger and withdrawn from the urethra.

The tray and equipment should be set aside, drapes should be removed, and the patient made comfortable.

The specimen should be labeled and sent to the laboratory. The urine in the basin should be measured and discarded.

CATHETERIZATION OF THE MALE PATIENT

Since catheterization involves exposure and handling of the external genitalia, it is usually done, not by the nurse, but by an orderly or by the intern or resident physician. The nurse sets up the tray and other equipment so that it is ready for use, and she assumes the responsibility of cleaning and caring for the equipment after use, of measuring the amount of urine obtained, and of recording the procedure on the patient's chart. However, if the nurse should be called on to do the procedure for a male patient, she should not hesitate because of false modesty or show reluctance to perform such a nursing service.

For the male patient, the equipment needed is essentially the same as that required for the female. Rubber gloves should be worn, and the procedure done with aseptic technique.

With thumb and index finger, the prepuce should be retracted and the glans penis cleansed. The penis should then be held firmly in the left hand and extended upward at an angle of 60 degrees. The catheter should be inserted with the right hand. After the catheter has been inserted 5 or 6 inches, an obstruction will seem to prevent its further penetration; after a few seconds, the constricted muscle causing the obstruction will relax and the catheter can then be inserted into the bladder. The flow of urine through the catheter indicates that the tip of the catheter has reached the bladder and further insertion is unnecessary.

TO OBTAIN A STERILE URINE SPECIMEN

When a sterile specimen of urine is needed for diagnostic purposes, it must be obtained by aseptic measures which prevent contamination of the specimen or of equipment used in catheterization.

The sterile specimen bottle with sterile cap or covering should be placed on the catheterization tray at the time the tray is being prepared.

When the catheter has been inserted and the flow of urine has been established, the end of the catheter should be held directly above the specimen bottle so that the urine flows into the bottle without coming in contact with the outer bottle surface or the gloved hands of the nurse who is doing the catheterization procedure.

The specimen bottle should be filled to approximately 75 per cent of its total capacity to insure an adequate amount of urine for examination. As soon as the specimen has been collected, the bottle should be covered with the sterile cap or covering provided.

When the catheterization procedure has been completed, the specimen bottle containing the urine should be properly labeled "catheterized specimen" and taken at once to the laboratory.

In extreme cases where catheterization may be difficult, as in the case of an operative patient who has had extensive repair of the vulvar area, the doctor may wish to perform the procedure for the patient. Even if the nurse does not perform the procedure, she should be sure there is a written order for catheterization before preparing the necessary equipment for use, or requesting intern or orderly to do the procedure.

THE RETENTION CATHETER

Because repeated catheterization may cause discomfort and result in cystitis, many physicians order use of a retention (indwelling, or mushroom) catheter to provide constant bladder drainage.

After insertion, the tip end of a retention catheter flares out into a collar-like structure, which prevents it from slipping out of the bladder. During insertion of the catheter, the flared portions are straightened out by being stretched over a probe. The probe is withdrawn, leaving the retention catheter in place, with the tip end well within the bladder.

A retention catheter should be irrigated twice during each 24 hour period to insure adequate drainage. After three or four days the catheter should be withdrawn and a different catheter inserted.

Retention catheters are used when there is obstruction in or around the urethra, to keep an incontinent patient dry, and to keep the bladder continuously drained of urine for a prolonged period.

Retention catheters may be held in place by being securely taped to the patient's thigh or to the penis. The end of the catheter is usually connected to a rubber tube through which the urine flows into a drainage bottle. The drainage bottle should be emptied and thoroughly cleaned several times each day, and each time the amount of urine that has been collected should be measured. A record should be kept so that total output of urine for each 24 hour period can be determined.

For intermittent drainage of the bladder by retention catheter, a clamp is placed on the end of the catheter and released at intervals, to empty the bladder of accumulated urine.

The Foley catheter is a specially made rubber catheter which has two lumina; the outer, of gum rubber, forms a bulb-like end at the tip of the catheter, the inner provides passageway for the drainage of urine. After the catheter has been inserted, the bulb is inflated with 10–30 cc. of air or solution. The catheter is prevented from slipping out of the bladder by the expanded bulb, and remains in place until the bulb is deflated.

Irrigation of a Retention Catheter. Retention catheters must be irrigated, to remove any pus, blood, mucus, or crystallized urine which might clog them and prevent free drainage of urine from the bladder.

Equipment needed for the procedure includes a tray containing a kidney basin, a 250 cc. graduate with normal saline solution at temperature of 100° F., two towels, and an Asepto syringe.

The tray should be placed at the bedside, a sterile towel put into place at the lower right side of the bed, and the tubing should be disconnected from the catheter, the end of the tubing being allowed to remain on the sterile towel. The irrigating solution should be drawn into the syringe and the tip of the syringe inserted into the catheter. About two ounces of solution should be gently injected into the catheter. The nurse should avoid injecting air or using force during injection of the solution. When the few ounces of solution have been injected into the bladder the syringe should be disconnected from the catheter and the solution allowed to drain out into the kidney basin. The bladder should not be aspirated if the solution does not return by gravity. Adding more solution will usually start the return flow. The irrigation should be repeated until the solution returns clear. When the irrigation has been completed, the catheter should again be connected to the drainage tube.

BLADDER IRRIGATION

Irrigation of the bladder is carried out in much the same way as irrigation of other body cavities. A small amount of solution (150–300 cc.) is introduced into the bladder and then allowed to drain out of the bladder into a receptacle. This is repeated several times until the prescribed amount of solution has been used.

Bladder irrigation is done to relieve cystitis, and to remove pus, mucus, bacteria, and waste products of decomposed urine from the bladder.

One of two methods may be used, the Y-tube method or the funnel method.

The Y-tube Method. The Y-tube method of bladder irrigation is ordinarily used when a large amount of solution has been prescribed. A reservoir or irrigating can is attached to a two-way, or Y-shaped, glass tube which is in turn attached to a catheter. The solution flows into the bladder through one tube and is drained from the bladder through the other. When the solution is flowing into the bladder, the outlet tube is clamped off. When drainage of the bladder is desired, the inlet tube is clamped off.

The Funnel Method. In the funnel method the solution is injected into the bladder through a funnel, attached to the catheter. To empty the bladder, the funnel is inverted and the solution allowed to drain into a receptacle. This process is repeated, each injection containing not more than 300 cc., until the prescribed amount of solution has been used or until the return flow is clear.

Equipment Needed for Bladder Irrigation. Equipment needed for bladder irrigation includes the completely set-up catheterization tray, a pitcher for the solution, a funnel, and a receptacle for the return flow of the solution. If the Y-tube method is used, the solution may be taken to the unit in the irrigating can. All articles used in bladder irrigation must be sterile, as the procedure is done under aseptic conditions.

Solutions Commonly Used. Solutions most commonly used for bladder irrigation include sterile boric acid solution 2–4 per cent, potassium permanganate 1:1000 solution, and a mild silver preparation, such as Argyrol.

Procedure. For irrigating the bladder the patient should be placed in position and draped as for catheterization. It is necessary to catheterize the patient before beginning the irrigation procedure, the catheter being left in place when the bladder is empty of urine. The irrigating solution is then injected through the catheter in an amount not exceeding 300 cc., which is then allowed to drain from the bladder. Approximately 300 cc. of solution is again injected and allowed to drain from the bladder, the process being repeated until the return flow is clear or the prescribed amount of solution has been used.

Care should be taken not to inject air into the bladder, and at no time during the procedure should the bladder be overdistended. Close observation of the return flow of the irrigating solution will enable the nurse to determine if the amount of return flow is approximately the same as the amount of solution injected, and by that means overdistention of the bladder can be prevented.

In irrigating the bladder the solution used should be introduced slowly, so that a minimum amount of pressure is exerted against the bladder walls and the procedure is not painful to the patient.

BLADDER INSTILLATION

Instillation is the slow dropping or pouring of a drug into a body cavity. Instillations are made into the bladder for the purpose of relieving inflammation, checking the growth of bacteria, and preventing cystitis.

Solutions or drugs commonly used are Argyrol 5 per cent, and other mild silver or mercury preparations. The amount of drug or solution instilled into the bladder usually does not exceed ½ to 1 ounce.

The drug is poured into the catheter, which has been left in place after catheterization, through a funnel, or it may be injected into the catheter by a large syringe. When the instillation has been completed, the catheter should be tightly pinched off and removed from the bladder. If it is not completely closed off, solution will continue to flow from the catheter as it is being removed, with possibility of staining the bed linen with the drug being instilled.

Drugs used for bladder instillation may change the color and appearance of the urine temporarily, and may cause a dark sediment in the next urine which is voided.

INSTILLATION INTO KIDNEY PELVES

If ureteral catheters have been placed in position for drainage of each kidney following cystoscopy, it may be necessary to instill a solution into the kidney pelves at regular intervals. Since the ureteral catheter is of extremely small diameter, a 5 cc. syringe and large hypodermic needle are used for the instillation procedure. All equipment must be sterile, and the instillation done by sterile technique.

Solutions used are boric acid 2 per cent, Mercurochrome 2 per cent, silver nitrate 1:2000, or potassium permanganate 1:8000. The solution should be injected very slowly, and not more than 5 cc. used at one time. If the patient complains of pain during the procedure, the instillation should be discontinued immediately.

Care of Equipment after Use

FOR CATHETERIZATION

Rinse the catheters with cold water, then wash with warm soapy water and rinse again.

Measure the amount of urine obtained.

Wash and rinse rubber gloves or finger cots.

Wash and clean all other articles on the tray.

Return tray and clean equipment to central supply to be made ready for use again.

FOR IRRIGATION AND INSTILLATION

The equipment should be washed and returned to central supply where it can be made ready for use again.

Summary of Important Factors

Do not catheterize a patient without a written order from the physician.

Before resorting to catheterization, try various methods which may help the patient to void.

Rubber catheters are considered more safe than those of glass or metal.

A good light is essential for catheterization.

Force should never be used in inserting a catheter.

The amount of urine obtained by catheter should be measured and recorded.

Approximately 1000 cc. of urine is the maximum amount which should be taken from the bladder at one time.

Privacy, careful draping, and explanation of the procedure will lessen embarrassment for the patient.

Catheterization is an aseptic procedure and sterile equipment is used.

Retention of urine exists when the bladder is not completely emptied at each voiding.

Suppression of urine exists when the kidney fails to secrete urine.

Residual urine is the urine retained in the bladder after voiding.

Catheterization is required when a sterile specimen of urine must be obtained.

Normal urine is yellow-amber, acid in reaction, aromatic in odor, and clear in consistency. It has a specific gravity of 1.015–1.025.

The nurse should, if the need arises, perform the catheterization procedure for a male patient.

Frequent irrigation of a retention catheter may be required to keep the catheter open.

Bladder irrigation is usually continued until the return flow of solution is clear or the prescribed amount has been used.

Not more than 300 cc. of solution should be injected into the bladder at one time during irrigation.

Bladder instillation is preceded by catheterization.

Factors To Teach the Patient

Pain or a burning sensation during urination may be caused by concentrated urine; additional fluid intake will dilute the urine and help relieve the cause of discomfort.

Elimination of waste products through the kidneys is largely dependent on intake of a sufficient amount of fluid.

Frequent urination may be caused by excitement, fear, or other emotional reaction.

Catheterization need not be painful if the patient is relaxed and has confidence in the skill of the nurse.

Patient cooperation is necessary, especially if a retention catheter is used.

Scientific Principles

Anatomy and Physiology. The urinary system consists of the kidneys, ureters, bladder, urethra. The kidneys are glandular organs which remove waste constituents from the blood in the form of urine. The ureters are tubelike structures conducting the urine from the kidneys to the bladder. The bladder is a hollow, muscular structure, capable of great distention, which acts as a reservoir for the urine. When approximately 300 cc. of urine has collected in the bladder, the desire to urinate is felt by the patient and urine is released from the bladder through the urethra. The external opening of the urethra is termed the *urinary meatus.*

Urine is retained within the bladder by action of the internal sphincter muscle, located at the site where the urethra enters the bladder.

The desire to urinate is caused by pressure of the accumulated urine, by the chemical composition of urine, and by reflex stimulation within the bladder. Normally the act of voiding is under voluntary control. The bladder is emptied by contraction of the muscles in the walls of that organ.

Chemistry. Urine is made up of about 95 per cent water and of organic and inorganic substances which include the waste products of metabolism.

The specific gravity of urine is the weight of a given volume of urine compared with the weight of an equal volume of water.

A device called the urinometer is used to measure the specific gravity of urine.

Urine is normally slightly acid in reaction. Disease in the urinary tract, the production of ammonia in urine that stands for some time, changes in diet, and certain drugs may cause a change in the reaction of urine.

Urea forms about 50 per cent of the solid organic matter in urine.

Sodium chloride is the most abundant inorganic matter in urine.

Abnormal constituents of urine include albumin, sugar, casts, calculi, acetone bodies, and pus.

Microbiology. Cystitis, or inflammation of the bladder, may be caused by highly concentrated urine, irritating drugs, bacteria, injury, and overdistention of the bladder walls.

To prevent germ transfer or contamination, the nurse should carefully wash her hands before and after a procedure involving treatment of the bladder.

Bacteria may be introduced into the bladder by an unsterile catheter.

If an infection appears in one part of the urinary system, it may readily affect another, as the organs are continuous.

Because the urinary tract is dark, moist, and warm, it is a favorable medium for the growth of bacteria.

Catheters are sterilized by boiling water or by steam under pressure.

The colon bacillus is the organism most commonly associated with urinary infections. Bladder infections are also caused by staphylococci, gonococci, and the typhoid and tubercle bacilli. Because the typhoid fever patient excretes typhoid bacilli in the urine, the urine must be disinfected where sewage disposal is not adequate.

Pharmacology. Sodium chloride solution 0.9 per cent has the same concentration as blood, so is nonirritating when used for bladder irrigation.

A 2 per cent boric acid solution is mildly antiseptic and is often used for bladder irrigations.

Argyrol 5–10 per cent solution is used for bladder instillation; the silver salts coagulate the protein of bacteria that might be present in the bladder.

Pyridium in a 0.3 per cent solution may be used in treating infections caused by the staphylococcus, gonococcus, and colon bacillus.

Diuretics are drugs which increase the flow of urine. Antidiuretics are drugs which decrease the flow of urine.

Physics. As urine accumulates in the bladder the muscles of the bladder wall tend to relax so that an even pressure is maintained. When the volume of urine has increased to about 300 cc. pressure in the bladder initiates nerve impulses which cause the desire to urinate.

The catheter acts as a siphon to drain the bladder, since fluid will flow in a siphon toward an area of less pressure.

The speed of flow of urine in catheterization depends on the diameter of the catheter being used.

The catheter is lubricated to reduce friction between it and the urethra at the time it is being inserted.

A hot water bottle over the lower abdomen or warm solution poured over the vulva may help a patient to void when voiding has been impossible because of tension or emotional upset.

Psychology. Frequency of urination may be caused by excitement, anxiety, or fear.

All treatments or procedures related to the bladder should be carefully explained to the patient so that he anticipates relief from pain or discomfort as a result of the treatment.

Dislike of using a bedpan and embarrassment because of the presence of other patients in a ward or of a nurse may cause temporary inability to void, even though the patient's bladder may be distended.

By seeing that the patient is given privacy, by proper draping, by keeping the body warm, and by distracting attention from bladder treatments, the nurse may help the patient to relax and thus minimize the discomfort and the danger of injury in catheterization.

A careless or thoughtless nurse who has caused pain to a patient in catheterization may make subsequent bladder treatments very difficult since the patient will be fearful and uncooperative.

Sociology. The public health nurse or visiting nurse may be called on to catheterize a patient in the home. She is also qualified to do bladder irrigation and instillation.

The nurse may need to interpret instructions given by the doctor and offer further explanation of the nature of various bladder treatments.

Situation Type Problems

1. A student nurse was asked to catheterize a patient who had not voided following major surgery and whose bladder was greatly distended. The catheter was easily inserted into the bladder and urine flowed freely so that soon the emesis basin provided to receive the urine was filled to capacity (850 cc.). Urine was still flowing freely from the catheter. There was no second emesis basin on the catheterization tray, there was no other nurse in the room, and the patient had been given a narcotic and was too drowsy to respond to instructions to turn on the signal light, which was out of reach of the nurse who was doing the catheterization. What would you have done?

2. A student nurse was assigned to carry out an order for catheterization as follows: "Catheterize at 10:00 A.M.—Send sterile specimen to laboratory."

The nurse properly prepared the tray, placing a sterile specimen bottle with other sterile equipment on it as she had been taught in the classroom. She carried the tray to the patient's room, draped the patient, explained the procedure, and, using aseptic technique, inserted the catheter into the bladder. As soon as urine began to flow through the catheter, she picked up the sterile specimen bottle and accidently dropped it to the floor. Not wishing to subject the patient to a second catheterization, she completed the procedure, collecting the urine in the emesis basin. Five minutes later she learned that the catheterization had been ordered for the sole purpose of obtaining the sterile specimen of urine. What would you have done?

Suggested Reference Reading

"Catherization of the male patient," Michael F. Lenkowski; American Journal of Nursing, June, 1951.

"Infections of the urinary tract," Philip R. Roen; Today's Health, February, 1952.

CHAPTER 32

Administration of Medicines

TOPICAL OUTLINE

IMPORTANT FACTORS IN ADMINISTRATION OF MEDICINE
CARE OF DRUGS AND MEDICINE CABINET
ACCURACY OF MEASUREMENT
PURPOSES OF MEDICINES
GENERAL INFORMATION
RULES FOR GIVING MEDICINES
A SYSTEM FOR ADMINISTRATION OF MEDICINES
METHODS OF ADMINISTRATION OF MEDICINES
- Orally
- Rectally
- Inhalation
- Instillation
- Inunction
- Local Application to the Skin

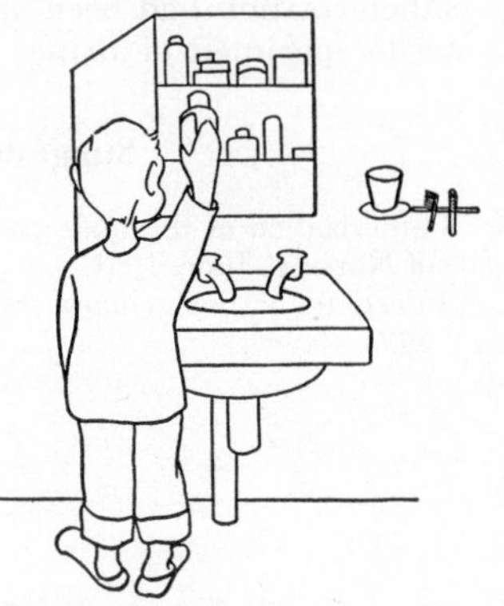

People indulging in self medication,
In order to save doctor's fees,
In due time discover, to their consternation,
Their hobby's become a disease!

Medicine may be defined as "A drug used to prevent, treat, or cure a disease." The various types of such drugs or remedies include: *compound medicine*—a remedy made up of several drugs; *patent medicine*—a publicly advertised remedy, usually of secret composition; *proprietary medicine*—a remedy marketed under a name to which the manufacturer has exclusive rights.

Medicine is a term also used to designate "The science of preventing or treating a disease or injury." Various types of medicine with reference to scientific study include: *aviation medicine*—the study of prevention or treatment of disease as concerned with aviation; *clinical medicine*—the study of medicine at the bedside of the patient, where symptoms and progress of disease can be observed; *domestic medicine*—home treatment of disease, without the advice of a physician; *forensic medicine*—medical jurisprudence, medicine as applied to questions arising in courts of law; *group medicine*—practice of medicine by a group of doctors who work together in diagnosing and treating disease; *internal medicine*—that branch of medicine not concerned with surgical treatment; *preclinical medicine*—that branch of medicine concerned chiefly with prevention of disease; *psychosomatic medicine*—consideration in treatment of disease of the interrelationship between the physical and mental or emotional processes; *socialized medicine*—the practice of medicine under the control of the government.

The administration of medicine is an important feature of the practice of medicine, and a grave responsibility is entrusted to the nurse when she is given the duty of carrying out orders of the doctor with reference to prescribed medication.

The doctor, by written order, will indicate the drug to be given, the number and frequency of doses, the amount of each dose, and, if necessary, the method of administration.

To intelligently carry out orders regarding medications, the nurse must know the expected effect of the drug, the minimum and maximum dosage, the most effective means of administration, and the signs and symptoms which would indicate that an idiosyncrasy to the drug exists. She is expected to carry out all medicinal orders promptly and with extreme accuracy, but is not expected to follow, without question, an order which would be injurious to the patient. If there is any doubt as to the kind or amount of drug ordered, the doctor should be consulted before the order is carried out.

To be adequately prepared to accept the responsibility of administering medications, the nurse should know the various factors which may modify the drug's action, and those which must be considered in determining the method and time of administration. In addition to the basic knowledge of drugs obtained from courses in pharmacology and therapeutics and through clinical experience in giving medicines, the nurse should also know of the new drugs which are continually appearing on the market. Information concerning the discovery, manufacture, and use of new drugs is available through informative literature published by pharmaceutical houses and through current articles on drug therapy that appear regularly in medical and nursing journals.

IMPORTANT FACTORS IN ADMINISTRATION OF MEDICINE

Many factors are capable of modifying the action of a prescribed drug and must therefore be given consideration in determining proper dosage. Such factors include age, weight and condition of the patient, and method of administration as well as factors related to tolerance or idiosyncrasy.

Age. Infants, young children, and aged persons require a smaller dosage of a drug than does an average adult. This is especially true with reference to the use of narcotics, to which children and old people may react with unexpected vigor.

Weight. A person who is considerably underweight will require less than the usual or average dose of a drug, and a person who is overweight, especially if he is extremely heavy, may receive little benefit from the drug unless the dose is markedly increased.

Sex. Since a person of female sex is usually lighter in weight than a male of the same age and height, the dosage of a drug may need to be modified according to the sex of the patient.

Physical Condition. The condition of the patient plays an important part in determining the dosage of drug to be given. If symptoms are severe, such as extreme pain, a larger dose may be needed to afford relief. In certain conditions, use of some drugs may be contraindicated. Laxatives or purgatives are not given if the condition of the patient indicates that abdominal surgery may be required. Drugs which might mask symptoms of serious complications, such as perforation or hemorrhage, should be withheld from the patient whose condition is such that serious complications may ensue.

Method of Administration. The effectiveness of a drug depends, sometimes to a great extent, on the method by which it is administered. Drugs given by rectum are absorbed slowly and only in part, so larger doses are required for a drug administered rectally. Drugs given intravenously have a very quick, almost immediate action, and may be given in doses slightly less than those required for oral administration. Drugs given subcutaneously and intramuscularly are absorbed readily and become effective in much shorter periods of time than when given orally.

Excretion of the Drug. Whether the drug will be excreted from the body in a few hours or remain for a much longer period needs to be considered in determining the size of the dose and the frequency of administration. Drugs such as penicillin and the sulfonamides, when first used in medicine, had to be administered every few hours, because they were excreted so rapidly from the body.

Patients who complain about being wakened at night to be given drugs will usually cooperate and willingly accept the necessary disturbance if they understand the action of the drug. If frequent and regular doses of the drug are necessary to maintain the desired level of concentration in the body, that fact should be made known to the patient.

Drugs such as digitalis and sodium bromide, usually excreted at a slower rate than that at which absorption takes place, can produce a toxic effect when repeated doses cause accumulation of the drug in the body. The nurse must know that such drugs have a "*cumulative action*," and she must observe the patient closely to recognize and report the first symptoms of toxicity.

Tolerance. Patients who possess a tolerance for a certain drug will require larger doses of the drug, if it is to be effective.

Habituation. Patients are said to be "habituated" to a drug when they have used it continuously for a long period of time and in addition to the development of a tolerance for the drug, have also developed a craving for it and will manifest definite symptoms if the drug is withdrawn. Persons who have resorted to sleeping pills or hypnotics over a long period of time may still be unable to sleep without them, even though there may be no definite cause for insomnia.

Addiction. Prolonged use of alcohol and of narcotics may produce an extreme form of habituation, and result in the condition termed *addiction*. The drug addict, suddenly deprived of the drug may display psychic craving for it and show definite organic symptoms.

These symptoms indicate that body cells have functioned for so long in the presence of the drug that they are unable to continue functioning without it. In such a patient, the dosage of the drug given to relieve pain may need to be several times that usually given, for the drug must be effective enough to overcome tolerance, satisfy the psychic craving, supply the additional physiological need created by addiction, and then afford relief from pain.

Idiosyncrasy. Idiosyncrasy has been defined as "an individual or peculiar susceptibility to some drug, protein, or other substance." Persons possessing such idiosyncrasy may react to a certain drug in some unusual way. The effect may be opposite to that ordinarily produced in other persons, or an average dose may have a toxic or poisonous effect. Symptoms of a serious nature may appear immediately after a drug is given should idiosyncrasy exist or may not occur until after several doses.

Effect Desired. A drug used for its local effect is applied directly to the site where the effect is desired, and its action is limited to the area to which it has been applied. A drug used for its general effect must be absorbed into the blood stream to produce the desired effect in various parts of the body remote from the site of application. The action of the drug may be on the body as a whole. The method by which a drug is administered, will help to determine its effect, so the nurse should know whether a drug is being given for a local effect or for a general or systemic effect.

Drugs given orally for local effect should not be diluted and should be given after meals so absorption is somewhat delayed and local effect is produced.

Drugs given orally for general effect should be diluted and given at a time when the stomach is comparatively empty. Under such conditions, the drug is more readily absorbed and general effect is obtained.

When the desired effect of the drug is known, the way in which it is to be given may readily be determined and through experience the young nurse soon learns the following should generally be applied.

Cough syrups are given undiluted, in small amounts, and in frequent doses.

Laxatives or cathartics are given between meals and on an empty stomach;

those that act quickly should be given just before breakfast, and those requiring a longer time for action should be given at night.

Bitter or unpleasant tasting drugs are given in capsule form, as a coated pill, or in effervescent preparations.

Oils are given in encapsulated form when possible. Oils taken in liquid form should be chilled, as cold lessens sensitivity of the taste buds and helps to disguise the unpleasant taste. Oils of a very disagreeable flavor, such as castor oil, should be mixed with lemon juice and a small amount (1/4 teaspoonful) of sodium bicarbonate. The mixture should be given to the patient while it is effervescing.

Drugs that will be destroyed by digestive juices are given in enteric-coated pills.

Drugs are given several hours after meals for rapid action.

Drugs to aid digestion are given one-half hour before meals.

Iron, arsenic, mercury, and iodide preparations are given well diluted. They should be given through a glass tube or a straw, as they discolor, and are destructive to, the teeth.

Sedatives are given with warm milk to increase and hasten the desired effect of the drug.

Bitter stomachics, given to stimulate the appetite, should be given undiluted and with no attempt to disguise their taste.

Drugs with a strong disagreeable taste may be diluted and should be followed immediately with a drink of cold water. Ice held in the mouth before and after medication will numb the taste buds and help overcome the disagreeable taste. Milk or other food should not be used to disguise the taste of such drugs. The dislike for the drug may be transferred to the food.

For patients who have difficulty in swallowing pills or tablets, drugs should be powdered and dissolved.

Medicines in clean, unchipped, or unbroken glasses or containers will be less distasteful to patients. The medicine tray should always be neat and attractive in appearance.

CARE OF DRUGS AND MEDICINE CABINET

Drugs. Bottles, boxes and other containers must be kept closed. Liquid medicines may evaporate if bottles are left open. Some pills and tablets tend to disintegrate if exposed to the air.

Ointments, salves, liniments, talcum powder, rubbing alcohol, and other similar supplies should be kept in a separate compartment of the medicine cabinet.

Oils, such as castor oil and viosterol, as well as serums, vaccines, and liver extracts should be kept in the refrigerator. Extreme cold prevents them from becoming rancid and makes the oil preparations a little less unpalatable.

Emergency drugs, such as stimulants, should be kept in a box or on a tray where they are readily obtainable for emergency use.

Labels that are defaced or soiled should be changed by the pharmacist.

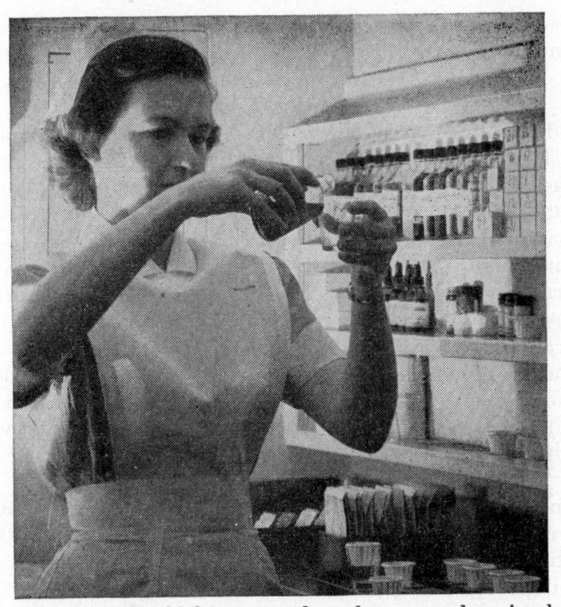

Fig. 189. The drug should be returned to the exact place in the medicine cabinet from which it was taken. (Buffalo General Hospital School of Nursing, Buffalo, New York.)

Each nurse who prepares a medication should be extremely careful to replace the bottle or container in the exact place from which she took it. Unauthorized rearranging of medicines is often responsible for mistakes made in giving medicines.

Drugs that are unusual in appearance, color, odor, or consistency should be returned to the pharmacy to be discarded.

Floor drugs should be checked twice daily so the supply remains constant. There should be two containers for each floor drug so that one is available while the other is in the pharmacy for refilling.

Unused drugs for a patient who is being dismissed should be sent to pharmacy so the patient's account may be credited for the drugs returned.

If medicines are sent home with a patient so he can continue to take them, complete directions for measuring and taking should be placed on the container.

Medicine Cabinet. To give proper care to drugs, each nursing department within the hospital should be provided with a suitable medicine cabinet. The cabinet should be large enough to accommodate all drugs to be stored there; should have a small sink with running water, and should be equipped with artificial lights to provide adequate lighting for the reading of labels. Shelves of the cabinet should be shallow, so that not more than two rows of bottles or other containers can be placed on them, thus facilitating location of a medicine when it is needed.

The medicine cabinet should be kept locked at all times and the key should be kept where only doctors and nurses will have access to it. These measures are necessary to prevent unknown drug addicts among the patients from gaining access to the drug they crave, to prevent patients with suicidal tendencies from obtaining drugs, to safeguard drugs from curious or dishonest visitors, to discourage self-medication on the part of unprofessional employees, and to prevent mishandling of drugs by persons untrained in their care and use.

Opiates and other narcotics should be kept in a separate compartment of the medicine cabinet, and the compartment should always be locked. The key to the narcotic compartment should be carried by the nurse in charge. These extra precautions are necessary to prevent drug addicts, who are often very sly and resourceful, from having access to the drugs.

If the medicine cabinet contains stock supplies for use by all patients, the containers should be arranged so that general classifications of drugs should be together, according to the form in which they are used, as pills, capsules, powders, ointments, liquids. If the different preparations in each category are arranged in alphabetical order, they may be located with ease.

If drugs are ordered on an individual basis for each patient, all medicines for one patient should be grouped together in the cabinet.

Drugs for internal use are usually placed in the medicine cabinet in the center just above the working space and sink compartment.

External remedies and poisons should be kept in a separate compartment or in a different cabinet. All poisonous drugs should bear a POISON label and should be kept in bottles or containers that have a distinctive shape and roughened surface, to warn of the danger involved in handling them.

The medicine cabinet should not be overstocked. Large quantities of drugs are not required, and many drugs deteriorate when left standing unused for more than short periods of time.

The medicine cabinet should always be neat and clean and all equipment, after use, should be thoroughly cleaned and returned to its proper place, ready for use again when needed.

Articles needed for administration of medicines, in addition to calibrated measuring devices, are small trays, glass drinking tubes, medicine glasses, and paper cups.

Since both metric and apothecaries systems of measurement may be used, suitable equipment for each will be needed and a complete table of equivalent values of the two systems should be prominently displayed in the medicine cabinet so that orders may be quickly and accurately transposed from one system to the other, when necessary.

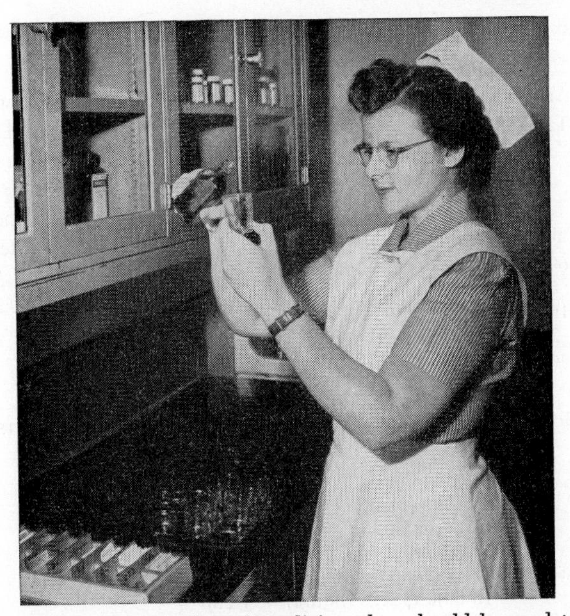

Fig. 190. The standard, calibrated medicine glass should be used to measure liquid medicine. (Presbyterian Hospital School of Nursing, Pittsburgh, Pennsylvania.)

ACCURACY OF MEASUREMENT

Accurate measurement of the dosage of a drug is of great importance in giving medicines.

For measuring liquid medicines, the standard, calibrated medicine glass should be used. Reading of the measured dose should be made at the lowest point of the meniscus, when held at eye level.

The minim glass, calibrated in minims, should be used to measure dosages ordered in minims. Minims and drops should not be used interchangeably, as they are not the same in amount.

The medicine dropper should be used for measuring drops when the dosage of medicine is ordered in drops. The nurse must bear in mind that the size of a drop varies according to the size of the bore in the medicine dropper, the angle at which the dropper is held, and the viscosity of the liquid.

Medicine in powder form may be measured in the calibrated medicine glass or by tablespoon or teaspoon. If measured with a spoon, a flat instrument should be used to level the amount of powder in the spoon. To measure a level teaspoon of powder, put more than that amount in a teaspoon and draw a tongue blade across the spoon, the edge of the blade resting on the upper edges of the side of the spoon.

Table 6. UNITS OF MEASUREMENT IN APOTHECARIES' AND METRIC SYSTEMS

APOTHECARIES' SYSTEM	METRIC SYSTEM
Table of Weight (Dry)	**Table of Weight (Dry)**
60 gr. = 1 dram	1000 mg. = 1 gram
8 dr. = 1 ounce	1000 gram = 1 kg.
12 oz. = 1 pound	
Table of Volume (liquid)	**Table of Volume (Liquid)**
60 minims = 1 dram	1000 ml. = 1 liter
8 drams = 1 ounce	(cubic centimeter—cc., which differs only slightly, is often used interchangeably with milliliter)
16 ounces = 1 pint	
2 pints = 1 quart	
4 quarts = 1 gallon	

HOUSEHOLD MEASURES AND WEIGHTS AND THEIR EQUIVALENTS IN THE APOTHECARIES' SYSTEM

1 teaspoon	= 1 dram
3 teaspoons	= 1 tablespoon
1 dessertspoon	= 2 dr.
1 tablespoon	= 3 dr.
4 tablespoons	= 1 wineglass
16 tablespoons (liquid)	= 1 cup
12 tablespoons (dry)	= 1 cup
1 cup (ordinary)	= 8 fl. oz., or ½ pt.
1 tumbler or glass	= 8 fl. oz.
1 wineglass	= 2 fl. oz.
16 fl.oz.	= 1 lb.
1 pint	= 1 lb.

EQUIVALENT MEASURES IN METRIC AND APOTHECARIES' SYSTEM

LIQUID MEASURE		DRY MEASURE	
Metric	*Apothecaries'*	*Metric*	*Apothecaries'*
.06 cc. =	1 minim	1 gram	= 15 grains
1 cc. =	15 minim	.5 gram	= 7½ grains
4 cc. =	1 dram	.3 gram	= 5 grains
30 cc. =	1 ounce	.2 gram	= 3 grains
500 cc. =	1 pint	.1 gram	= 1½ grains
1000 cc. =	1 quart	.06 gram	= 1 grain

METRIC			APOTHECARIES'	
Dry	Liquid		Dry	Liquid
.06 gram	= .06 cc.	=	1 grain	= 1 minim
1 gram	= 1 cc.	=	15 grains	= 15 minims
4 grams	= 4 cc.	=	60 grains	= 60 minims (1 dram)
30 grams	= 30 cc.	=	480 grains	= 480 minims (1 oz.)

The amount of powder remaining in the spoon is a level teaspoonful.

Medicine ordered to be taken in dosage of "powders" is prepared by a pharmacist, who measures the proportion of drug to be contained in each powder and then folds it within a paper container; each folded container is said to be a *powder*.

In measuring oils or heavy liquids, every effort should be made to get all the medicine transferred from the container in which it is measured to the glass tumbler or other container in which it will be presented to the patient. A tongue blade or spoon may be needed to scrape the thick liquid from the end and sides of the container calibrated for measurement.

If dosage must be computed, this should be done with utmost care. Paper and pencil should be used, and the result should be verified by a clinical instructor or by the nurse in charge.

Table 6 gives units of measurements in the apothecaries' and metric systems, and their equivalents, as well as equivalents of various household measurements.

THE PURPOSES OF MEDICINES

There are four chief purposes of administering medicine to a patient. Each order for medication is given to achieve one or more of those four purposes which include: to diagnose disease; to treat disease; to cure disease; to prevent disease.

Drugs given for diagnostic purposes are those which aid in diagnostic procedures or help, by their action to determine the cause of physical impairment or of disease. Such drugs include barium, used to render a part opaque to x-rays, and phenolsulphonphthalein, used as a means of testing kidney function.

Drugs used in treatment of disease may be classified according to the desired effect, as: (1) a drug which is given for palliative effect or for temporary relief of distressing symptoms, but does not relieve the cause or effect a cure; (2) a drug used to help restore normal functioning, such as digitalis to slow a rapidly beating heart; (3) a drug used to supply a substance which is deficient in the body, such as insulin in diabetes mellitus.

Drugs used to cure diseases are known as *specifics* and have been proved effective against the disease for which they are used. Quinine is a specific used to cure malaria.

Drugs given to prevent disease are the vaccines and serums known to be active in preventing the development of certain diseases. Smallpox vaccine and typhoid serum are examples of such drugs.

GENERAL INFORMATION

Before taking up definite rules or regulations pertaining to the giving of medicine, several factors related to that procedure should be impressed on the mind of the nurse assigned to medications.

Each dose of medicine to be administered must be considered as offering opportunity for a potential mistake in medication.

Doctors should order in *writing* the name of the drug, the dosage, the time and frequency of giving, and the method of administration.

Verbal orders should be accepted only in extreme emergencies. The doctor is obligated to put the verbal order in writing and to sign it at his earliest convenience.

The nurse should know the diagnosis and the age of the patient, as well as his mental condition.

The nurse must inform the doctor if the patient is allergic or shows symptoms of an idiosyncrasy which would contraindicate use of a certain drug.

The nurse should know the usual effect of each drug being handled.

The nurse should be able to recognize all abbreviations and symbols used in ordering medicines.

The use of a medicine dropper is inaccurate in measuring. The bore of the dropper, angle at which dropper is held, and viscosity of the solution can significantly alter the size of the drop.

The nurse should be able to use either the apothecary or the metric system of measurement.

RULES FOR GIVING MEDICINES

To guard against inaccuracy in handling and dispensing drugs and to protect the patient from injurious effects of a mistake in medication, the following regulations must be learned, understood, and practiced by each nurse assigned to the care of the patient.

General Rules. 1. Observe the "five rights" in giving each medication: the *right patient*, the *right time*, the *right medicine*, the *right dose*, and the *right method* of administration.

2. Consult the head nurse if a written order is not clear as to meaning, not legible, or not signed by the doctor.

3. Wash hands thoroughly before measuring or preparing a medication.

4. Make certain that all equipment is clean.

5. When giving pills or tablets, place in proper container directly from bottle. Do not touch them with your hands.

6. Determine if medication is to be delayed or omitted for a specific length of time, as for x-ray examination or basal metabolism test.

7. Never leave the medicine cabinet unlocked.

8. Do not return to stock supply excess medicine or medicine refused by a patient.

9. Do not use a drug that differs from normal in color, odor, or consistency.

10. Provide drinking tubes for irritating drugs and for those likely to stain the teeth.

11. Do not pour a drug from one bottle to another.

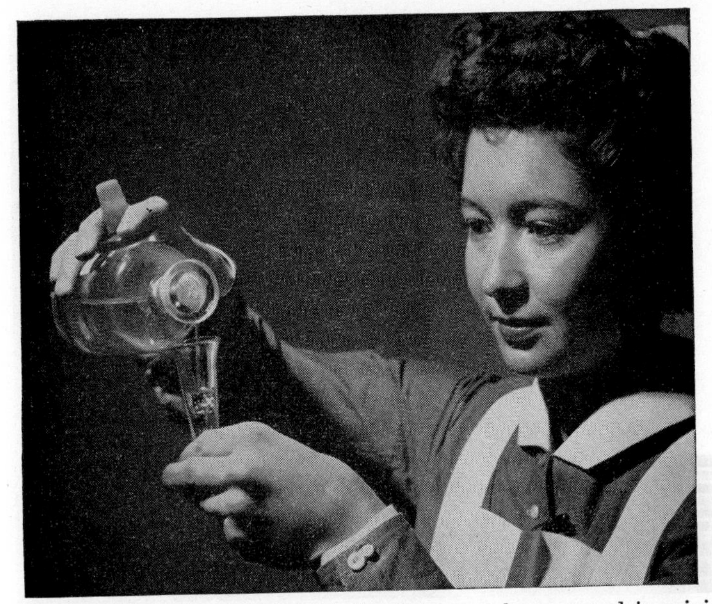

Fig. 191. When minims are ordered, the drug must be measured in minims. (Michael Reese Hospital School of Nursing, Chicago, Illinois.)

12. Never give two or more drugs at one time, unless they are so ordered.

13. Do not permit one patient to carry medicine to another.

14. Know the minimum and maximum dose for the medication being given.

15. An error in medication must be reported immediately to the nurse in charge.

16. Always provide a drink of fresh water to the patient immediately after giving an oral medication, unless water is contraindicated.

Rules for Measuring Medications. 1. Measure the exact amount of drug ordered, using a calibrated measure.

2. Do not converse with anyone while preparing a medication.

3. Make sure that medicine glasses are dry before pouring or measuring a medication.

4. Cleanse the mouth of every bottle before replacing it after use.

5. Measure drops, if drops are ordered. If minims have been ordered, measure the drug in minims.

6. Hold the medicine glass at eye level and place thumbnail (of the hand holding the glass) at the height on the glass to which medicine is to be poured.

Rules Regarding Labels. 1. Give medications only from clearly labeled containers.

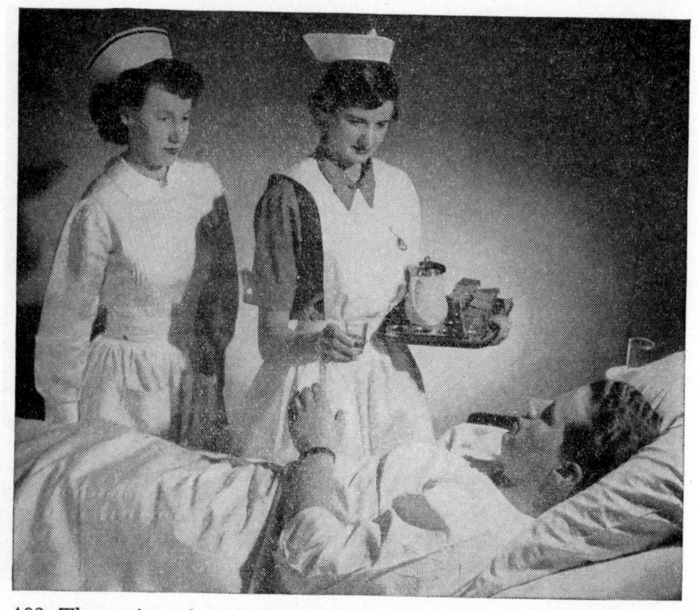

Fig. 192. The patient should always be identified before a medication is given. (Presbyterian Hospital School of Nursing, Chicago, Illinois.)

2. For each dose of medicine prepared, read the label three times: before removing the bottle from the medicine cabinet, before pouring the measured amount of the drug, before replacing the bottle in the medicine cabinet.

3. Never give a drug from an unmarked bottle or box.

4. Pour medicine from the bottle on the side opposite the label.

5. Labels on medicine containers should be changed only by the pharmacist.

6. If a drug has two commonly used names, both names should appear on the label.

Rules for Giving Medications. 1. Give the medication at the time for which it is ordered.

2. Always identify the patient before giving the medication.

3. If medication is refused, or cannot be administered, notify the head nurse.

4. Remain at the bedside until the patient has taken the medication.

5. Administer only those medicines which you have measured and poured.

6. Never give two drugs together, unless specifically ordered to do so. Different drugs taken at the same time may form a chemical compound that can be injurious to the patient.

7. When a patient goes to the operating room, all orders for medication are discontinued. New orders for postoperative medications will be written by the doctor.

8. When special tests are being done, medications due at that particular time are omitted; they are resumed when next due.

9. A mistake in medication must be reported immediately to the nurse in charge.

Rules for Recording Drugs Administered. 1. Record if an ordered medication is refused or if it cannot be administered.

2. Record each dose of medicine soon after it is administered.

3. Use standard abbreviations in recording medications (see Table 7).

4. Record only those medicines which you have administered.

5. Record time, kind, and dose of drug given.

6. Record effect, especially any unusual effect, of medication.

7. Never record a medication as given before it has been administered.

A SYSTEM FOR ADMINISTRATION OF MEDICINES

Although hospitals differ in the details of the system used in administering medicines, most of them will use some form of doctor's order book, and a card filing system where medicine cards and treatment cards are in use.

All orders are written in the doctor's order book by the doctor or by the nurse in charge, who may write an order over the doctor's signature at his request.

The nurse in charge is then responsible for placing the order on the patient's card in the proper file. When the order has been transcribed to the patient's card, the nurse signs her initials after the order in the book. This signifies that the order has been checked and placed on the file card.

When the order is placed on the file card, the nurse in charge should make out the medicine card which will be used in administering the medicine to the patient.

Information contained on each medicine card includes: Name of patient, room number, name of drug, dosage of the drug, time of administration, and frequency of dosage.

Various colored cards are used, each color indicating a certain time or frequency of administration. Medicine cards are usually about 2 inches square in size. All information on the card should be printed clearly, with legible numbers and letters. As soon as the card has been printed it should be placed in a transparent cover to protect it from dust and moisture and keep the printed information plainly legible.

Medicine cards are used when medicines are poured or measured. They should be placed on the medicine tray beneath the medicine glass containing the medication and used to identify the patient when the medication is taken to the bedside.

Table 7. STANDARD ABBREVIATIONS PERTAINING TO MEDICATIONS

Abbreviation	*Definition*	*Abbreviation*	*Definition*
a or $\overline{aa}$	of each	mg	milligram
a.c.	before meals	mist	mixture
ad lib	as desired	mm	millimeter
alt. dieb	every other day	no	number
alt. hor	every other hour	O	pint
alt. noc	every other night	ol	oil
aq	water	os	mouth
aq. dest	distilled water	oz	ounce
b.i.d	twice a day	p.c	after meals
$\bar{c}$	with	per	by
C	centigrade	pil	pill
cap	capsule	p.r.n	as needed
cc	cubic centimeter	pt	pint
cg	centigram	pulv	powder
chart	powder	q.h	every hour
cm	centimeter	q.2h	every two hours
comp	compound	q.3h	every three hours
dil	dilute	q.i.d	four times a day
dr	dram	q.s	a sufficient quantity
elix	elixir	qt	quart
emp	a plaster	℞	take
ext	extract	$\bar{s}$	without
F	Fahrenheit	S	mark
fld	fluid	sat	saturate
fl.dr	fluid dram	sig	write
fl.oz	fluid ounce	sol	solution
fract. dos	divided doses	solv	dissolve
gm	gram	s.o.s	if necessary (one dose only)
gr	grain	sp. gr	specific gravity
gtt., gtts	drop, drops	spt	spirit
H	hour	$\overline{ss}$	half
h.s	at bedtime	stat	immediately
hypo	hypodermically	syr	syrup
I.M	intramuscularly	tab	tablet
inf	infusion	t.i.d	three times a day
I.V	intravenously	tr., tinct	tincture
kg	kilogram	ung	ointment
lb	pound	V	volume
liq	liquid; fluid	V.O	verbal order
M	mix	wt	weight
m	minim		

When not in use, medicine cards should be kept in the medicine cabinet in a file divided into compartments and marked with the various hours of administration. When the medicine has been given and proper recording done on the patient's chart, the medicine card should be placed in the compartment of the box marked with the hour at which the medicine is next due.

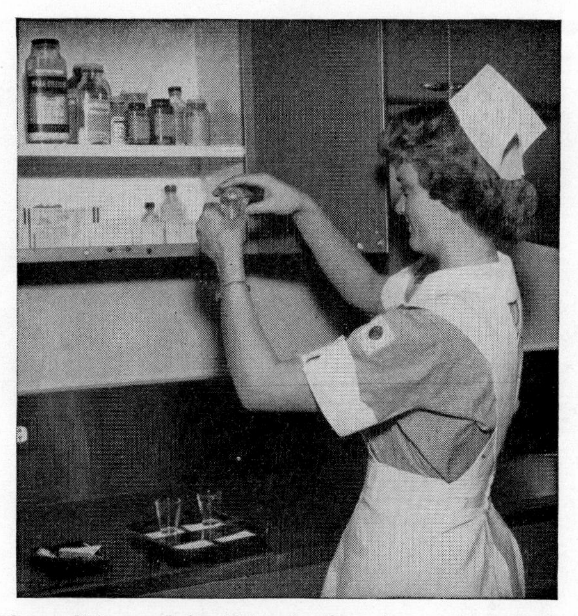

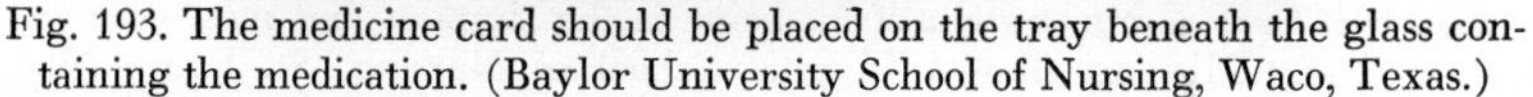

Fig. 193. The medicine card should be placed on the tray beneath the glass containing the medication. (Baylor University School of Nursing, Waco, Texas.)

The medicine card box can be checked at frequent intervals during the day by the nurse in charge. A medicine card that has not been moved ahead to the hour for the next administration is a reminder that the medicine has not been given.

METHODS OF ADMINISTRATION OF MEDICINE

Drugs may be administered by various methods, many drugs can be given by more than one method. Through common practice, if the doctor has not indicated a specific method, the drug is given orally.

The methods of administration which the nurse will need to know and use, include *orally* (by mouth); *sublingually* (the preparation is held beneath the tongue until it dissolves); *rectally* (by retention enema, suppository, or proctoclysis); by *inhalation* (the drug is inhaled and absorbed through pulmonary mucous membrane); by *instillation* (the drug, in liquid or dry form, is directed into a wound or body cavity); by *insufflation* (the drug, in powder form, is blown into a wound or body cavity); by *inunction* (the drug, in the form of an ointment, is rubbed into the skin), or by *local application to the skin* (the drug is applied to the surface of the skin).

A drug may also be given *parenterally* (injected by means of a syringe and needle). The drug may thus be given: *subcutaneously* (into

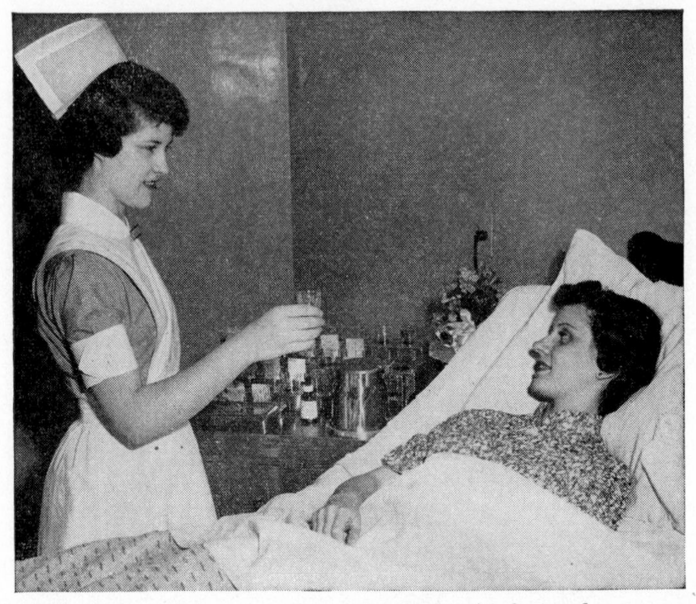

Fig. 194. Oral administration of medicine is the simplest and most economical method. (Missouri Baptist Hospital School of Nursing, St. Louis, Missouri.)

subcutaneous tissue), *intradermally* (into the superficial layers of the skin), *intramuscularly* (deep into muscle tissue), *intravenously* (into a vein), *intraspinally* (into the subarachnoid space of the spinal canal), or *intraperitoneally* (into the peritoneal cavity). Parenteral administration is discussed in Chapter 33.

Orally. Giving drugs by mouth is the simplest and most economical method of administration. Drugs may be given by this method for a local effect, as cough syrup to relieve throat irritation, or for a systemic effect, such as that produced by digitalis to influence heart action.

The three chief disadvantages to oral administration of drugs are: (1) nausea and vomiting may be produced if the drug has an irritant effect upon the stomach; (2) the digestive juices may act on the drug in the stomach and render it ineffective; (3) absorption of the drug from the intestines may be inadequate.

Effective means of overcoming or offsetting the disadvantages of administering the drug orally have been discussed earlier in the chapter, under the heading "Effect Desired."

If the drug is in tablet, pill, or capsule form, it should be gently shaken from the bottle into the bottle cap, then transferred to the paper container or medicine glass in which it will be taken to the patient. Most tablets, pills, and capsules can be removed one at a time from the container by holding it at an angle and gently tapping the top or side with the index finger.

If a pill or tablet must be crushed to be administered (some children have difficulty in swallowing pills), it should be placed in a small porcelain mortar and crushed with the pestle. If this equipment is not available, the pill may be placed in a tablespoon and crushed by applying pressure with the bowl of a teaspoon.

Powders should be packaged in the pharmacy. When time to give the medicine has arrived, the folded paper containing the powder should be opened at one end, held over the medicine glass and tapped with the index finger until the powder has been shaken into the glass. If the powder is sent to the nursing department in bulk, the dose must be accurately measured each time.

A small amount of water added to the powder in the medicine glass will make a solution that can be easily administered to the patient.

To measure liquid drugs, the nurse should hold the calibrated glass in her left hand, place the thumb nail on the line of the glass designating the required amount of the drug, hold the glass at eye level, and pour the medicine, holding the bottle with the label toward the palm of her hand. In measuring liquids in drams or minims, the lowest part of the meniscus should be at the line of measurement.

The mouth of the bottle should be thoroughly cleaned and dried before the bottle is replaced on the shelf.

Unless contraindicated, as for cough syrup, oral medications should be followed immediately with a drink of water, which will rinse the medicine from the mouth and remove any unpleasant after-taste of the drug.

Oily drugs should be followed with citrus fruit or fruit juice, if the diet permits.

Carminatives may be more effective if they are given in hot water.

Rectally. Medications administered by rectum are usually in the form of retention enemas or suppositories. To insert a rectal suppository, the nurse should wear a rubber glove or finger cot. The suppository should be inserted well into the rectum. Pressure should then be applied against the anal region to help overcome the impulse to defecate which insertion of the suppository will produce.

If medication is to be given by vaginal suppository, the patient should first be asked to void. The nurse should wear sterile rubber gloves to prevent contamination in inserting the suppository. The labia should be separated with one hand and the suppository inserted high into the vagina with the other, extending into the canal for a distance of about 2½ inches.

Aseptic technique should be used in inserting a urethral suppository. The suppository should be inserted in the same manner as a catheter is inserted for catheterization.

Inhalation. Drugs may be administered by inhalation for their general effect or to produce a local reaction.

Drugs commonly given by inhalation for systemic effect are smelling salts, ammonia, amyl nitrite pearls, Adrenalin, penicillin and streptomycin.

Ammonia and smelling salts are used as respiratory stimulants and to stimulate heart action in such conditions as fainting.

Amyl nitrite pearls, crushed between thumb and fingers, give off fumes that may be inhaled to relax spasmodic contractions of the coronary arteries, thus relieving attacks of angina pectoris, or to relax the spasm of involuntary muscles in the walls of the bronchi to relieve asthmatic attacks.

Oxygen therapy, an important inhalation procedure, is discussed in detail in Chapter 35, on "Inhalation Therapy."

Instillation. Instillation is the procedure of pouring a liquid medicine drop by drop, into a body cavity. Instillation of medicine into the bladder is discussed in Chapter 31, on "Catheterization." Instillation of medicine into the eye or nose is discussed in Chapter 30, on "Eye, Ear, Nose, and Throat Procedures."

Inunction. Administration of medications by inunction (rubbing into the skin) has been discussed in Chapter 24. For systemic effect, the drug should be applied to a large area of skin, which has been made thoroughly clean with soap and water, and rubbed in so that absorption takes place. Medicines commonly applied by inunction are liniments, oils, cocoa butter, and a variety of ointments, including those containing mercury.

Local Application to the Skin. Various antiseptic solutions may be applied locally in treating minor cuts or injuries. The medicine should be applied with a cotton applicator touched lightly against the skin surface at the site of injury. Ointments and salves applied as a dressing may be spread on several layers of gauze with a tongue blade, applied to the affected area, and held in place with adhesive or a bandage. Lotions are applied directly to the skin to soothe the local lesions or to relieve itching. The lotion should be liberally applied and allowed to dry.

Care of Equipment after Use

All medicine glasses should be washed, rinsed, and sterilized after each use to prevent cross-infection among patients.

The mouth of each bottle containing liquid medicine should be cleaned with a dampened gauze square after medicine has been poured and before the cap is replaced on the bottle.

Small paper containers used for administering pills and capsules should be discarded after use.

Summary of Important Factors

To administer medicine intelligently the nurse must know the minimum and maximum dose, the expected effect, and symptoms of idiosyncrasy to a drug.

Dosage of a drug is determined by age, weight, size, condition of the patient, and method of administration.

All members of the nursing staff should be familiar with the placement of drugs in the medicine cabinet and when preparing medications should return containers to their proper place in the cabinet.

Correct measuring devices should be used as indicated so drugs will be accurately measured.

Both the metric and the apothecary system of measurement should be known by the nurse.

Abbreviations used in administration of medicines should be known by all nurses.

Medicines are given to diagnose, treat, cure or prevent disease.

General and specific rules for giving medicine should be known and observed, especially the five rights of giving medicines to prevent mistakes: the *right patient*, the *right dose*, the *right time*, the *right medicine*, and the *right method* of administration.

Factors To Teach the Patient

How to prepare, measure, and administer medicines he will need to take after leaving the hospital.

The correct use of household measuring devices, such as teaspoon, tablespoon, and medicine dropper.

The dangers involved in overdose of medications.

That the only safe prescriptions are those written by a competent physician.

That self-medication can be dangerous and costly.

Drugs prescribed for one person should not be used by another.

Drugs "left over" when a patient has recovered from an illness should be discarded; many drugs deteriorate or undergo chemical changes when kept for a long time.

Patent medicines may be expensive and are very likely to be ineffective.

Poisonous drugs should be clearly labeled and kept in a place other than the bathroom medicine cabinet where ordinary drugs are kept.

All drugs should be kept out of reach of young children.

The amount of drug taken should be that ordered by the physician; it does not follow that if the usual dose or amount is effective a greater amount will be even more effective.

Water should not be given after cough syrup.

Oily substances or medicines should be kept in the refrigerator.

Several different drugs should not be taken at the same time.

When taking hypnotics or drugs to induce sleep, environmental factors should also be conducive to sleep, as quiet, darkened room, comfortable bed, relaxing bath, etc.

Scientific Principles

Anatomy and Physiology. Taste buds, nerve endings for the sense of taste, are more numerous at the tip and sides of the tongue; bitter or unpalatable drugs given through a tube are not so readily tasted by the patient.

Only substances in liquid form can be tasted. If pills or tablets taste it is because the patient does not swallow them at once and they have started to disintegrate.

A drink of ice water may help to minimize the unpleasant taste of drugs. Nausea and vomiting may be caused by drugs with a very disagreeable taste.

Drugs are absorbed in the stomach and in the small intestines. The more diluted the drug, the more rapid the absorption.

Chemistry. Systemic action of drugs is dependent on chemical reaction. The drug must be dissolved so chemical action between molecules can occur.

A chemical antidote for poison is one that reacts chemically with the poison to make it inert. An antidote for an acid poison is a mild alkali. An antidote for an alkali poison is a mild acid.

Drugs that combine chemically with foods are not effective if they are given when there is food in the stomach.

Microbiology. The nurse should wash her hands before measuring or pouring medicines.

Pills, tablets, and capsules should never be placed in the nurse's hand. They should be transferred from their container directly to the paper cup in which they will be taken to the patient.

Bottle mouths and caps should be cleaned after medicine has been poured, so they remain free from an accumulation of dried or sticky deposit.

Medicine glasses from which various patients may drink should be sterilized after use to prevent cross-infection.

Liquid medicines for the patient in isolation may be measured in the standard medicine glass, then poured into a paper cup to be given to the patient. The paper cup can then be burned.

Pharmacology. Dilution of a drug hastens its absorption. Liquid drugs, with the exception of cough syrup and oils, are diluted before being given. Water, milk, chocolate, and fruit juices may be used to dilute liquid drugs.

The dosage of medicine for children up to 12 years of age is only a fractional part of the usual adult dose.

Drugs to increase appetite or aid in digestion should be given before meals.

Drugs to neutralize digestive juices and prevent gastrointestinal irritation are given after meals.

Calibrated measuring devices should be used to insure accurate dosage of the drug.

The patient should not be wakened at night for medications, unless the doctor has specifically ordered that medicine be given during the night.

Physics. Because liquid adheres to glass, the meniscus on the liquid in a minim glass is concave.

Pills, tablets, and capsules are more easily swallowed when taken with water because friction between the pill, tablet or capsule and the mucous membrane of the throat is reduced by the water.

Radioactive drugs, given orally, must be carefully controlled as they are hazardous to patient, nurse, and doctor.

Psychology. Patients are unusually sensitive to the sight, odor, and taste of medicines. Drugs with unpleasant tastes should be given so the taste is disguised.

Since the ill person is very apt to accept suggestions in regard to medications, the nurse should indicate that drugs are given to "relieve discomfort," to "induce sleep and rest," to "relax," or to "help" them.

Sociology. Teamwork and cooperation is the basis for successful administration of medicine. The medicine is prescribed by the doctor, prepared by the pharmacist, and administered by the nurse.

The sale of drugs and the manner in which they are advertised is regulated by the federal Food, Drug, and Cosmetic Act.

Situation Type Problems

1. A student nurse giving H.S. medications in a ward on a medical department discovered that one patient had been accepting a hypnotic tablet each night for the past week but had not taken any of the tablets and had seven of them in her possession. The nurse, despite vigorous protests from the patient, took the seven tablets away to discard them.

The patient insisted that she had been charged for the medication and that the tablets belonged to her. She threatened to have the nurse arrested, and refused to take the tablet which the nurse had prepared for her in accordance with the doctor's orders. What would you have done?

2. A student nurse was bathing a patient when the attending physician came into the room. During their conversation the patient complained that she had been unable to sleep the night before and had a severe headache as a result. As he left the room the doctor said to the nurse, "See that Mrs. Smith gets three grains of amytal tonight and

give her some aspirin now for the headache." The student followed the doctor into the corridor and explained to him that she was unable to take the verbal order. The doctor told her to give the usual dose of aspirin at once and said he would write the order.

The student did not find the head nurse at her desk so she asked a private duty nurse how much aspirin is considered a "usual dose." The private duty nurse told her to give 15 grains for a severe headache. The student gave the patient 15 grains of aspirin and recorded it on the chart.

Twenty minutes later the head nurse questioned the student about the medication. The doctor had ordered the amytal but had written no order for aspirin. The head nurse was unable to reach the attending doctor by telephone so she asked the intern to write an order for aspirin for the patient. The intern wrote on the doctor's order record that the patient was to be given 10 grains of aspirin, for headache. What would you have done?

Suggested Reference Reading

"What you don't take won't hurt you," Roy R. Kracke; Hygeia, December, 1947.

"Drug reactions," Windsor C. Cutting; American Journal of Nursing, March, 1948.

"Taste, the trickiest sense," George Mann; Science Digest, September, 1948.

"Some recent developments in drug therapy," Elizabeth S. Gill; Public Health Nursing, May, 1949.

"The development of new drugs," Harold D. Kautz; American Journal of Nursing, January, 1953.

CHAPTER 33

Parenteral Administration of Medicines

TOPICAL OUTLINE

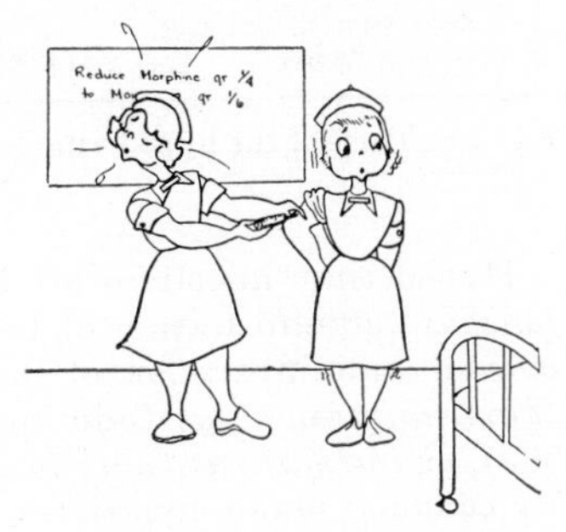

We learn to do by doing!

Parenteral has been defined as meaning "by some route other than the intestinal tract, as subcutaneously or intravenously." Through common usage, it has come to mean the administration of a drug or fluid by needle injection and includes subcutaneous, intramuscular, intradermal, and intravenous injections. The term "injection" is defined as "the forcing of a fluid into a cavity, the tissues, or a blood vessel through a hollow tube or needle."

HYPODERMIC INJECTION

The purpose of the hypodermic injection of a drug is threefold: (1) to obtain a rapid and systemic effect of the drug; (2) to prevent the drug from being destroyed or rendered ineffectual by action of digestive juices in the stomach; (3) to administer the drug when it cannot be given orally, as for the unconscious or uncooperative patient, the patient for whom gastric suction is being used, or the patient with nausea and vomiting.

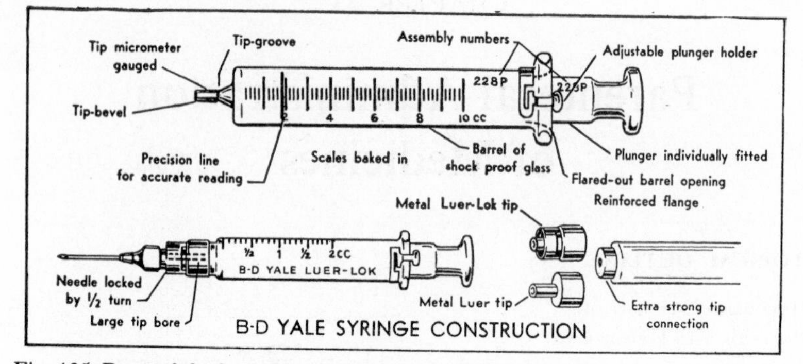

Fig. 195. Parts of the hypodermic. (Becton, Dickinson and Company, Rutherford, New Jersey.)

Hypodermic injections are given in various ways, including *subcutaneous* (administration of the drug into subcutaneous tissue), *intradermal* (administration of the drug within the surface layers of the skin), *intramuscular* (administration of the drug deep in muscle tissue), or *intravenous* (administration of the drug directly into a vein). By common usage, hypodermic injection implies administration of the drug by subcutaneous injection.

PARTS OF THE HYPODERMIC

The various parts of the hypodermic include: the syringe (barrel)—the part which contains the drug in solution; the plunger—used to draw the solution into the syringe and supply the pressure when the solution is injected; the needle—through which the drug is injected into body tissues; the stylet—a fine wire passed through the lumen of the needle to keep it open.

The Hypodermic. Hypodermic syringes are made of glass in sizes 2 cc., 5 cc., 10 cc., 20 cc., 30 cc., and 50 cc., and are calibrated in cubic centimeters and minims for accurate measurement of the drug. The 2 cc. (30 minim) size is most commonly used. The average amount of solution given ranges from 12 to 20 minims.

Special syringes are made for insulin and tuberculin. The insulin syringe is calibrated in units instead of cubic centimeters and minims. The tuberculin syringe is calibrated in tenths and hundredths of a cubic centimeter, as the drug is given in minute amounts.

The Hypospray, a device used in place of the hypodermic, sprays the drug through the skin under high pressure. No needle is needed. A cylinder (into which a cartridge of drug is inserted) is used. Pressure of more than 100 pounds per square inch is created in the device and forces the drug into the tissues in a very rapid spray. The

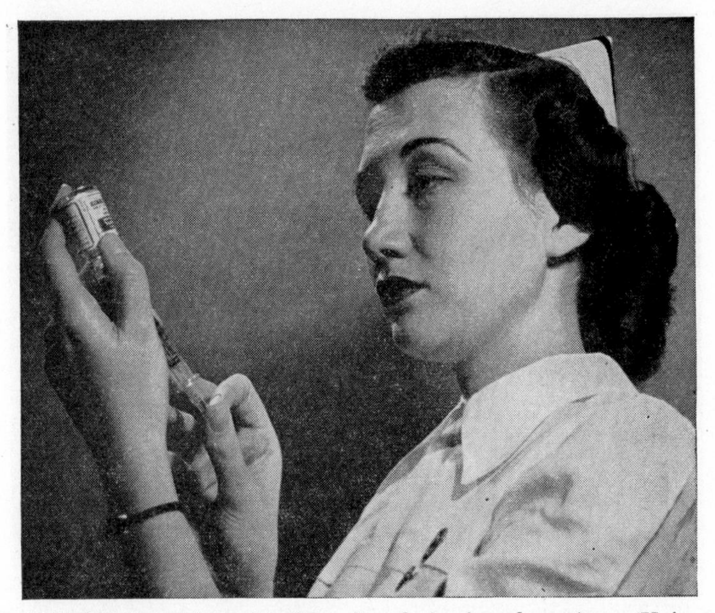

Fig. 196. The plunger is used to draw the solution into the syringe. (University of Michigan School of Nursing, Ann Arbor, Michigan.)

patient feels no pain when the drug is administered and no visible marks appear on the skin at the site of injection.

The plunger, used to draw the solution into the syringe, may be frosted or colored to facilitate reading of the calibrations on the syringe for accurate measurement. The syringe and plunger each bears the same number, and numbers should be matched to assure that the plunger fits the syringe exactly, thus eliminating the danger of losing some of the drug in administration. Syringes are now available in which the parts are interchangeable. The syringe may have a plain glass tip or a metal tip. With the metal tip the needle may be locked in position so it cannot come loose from the syringe.

To avoid unnecessary breakage of syringes, they should be boiled no longer than is necessary for sterilization. The plunger should not be inserted into the syringe at an angle, and it should not be left in the syringe after the medication has been given. Syringes may be broken by having a heavy object dropped on them; being dropped; being boiled without having been thoroughly cleaned; by efforts to insert a plunger that does not fit or to insert plunger at an angle; by holding a finger over the tip and suddenly releasing the plunger; by efforts to remove a needle that is stuck. Syringes may be sterilized by

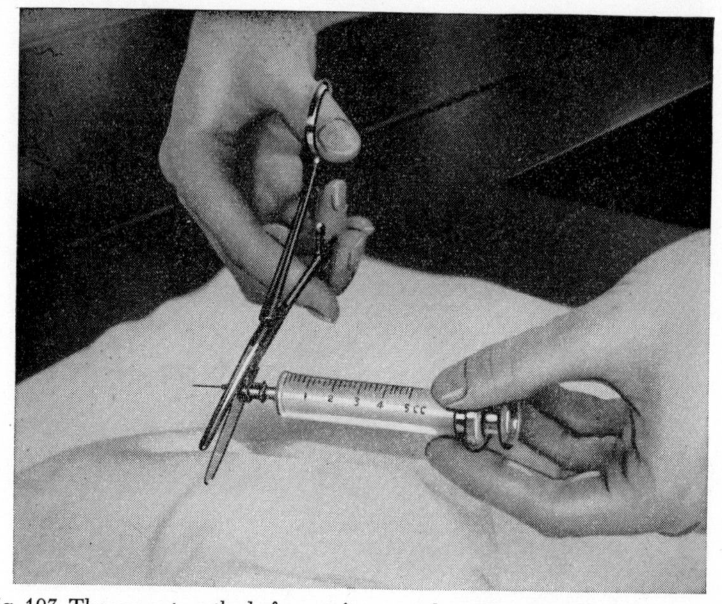

Fig. 197. The correct method of removing a stuck needle. (Becton, Dickinson and Company, Rutherford, New Jersey.)

boiling in distilled water for 20 minutes; by wrapping between layers of gauze and muslin and placing in an autoclave for 20 minutes; by immersion for the required time in a chemical agent; by exposure to dry heat or the hot air sterilizer for one hour.

The Needle. The needle used in giving a hypodermic injection should always be clean, sharp, and straight. With the needle in good condition, the procedure is not painful to the patient and may be done by the nurse without difficulty. Four factors which usually need to be considered in selection of the size of needle to be used for various injections are: the safety with which a needle can be used, the rate of flow of medicine to be administered, the comfort of the patient, and the depth to which the needle must penetrate.

Parts of the needle are: the lock flange—the part that fits on the tip of the syringe; the hub—the larger part of the needle; the cannula—the stem, or long slender portion of the needle; the point—the beveled opening of the needle ending in a sharp point.

The length of the needle is determined by the length of the cannula and point. The diameter size of the needle is indicated by gauge numbers, which range from 13 to 27. The larger the gauge number, the smaller the diameter of the lumen of the needle. Needles used for subcutaneous injection are usually 24–25 gauge and ¾–1 inch in length.

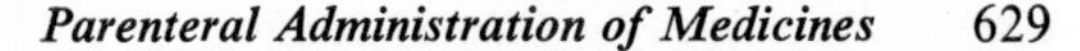

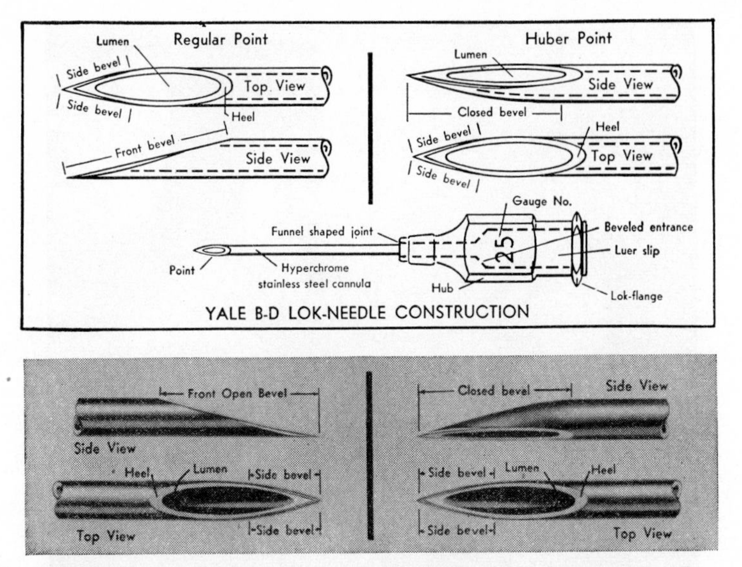

Fig. 198. Parts of a hypodermic needle, including the sharp point. (Becton, Dickinson and Company, Rutherford, New Jersey.)

The best method of cleaning a hypodermic needle is to flush it with cold water immediately after use, wash it in soap and water, then rinse with alcohol or ether. For sterilization hypodermic needles may be placed on several thicknesses of gauze and boiled 10–20 minutes, or they may be placed in a test tube which contains a small cotton pledget in the end and autoclaved for 10–20 minutes. A large number of needles may be placed in a circle on a layer of gauze inside a glass laboratory dish, covered, and autoclaved for the required period of time.

TO ASSEMBLE STERILE NEEDLE AND SYRINGE

It is essential that a sterile syringe and needle be handled without contamination of parts which must remain sterile if the drug is to remain sterile. Parts to be kept aseptically clean are the needle, the tip end of the syringe, the inside of the syringe, and the plunger, with the exception of the handle.

The syringe should be lifted from its container in the nurse's left hand, only its outer surface being touched as she holds it at the center of the shaft. The plunger, with handle only being touched, should be removed from the container. The end of the plunger is then inserted into the opening of the syringe with both pieces held as indicated

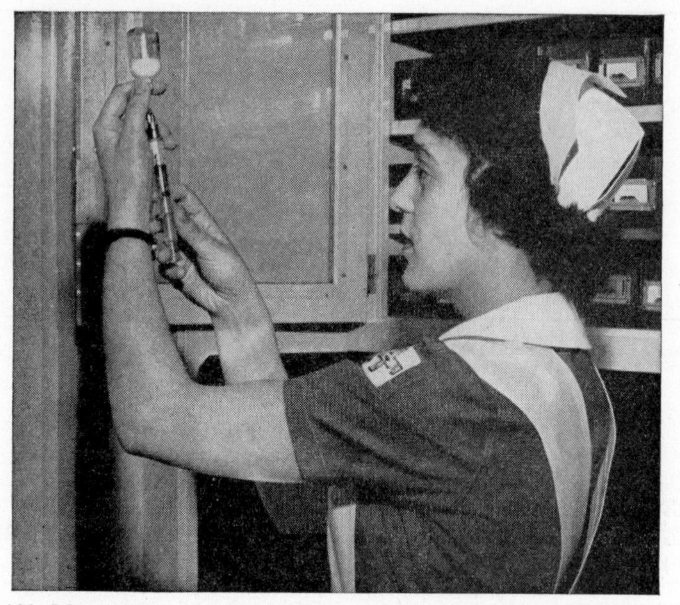

Fig. 199. Measuring penicillin for parenteral administration. (Bridgeport Hospital School of Nursing, Bridgeport, Connecticut.)

above. While the syringe with plunger inside is held in the left hand, the right hand should be used to handle sterile forceps which grasp the hub portion of the needle to remove it from its container and place it firmly on the syringe. Turning the syringe part way will tighten the needle on the tip so that it remains securely in place while the drug is being measured and administered.

As the needle is removed from its container with the forceps, it should be closely inspected. The point should be sharp and the cannula or stem of the needle should be straight. A bent needle may break while being inserted, and it may be difficult to locate and remove the part remaining in the patient's body.

All necessary equipment for the giving of a hypodermic injection is kept on a tray in the medicine cabinet near the narcotic box. The tray should always be ready for use with all supply containers kept properly filled. Articles found on the tray include: A container for the syringe and plunger. A container of sterile needles, alcohol, alcohol lamp with large spoon attached, sterile cotton sponges, sterile distilled water, matches, small thumb forceps in a container of disinfectant solution, a small file for opening ampules. A container for used syringes and needles may be kept conveniently at hand in the utility room. A wastebasket should be near the medicine cabinet for discarded empty ampules or soiled sponges.

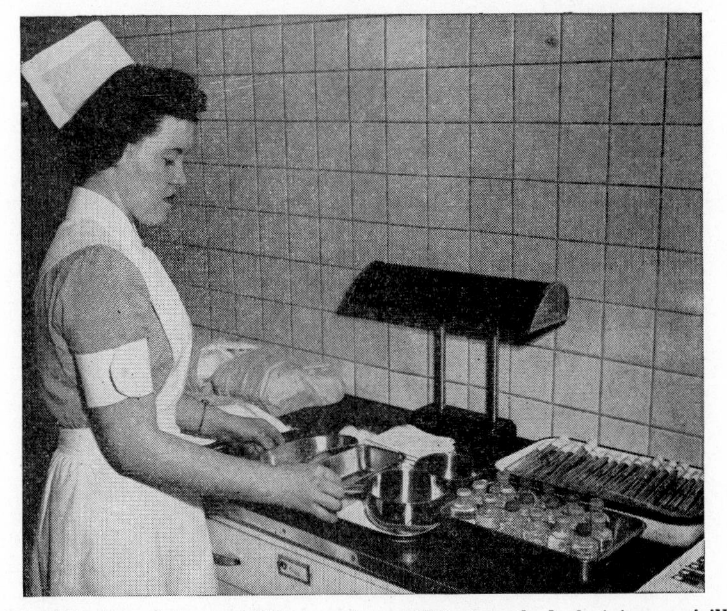

Fig. 200. Use of the penicillin tray is an efficient method of giving penicillin to large numbers of patients. (Missouri Baptist Hospital School of Nursing, St. Louis, Missouri.)

CALCULATION OF DOSAGE

Calculation of dosage may be required before the solution can be prepared. Dosage must be computed accurately. The nurse should know exactly how to prepare the amount of drug needed from the tablet or powdered drug on hand. She must know how to measure 50,000 units of penicillin from a vial containing many times that amount. She not only must compute accurately the amount of drug to use, but must know the amount of solvent to be used in dissolving the drug. The amount of solvent for a hypodermic injection should be not less than 4 minims and not more than 20 minims. If less than 4 minims is used and a drop or two should be spilled, much of the drug would be lost. If the amount given exceeds 20 minims it may cause discomfort or pain to the patient.

PREPARATION OF THE DRUG

Drugs that are in solution need no special prepartion prior to administration. Drugs that are not stable in solution and are supplied in powdered or crystalline form must be dissolved before they can be injected. Such drugs as penicillin, streptomycin, some barbiturates,

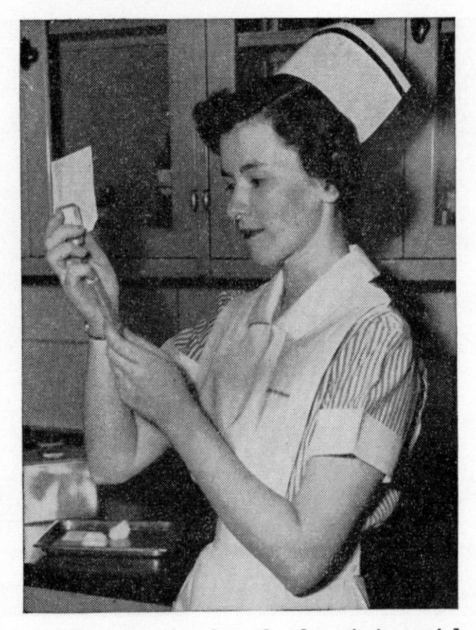

Fig. 201. Preparing a hypodermic when the drug is in a vial with rubber diaphragm. (Delaware Hospital School of Nursing, Wilmington, Delaware.)

and vitamin concentrates are in this classification. Sterile distilled water and sterile normal saline solution are usually used to dissolve hypodermic tablets and powdered drugs. The method of preparation of the medication depends on the form in which the drug is supplied.

If the drug is in tablet form: fill tablespoon two-thirds full of sterile distilled water; place spoon over flame of alcohol lamp; place needle in spoon and boil for 1 minute; place needle on syringe and tighten so that it is held securely; draw 1 cc. water from the spoon into the syringe; discard remainder of water from the spoon; put the tablet form of drug in the spoon—expel water from syringe on the drug to dissolve it; draw solution into syringe to the desired amount; place needle on top of alcohol sponge and fold lower portion of sponge over the needle; place hypodermic with needle and sponge on small medicine tray for carrying to the patient's room.

If the drug is in ampule form: remove sterile syringe and needle from container and place needle on syringe; place on tray so needle is protected by an alcohol sponge; snap tip of ampule lightly with fingers to dislodge solution that might be there; file neck of ampule evenly on three sides; break tip from ampule, holding with dry alcohol sponge, so fingers will not be cut; introduce needle into ampule without touching its sides, thus keeping needle sterile; withdraw desired dosage of the solution from ampule into syringe.

If the drug is in powder form: If an ampule contains a drug in powder form, the ampule should be opened and sterile distilled water injected. After the powder has dissolved, the proper amount of solution should be drawn into the syringe.

If the drug is in a vial with rubber diaphragm: remove sterile syringe and needle from their container; place needle on syringe and place on tray so needle is protected by an alcohol sponge; cleanse top of vial with another alcohol sponge; draw air into syringe to equal the amount of solution to be given; insert needle into diaphragm (at center), hold vial vertically, and force air from syringe into vial; withdraw solution until desired dosage has been obtained; withdraw needle from vial—the opening made by needle seals itself when needle is withdrawn.

HARRISON NARCOTIC LAW

All nurses given the responsibility of handling narcotics should be instructed regarding provisions of the Harrison Narcotic Law effective since 1915. This law requires: that each physician prescribing narcotics put his registry number on each prescription; that each hospital keep a record of the amount of each narcotic purchased and of each narcotic given to patients, so that at all times the record of narcotics purchased, narcotics used, and narcotics on hand must tally; that a prescription containing an opiate cannot be refilled; that all doses of narcotic given by each nurse must be recorded.

PREPARATION OF THE HYPODERMIC

When the dosage of the drug has been accurately calculated and the solution prepared, the amount to be given must be measured in the syringe. To do this, the syringe must be held in vertical position at eye level to permit accurate observation of the calibrations.

After the correct measurement has been made, the hypodermic should be placed on a small medicine tray. The needle should be placed on an alcohol-saturated cotton pledget which is then folded over it and held in place with the index finger of the hand which carries the tray. If the thumb is placed over the syringe, as tray and hypodermic are being carried to the patient, the syringe will not roll about on the tray.

ADMINISTRATION OF THE HYPODERMIC

On entering the room, the nurse should identify the patient by repeating his name clearly and distinctly. Identification of the patient prevents mistakes in medication. The procedure should always be explained to the patient, and he should be assured that it is no more painful than an ordinary pin prick.

Subcutaneous Injection. The site chosen for administration of a subcutaneous injection is usually the outer surface of the upper arm about two inches below the shoulder or the muscular anterior portion of the thigh. Care should be taken to avoid striking bone tissue with the needle. The site of large blood vessels and proximal areas of a nerve should be avoided in giving a hypodermic injection.

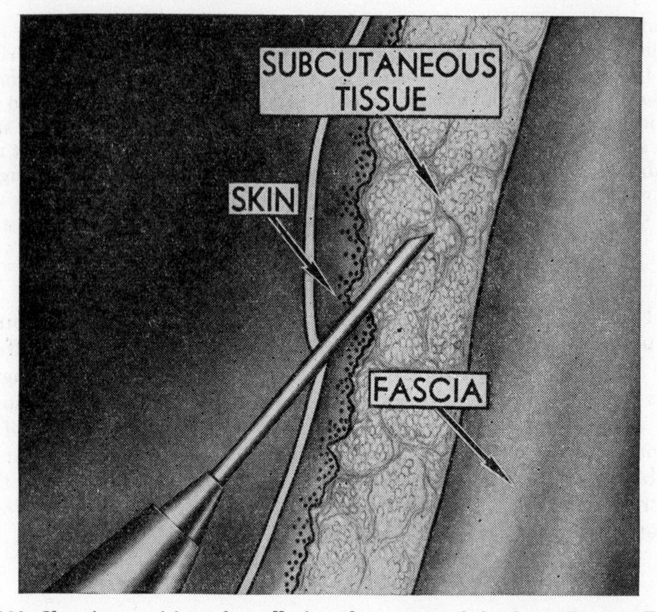

Fig. 202. Showing position of needle in subcutaneous injection. (Becton, Dickinson and Company, Rutherford, New Jersey.)

The site of injection should be cleansed with the alcohol sponge and all air should be expelled from the syringe and needle, by holding the syringe in a vertical position at eye level and very slowly rotating and moving the plunger upward. As air is expelled from the syringe it may cause a very little amount of spraying of tiny droplets from the needle tip. When all air has been removed, the spraylike action ceases and one complete drop of solution will form at the tip of the needle. This indicates that all air has been removed from the syringe and needle and the hypodermic is ready to be administered.

The area of injection should be pinched firmly between thumb and forefinger of the nurse's left hand and the needle inserted at a 45 degree angle. If the needle is pushed through the skin with a firm, even, rapid movement it is less painful than if inserted slowly. When the needle has been fully inserted it should be withdrawn slightly and the drug injected gently and steadily into the tissues. All of the drug must be injected so that the patient receives the desired dosage. While the needle is inserted into the tissues, it should be held steady. Movement of the hypodermic syringe during injection of the drug causes the tip of the needle to move and injury to tissue will result.

When the medication has been injected, the cotton pledget should be placed over the site of injection and the needle withdrawn

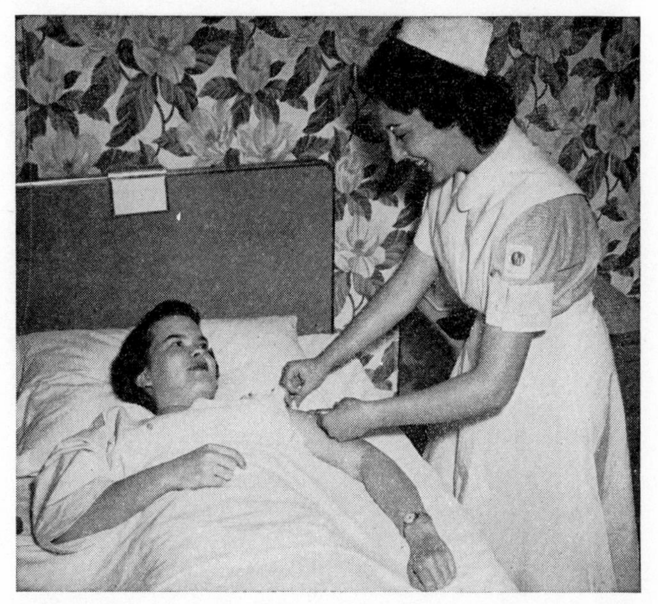

Fig. 203. Removing the needle after hypodermic injection. (Baylor University School of Nursing, Waco, Texas.)

smoothly. After the needle has been withdrawn, the area should be gently massaged with the alcohol pledget to aid absorption by stimulating circulation in the part.

Intramuscular Injection. When the prescribed drug might be very irritating to subcutaneous tissue or when a more rapid action is desired, it may be given intramuscularly. The drug is usually measured in a 5–10 cc. syringe, and a 22-gauge needle about 1½ inches long is used. The site of injection is usually the gluteal muscles, although intramuscular injections can be given in the deltoid muscle of the arm. The patient should be lying on his abdomen with buttocks exposed when ready to receive the medication in the gluteal muscles.

The needle should be inserted with a rapid sure motion which causes it to penetrate skin and muscle without causing undue pain. With the syringe held perpendicularly to the skin surface, the needle is inserted straight downward into the muscle. Before injecting the drug, the plunger should be withdrawn slightly to make sure the needle is not in a blood vessel. The presence of blood in the lower portion of the syringe as the plunger is withdrawn indicates that the point of the needle is in a blood vessel. If blood appears, the needle should be withdrawn and inserted again at a different site. When the drug has been injected, the area should be gently massaged to aid absorption.

Intravenous Injection. Although injection of a drug directly into a

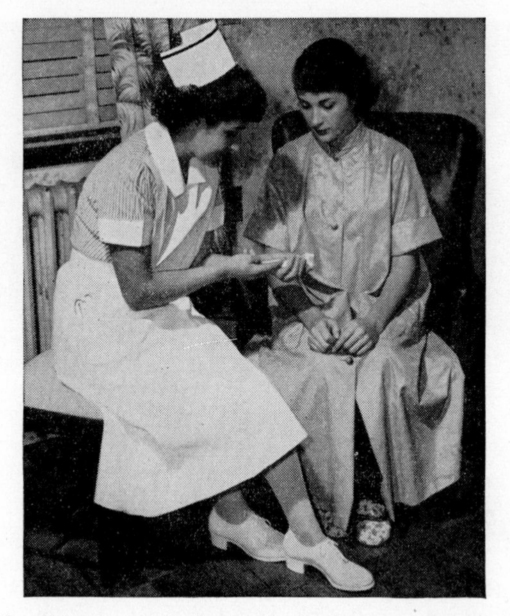

Fig. 204. The diabetic patient should be taught to prepare, measure, and administer her own insulin. (Delaware Hospital School of Nursing, Wilmington, Delaware.)

vein is usually done by the doctor, preparation of the drug and the hypodermic is the responsibility of the nurse. To avoid mistakes in medication the container from which the drug is taken should be shown the doctor so he may make sure the correct medicine is being administered. Drugs are injected intravenously when a very rapid action is desired, for certain diagnostic tests, and when the drug cannot be tolerated when given by other methods.

The size of the syringe used for intravenous injection of a drug may range from 2 to 50 cc., depending on the amount of solution to be administered. A 20–22-gauge needle about 1½ inches in length is most commonly used.

Before intravenous injection, the procedure should be explained to the patient. A slight degree of pain may be experienced by him, since veins contain sensory nerves and the needle must pierce the blood vessel wall. Veins usually selected for intravenous injection are the cephalic or the median basilic inside the elbow. A tourniquet is applied to the arm to make the vein more accessible to the doctor. After the needle has been inserted, the tourniquet should be released. The plunger should be pulled back slightly to make sure the needle is in the blood

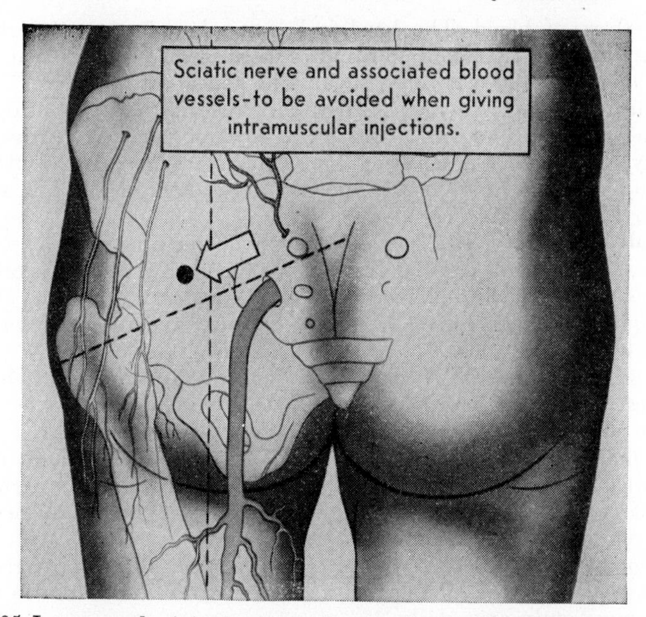

Fig. 205. Intramuscular injection is usually given in the gluteal muscles. (Becton, Dickinson and Company, Rutherford, New Jersey.)

vessel. If blood appears in the syringe, the drug may then be injected. When the needle is withdrawn, slight pressure should be exerted over the site of injection to prevent bleeding from the vein.

Intradermal Injection. Intradermal injections, used chiefly for diagnostic purposes, as in Schick tests and skin tests for specific allergic reactions, are usually given by the doctor. The tuberculin syringe is used, since the amount of drug given is very small. A 26-gauge needle about ⅜ inch long is usually used. Injections may be made on the inner surface of the forearm, midway between wrist and elbow, on the upper arm, or on the back. The needle is inserted at an angle of approximately 15 degrees, with the bevel of the needle turned upward. A very small amount of drug is injected just under the outer layer of skin, producing a small bleb.

INSULIN ADMINISTRATION

When the body fails to supply enough insulin to utilize the sugar taken in through food, insulin must be administered to supply the deficiency. The insulin given by hypodermic injection acts in the same way as that normally supplied by the body, helping to maintain blood sugar level within normal limits. Normal blood sugar is 80–120 mg.

per 100 cc. of blood. The level is lowest when fasting (just before eating) and highest about 30 minutes after eating. When blood sugar level increases above normal, sugar will appear in the urine.

Insulin was discovered in 1921 by Sir Frederick Grant Banting, Dr. Charles H. Best, and Dr. J. B. Collip, working together at the University of Toronto. One of the greatest medical discoveries of all time, it resulted in the first effective means of treatment of diabetes, which earlier had inevitably resulted in death.

Kinds of Insulin. The four chief kinds of insulin are:

Regular Insulin. Regular insulin was the form first made available for use: it is a clear liquid and has its greatest effect 2 or 3 hours after it is administered. The effect lasts 6 to 8 hours, and the drug must be given before each meal.

Crystalline Insulin. A clear liquid form of insulin which has its greatest effect in 2 or 3 hours, lasts 6 to 8 hours, and must be given before each meal.

Protamine Zinc Insulin. A form of insulin that is cloudy in appearance. The effect is greatest 12–16 hours after administration, and the effect lasts slightly more than 24 hours. This type insulin needs to be given only once each day.

Globin Insulin. A clear liquid form of insulin that has its greatest effect in 8 to 16 hours. The effect lasts 20 hours, and the insulin needs to be given only once daily.

Measuring Insulin. A *unit* of insulin is the amount of insulin used as the standard for its measurement. Insulin solutions are of various strengths and are classified according to the number of units in each cubic centimeter: yellow label (U. 20 insulin) contains 20 units of insulin in each cc.; red label (U. 40 insulin) contains 40 units of insulin in each cc.; green label (U. 80 insulin) contains 80 units of insulin in each cc. Each bottle of insulin contains 10 cc.

The Insulin Syringe. The insulin syringe is a 1 cc. syringe marked off into 10 equal parts. For U. 20 insulin there is 20 units of insulin in each 1 cc., therefore each part contains 2 units of insulin. For U. 40 insulin there is 40 units of insulin per cc. and each part contains 4 units of insulin. For U. 80 insulin there is 80 units per cc. and each part contains 8 units of insulin.

In ordering insulin for a patient, the doctor will prescribe the strength of insulin to be used and the number of units to be given for each dose. If a large amount of insulin is ordered U. 80 insulin may be used so the amount to be administered will not be such that discomfort is caused the patient.

The calibrations on the insulin syringe are U. 10 to U. 20: U. 20 to U. 40: U. 40 to U. 80. The scale on the syringe which is used must correspond to the strength of insulin used. If U. 40 insulin is used, the U. 40 scale on the syringe must be used to measure the amount of insulin to be given.

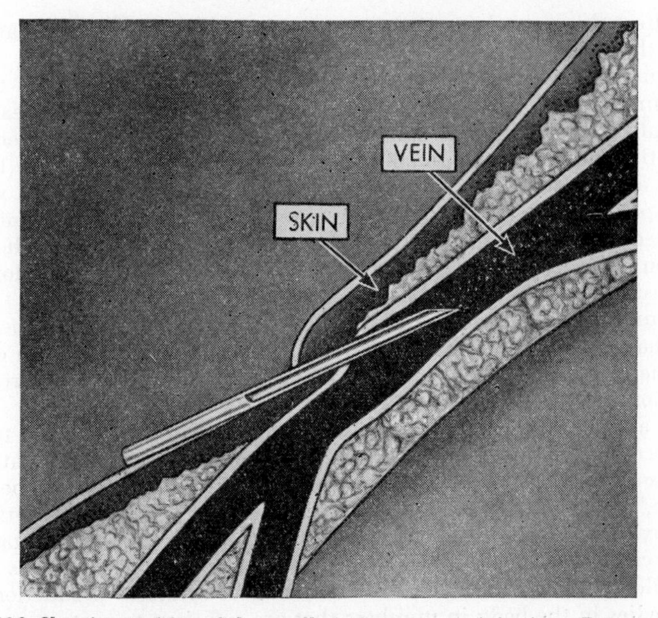

Fig. 206. Showing position of the needle in intravenous injection. (Becton, Dickinson and Company, Rutherford, New Jersey.)

Preparation of a Combined Dose. The procedure for preparing regular insulin and protamine zinc insulin to be given in one injection. Check the medicine card and the label on each bottle of insulin; mix protamine zinc by rolling bottle between hands gently; assemble hypodermic; cleanse top of each bottle with sterile cotton pledget dampened with Zephiran solution; draw into syringe amount of air equal to dosage of protamine zinc insulin desired; inject air into protamine zinc bottle; *do not withdraw insulin;* draw into syringe the amount of air equal to dosage of regular insulin desired; inject air into the bottle, then withdraw regular insulin; reinsert needle into protamine zinc insulin; withdraw protamine zinc insulin; draw a small amount of air into syringe and tip the syringe back and forth several times (gently) to mix the two types of insulin; administer to the patient by subcutaneous injection.

All diabetic patients should be taught how to prepare, measure, and administer their own insulin before they are dismissed from the hospital. The nurse should supervise the procedure until she is certain the patient understands it and is capable of doing it for himself.

SERUM AND VACCINE ADMINISTRATION

The physician usually administers serums or vaccines to the patient. The nurse needs to know the purpose of these biological products and the effect they may have if she is to give adequate care to the patient after the injection.

Serum is the clear portion of blood that has been withdrawn from an animal or a human being. Normal serum is serum from a healthy animal or human. Antibodies are substances which will fight certain causative organisms of infection. They are manufactured in the body of an animal that has been injected with the bacteria, toxin, or virus of a specific disease. The antibodies remain in the bloodstream of the injected animal for a time to protect against a recurrence of the infection. The invading agent or factor that causes the production of antibodies is termed *antigen.*

Human convalescent serum, obtained from the blood of a person who has recovered from a disease, contains antibodies which can combat the disease so is of benefit in helping another patient to overcome invasion by the same kind of bacteria.

An antitoxin is a substance in serum that helps overcome the toxin produced by a pathogenic microorganism and is used to combat the disease caused by the particular organism. It is also termed a "specific serum," since it acts against only one type of organism, as tetanus antitoxin, which is effective only against the organism causing tetanus.

Vaccines are suspensions of dead or weakened bacteria or virus in a suitable fluid. Administration of a vaccine stimulates production of antibodies in the body in numbers that are sufficient to protect against an ordinary attack of the disease so that illness does not follow exposure to the causative organisms.

Toxoid is a mild toxin preparation containing antibodies which were produced by a small dose of the toxins of bacteria which cause disease. Toxoid may be used to effectively immunize young children against such diseases as diphtheria.

Injection of vaccines and toxoids causes production of antibodies in the body of the recipient. Specific serums and antitoxins contain the antibodies which are transferred to the patient receiving the injection. Serums and antitoxins must be manufactured by living animals or human beings. Vaccines and toxoids may be made from bacteria grown in the laboratory, except for smallpox vaccine, which is produced in the bodies of healthy calves.

Serums and vaccines are used for various purposes, including susceptibility tests, diagnostic tests, immunization, and treatment. The Schick test is used to determine susceptibility to diphtheria. The Dick test is used to determine susceptibility to scarlet fever. The Wassermann and Kahn tests are used to diagnose syphilis. Von Pirquet and Mantoux tests are used to diagnose tuberculosis. The Widal test is used to diagnose typhoid fever.

Immunization against diphtheria is accomplished by a toxoid; against scarlet fever by a toxin or toxoid; against smallpox by a vaccine which contains virus; and against typhoid by a series of injections of vaccine.

Diseases or conditions treated by serum therapy include acne, boils, anthrax, colds, diphtheria, dysentery, measles, pertussis, and tetanus.

Serums are given subcutaneously, intramuscularly, intravenously, or intraspinally. The size of the dose is determined by the age of the patient, the concentration of the serum, and the severity of the disease. The prophylactic dose is usually much smaller than that given for treatment.

Vaccines are given hypodermically, intradermally, or by very fine scratches made on the skin surface.

Unfavorable reaction to serum or vaccine is due to abnormal sensitivity of the patient to the protein substance it contains. The proteins taken into the body in foods that are eaten undergo chemical changes in the digestive tract and are absorbed into the blood stream as amino acids rather than as proteins. Proteins of serum and vaccines are introduced directly into the blood stream without having been changed by chemical processes. Such proteins are termed "foreign proteins," since they act as a foreign substance to the blood and may cause undesirable reactions, termed anaphylactic reactions. Anaphylaxis is defined as "an unusual or exaggerated reaction to a foreign protein, due to sensitization."

Allergy is a mild form of anaphylaxis. Allergic reactions vary from a mild form, as slight urticaria, to severe and distressing asthma.

To prevent anaphylactic shock a test for protein sensitivity is done before administration of the required dosage of serum, if there is sufficient time to do so. A patient with a history of food allergy or of asthma may be more sensitive to foreign protein substances.

Reaction to vaccine is usually much less severe than that to serum and many patients can be vaccinated without more than minor discomfort.

Care of Equipment after Use

Immediately after use, the syringe and needle should be rinsed in cold water, washed in warm soap and water, and rinsed again.

Syringes and needles should be sent to central supply to be cleaned, inspected, and resterilized.

All hypodermic needles should be inspected periodically. Points of the needles should be sharpened when necessary, and needles that are bent should be discarded. Needles should be autoclaved at frequent intervals during the day so that an adequate supply is available in the various departments of the hospital at all times.

Summary of Important Factors

Drugs are given by parenteral injection to assure rapid action; to prevent the drug being acted on by digestive juices; to give a drug when it cannot be given orally.

The method most commonly used is subcutaneous injection.

The amount of solution injected subcutaneously should not be more than 20 minims or less than 10.

Syringes and needles require careful attention and should always be cleaned immediately after use.

A drug should not be administered hypodermically without first expelling all the air from the syringe and needle.

By aspiration it can be determined if the needle is in a blood vessel.

The insulin syringe is a special device for giving insulin.

Insulin is measured in units and comes in strengths of U. 20, U. 40 and U. 80.

The procedure for giving combined regular and protamine zinc insulin is relatively simple, when adequately explained.

Intramuscular injections should be given where there are no large blood vessels, as in the lower inner corner of the upper outer quadrant of a buttock.

The tourniquet will be needed for an intravenous injection.

Sensitivity to foreign proteins may make serum therapy a hazardous means of treatment.

Factors To Teach the Patient

The reasons for giving a drug hypodermically when the patient would prefer to take it orally.

The proper diet, administration of insulin, and other measures necessary for the protection of the diabetic patient. He should be instructed to carry an identification card stating that he is a diabetic patient and taking insulin.

Aseptic technique must be used for hypodermic injections, if infection is to be avoided.

Scientific Principles

Anatomy and Physiology. Because the skin contains numerous nerves that convey pain, a hypodermic injection may cause pain to the patient. Only an extremely small amount of medicine may be given intradermally since the injection is made very near the surface of the skin and is more painful.

Drugs given subcutaneously become effective in a very short time since complete circulation time is about 20 seconds.

Because muscles are well supplied with blood vessels, caution must be used to prevent the needle from entering a blood vessel when an intramuscular injection is being made. The lower inner corner of the upper outer quadrant of the buttock is the area usually selected.

For immediate effect drugs may be given intravenously, the cephalic or median basilic vein usually being chosen as the site for injection.

Chemistry. Laboratory tests may be used to determine the proper frequency of dosage. Chemical tests may be made on blood to ascertain the amount of a certain drug that may be present in the blood.

Microbiology. To prevent infection, all parts of the hypodermic needle or syringe with which the drug will come in contact must be sterile. The part of the needle which penetrates the skin must also remain sterile.

All solutions of drugs given hypodermically are sterile. The preparation and administration of a hypodermic must be done with strictly aseptic technique.

After use all needles should be boiled or autoclaved long enough to make them absolutely sterile.

Pharmacology. Drugs given hypodermically to prevent disease include serums and vaccines.

Antibiotics and specifics are given for their remedial action.

Drugs given to relieve pain and produce sleep or rest are narcotics, sedatives, and anesthetics. General anesthesia is commonly given by intravenous injection.

Drugs given in substitute therapy include insulin, thyroid extract, liver extract, minerals, and vitamins.

The standard insulin measurement is called a *unit*. A unit of insulin is the amount that will be used to metabolize about 1.5 gm. of dextrose.

Drugs may be given hypodermically for diagnostic purposes.

Physics. The factor of pressure is important in making all hypodermic injections. When the plunger is pulled back pressure is lowered in the syringe and the solution enters the barrel. Air injected into a rubber-capped vial raises the air pressure in the vial, which forces the solution through the needle into the syringe.

In giving a hypodermic injection, pressure against the plunger causes pressure against the solution, forcing it into the tissues. Pressure is greater in the tissues than in the capillaries, so the drug enters the circulatory system.

The tourniquet applied to the arm for intravenous injection obstructs the flow of blood; pressure of blood not able to escape pushes the elastic walls of the vein outward, making the vein more clearly visible.

To hold the syringe firm and steady with the fingers, friction is required. Water reduces friction so a syringe that is wet is much more difficult to hold.

Psychology. All procedures in which a needle is used as a means of injecting medicine or fluids may produce fear in the patient because the insertion of the needle causes pain.

The nurse should explain to the patient that the pain is only of very short duration. Children are especially fearful of needle injections and that psychological factor should be given careful attention by the nurse.

If the needle for injection is very sharp, the pain experienced by the patient will be lessened.

Sociology. The diabetic patient may need to administer his own insulin and will need to be instructed in the procedure and informed as to needed equipment.

The American Diabetic Association is an organization that can be helpful to the diabetic patient.

Hypodermic injections may be given in emergency situations at a doctor's office, clinic, or hospital, or at the place of the accident.

Patients should be informed as to where they may go for additional treatment. They may not be aware that the services of the Visiting Nurse Association are available to them.

The Harrison Drug Act controls the manufacture and sale of narcotics.

Situation Type Problem

1. A student nurse assigned to duty in the Pediatrics department was asked to give an intramuscular injection to a patient 4 years of age. The child seemed unusually fearful of her and began to cry when she attempted to explain the necessity for the hypodermic injection. When she attempted to turn him on his abdomen to expose the buttock, the youngster began to kick and scream. The mother came into the room and was very indignant because the nurse had "upset" the child.

The mother requested that another nurse on the department, a younger student, be asked to give the injection, since she seemed to be the only nurse with whom the patient would cooperate. What would you have done?

Suggested Reference Reading

"Needles, their care and sterilization," Lillian Ruth Roy; American Journal of Nursing, September, 1936.

"Hypodermic techniques that save time," Pauline S. Buechel; American Journal of Nursing, November, 1944.

"Narcotics in sterile solutions," Sister Henrietta; American Journal of Nursing, February, 1948.

"Care is important" (a pamphlet of instructions on care of needles and syringes); Becton, Dickinson, and Company, Rutherford, New Jersey, 1951.

"The technique of venipuncture and intravenous injection," Elliott V. Newman; American Journal of Nursing, April, 1952.

CHAPTER 34

Administration of Fluids

TOPICAL OUTLINE

KINDS OF BODY FLUIDS
SOURCES OF FLUID INTAKE
MEANS OF FLUID OUTPUT
FLUID BALANCE
MINIMUM FLUID REQUIREMENTS
REPLACEMENT OF BODY FLUIDS
- Gastric Gavage
- Rectal Feeding
- Proctoclysis
- Hypodermoclysis
- Intravenous Infusion
- Blood Transfusion

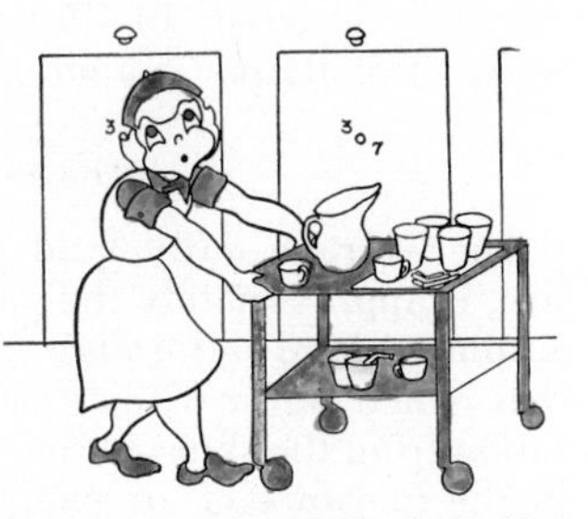

"When he ordered 'Push Fluids,' I thought he had the patient in mind. I didn't know he meant me!"

To help maintain fluid balance for a patient the nurse must know fluid requirements and principles underlying the metabolism of fluids.

An understanding of the important role played by water, normal saline, and glucose in the body enables the nurse to see that adequate fluid balance is maintained, that accurate records are made of fluid intake and output, and that symptoms of clinical significance are reported to the physician.

KINDS OF BODY FLUID

The fluids of the body can be classified into three main groups, according to the kind and amount of each fluid and the body space which each occupies.

Intracellular fluid—this fluid, approximately 35,000 cc. in amount, is the fluid found within cells that are separated from the rest of the body by cell membranes, such as muscle cells.

Interstitial fluid—about 10,000 cc. in amount, is the fluid between cells.

Blood—about 7,000 cc. in amount, is made up of red blood cells and plasma, each about 3,500 cc.

SOURCES OF FLUID INTAKE

The average daily fluid intake, for the normal adult of average size, is approximately 3000 cc. Liquid taken by mouth is the chief source of fluid intake, although fluid contained in solid food is another source. It is estimated that about every gram of solid food contains 0.9 cc. of fluid. During metabolism, when food is burned in the body, water of oxidation is freed. In the average diet the daily intake of potential water of oxidation is approximately 250 cc.

MEANS OF FLUID OUTPUT

The average daily fluid output, for the normal adult of average size, is approximately the same as intake, 3000 cc. About half the total output of fluid is through "insensible loss." Insensible loss of fluid is that which is lost without being noticed. It includes that lost by evaporation from the skin (in some instances visible perspiration occurs) and in the moisture of air exhaled from the lungs. The insensible loss of fluid (about 1500 cc. per day) remains fairly constant regardless of increased intake or decreased urinary output.

The output of urine (about 1500 cc. per day) is an important means of fluid output. The kidneys secrete urine which holds in solution the waste products of metabolism so they may be excreted from the body. To carry out this vital function, the urinary output must be maintained at a minimum of 600–700 cc. per day.

Fluid is lost from the body in lesser amounts through feces; 100–200 cc. per day may be lost in this manner.

Fluid may also be lost from the body through excessive perspiration, vomiting, diarrhea, or hemorrhage.

FLUID BALANCE

Fluid balance is disturbed when an unusual amount of fluid is lost, and the only means of restoring fluid balance is to replace the fluid that was lost.

If the fluid has been lost in the form of perspiration, it also contains a mixture of salts, and an attempt is made to restore the salts as well as the fluid which was lost.

If fluid is lost through long continued vomiting, other elements lost from the body, such as potassium and calcium, will need to be replaced.

When whole blood has been lost by hemorrhage, it may be necessary to replace it with blood taken from another person, or blood plasma may be a satisfactory means of replacing the fluid lost.

MINIMUM FLUID REQUIREMENTS

Water is essential for life; without it, dehydration and death will occur in a relatively short period of time. Water is needed by the body to replace the insensible loss of fluid through evaporation from the skin and exhalation of moisture-laden air from the lungs. Under normal conditions of temperature and humidity, the fluid lost may be 1000–1500 cc. per day. That amount is increased when the temperature of the body is increased or when the environmental temperature is high and the humidity is low.

Water is needed, too, so the kidneys can function normally in their work of excreting body wastes. Salt and protein intake bear a direct relationship to the amount of water that is needed. For secretion of 1000–1500 cc. of urine per day approximately that amount is required as fluid intake, in addition to the amount needed for replacing the insensible loss of fluid.

The minimum fluid requirement for the adult of average size is 2000–3000 cc. per day. There is little indication that patients should be encouraged or "forced" to drink larger quantities of water.

Under normal conditions the average adult needs at least 200 grams of glucose per day to supply the basic energy requirements of about 1600 calories.

The administration of 2000 cc. of 5 per cent glucose in saline affords approximately 100 grams of sugar or 800 calories of needed carbohydrate.

Salt intake of 1 gram per day is considered sufficient to maintain normal functioning of the various organs of the body. The kidney excretes about the same amount of salt as that taken into the body. When abnormal conditions exist and the kidney does not excrete the usual amount of salt, that retained in the body causes an accumulation of water in the tissues and eventually produces edema. Salt, in an amount of more than 2 or 3 grams per day, should be given only to patients who have lost salt through excessive perspiration, diarrhea, or vomiting.

At least 70 grams of protein should be included in the diet each day. Protein may be given by mouth or intravenously in the form of amino acid.

Special fluids may be given as a corrective measure for some abnormal condition, as sodium lactate for the correction of acidosis.

REPLACEMENT OF BODY FLUIDS

Normally, enough fluid is taken into the body by mouth to supply the body's needs. When fluids cannot be given orally, or when oral intake is inadequate or undesirable, other means of supplying fluids must be used, especially when fluid loss is increased.

The doctor will determine the method of replacing the fluid lost, depending on the condition of the patient and the purpose for which fluid is given. Methods usually used include: gastric gavage, rectal feeding, hypodermoclysis, intravenous infusion, and blood transfusion.

Gastric Gavage. Gavage is the process of feeding the patient by means of a tube passed into the stomach by way of the mouth or nose.

Food or fluid is usually supplied in this manner to adults unable to take nourishment by mouth and to premature babies who may be so weak they are unable to nurse. Conditions in which gavage may be indicated are unconsciousness, fracture of the jaw, cleft palate, delirium, and psychosis. Gavage may be necessary for premature infants and for patients who have had surgery of the mouth, lips, or throat.

A stomach tube or small catheter is used in giving gavage, the size of tube depending on whether the patient is an infant, child, or adult, and whether the tube is to be inserted through the mouth or the nose. A very small tube is easier to swallow and less irritating to the throat, but is more apt to become clogged with the fluid used for feeding. A tube with side opening just above the tip is preferable to one with end opening. A small funnel attached to the tube facilitates the pouring of the fluid or formula which is to be given.

The patient is usually placed in a sitting position, although the procedure may be done with the patient lying down. Children and delirious or psychotic patients will need to be restrained, and help will be needed for the treatment.

Passage of the Tube through the Mouth. The tube should be immersed in ice water for half an hour so it will be chilled and hardened and thus made easier for the patient to swallow.

Before beginning the procedure, dentures the patient may be wearing should be removed. The procedure should be explained to the patient, and he should be assured that it is not painful, and that discomfort he may experience in swallowing the tube will be temporary.

The patient's clothing and the bed linen should be protected with a rubber or plastic covering. Old newspapers may be used to protect the floor, as it is not unusual for swallowing of the tube to cause sudden emesis.

The doctor or nurse may insert the tube, holding it in an arched position slightly above the level of the patient's mouth so that the patient's head is lifted upward and the tube can enter the esophagus in a straight line. When the tube is introduced into the throat, it is necessary to avoid touching the posterior wall of the pharynx since to do so will cause the patient to gag.

As the tube is passed into the esophagus, the patient should be instructed to swallow constantly. A drink of water given at this time may help the patient to keep up continuous swallowing action.

The tube is marked to indicate when it has reached stomach or duodenum, and when the appropriate marking has reached the teeth the tube is in proper position.

The tube must be in the stomach and not in the trachea before fluid can be administered. If liquid is poured into the tube and allowed to enter the respiratory tract, asphyxiation of the patient may result. The same precautions must be observed as in passing the tube for gastric lavage, discussed in Chapter 29. During the treatment if coughing occurs or if the patient becomes cyanotic, the tube should be clamped tight and removed immediately.

The feeding should require about 10 minutes, as the fluid should be poured slowly into the funnel and allowed to flow slowly through the tubing. Care should be taken to see that the funnel remains partially filled at all times during the feeding so air will not enter the tube. The rate of flow of the feeding can be regulated by raising or lowering the funnel.

When the feeding has been completed, the tube should be clamped tightly and withdrawn from the esophagus and from the mouth. If the tube is securely clamped, no fluid will flow from it as it is being removed, and no fluid will pass into the trachea.

The patient should be instructed to remain in the same position for a short time and be quietly relaxed, to avoid the possibility of nausea and vomiting.

The amount and kind of fluid given by gavage is prescribed by the doctor. Usually the feeding is highly nutritious, since only small amounts can be given. Fluids usually given are milk, malted milk, peptonized milk, milk with cocoa, milk with eggs, beef juice, liver juice, fruit juice, and thin gruels or purées. Vitamins and additional carbohydrates in the form of glucose may be added to the regular feeding.

Temperature of the fluid should be about 105° F. The exact amount given the patient should be noted and recorded.

Feedings are calculated and planned on a 24-hour basis, and the total quantity divided into the desired number of feedings. The doctor will decide if feedings are to be given during the night, and will indicate the interval of time which should elapse between feedings.

Passage of the Tube through the Nose. For insertion through a nostril the tube should be smaller than that used for passage through the mouth. If there is difficulty in passing the tube through one nostril, the other may present a better passageway.

The same care must be taken to insure that the tube is in the stomach so that no fluid enters the respiratory tract. The temperature of the fluid, the amount, and the method of administration is the same as described for oral gavage.

Gavage for Infants. A number 14 or 16 French catheter is used for gavage for infants. The fluid is poured through a small funnel attached to the catheter. The baby should be wrapped securely in a blanket and placed on the treatment table.

The distance, measured just above the body surface, from the lips to the stomach should be determined and the catheter marked. (The distance should be approximately seven inches.) The end of the catheter should be moistened with warm water and passed over the tongue and down into the esophagus.

After the catheter is inserted the desired distance, the same tests

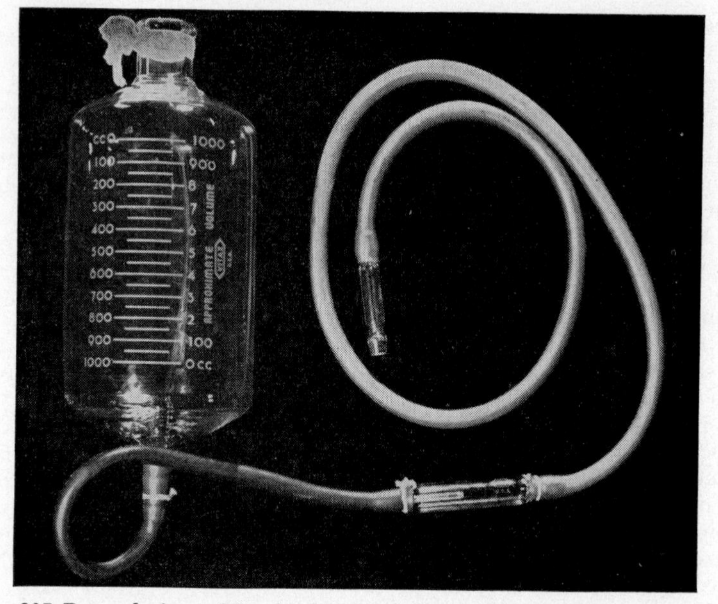

Fig. 207. Proctoclysis set (Murphy drip set). (Nursing Service Department, New England Center Hospital, Boston, Massachusetts.)

should be made as in the adult, to make sure the end of the catheter is in the stomach.

The fluid should be given slowly, and in the same manner as for the adult. The catheter is removed in the same manner, with care being taken to pinch the catheter tightly so no fluid will escape into the respiratory tract.

Rectal Feeding. Rectal feeding by means of the nutritive enema is of questionable value since little if any absorption takes place in the large intestine. The procedure has been discussed in detail in Chapter 18, on "Enemas and Other Rectal Treatments."

Proctoclysis, or the slow, continuous injection of a solution into the rectum, known also as the "Murphy drip," since it was first put into use by the famous Chicago surgeon, Dr. John B. Murphy, was also discussed in Chapter 18.

Hypodermoclysis. Hypodermoclysis, or the injection of a large quan-ity of fluid into subcutaneous tissue, supplies fluids in a relatively short time to replace those lost in hemorrhage, diarrhea, or other abnormal conditions in which fluids cannot or should not be given by mouth. The treatment may be used to dilute toxins in conditions of toxemia or septicemia, and to stimulate circulation in shock or collapse.

Hypodermoclysis is contraindicated in an edematous patient. Dangers of treatment include possible infection with abscess formation, puncture of a large blood vessel, and death and sloughing of tissue which may result from lack of absorption of the fluid given.

The solution most commonly used is normal saline solution, which is isotonic with the blood. The large number of solutions which may be given intravenously are not usually given by hypodermoclysis.

The equipment needed consists of the container with solution which has been made up and sterilized in the manufacturer's laboratories and is marketed ready for immediate use. A connecting length of tubing from the container to a glass Y-tube is equipped with a Murphy drip glass connector and clamp which can be adjusted to regulate the flow of solution. Two smaller pieces of tubing are connected to the Y-tube, each with a clamp attached. At the end of each smaller piece of tubing is a hypodermoclysis needle, which is introduced into muscle tissue at a 30 degree angle.

The solution should be warmed to 105–110° F. and should be kept at body temperature while being injected. This may be accomplished by placing the tubing through which the solution must flow between two hot water bottles.

The most common sites of injection for hypodermoclysis are the front of the thighs and the loose tissue below each breast. Other possible sites are the buttocks, below the axillae and beneath the skin of the abdomen midway between the navel and the anterior superior spine.

The articles and solution used in giving the treatment should be sterile, and the procedure should be done with aseptic technique.

The skin is prepared by being cleansed with an antiseptic solution. Air can be removed from the tubing and needles by allowing a small amount of solution to run through the tubing.

The needles are introduced into muscle tissue, and when the solution is flowing properly through both needles they may be fastened in place with strips of adhesive tape.

The rate of flow of the solution is regulated by the stopcock above the Murphy drip connector and can also be regulated by the clamp on each of the sections of smaller tubing attached to the arms of the glass Y-tube.

The procedure requires almost continuous attention on the part of the nurse, since the solution must be kept warm, the flow from each needle regulated so it is neither too slow nor too fast, and the patient must be watched for symptoms of discomfort.

Time required for 1000 cc. of solution to be given should be about 30 to 45 minutes. As much as 2000 cc. may be given at one time, depending on the doctor's orders.

Just before all the solution has left the flask or container the clamps should be tightened to stop the flow of solution and the needles should be quickly withdrawn. A small sterile dressing should be held over the site of injection as the needle is withdrawn and should be immediately secured in place with a strip of adhesive tape.

Within a few hours after the solution has been given it should be completely absorbed from the tissues without any ill effects resulting from the treatment.

Fluids are given much less frequently by hypodermoclysis than by intravenous infusion.

Intravenous Infusion. An intravenous infusion is the slow introduction of a large quantity of fluid into a vein.

The purposes of intravenous infusion and the reasons for its wide use in hospitals throughout the country include: more rapid absorption of the fluid; the means of giving a large quantity of fluid; the fact that fluids may be given continuously over a long period of time, and to give fluids when they can't be given orally or by other methods. Infusion also serves to increase blood volume following hemorrhage.

One advantage of intravenous infusion over other methods of giving fluids is that it is painless. Solutions which might be irritating when given by other methods are introduced directly into the blood stream so rapidly that no local pain is experienced by the patient. Infection and abscess formation are not apt to occur when fluids are given intravenously.

Solutions most commonly used for intravenous infusion include normal saline, glucose 5–10 per cent in normal saline, and glucose 5–10 per cent in distilled water. Drugs commonly added to the intravenous solution are vitamins, aminophyllin, amino acids, insulin, and various forms of the sulfa drugs.

The site of injection chosen for intravenous infusion is usually the median basilic vein on the inner surface of the arm, a vein on top of the foot, or, in an infant, the jugular vein.

Equipment needed for the treatment includes the container of solution, a disposable sterile recipient set, intravenous needles, and the arm board, adhesive tape, scrub tray, and a standard.

The procedure should be explained to the patient, and he should be placed in a comfortable, reclining position. Care must be taken that the correct solution is being used; if drugs are being administered at the same time, the labels must be carefully checked so no mistake will occur. The solution should be warmed to body temperature by placing the container in a basin of water at 120° F. for a reasonable length of time.

When the site of injection has been determined, the sleeve of the patient's gown should be removed from the arm (if the median basilic or cephalic vein has been chosen) and the arm should be fastened securely to an arm board. Slight movement by the patient will not dislodge the needle from its place within the vein and thus interfere with injection of the fluid if an arm board is used.

The metal identification disc on top of the container identifies the solution and, when removed at the time the solution is to be used, should be saved for use as a clamp on the plastic tubing.

The end of the plastic tubing is inserted into the free hole in the

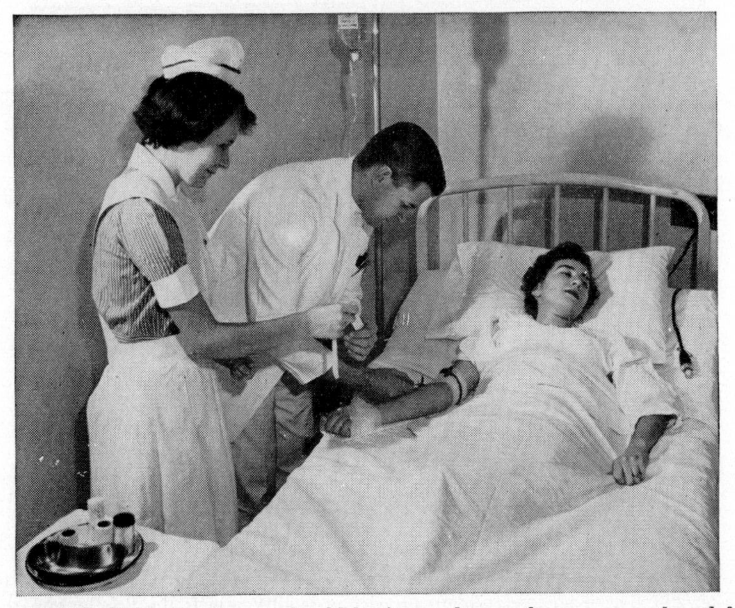

Fig. 208. The patient's arm should be fastened securely to an arm board for intravenous infusion. (Lenox Hill Hospital School of Nursing, New York, New York.)

rubber top of the container. The metal disc can be folded over the tubing as a clamp to regulate the flow of solution.

The solution container is then suspended on the standard, the rubber covering removed from the needle adapter at the end of the tubing, and the solution allowed to enter the tubing to where the metal disc is fastened.

The plastic drip connection should be half filled with solution. This can be accomplished by alternately pinching and releasing the tubing, in a milking action, between the connector and the metal disc. The remainder of the tubing should then be filled with solution so all air will be expelled.

The needle is then attached to the tubing and placed again inside the sterile needle holder (with tubing attached), which is taped to the standard until it is needed.

The patient's arm, fastened securely to the arm board, should be extended on the bed. A tourniquet is applied well above the elbow and the patient instructed to open and close his hand several times.

The site of injection should be cleansed with alcohol, the arm properly draped, and the needle inserted into the vein. If blood is drawn into the glass adapter, the needle is in the vein, and the tourniquet can be released.

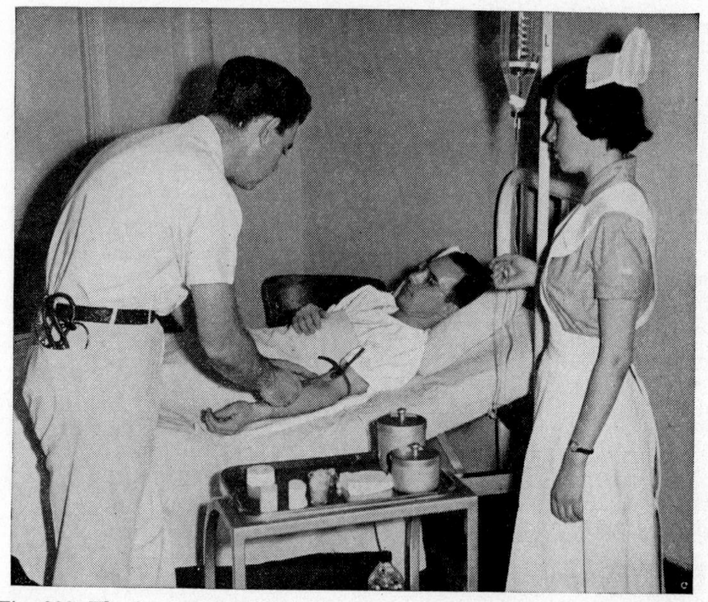

Fig. 209. The intern or resident physician usually inserts the needle into the vein for an intravenous infusion. (Kansas City General Hospital School of Nursing, Kansas City, Missouri.)

The rate of flow of the solution can be regulated by gradually unbending the metal disc until it lets the desired amount of solution through the tubing.

An intravenous infusion of 1000 cc. of solution should require 1–2 hours for administration. Infusions containing amino acids (protein) may require 2–4 hours. After the solution has been given, the tube should be clamped off and the needle should be removed from the arm. A sterile dressing, applied with pressure, should be placed over the site of injection to prevent bleeding from the vein.

If the patient complains of pain at the site of injection or shows symptoms indicating an unfavorable reaction to treatment, a report should be made to the doctor at once. Symptoms of an undesirable reaction might include increased pulse rate, dyspnea, chilliness, increased body temperature, and pain in the cardiac region.

BLOOD TRANSFUSION

In hospitals throughout the country the giving of blood and plasma transfusions has become part of daily routine, with blood transfusion becoming a relatively safe and minor procedure. The therapeutic value of whole blood has long been known to medicine, and when

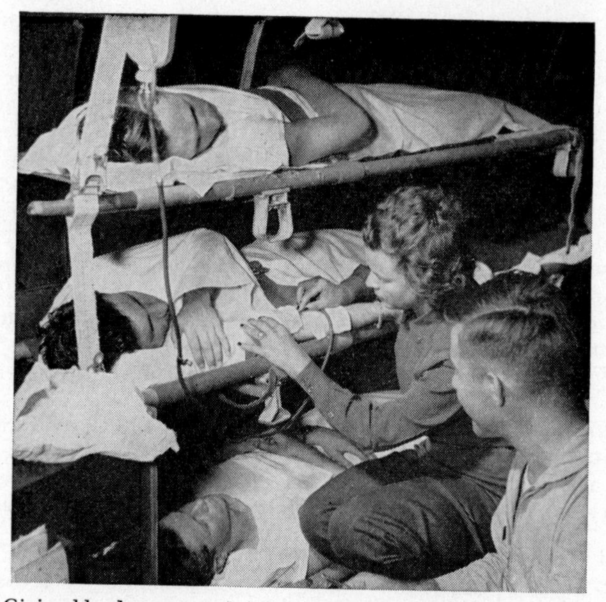

Fig. 210. Giving blood to a wounded G.I. as he is being evacuated by air. (Bureau of Medicine and Surgery, Navy Department, Washington, D.C.)

blood is needed there is no real substitute for it. Whole blood is now used in about 90 per cent of all transfusions. When whole blood is given, grouping and cross-matching are required to prevent serious or fatal reactions. Errors made in performing these tests may have fatal consequences for the patient, so extreme care must be used in all laboratory tests or procedures pertaining to blood.

Blood. Blood is the nutritive fluid of the body which circulates through heart, arteries, capillaries, and veins. It carries food and oxygen to the tissues and carries away carbon dioxide and other waste products.

Blood is made up of about 78 per cent water and 22 per cent solids. The fluid part of blood is termed plasma. The blood cells, suspended in the plasma, include red corpuscles, white corpuscles, and platelets. Blood serum is the liquid portion of blood with the clotting substances removed.

The adult person of average size has a total blood volume of approximately 5.5 liters. Blood has a specific gravity of 1.055–1.062. In circulating through the vascular system, it makes the complete circuit in about twenty seconds. Arterial blood is bright red in color and venous blood is dark red.

Blood to be used in transfusion may be classified as *fresh*, *stored*, or *preserved*. Fresh blood is kept in liquid form by the addition of sodium citrate, which is an anticoagulant. In this form the blood should be given to the recipient very soon after it has been withdrawn and, if not used immediately, it should be kept in the refrigerator. Stored blood contains sodium citrate, should be kept in the refrigerator, and should be used within five days after its withdrawal. Preserved blood contains sodium citrate and dextrose, which helps to prolong the survival time of the red cells. Preserved blood is refrigerated and can be used for transfusion with satisfactory results any time within 21 days.

Blood Grouping. The blood of all human beings may be classified into one of four groups, O, A, B, or AB, based on the phenomenon of agglutination. If the red cells of blood of one group clump together when mixed with the serum of blood of a different group agglutination has occurred.

Agglutinogen is a substance which, acting as an antigen, stimulates the production of agglutinins.

Agglutinin is a sensitizing antibody, which causes agglutination or clumping of red blood cells in a suspension.

The action of agglutinogen in red cells and agglutinin in serum for the various blood groups may be explained by the table below:

Blood Group	Agglutinogen in red cells	Agglutinin in serum	May give blood to	May receive blood from
O	O	ab	all	O
A	A	b	A and AB	O and A
B	B	a	B and AB	O and B
AB	AB	o	AB	all

In blood transfusion the donor should be from the same blood group as the patient. In an emergency when a donor of the same group may not be available another group may be chosen providing the serum from the patient's blood will not agglutinate cells in the blood of the donor. Because of the above characteristics a person with blood of group O is spoken of as a universal donor (may give blood to all other groups), and one with group AB blood is termed a universal recipient (may receive blood from all other groups). Generally speaking, however, only blood of the same group as that of the patient should be given in transfusion.

Blood Typing. In selecting a donor the patient's blood should be typed and a donor chosen on the basis of the blood type of the patient. Cross matching should be done, and the Rh factor should be known for both donor and recipient.

Rh Factor. When, in experimental laboratories, red cells of the Rhesus monkey were injected into rabbits, it was found the serum of the rabbits caused agglutination of red cells in a high percentage (85%) of humans, regardless of their blood groups. This agglutinin became known (by the first two letters of the word Rhesus) as the Rh factor. When the Rh factor is present in red blood cells, the person is said to be Rh positive. When the red cells lack the Rh factor the person is termed Rh negative.

The Rh factor is important in pregnancy. If the father should be Rh positive and the mother Rh negative, the mother's blood may develop anti-Rh agglutinins and cause abortion or a stillbirth, or the infant may have erythroblastosis fetalis, a condition marked by an excess of rudimentary cells in the blood. The anti-Rh agglutinins may also occur as the result of transfusion of Rh-positive blood given to an Rh negative recipient. For this reason the Rh type of both donor and recipient should be determined, and only blood of the same type should be used in blood transfusion.

Purpose of Blood Transfusion. Whole blood transfusions are used chiefly to combat shock (operative, traumatic, or hemorrhagic) and to overcome acute and chronic anemia. It is now a common procedure to give whole blood in the operating room during an operation to replace blood, volume for volume, as it is lost. Such transfusion helps to prevent shock and to maintain normal blood pressure.

Whole blood is also given as part of the early treatment of severe burns, to prevent anemia which may occur about the third day after the burn. The transfusion helps to reduce toxicity and to increase resistance to infection which may be a complication of the burn.

Technique of Transfusion. Blood transfusion may be given by the "indirect" method. The blood is withdrawn from the donor, stored or preserved by special techniques, then administered to the recipient in the same manner as that described for intravenous infusion. The usual amount given at one time is 500 cc., although the amount may vary, depending on the condition of the patient and the need for blood. In most hospitals blood is collected and stored for several days or weeks in the "blood bank." The bank functions by an exchange system which makes blood of any desired group available as it is needed. Friends or relatives of the recipient may donate blood to replace that used from the bank.

Although the method of giving blood has been simplified and the procedure is a matter of routine, there is still an element of risk for the patient. To eliminate as much as possible the dangers involved in the treatment, the following precautions should be observed.

All equipment and supplies used should be sterile and the procedure should be performed with strict, aseptic technique.

The donor should be a person in good health and should have fasted for several hours before giving blood. (This last precaution prevents a possible allergic reaction on the part of the patient to food that might have been eaten by the donor.) He should have a negative Wassermann at the time of giving blood and should be free of malaria.

Cross-matching of the donor's cells with serum from the patient who will receive the blood is needed to insure compatibility of the blood.

The rate at which blood is given should be carefully regulated. The usual transfusion of 500 cc. of blood requires about 2 to 3 hours for administration. Blood is sometimes introduced very slowly and for a long period of time.

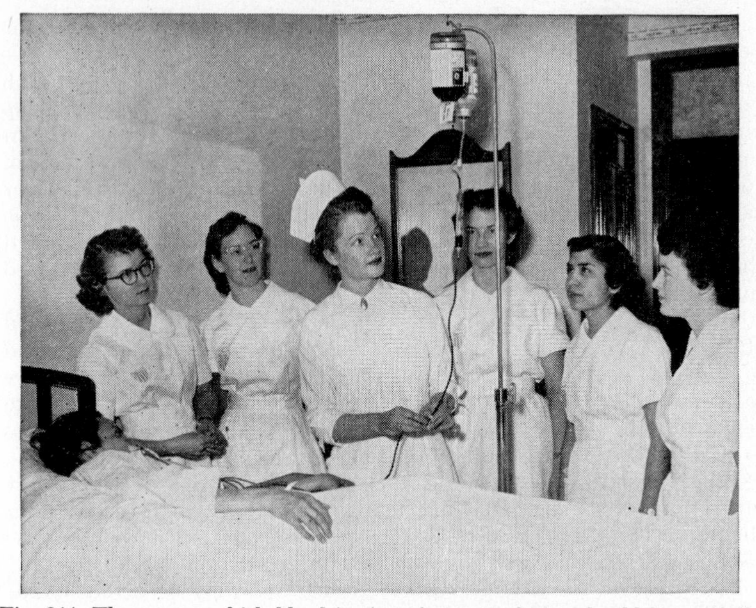

Fig. 211. The rate at which blood is given in a transfusion should be carefully regulated. (Mercy Hospital School of Nursing, Denver, Colorado.)

The Rh factor should be known for both donor and recipient.

If the blood has been refrigerated, it should have been kept at a temperature of 39.2° F. The blood should not be heated before being used for transfusion; if it has been kept in the refrigerator, it should be allowed to remain at room temperature for an hour or more before being administered to the patient.

During the transfusion the patient should be watched carefully for symptoms of reaction. The doctor or technician who starts the transfusion should remain with the patient for a short time until assured that no untoward reaction is likely to occur. The temperature of the patient should be taken before transfusion as a basis for comparison should the temperature rise after the treatment.

Reactions and Complications. Although the administration of blood is now considered relatively safe, it can sometimes be a dangerous form of therapy. All nurses who assist with a transfusion should be aware of the possible reactions and complications and of the serious consequences they may have.

Pyrogenic Reaction. The most frequent reaction is the pyrogenic reaction, characterized by fever, or by chills and fever which may occur during or immediately after the transfusion.

This reaction is caused by substances produced by bacteria or dried plasma proteins called pyrogens which may have been present because of inadequate or improper cleansing of equipment or preparation of solution. The reaction is not serious except for the patient who may be critically ill.

Hemolytic Reaction. The hemolytic reaction is perhaps the most feared reaction and is serious in nature. It is caused by incompatibility between the red cells of the donor and the serum of the recipient, or by the red cells of the recipient being hemolyzed by serum of the donor. The basic cause of the hemolytic reaction is the presence of free hemoglobin in the circulating blood stream. If a large amount of free hemoglobin is present, the kidneys are damaged and death may ensue because of renal failure. The chief symptoms are chills and fever, and pain in the lumbar region and in the loins. The patient may complain of a sensation of constriction in the chest and may have the appearance of extreme prostration. If the patient recovers from the acute and immediate reaction he may become icteric in appearance. Oliguria and anuria may develop, with death occurring in 5 to 12 days.

Because the early symptoms of this serious reaction, chills and fever, are the same as symptoms of the mild form of reaction, their appearance should not be taken lightly. Since there is danger of the serious reaction, transfusion must be stopped immediately if chills and fever occur.

The number of hemolytic reactions to blood transfusion has been reduced by the discovery of the Rh factor and of substances used to neutralize the agglutinins in universal donor blood.

Proteolytic Reaction. Proteolytic reaction is allergic in nature and usually characterized by urticaria. It can be controlled and relieved by appropriate use of antihistaminic or adrenergic drugs.

Circulatory Overload. Circulatory overload is caused by an excessive increase in blood volume. It may result from giving blood too fast or giving too much blood. The condition is characterized by dyspnea, cyanosis, orthopnea, gurgling sounds, and the coughing up of red, frothy liquid. The left side of the heart becomes dilated, with subsequent heart failure, followed in rapid sequence by pulmonary congestion and edema.

Phlebotomy may be necessary and other means of treatment include oxygen, morphine, and intravenous administration of aminophylline. Death may occur within a short time. The reaction can be prevented by correct regulation of rate of flow and the amount of blood administered.

Air Embolism. Air embolism, which may have serious consequences, can be prevented by eliminating all air from the tubing before the flow of blood is started.

Transmission of Disease. Transmission of disease by blood transfusion is uncommon, although syphilis and malaria have been transmitted in this way.

Giving of Contaminated Blood. Careful checking of blood supply and of refrigeration of the blood will eliminate the possible complication of administering contaminated blood.

Phlebotomy. Phlebotomy is the withdrawal of blood from a vein, done usually to obtain blood for use in transfusion. On rare occasions it may be done to decrease blood volume as a means of treating hypertension, congestive heart failure, or polycythemia.

The nurse assembles the necessary equipment and assists the doctor in the procedure. Novocain may be used before the procedure is started to lessen pain caused by introduction of the needle into the vein. The tourniquet should be applied and skin cleansed at the site of puncture, as for an intravenous infusion.

The bottle in which the blood is collected contains sodium citrate and should be gently rotated so that the blood mixes readily with the anticoagulant solution and clotting is prevented.

The patient may be instructed to alternately open and close his fist to aid in the withdrawal of the blood.

When the desired amount of blood has been obtained, the tourniquet is released and the needle withdrawn. A sterile sponge applied with pressure at the site of puncture will stop bleeding from the vein.

Care of the Donor. The after-care of the donor of blood is the responsibility of the nurse.

A small sterile dressing should be applied to the arm to keep the site of puncture clean and protected for a short time after the procedure.

The donor should be given a nourishing drink, such as eggnog or orange juice, to partially replace the fluid lost. He should be instructed to remain in the dorsal recumbent position for 15 to 20 minutes.

Before being permitted to leave, he should have his pulse rate checked, his color should be natural, and he should be questioned as to vertigo or a feeling of faintness. Any indication that he is not completely recovered from the weakening effect of the loss of blood should be sufficient reason for requiring him to remain under close observation.

Professional donors or persons who have blood withdrawn frequently for transfusion purposes are restricted as to the amount that can be given and the frequency of donation. A second withdrawal should not be made until the blood volume and its constituents have returned to normal. Too frequent withdrawals of blood may result in harmful effects to the health of the donor.

Care of Equipment after Use

FOR GASTRIC GAVAGE AND RECTAL FEEDING

Catheter or rectal tube should be rinsed with cold water, washed with warm water and soap, boiled for five minutes, rinsed in cold water, dried, and returned to storage place.

Small pitchers, funnels, and other articles used should be washed in soap and water, rinsed, dried, and returned to central supply to be used in making up another tray.

FOR HYPODERMOCLYSIS, INTRAVENOUS INFUSION, AND BLOOD TRANSFUSION

Tubing should be rinsed with clear, cold water. (If disposable pack has been used, tubing may be discarded.) Tubing should be washed, rinsed, and hung to dry.

Needles should be rinsed with cold water immediately after removal from the site of insertion, cleansed, and sterilized. To thoroughly clean needles, a detergent solution should be forced through them. All traces of blood must be removed. Incomplete cleaning of the needle may cause a pyrogenic reaction in the next patient.

Equipment used to set up trays (bottles, tubing clamps, etc.) should be thoroughly cleaned, then set up for use again. Trays should be wrapped securely and autoclaved.

All hypodermic syringes should be separated, washed with a detergent, and allowed to dry thoroughly before being autoclaved.

Summary of Important Factors

Fluids of the body are intracellular fluids, interstitial fluids, and blood.

Sources of fluid intake—water by mouth, food.

Means of fluid output—urine, perspiration, feces; abnormal loss may occur through vomiting, diarrhea, hemorrhage.

Minimum fluid requirement—average adult, per day, 2000–3000 cc.

Fluid loss—average adult, per day, about same as intake.

Body fluids replaced by gavage, rectal feeding, hypodermoclysis, intravenous infusion, and blood transfusion.

In gavage, tube must be in stomach before giving fluids.

Because the lower colon does not absorb fluids readily, proctoclysis is no longer an efficient means of replacing body fluids.

In conditions of edema, the use of hypodermoclysis is contraindicated.

Intravenous infusion is used to increase blood volume, to give large quantity of fluid, to give fluids over a long period of time when they cannot be given by other methods, and for rapid absorption.

The median basilic vein is usually chosen as the site of injection in intravenous therapy.

Proper identification of patient and of drugs being given is essential to avoid mistakes.

The rate of flow of solution should not be more than 60 drops per minute.

Blood transfusion is still a dangerous procedure for the patient.

When whole blood is given, blood grouping and cross-matching are required.

Stored blood should not be used after 5 days. Preserved blood should not be used after 21 days.

The four blood groups are O, A, B, AB. Group O is the universal donor group. Group AB is the universal recipient group.

The Rh factor should be known in pregnancy and for blood transfusion.

Whole blood transfusion is needed to combat shock and anemia.

Reactions and complications in blood transfusion include pyrogenic reaction, hemolytic reaction, proteolytic reaction, circulatory overload, air embolism, transmission of disease, and the giving of contaminated blood.

Factors To Teach the Patient

The importance of drinking water and other fluids in sufficient amount to supply body needs.

The fact that salt water, as such, cannot be used by the body so is not effectual in quenching thirst.

Explanation of all procedures used as means of replacing body fluids. The patient is much more cooperative when he understands the purpose of a procedure.

In swallowing the tube for gavage, a drink of water may be helpful.

To remain in recumbent position for a short time after gavage so feeding will not be vomited.

Rectal feedings or proctoclysis are meant to be retained.

That "swelling" caused by hypodermoclysis is not in any way injurious to the tissues when the administration of the fluid given in this manner is controlled properly.

That only slight pain is experienced when the needle is inserted into the vein for intravenous therapy.

That for long continued procedures, as for intravenous, some movement is permitted, care being taken not to dislodge the needle from the vein.

The benefits to be derived from a treatment being given.

In event of undesirable reaction or complication, reassurance that no serious consequences need result.

The need for donors so that blood used from the bank can be replaced.

The value of rest and nourishment for the donor immediately after blood has been withdrawn

The need to restrict the number of times blood can be withdrawn as a means of safeguarding the health of the donor.

Scientific Principles

Anatomy and Physiology. Equipment used in intravenous therapy must be clean, free from foreign matter, and sterile to prevent the formation of an embolus, a clot floating free in the blood stream, or a thrombus, a clot adhering to the wall of the blood vessel. The thrombus may partially close the blood vessel or close it entirely, causing necrosis of the surrounding tissues. Emboli may be carried into a small blood vessel or into the valves of the heart, causing sudden death.

Fluids can be given intravenously at the rate of 30–60 drops per minute. More rapid administration may cause an unfavorable reaction.

Infusion solutions tend to increase pulse rate, relieve thirst, and increase the output of urine.

Glucose given intravenously can be rapidly absorbed by body cells and serves as nourishment to the cell, thus tending to relieve hunger.

Chemistry. Because the molecules of glucose are smaller than those of other sugars, allowing them to pass through the walls of cells readily and to be rapidly absorbed, glucose is used for intravenous infusions.

Fluids of different concentrations separated by a semipermeable membrane tend to equalize their concentrations by osmosis and dialysis. The direction of passage through the membrane is from the fluid of lesser concentration to that of greater concentration. Hypotonic solutions are of lesser concentration than blood and if used intravenously will destroy the cells of the blood by hemolysis. Hypertonic solutions are of greater concentration than blood and may draw out the cell substance, causing plasmolysis. Isotonic solutions are of the same concentration as blood.

Microbiology. The skin protects the body from bacteria, although the skin itself may not be free of bacteria. Intravenous therapy requires that the skin be disinfected at the site of injection and that needles used in penetrating the skin be sterile.

Hemolysis is destruction of the red blood cells with liberation of hemoglobin. This part of the red cell which carries oxygen to the tissues cannot be re-united with other red cell constituents once it has been separated from them. Hypotonic solutions, water, certain drugs, and snake venom are hemolytic agents.

Water used in making solutions for intravenous infusion is freshly distilled and sterilized.

Pharmacology. Fluids commonly given to replace or supply body fluids are saline solution, glucose solution, whole blood, and plasma.

Transfusions of blood and plasma are given to increase the volume of blood. Whole blood is used when it is desirable to increase the number of red blood cells.

Physics. The tourniquet is applied in intravenous therapy to cut off the return of venous blood. Not being allowed to escape from the arm, the blood pushes outward on the elastic walls of the blood vessel and thus distends the vein, which is then more clearly outlined to view.

Collecting blood from the donor into a vacuum bottle depends on differences in pressure. Pressure within the bottle is lowered when air is removed from the bottle. When the bottle is connected to the vein of the donor, the blood runs into the collecting bottle because there is greater pressure in the veins.

Psychology. Before beginning the procedures of intravenous infusion or blood transfusion, the patient should be given opportunity to use urinal or bedpan and should be placed in a comfortable position. He should understand that the procedure may be of rather long duration but that danger is minimized by careful laboratory tests, by aseptic technique, and by the watchfulness of the nurse. He should be informed that there is only slight pain connected with the penetration of the needle into the vein. The nurse should divert the patient's thoughts from the procedure and should relieve apprehension as to the effect of the treatment.

Sociology. The exchange system on which banks function makes it necessary that donors be procured when needed. Friends and relatives of patients usually respond when asked to give blood to replace that used from the blood bank. Planning and organization are required to maintain a sufficient quantity of all types of blood in the bank. The Red Cross and similar organizations help by appealing to the public for donors when the need becomes imperative.

Situation Type Problem

1. The resident doctor on the surgical department in a hospital had a difficult time getting a needle into the median basilic vein to give intravenous solution to a patient. After several attempts to insert the needle, he finally succeeded in getting it into the vein. He remarked to the student nurse assisting him that starting an intravenous for this particular patient was very difficult because the patient was undernourished and dehydrated and the veins were hardly perceptible. He ordered the nurse to stay with the patient because he seemed very restless and might inadvertently cause the needle to penetrate the wall of the vein.

Soon after the doctor left, the head nurse came into the room and asked the student to give a hypodermic injection to a patient in the adjoining room. The student explained that the doctor had ordered her to remain with the patient getting intravenous fluids. The head nurse said *she* would remain with the patient while the student gave the hypodermic medication to the other patient.

The student left the room, prepared and administered the hypodermic injection for the other patient, then returned to the patient being given intravenous fluids. The head nurse was not in the room, the patient had turned to a different position and, despite the arm board and other precautions that had been taken to keep the needle in place, it had penetrated the wall of the vein and the solution was entering the tissues of the arm. A large amount of solution had already entered the tissues and caused a marked swelling of the involved area.

The student withdrew the needle from the patient's arm and as she did so the resident doctor appeared. He noted what had happened and was criticizing the student for having left the patient when the head nurse returned to the room. The doctor reported to the head nurse that he had given specific orders for the student to stay with the patient. The head nurse assured him that the student's negligence would be reported at the nursing office and that if he wished to start the intravenous again *she* would remain with the patient herself to make sure that he received proper attention. What would you have done?

Suggested References Reading

"Fluid balance from the nurse's point of view," Robert Elman; American Journal of Nursing, April, 1949.

"Legal use of blood typing," Beatrice Goldsmith; American Journal of Nursing, November, 1949.

"Clinical use of blood and blood derivatives," Charles K. Kirby; American Journal of Nursing, February, 1950.

"Nasal gavage," Students at Teachers College, Columbia University; American Journal of Nursing, January, 1951.

"Blood transfusions for geriatric patients," Victor Ginsberg; Journal of American Medical Association, December, 1951.

"Newer methods of blood collection," Karl W. Walter; Hospital Management, June, 1952.

"Whole blood preservation," Robert B. Pennell; Hospital Management, July, 1952.

"Technique of venipuncture," Madge L. Crouch; Nursing World, August, 1952.

"Taking food and fluids through a tube," Bertha I. Taylor; American Journal of Nursing, March, 1953.

CHAPTER 35

Inhalation Therapy

TOPICAL OUTLINE

STEAM INHALATIONS
OXYGEN THERAPY
    Concentration of Oxygen
    Requirements for Administration of Oxygen
    The Oxygen Regulator
    Methods of Administration of Oxygen
CARBON DIOXIDE THERAPY
AEROSOL THERAPY
THE MECHANICAL RESPIRATOR

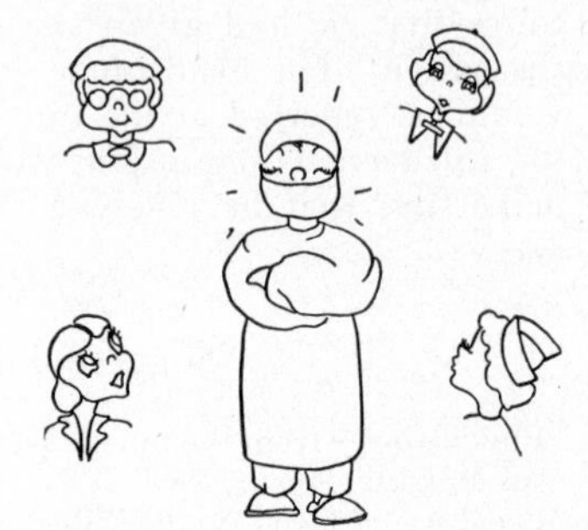

Flattery won't hurt a man, so long as he doesn't inhale!

Inhalation is defined as the drawing of air or other vapor into the lungs. An *inhalant* is a medicine or substance which may be breathed or inspired into the lungs. An *inhalator* is an apparatus used for administering gas or vapor into the respiratory tract as a means of treating disease.

When medication is administered by inhalation, it is for the purpose of giving volatile substances or gaseous drugs to the patient. Those most frequently used are anesthetic drugs, such as ether and nitrous oxide, drugs used for relief of inflammation in the upper respiratory tract, as tincture of benzoin, thymol, creosote, oil of pine, oil of peppermint, eucalyptus, and menthol, or antibiotics, such as penicillin.

Drugs given by inhalation for local effect are usually mixed with steam and administered as a moist inhalation. An electric steam inhalator, a croup kettle, or an improvised inhalator made of a teakettle with a paper cone fitted over the spout may be used. Medicated steam inhalations are used in treatment of respiratory infections to relieve inflammation and congestion of the mucous membrane, to relieve persistent coughing by loosening secretions and promoting productive coughing, and to relieve dyspnea and lessen irritation by warming and moistening the air. Although rarely used, the fumes from stramonium leaves may be inhaled through a cone held over the burning leaves, or they may be made into cigarettes and smoked by the patient for treatment of asthma.

Drugs given by inhalation for general effect act very quickly, due to the large surface of the lungs where absorption takes place. Drugs most frequently used are ammonia, which acts as a stimulant to overcome fainting; amyl nitrite, which is inhaled from the crushed pearl to relieve angina pectoris. In general drugs given as palliative treatment for respiratory conditions are administered parenterally rather than by inhalation. Oxygen, helium, and carbon dioxide gases are administered by inhalation for their general or systemic effect.

STEAM INHALATIONS

Steam inhalations are given for their local effect in relieving symptoms of upper respiratory infection and as a part of treatment after surgery involving the larynx, trachea, and bronchi.

Best results are obtained when humidity is maintained in the room at approximately 70 per cent. Most hospitals now use electric inhalators, although the footstool, hot plate, and teakettle with a paper cone made of newspaper may still be used effectively if care is observed in preventing the teakettle from boiling dry.

The Steam Inhalator. The electric inhalator provides for addition of the desired drug in the attached receptacle. The large glass bottle is filled with water and inverted into position in the apparatus. The inhalator is then attached to an electric socket at the patient's bedside. The switch should be turned to high until steam is produced from the extended spout, which is then placed in position near the patient's face. The patient should be in a comfortable position and the moisture from the inhalator should surround his head so that he breathes the medicated vapor. During inhalation treatment windows to the room should be closed. When the humidity has reached approximately 70 per cent, the switch may be turned to medium or low, to maintain the desired degree of moisture.

Length of treatment will depend on the purpose for which it is given, the condition of the patient, and the wishes of the physician. Inhalations are usually given for 15–20 minutes, every 3 or 4 hours. Care must be taken to prevent the patient from being burned and to make sure he is kept warm to prevent chilling.

If steam inhalations are being given to an infant or child, the spout of the inhalator must be placed so that the patient cannot touch it with his hands or put his face in direct contact with the steam.

The Croup Tent. For patients who must have inhalations continued for a long period of time, and for children, the croup tent is sometimes used.

A canopy is made from woolen blankets fastened at the top across two tall screens, for the adult patient, and stretched across the top of

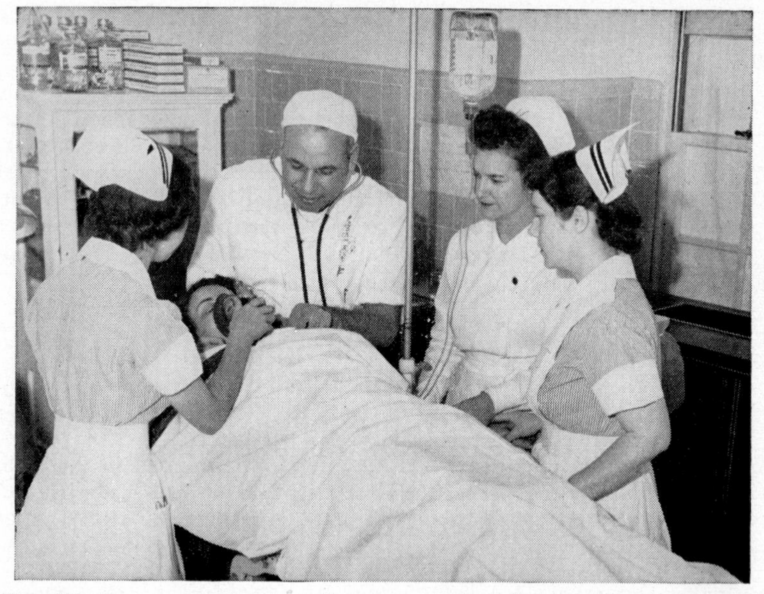

Fig. 212. Oxygen is given to relieve anoxemia. (Mississippi Baptist Hospital School of Nursing, Jackson, Mississippi.)

the crib, for a child. The blankets hang freely at the sides and form a tent across the upper third of the bed so that it is open only across the front. The outside may be covered with sheets to enhance the appearance. Wool blankets are used because wool material will absorb a great deal of moisture without danger of water dripping from the canopy. Steam should never be directed toward the patient, and, in the case of a child, the inhalator should be placed so that it is out of reach.

The Steam Room. In some pediatric hospitals, steam rooms are provided for the treatment of children with respiratory infections. The room is continuously filled with medicated steam from a vaporizing apparatus. Nursing care is simplified since several cribs can be placed in the room at one time. The children enjoy freedom of movement which is not possible when they are confined in a croup tent. Without the hindering tent canopies nursing procedures can be done in less time and with more efficiency.

Improvised Inhalation Apparatus for Use in the Home. If the patient being cared for at home requires steam inhalations, a canopy can be made by placing floor lamp stands, hall trees, or other tall objects beside the bed and covering them with woolen blankets, enclosing all but the front of the area.

Inhalators can be purchased for home use but can also be improvised. A boiling teakettle with a paper cone of heavy wrapping paper placed over the spout, a piece of rubber tubing, or a cardboard mailing tube will also serve.

If a drug is used for the inhalation, it should be contained in a cotton pledget which can be fastened inside the cone or tube, so that steam passes through it to release the desired medicated vapor.

OXYGEN THERAPY

Oxygen is administered by inhalation to relieve *anoxemia* (a deficiency of oxygen in the blood) and *anoxia* (a condition in which body cells and tissues obtain insufficient oxygen to carry on normal functioning). Oxygen inhalations are needed to supply oxygen in treating such diseases as congestive heart failure, coronary thrombosis, pneumonia, atelectasis, emphysema, and other conditions that interfere with normal breathing and normal oxygenation of the blood. Carbon monoxide poisoning also causes anoxia; when the body fails to get sufficient oxygen to supply its needs, cyanosis and dyspnea occur as characteristic symptoms.

Air normally contains approximately 20 per cent oxygen, which is absorbed through the lungs and united with the hemoglobin of red blood cells. Oxygen, to be effective when anoxia exists, must be given in concentrations of 40–50 per cent or even higher. Oxygen is not a stimulant and, when given in higher concentrations, will have no effect on the normal person. Its administration serves only to restore normal oxygen concentration in the blood, thus relieving anoxemia.

The nurse should understand the significance of oxygen therapy in the treatment of patients displaying marked cyanosis and dyspnea in order to evaluate the effect of oxygen administration. Soon after oxygen treatment is instituted, the patient's temperature may suddenly drop 2–4 degrees, with an almost equally sudden decrease in general clinical symptoms. The patient's color may immediately improve and the former lethargic or stuporous condition give way to alert awareness of his surroundings and the activity going on about him.

Oxygen itself does not burn, but it supports combustion. A tiny flame, in the presence of oxygen, will burst into a huge fire, enveloping a large surrounding area. Because of this, the patient must not have matches or smoke while oxygen is kept in the room. The electric signal cord should be replaced with a hand bell, to eliminate danger of fire from the electric circuit. To prevent possible combustion from oil or alcohol, such substances should not be used in providing general care to the patient. The backrub should be given with lotion or with powder. Oil or grease should never be applied to the regulator or to any part of the oxygen equipment; the large size, 244–cubic foot oxygen cylinder, frequently used, should not be stored near oil, grease, or other flammable material. Oxygen cylinders should not be

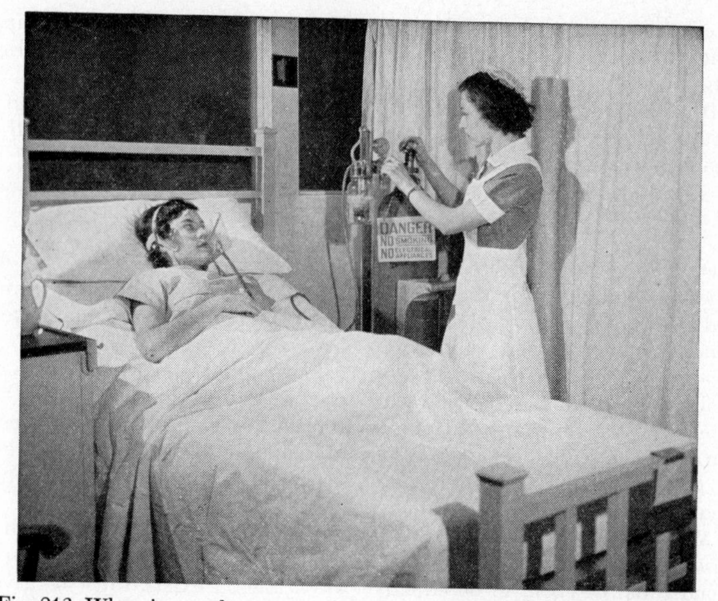

Fig. 213. When in use the oxygen cylinder should stand upright and be firmly anchored to a substantial support. (Massachusetts General Hospital School of Nursing, Boston, Massachusetts.)

stored near boilers, furnaces, radiators, steam pipes, autoclaves, and other heating devices, because heat from such equipment may cause an excessive rise in pressure of the oxygen in the cylinder. Most cylinders are equipped with safety disks, so the rise in pressure could not cause an explosion, but it could and does result in loss of oxygen from the cylinder. Full cylinders of oxygen should be stored apart from empty cylinders, and as a cylinder is emptied it should be marked "empty" and returned to the distributing station.

When in use, the oxygen cylinder should stand in an upight position and should be securely fastened to a substantial support. If a cylinder is knocked over accidentally, there is danger of injury to persons in the room and there is probability of damage to the equipment which may necessitate costly repair or replacement.

The large cylinder contains approximately 2,200 pounds or 6,900 liters of oxygen, and when regulated to the usual rate of flow (6 liters per minute) will provide oxygen for the patient for a 19-hour period. The amount of oxygen contained in the cylinder and the rate of flow to which it is regulated will determine the length of time the cylinder will provide oxygen.

Concentration of Oxygen. As the effectiveness of oxygen administration is largely determined by the per cent of concentration, the

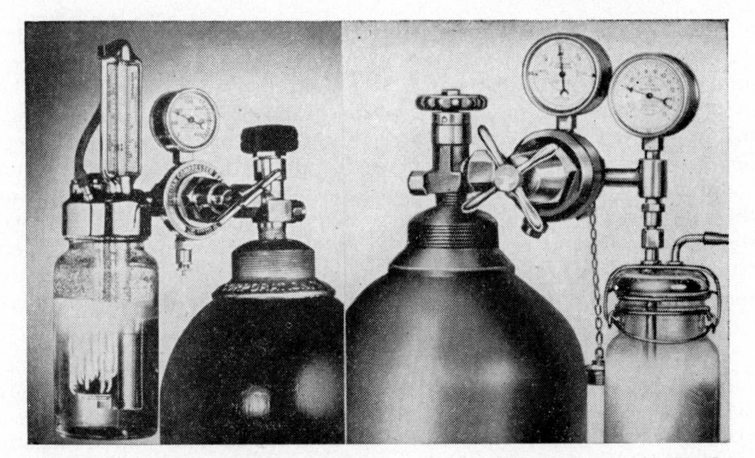

Fig. 214. The oxygen regulator and the oxygen humidifier. (Linde Air Products Co., New York, New York.)

oxygen concentration must be sufficiently high to benefit the patient. To supplement the 20 per cent contained in air, a higher concentration (40–60 per cent) is required. An oxygen analyzer is necessary to determine the concentration of oxygen administered by tent or in the oxygen chamber. Tests should be made regularly about every four hours to maintain the desired concentration and to determine if oxygen is being wasted. Most analyzers are simple to understand and operate, so periodic checking of the oxygen concentration in the tent or in oxygen rooms may be readily accomplished.

A known quantity (10 cc.) of the atmosphere to be tested is injected into a pipette, where it is measured as to volume. All the oxygen will be absorbed from the test sample then the remaining volume is measured. The difference between the reading on the pipette and the reading on the original sample will represent the percentage concentration of oxygen. Standard analyzers are calibrated directly and no calculation is necessary to determine the oxygen concentration. If there should be any doubt as to accuracy of the oxygen analyzer, room air should be tested. If the analyzer is functioning accurately, the room air will show approximately 20 per cent oxygen content.

Requirements for Administration. The four basic requirements for effective administration of oxygen are: (1) sufficient supply of U.S.P. oxygen; (2) a safe and dependable regulator that will deliver oxygen to the patient at the desired constant rate of flow; (3) proper apparatus for administering oxygen, whether by tent or other method; (4) all persons assisting in care of the patient to have a thorough knowledge of the handling of oxygen and of the apparatus being used in its administration.

The Oxygen Regulator. A 244 cu. ft. cylinder of oxygen is under 2,200 pounds pressure per square inch. That pressure must be reduced and controlled before oxygen can be administered to a patient. The oxygen regulator is used for that purpose, and no oxygen should be administered without the use of a regulator. The oxygen regulator performs two very important functions: it reduces the pressure of oxygen coming from the cylinder and insures a steady, even flow of oxygen at the rate desired. The regulator most commonly used is termed a two-stage regulator and is actually two regulators in one. As the oxygen enters the first stage, pressure is automatically reduced; in the second stage, the flow of oxygen is regulated to the desired number of liters per minute.

The following basic rules should be observed in using oxygen regulators: (1) Any person handling an oxygen regulator should first wash his hands thoroughly in soap and water to remove any oil or grease. (2) Before the regulator is attached to the cylinder of oxygen, the cylinder valve should be "cracked" (opened slightly and quickly closed again) to blow out any dust that may have lodged in the opening. (3) The regulator should be attached to the cylinder and the flow-adjusting screw turned to the left (OFF) before the cylinder valve is opened. (4) The cylinder valve is opened slowly; when the pointer on the cylinder-contents gauge of the regulator stops moving, open the cylinder valve completely. (5) The flow-adjusting screw is turned to the right (ON) until the needle on the flow-indicator gauge indicates the desired rate of flow in liters per minute. (6) Oil or grease should never be used on any part of the oxygen apparatus or mechanism.

Methods of Administration. Regardless of the method used in administering oxygen, the apparatus or equipment used must meet the following three requirements: (1) it must be able to maintain a continuous and steady flow of oxygen at a desired rate of flow; (2) it must provide oxygen without causing great discomfort to the patient; and (3) it must be safe and economical in operation.

Six types of oxygen therapy equipment are available for use at the present time: the oxygen tent, face mask, nasal catheter, nasal inhaler, helium-oxygen apparatus, and the oxygen room.

The choice of equipment to be used in administering oxygen may well determine the effectiveness of the treatment. For general use, where only a moderate concentration of oxygen is required, the tent, inhaler, or catheter may be used. If higher concentration is desired (above 60 per cent), the patient must wear some type of mask. The patient's comfort should be considered in selecting the equipment, too, since discomfort and subsequent objection to treatment will markedly reduce the benefit derived from oxygen administration.

Each nurse responsible for the care of the patient receiving oxygen should understand the importance of gaining the patient's cooperation by carefully explaining the procedure and by relieving him of fear or anxiety concerning the treatment. Only through the patient's accept-

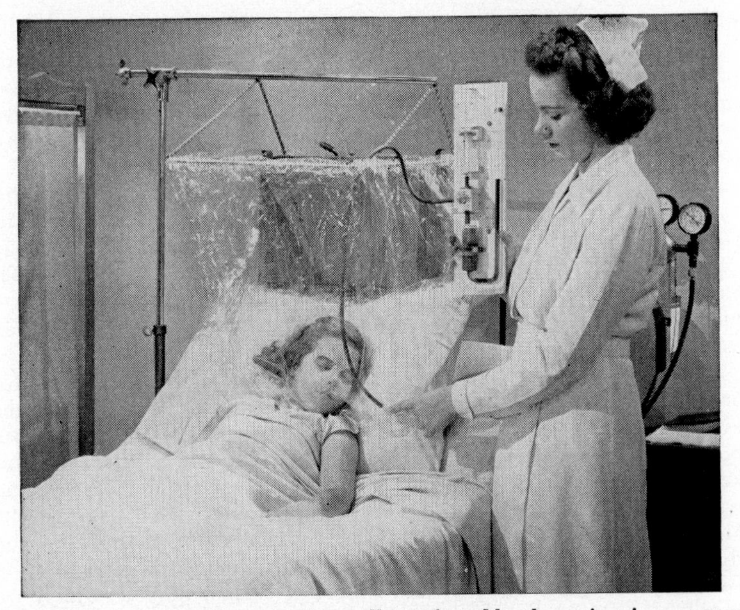

Fig. 215. The transparent canopy is usually preferred by the patient in an oxygen tent. (Linde Air Products Co., New York, New York.)

ance of the treatment and his cooperation in carrying it out can maximum benefit be obtained.

The Oxygen Tent. The oxygen tent is frequently chosen for administration of oxygen since it is more economical than the oxygen room. A number of different types of oxygen tents are available and the nurse will need to read and understand the instructions supplied by the manufacturer of the tent which is in use. Directions for operation are not difficult to understand and, although the various tents differ in detail, they are basically the same.

The oxygen tent consists of a canopy which encloses, usually, the head and upper part of the patient, and a cabinet that provides the means of controlling humidity and temperature. The oxygen passes through the ice chamber in the cabinet to be cooled and humidified before being circulated through the canopy to be utilized by the patient. Tents with an electric air-conditioning device do not, of course, require the ice chamber for regulating temperature and humidity.

The canopy should be made of a fabric that is impervious to the gas. It may be made entirely of transparent material or contain large windows of a transparent non-inflammable material so visibility is sufficient to prevent a feeling of restriction being imposed on the patient. Some canopies fit over the entire mattress and are tucked in at top and bottom and at both sides. Such canopies are not especially expensive and can be discarded after use. Other canopies cover the patient's head and upper part of his body only, and must be tucked under the mattress at head and sides, then the edge across the front is sealed or made air tight by being enfolded in the top sheet which is tucked under the side of the mattress.

The tent may be closed with zippers which can be opened to give care to the patient. It may have sleeve-like attachments through which the nurse may put her arms to care for the patient. A few tents are "open-top," facilitating the carrying out of nursing procedures. The canopy is supported on an adjustable metal frame which extends well above the bed and permits elevation of the backrest so that the patient may be in an upright position.

The oxygen in the tent is kept in circulation by the motor blower or is dependent on the principle of warm air being lighter than cool air. The cooled oxygen, which is heavier than air, is continuously blown into the tent to become warmer and rise to the surface, thus keeping the air inside the tent in circulation. The cabinet or device which provides for the regulation of temperature and humidity may also provide for removal of carbon dioxide from within the tent through the use of soda lime. With this equipment, the air which has circulated through the tent and absorbed carbon dioxide which was exhaled by the patient may be recirculated through the tent after the carbon dioxide has been removed.

The nurse is required to maintain the desired concentration of oxygen in the tent, give needed care to the patient, and safeguard the patient and others who may not be aware of the danger of fire where oxygen is in use.

To bring the concentration of oxygen to the desired level, the oxygen flow is set at 15 liters per minute for the first half hour. After that time, the flow is regulated to 10–12 liters per minute, depending on the doctor's orders. Concentration of oxygen within the tent should be tested at intervals during the day, so that it remains constant. Use of a rubber sheet over the mattress will help conserve oxygen in the tent, by preventing its escape into the hollows and air spaces of the mattress.

Nursing care should be carefully planned so that the number of times the tent must be opened to give care to the patient is kept at a minimum.

Temperature in the tent should be maintained at approximately 60–68° F. In summer the temperature may be slightly higher, as ordinary room temperature may be increased beyond the usual 70–76° F. Because temperature in the tent is somewhat lower than ordinary room temperature, the patient should be kept warm with sufficient clothing and blankets. The patient's head should be protected from the draft that may be created by the flow of oxygen into the tent.

In giving fluids, taking temperature, giving medicine, and doing

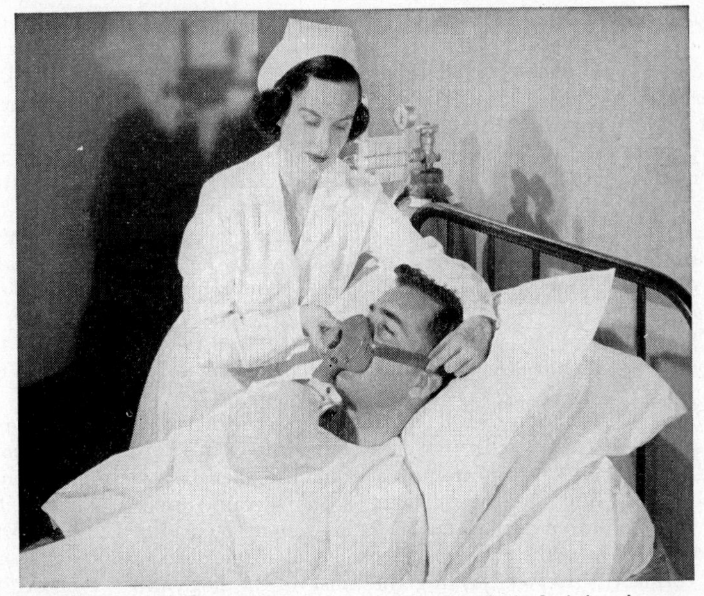

Fig. 216. The face mask provides an inexpensive method of administering oxygen. (Linde Air Products Co., New York, New York.)

other ordinary procedures, the canopy may be opened to permit entrance of the nurse's hands and arms. For procedures requiring a longer time, such as the bath, the canopy may be tucked securely under the edges of the pillow so that only the patient's head remains inside. The rest of the patient's body can then be bathed, without disturbing the concentration of oxygen in the tent.

Because oxygen supports combustion, the danger of fire is ever present where oxygen is in use. The patient should be told of the danger involved so that he will understand the necessity to refrain from smoking. "No Smoking" signs should be placed on the oxygen cylinder, and all visitors should be informed of the danger from lighted matches, cigarettes, or other possible fire hazards. Electrical appliances should not be used; heating pads, electric blankets, electric razors, etc. are all hazardous because a spark from any such appliance may cause a fire when in the presence of oxygen. The electric signal cord for the patient in an oxygen tent should be replaced with a small hand bell for summoning the nurse. Catholic patients and their friends may need to be warned that lighted candles must never be used in a unit where oxygen is being given.

The Face Mask. Many doctors favor use of the face mask because it is inexpensive, portable, and capable of administering oxygen in concentrations as high as 95–100 per cent.

In using a face mask, the following instructions are important: (1) Select a suitable size and type of mask. (2) Start the oxygen with rate of flow slightly higher than that desired. (3) Adjust the mask to the patient's face so that it fits snugly, fasten head strap so it fits well but is not tight around the head. Make certain that air from top of the mask isn't being blown into the patient's eyes. (4) Wait until the patient relaxes and is breathing normally before adjusting the liter flow to the desired rate. (5) At least every two hours remove the mask. Wash and dry the patient's face and apply powder or vanishing cream to areas where the mask rests against the face. This is especially necessary in hot weather, to lessen the discomfort of wearing the mask.

During use of the mask the air is kept at suitable humidity by the deposit of moisture, within the mask, from the air exhaled by the patient.

B.L.B. Mask. The B.L.B. mask is available in two types: the nasal mask which covers only the area immediately surrounding the nose, and is generally the most comfortable, and the oronasal mask, which covers nose and mouth, is required for the unconscious patient, for the uncooperative patient, and for the patient accustomed to breathing through the mouth. Each mask consists of three parts: the mask itself, the connective device, joining the mask to the bag, and the breathing bag.

The oxygen concentration in the mask is controlled by the control of liter flow. A control of 4 liters per minute will supply approximately 40–50 per cent oxygen, while a control of 6 liters per minute supplies an oxygen concentration of 50–60 per cent. When giving high concentrations of oxygen, the liter flow should be high enough that the bag does not collapse completely during inspiration. When giving lower concentrations of oxygen, the bag should collapse during each respiratory cycle. The longer the bag remains collapsed, the lower will be the concentration of oxygen in the inspired air.

The plug in the bottom of the breathing bag may be removed to drain off excess moisture. The plug in the mask proper is removed if it is necessary to insert a Miller-Abbott tube or a suction tube.

Positive Pressure Mask. When oxygen needs to be administered under slight positive pressure, as in the treatment of pulmonary edema, the special type O.E.M. meter mask should be used. By adjusting the dial on the front of the mask, oxygen can be given under 1, 2, 3, or 4 centimeters of water pressure. The largest opening in the disk is for administering oxygen at normal atmospheric pressure.

The O.E.M. mask operates in much the same manner as the B.L.B. mask, except for one important factor. Regardless of the concentration of oxygen being given, the breathing bag should never be allowed to completely collapse during the respiratory cycle.

Nasal Catheter. Use of a nasal catheter permits oxygen to be delivered directly into the oropharynx. A special catheter for oxygen

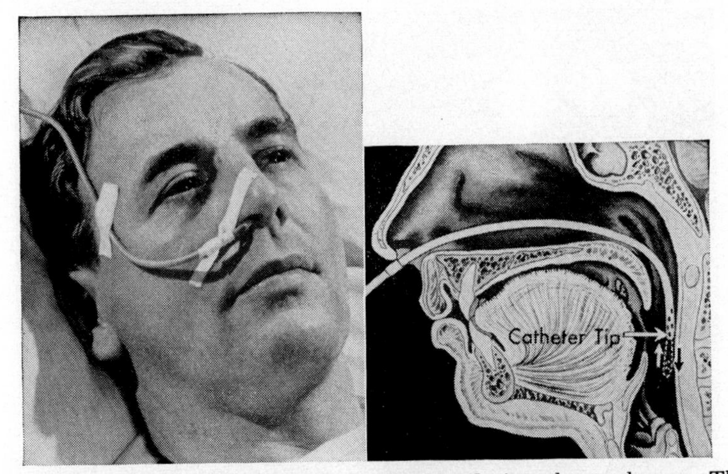

Fig. 217. A nasal catheter delivers oxygen directly into the oropharynx. The catheter is fastened in place by adhesive tape. (Linde Air Products Co., New York, New York.)

therapy, made of soft rubber and perforated with several holes near the end, prevents the stream of oxygen being directed entirely in one spot in the throat. To avoid dryness and irritation of the mucous membrane of the throat, the oxygen must be passed through a suitable humidifier, which breaks the oxygen stream into tiny bubbles and thus the oxygen is moistened.

For insertion and correct placement of the catheter, the following suggestions should be followed: (1) Measure the distance from the external nostril to the tragus of the ear on the catheter and mark this distance on the catheter with a narrow piece of adhesive tape. (2) Turn on the oxygen to a rate of flow approximately 5 liters per minute. (3) Lubricate the catheter, using a moderately heavy lubricating medium rather than a lighter oil, which is soluble in water and soon leaves the catheter dry and harsh. (4) Insert the catheter through the nostril into the pharynx until the tip of the catheter can be seen through the mouth, hanging just opposite the uvula. (5) Fasten the catheter in place with an adhesive strip wound around the catheter, the two ends being brought horizontally across the nose just slightly above the nostril, and across the forehead. (6) Insert a clean, freshly lubricated catheter in the alternate nostril at least once every 12 hours to prevent the catheter from adhering to the inside of the nose.

With the nasal catheter, oxygen concentration will depend on placement of the catheter, the liter flow rate, and the patient's tolerance. The most satisfactory method is to adjust the rate of flow to 5, 6, or 8 liters per minute, maintaining it at the rate which best overcomes the patient's symptoms.

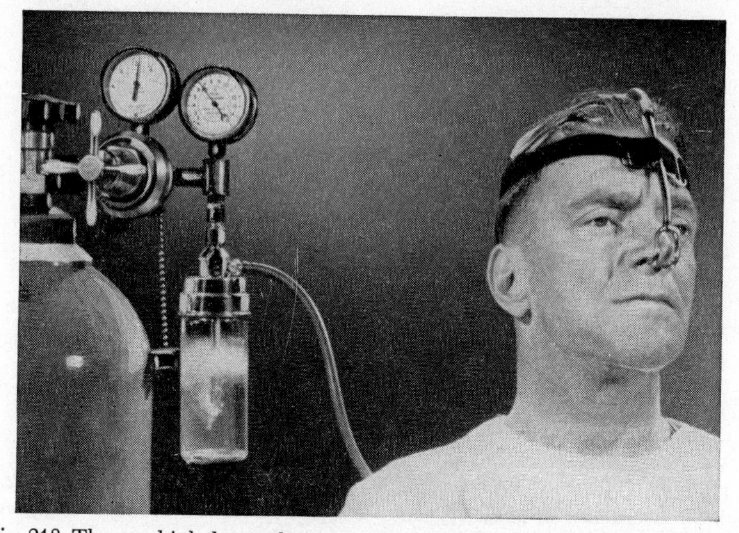

Fig. 218. The nasal inhaler method of administering oxygen. (Linde Air Products Co., New York, New York.)

Nasal Inhaler. The metal nasal inhaler is a hollow two-pronged tube with tips that fit into the nostrils, through which oxygen is supplied to the patient. It is held in position by means of a head band. The tips of the inhaler can be bent slightly inward or outward to a position that will be most comfortable for the patient. A short piece of rubber tubing placed on the end of each tip and lubricated before the tips are inserted into the nostrils may make the device more comfortable and will not interfere with administration of oxygen.

A length of rubber tubing connects the inhaler to the oxygen regulator, which is attached to the oxygen cylinder. The tubing should be pinned to the pillow or back of the mattress in such a way that movement of the patient's head is not restricted. A flow of 9 liters per minute gives about 50 per cent oxygen concentration to the inspired air.

Helium-Oxygen Apparatus. Because nitrogen, which makes up about four fifths of the total volume of air, is a heavy gas, effort is needed to expel ordinary air from the lungs. In cases of obstructive dyspnea, as in bronchiectasis, the effort may be too great for the patient. Oxygen may be given, but when it is mixed with air which is largely nitrogen the dyspnea persists. Helium, which is a light gas weighing only one-seventh as much as nitrogen, can be substituted for the latter to bring relief to the patient. A mixture of 75 per cent helium and 25 per cent oxygen is used for patients with asthma and other respiratory conditions. Helium is not explosive and is not harmful to tissues. The helium-oxygen mixture can be inhaled and exhaled with about one-third the effort required to inhale and exhale the oxygen-air mixture.

Equipment usually used is a special hood with a soft removable collar that fits over the head and can be fastened snugly about the neck. The mixture is passed through an air-conditioning cabinet before entering the hood, and because helium is an expensive gas the principle of rebreathing is employed. Helium may be purchased in cylinders where it is already mixed with oxygen in the proportion desired.

The Oxygen Room. The ideal, and most expensive, method of administering oxygen is by means of the oxygen room. The room is air tight and oxygen is introduced by pipes so that the concentration of oxygen in the room is maintained at the desired level. Several patients may be accommodated in the room at one time. The movements of patients are not restricted and the administration of oxygen is not interrupted when treatment or nursing care is necessary. Portable oxygen chambers, made of rubberized fabric, large enough to provide for requirements of one patient unit, are available and are being used in some hospitals.

CARBON DIOXIDE THERAPY

Carbon dioxide is sometimes given in conditions of respiratory depression. It is used in resuscitation of the newborn or of a drowning patient, and in anesthesia when the patient is too deeply anesthetized. It has been used effectively as a nonspecific remedy for hiccups.

Carbon dioxide may be administered by mask in combination with oxygen or it may be used from a tank containing 100 per cent carbon dioxide and administered by being held at least 6 inches from the patient's face so it is mixed with air. Hyperventilation of the lungs (increasing the carbon dioxide content of inspired air) may be accomplished by placing a paper bag over the face of the patient. Expired air containing about 4% carbon dioxide is rebreathed and the amount of carbon dioxide in the inspired air is thus increased.

Carbon dioxide therapy is hazardous for the patient and should be given only by persons trained in its administration or under their direct supervision. If hyperpnea does not occur within 20–30 seconds, carbon dioxide should be discontinued, as serious depressant effects may result.

Aerosol Therapy. The terms *nebulin* and *aerosol* mean "very fine mist or spray." A *nebulizer* is an atomizer or other device used to transform a prescribed drug or solution into a fine mist or spray. For antibiotic drugs, such as penicillin, which cannot be given by steam inhalation because they are not volatile, the nebulizer provides an effective method of administration. The penicillin solution is placed in a glass or plastic nebulizer and a stream of oxygen under pressure is passed through it, producing a very fine mist which can be inhaled by the patient.

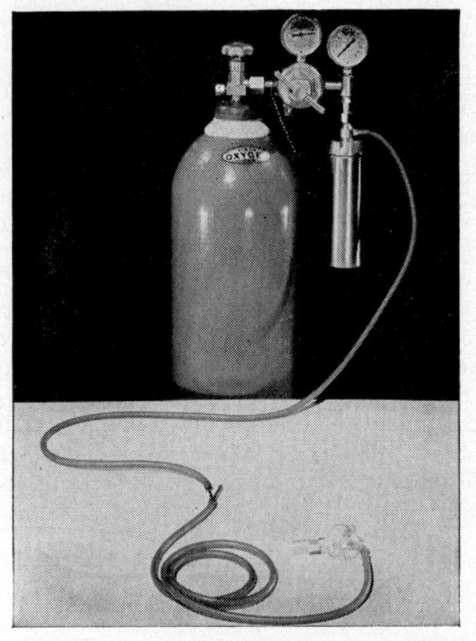

Fig. 219. The nebulizer for penicillin inhalation. (Linde Air Products Co., New York, New York.)

One end of the nebulizer is shaped to form a mouthpiece which the patient holds in his mouth; the other end is attached to a rubber tube leading to the tank of oxygen. The humidifier on the tank of oxygen should be empty when the oxygen is used with the nebulizer. The lower, bulb-shaped part of the nebulizer contains the penicillin solution. Oxygen enters through a very fine tube, and by placing his finger on an opening in the glass nebulizer the patient can regulate the flow of the mist or spray. If the glass nebulizer has no opening, the rubber tubing is connected with a Y-tube, one of the Y stems or piece of tubing is open. By opening and closing this tube the flow of mist may be regulated. The oxygen is introduced into the nebulizer under low pressure, at the rate of 4–6 liters per minute. The very fine particles of the penicillin solution penetrate to the smaller bronchioles and alveoli of the lungs and are absorbed into the blood stream so that both local and systemic effects are obtained. Each treatment requires 20–30 minutes.

The aerosol form of treatment may be used effectively in chronic or acute infections of the respiratory tract

In sinusitis, use of a nasal aerosol with alternating negative pressure apparatus has been successful in withdrawing air from the paranasal sinuses to insure penetration into the sinuses of the antibiotic drug. Bronchiectasis and lung abscess may also be treated by aerosol therapy.

In using the nebulizer, the patient should be told to close the opening or the open end of the tubing to inhale, to hold his breath momentarily at the end of each inspiration, then to remove his finger from the opening or release the open end of tubing while exhaling through his nose. The process is repeated until the desired dosage of drug has been used. The frequency of treatment should be determined by the doctor. After each treatment, the patient should be encouraged to wash his mouth thoroughly with clear water to prevent soreness of the tongue.

THE MECHANICAL RESPIRATOR

In certain conditions, notably poliomyelitis, the patient may be unable to breathe normally and it becomes necessary to provide mechanical aid to insure continued functioning of the respiratory system. The respirator or *iron lung* is such a mechanical aid. To understand the action and use of the respirator the nurse must understand the mechanics of respiration.

Mechanics of Respiration. The lungs are enclosed in a bony cavity made up of the ribs, which are linked together by opposing layers of muscles. At the back, the ribs are connected with vertebrae of the spinal column by joints which permit only slight movement. At the front of the chest the ends of the ribs are free and when certain chest muscles contract the ribs are pulled upward and outward, the sternum is raised, and the chest cavity is enlarged. At the same time, the diaphragm contracts and flattens so that the chest cavity deepens. When this occurs, air rushes into the expanded lungs (inspiration). When the muscles relax and the diaphragm expands, the chest cavity is narrowed and shortened, and air is forced out (expiration).

In paralysis of the respiratory muscles the contraction and relaxation necessary for breathing do not occur, and the patient must be placed in the mechanical respirator so respiration may be continued. In the respirator, a partial vacuum or area of low atmospheric pressure is created, pulling the chest walls outward so air enters the lungs. When the negative pressure is discontinued in the respirator, the chest walls fall again, forcing air out of the lungs. By alternate application and removal of negative pressure the rhythm of normal respiration can be maintained.

The Respirator. The mechanical respirator is a large cylindrical, metal tank which can be opened at one end to admit the stretcher or frame bearing the body of the patient. The patient's head is passed through a hole in the door. A large sponge rubber collar in the opening fits closely around the neck of the patient to prevent escape of air from the tank. When the door is clamped shut the interior of the tank is air tight.

The inside of the tank is illuminated by electric lights, and small windows along the sides of the tank enable the nurse to see the body of the patient. The electric lights also provide warmth, and a light blanket is the only covering required. Larger openings or portholes with small sponge-rubber cuffs on each side of the tank permit entrance of the nurse's hand and arm to provide care for the patient. The cuffs, fitting snugly about the nurse's arms, prevent entrance of outside air. Large doors at the side permit passing the bedpan and other articles used in caring for the patient into the tank. The stretcher inside the tank can be tilted from head to foot and from side to side to change position for the patient.

Pressure inside the tank is maintained by an electrically operated bellows. An attachment provides for hand operation, should the electricity fail. The tank is equipped with various gauges to provide information on the amount of pressure being maintained and the rate of change of pressure which controls the rate of respiration for the patient.

Each respirator is equipped with detailed directions for its operation; in some models directions are posted on the side of the respirator for all to read. If the directions are carefully observed, the machine will function satisfactorily.

Placing the Patient in the Respirator. Before bringing the respirator into the room, the nurse should explain to the patient the necessity for its use and should describe the size and appearance of the mechanism, which may be frightening when viewed for the first time.

All necessary equipment should be assembled in the room before the machine is brought in. The machine should be tested to make sure it is in good working order. Rubber gaskets should be inspected. Sponge-rubber collar and cuffs should be in good condition and the machine, inside and out, should be clean. The stretcher should be made up with clean linen and persons who are to help should be told what they are to do to help place the patient in correct position. Four or five persons will be needed to place the patient inside the respirator.

With the stretcher pulled almost completely out of the respirator, two or more persons lift the patient's body and place him with head against the rubber cuff at the door of the cylinder. Two persons open the diaphragm neck pieces, and the nurse standing at the head of the patient reaches hands and arms through the sponge-rubber collar. One hand supports the patient's head, the other covers his face to protect nose and mouth as the head is brought through the small opening. The patient's head should be turned to one side, with chin kept down. Persons holding the patient's body ease it into position high on the stretcher so that the rubber collar fits low on his neck. If necessary, the mattress should be raised so that the patient's neck is on a straight line with the opening of the collar.

The stretcher is then pushed into the respirator and the door is clamped shut. The motor should then be started and adjustments made so that the rate of mechanical respiration is the same as the patient's normal respiration rate.

Position of the Patient inside the Respirator. Inside the respirator the patient will need to be placed in a position that will be comfortable and will prevent complications, such as footdrop. The shoulders should be well supported and, if necessary, padded across the top to prevent rubbing against the door of the respirator. The bed linens should always be free of wrinkles so there will be no undue pressure on shoulders or back. Arms should be extended at the patient's sides and the hands should be gently curved about a small roll of cotton wrapped in several layers of gauze. A knee roll should be placed under the knees to prevent strain in the muscles at the back of the legs. A hard pillow or padded board should be placed at the foot of the respirator to support the feet in an upright position. If the patient is to remain in the respirator for some time, buttocks and heels may need to be padded to prevent pressure sores.

Outside the respirator, the patient's head should be supported and made comfortable by placing a small pillow on the head shelf. A mirror placed on the door of the respirator above the patient's head will enable him to see the room and to see persons who are in the room.

Exercise for the Respirator Patient. The patient in the respirator is unable to move his body voluntary, so exercise of a passive nature is necessary if body tissues are to remain in good condition. The neck should be gently massaged at frequent intervals to prevent strain in neck muscles. During the bath, arms and lower limbs should be exercised gently. The entire surface of the body should be massaged at intervals, with special attention to areas where pressure sores may develop.

Change of position is extremely important, even though the change is only slight. If two nurses work together the position of the patient may be changed without removing him from the respirator.

Nursing Care for the Respirator Patient. The patient in the respirator is completely dependent on the nurse. Keeping the throat and nose clear of mucus is an important factor in nursing care. Removal of mucus is best accomplished with the electric suction device but can be done with an ordinary rubber bulb syringe.

Treatments such as enema, catheterization, and hypodermic injections may be given without removing the patient from the respirator, although they may be difficult. If the patient in the respirator requires oxygen, it is usually administered by the nasal catheter method.

Nursing care must be modified to meet the needs of the patient, and is usually adapted to satisfy one of the three following conditions.

1. When the patient can be removed from the respirator for a short period: With all equipment or articles that will be needed assembled and the room made comfortable, the respirator door is opened and the stretcher removed from the tank. Nursing care is given as for other patients and the patient's position is changed. The stretcher is then returned to the tank and the door closed and securely locked.

2. When the patient can be removed for only an extremely short period: All articles and equipment should be assembled. Two to four

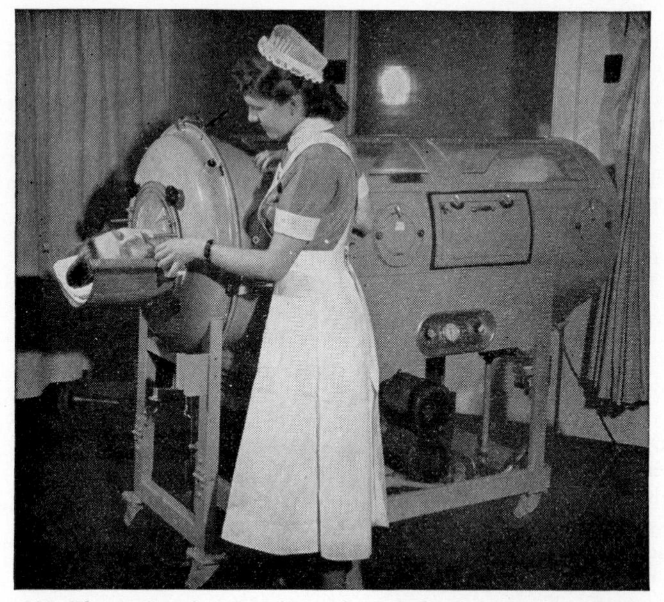

Fig. 220. The patient in a respirator is entirely dependent on the nurse for daily care and for constant reassurance. (Massachusetts General Hospital School of Nursing, Boston, Massachusetts.)

nurses should be available to perform the necessary procedure. The doctor should hyperventilate the patient. The stretcher should be withdrawn quickly and the nurses should work together very rapidly and in unison to complete the nursing care in the shortest possible time. The stretcher should be replaced and the door securely locked.

3. When nursing care can be given through portholes: Procedures such as giving bedpan or urinal, taking pulse, and massaging a part can be done by reaching through portholes. Such care should be done quickly and portholes should always be closed tightly after care has been given.

The nurse should carefully watch the patient in a respirator for cyanosis or other indications that the machine is not functioning properly.

The patient in a respirator must learn to talk in rhythm with the pull of the machine. Food and fluids must be given with care to prevent aspiration into the lungs during forced inspiration produced by the machine.

Diversion for the Patient in a Respirator. As the patient in a respirator recovers from the acute stage of disease and becomes used to being in the machine, he will need certain forms of entertainment or diversion to help maintain an optimistic state of mind.

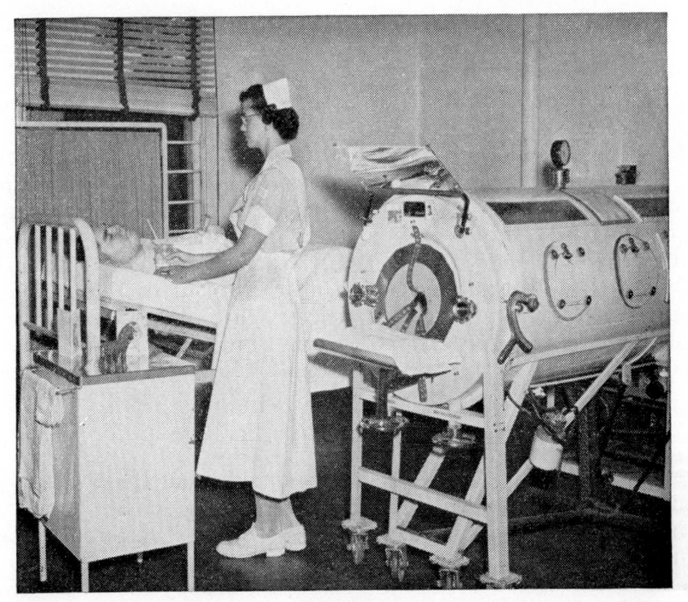

Fig. 221. To re-establish normal breathing the patient is removed from the respirator for gradually increasing periods of time. (Indiana University School of Nursing, Indianapolis, Indiana.)

Reading may be done by the patient with the aid of mirrors and a nurse or attendant to turn the pages of the book or magazine.

Television and radio are good means of keeping the patient entertained. Ingenious friends and relatives of patients required to spend a long period of time in a respirator have invented many gadgets that can be used by the patient, even though use of the hands is not possible.

Many patients, through use of the telephone, have been able to keep in close touch with family and friends. Some have even managed a small business while confined to the respirator.

When Use of the Respirator can be Discontinued. The patient who has been in a respirator for a long time may be frightened at the thought of being without its steady rhythmic help in breathing, and he may resent any word or action from doctor or nurse which indicates that use of the respirator could be given up for short intervals. The nurse must be very considerate and offer continual reassurance to dispel the patient's fear and to begin the process of discontinuing use of the respirator.

The effort to re-establish natural breathing by the patient may be made in one of two ways. He may be removed from the respirator for gradually increasing periods as he learns to breathe again for himself.

As an alternative method, pressure in the machine may gradually be decreased so the patient is forced to put forth an effort to maintain normal respiration. If the patient's attention is diverted during the time he is out of the machine, or not depending entirely on it, he may be less apprehensive.

Most patients look forward eagerly to the time when they can leave the machine during the day but are very hesitant about remaining out of it at night. No attempt should be made to hurry the patient into being entirely on his own. If given understanding and encouragement, he will gradually overcome anxiety about being away from the machine and will eventually learn to do without it. Work done by the nurse in helping the patient regain self-confidence and develop the desire to once again resume normal activities in living is a very important part of the nursing care given to the patient in a respirator.

Care of Equipment after Use

Steam Inhalator. Water should be emptied from the bottle in the inhalator. The cup which contained the drug should be washed and cleaned. The inhalator should be washed with a disinfectant solution and returned to central supply for proper storage until needed again.

Croup Tent. Blankets used in making the canopy should be sent to the laundry or cleaner. Inhalator or improvised equipment should be cleaned with a disinfectant solution. Paper bags or cardboard mailing tubes should be burned.

Oxygen Tent. If the transparent canopy which is fairly inexpensive has been in use, it should be discarded when no longer needed for the patient. The fabric tent with transparent windows should be washed thoroughly with a strong disinfectant solution. The windows should be cleaned with soap and water. The tent should be hung for storage without folding or creasing, which might cause it to be broken so that it would not be air tight. In storage it should be covered to protect it from dust and dirt.

At frequent intervals the tent should be thoroughly inspected for leaks or possible need for repair. Zippers on the tent should be kept in good working order and should always be closed while the tent is in storage.

The cabinet should be washed in disinfectant solution. All ice and water should be removed. Mechanical parts should be inspected and soda lime renewed or replaced or made available for immediate use, should the tent be needed for another patient.

Oxygen cylinders should always be stored in a room where temperature is relatively low. They should not be placed near hot radiators or pipes, electrical appliances, or inflammable material. They should be clearly marked "FULL" or "EMPTY," and should not be placed where they may be knocked over.

Face Mask. After use, the mask, bag, and connecting bag should be washed in soap and water, rinsed well, then cleansed with disinfectant solution. The two small rubber sponges in the mask which absorb carbon dioxide exhaled by the patient should be removed, washed, and cleansed in disinfectant solution, and thoroughly dried. When dry, they may be replaced in the mask. The mask should then be thoroughly dried, placed in a labeled box, and stored until needed again.

Nasal Catheter. Used nasal catheters should be washed and boiled, to be ready for use again.

Nasal Inhaler. Tubing and inhaler should be washed in a disinfectant solution, rinsed and dried, and returned to storage.

Helium-Oxygen Apparatus. The hood and collar should be washed in disinfectant solution, dried, and stored until needed again.

Nebulizer. When treatment is discontinued, the nebulizer should be washed with distilled water, dried, and put away until needed again. If the nebulizer becomes clogged while in use, it should be disconnected from the tubing and a new nebulizer substituted.

Mechanical Respirator. After each use, the respirator must be thoroughly cleaned with soap and water and washed in a disinfectant solution.

The mechanism should be checked by a competent engineer at frequent and regular intervals. Collars of various sizes should be kept on hand at all times. When the respirator is needed it is usually for emergency treatment and delay in getting it into operation because of needed repairs or cleaning could result in death of the patient for whom it was to have been used.

Summary of Important Factors

For best results in steam inhalation, a tent should be constructed and humidity in the tent maintained at about 70 per cent.

Precautions must be taken to avoid burning the patient, especially if the inhalations are for a child.

Inhalations are usually continued for 15–20 minutes, every 3 or 4 hours.

Inhalation apparatus can be devised at home for effective treatment.

Oxygen must be given in concentrations of 40–50 per cent to be effective.

Where oxygen is being used, because of the increased fire hazard, there should be strict observance of the following rules: No smoking—no open flame near the oxygen tent; the patient should not have an electric signal bell; flashlight should not be used near oxygen.

All persons helping in oxygen administration must understand handling of oxygen and correct operation of equipment being used.

Correct instructions must be given the patient who uses the nebulizer.

To understand the principle of operation governing the use of the mechanical respirator, the mechanics of respiration must be clearly understood.

The complete dependence on the nurse of the patient in the respirator requires that the nurse continually offer reassurance to the patient.

The nurse should be very considerate of the patient who must adjust to the rather frightening experience of learning to breathe normally outside the respirator when its use is to be discontinued.

Factors To Teach the Patient

How to improvise equipment needed to give steam inhalations.

The proper method of disposing of paper mouthwipes and expectorated material.

Precautions necessary to prevent burns from steam in giving inhalations.

The advantages of moist, warm air in relieving difficult breathing.

That oxygen therapy need not be feared and is used usually as a temporary measure.

The dangers of fire that are increased where oxygen is being used. Why no smoking, no flame, no electrical appliance should be permitted near a source or supply of oxygen.

Services of the Visiting Nurse are available and she may be called to help in the operation of devices used in inhalation therapy.

The correct method of using the penicillin nebulizer.

Diversional activities for the patient in the respirator.

How to eat and talk in rhythm with the mechanical respirator.

How to cooperate in receiving nursing care.

Method of overcoming apprehension on being removed from the respirator for short periods when treatment is to be discontinued.

Scientific Principles

Anatomy and Physiology. The respiratory tract, composed of nose, pharynx, larynx, trachea, bronchi, and lungs, is lined with ciliated mucous membrane. Some body heat is eliminated through vaporization of moisture from the mucous membrane.

Internal respiration, or the exchange of carbon dioxide and oxygen occurs in the alveoli of the lungs. Red blood cells transport oxygen to the tissues of the body.

External respiration is a mechanical process, accomplished through the combined action of the diaphragm and the muscles of the chest and abdomen. Regulation and maintenance of rhythmic respiration depends on the respiratory center in the medulla, nerve fibers of the autonomic nervous system, and the chemical composition of the blood.

Normal rate of respiration for the average adult is 18–20 per minute.

Chemistry. In many respiratory conditions the lung loses much of its normal surface area for absorbing oxygen from the air so a high concentration of oxygen must be administered to supply the body needs.

Oxygen is not inflammable in itself, but it supports combustion so that where oxygen is in use the danger of fire from a spark or flame is greatly increased.

Oxygen comprises about 20 per cent of the air.

Oxygen deficiency causes increased respiration.

Excessive amounts of carbon dioxide will cause death by asphyxia.

Nitrogen has a molecular weight of 28; helium, a molecular weight of 4. In respiratory conditions breathing of the heavier gas causes dyspnea and fatigue.

Microbiology. The cilia of the mucous membrane of the nose entrap dust, dirt, and bacteria and with their wavelike motion propel it in an outward direction away from the respiratory tract.

Inhalation apparatus must be sterilized or disinfected after use. Very large devices or articles, as an oxygen tent, may be made completely safe for use again by washing with a strong disinfectant solution.

Pharmacology. The most commonly used respiratory stimulants are carbon dioxide, caffeine, atropine, strychnine, and ammonia.

Opiates are respiratory depressants.

Drugs given to act on mucous membrane of the respiratory tract are demulcents, expectorants, and antiseptics. They may be given by inhalation or by mouth.

Penicillin may be given by means of a nebulizer.

Oxygen is used when there is a deficiency in the supply to body tissues. The flow of oxygen is usually regulated to 6–12 liters per minute for the average adult patient.

Physics. The movement of gases is affected by their weight or specific gravity. Oxygen is heavier than air and will sink into the air spaces of the mattress unless the bed is covered with a rubber sheet.

In giving nasal oxygen by funnel the patient will get more oxygen if the funnel is held above the nose and mouth, rather than below it.

The diffusion of oxygen through the walls of the alveoli of the lungs into the blood stream and the diffusion of carbon dioxide from the blood into the alveoli depend on a difference in pressure of the two gases.

The mechanics of respiration depend on atmospheric pressure and intrapleural pressure, as explained in discussion of the mechanical respirator.

In a tent where steam inhalations are being given, a wool or porous blanket, which will absorb the condensed water and the vapor of the drug by capillary attraction, thus preventing its accumulation, should be used for a canopy.

Each cylinder of 220 cu. ft. capacity contains 6000 liters of oxygen under 2000 pounds of pressure per square inch. One gauge on the cylinder measures the pressure in pounds and indicates the amount of oxygen in the cylinder. The other gauge is on the oxygen regulator. The regulator reduces the pressure from 2000 pounds to 20, which can be tolerated by the patient, and measures the discharge of oxygen from the cylinder in liters per minute.

Oxygen has a drying action on mucous membrane because it flows into the lungs under greater than atmospheric pressure and surface fluids evaporate more rapidly. Oxygen administered to a patient must be humidified by being passed through water or over ice.

The penicillin nebulizer operates on the principle that a moving stream of air reduces the air pressure about it. The air pressure in the nebulizer is lower than upward pressure of the fluid. The fluid is forced into the area of lowered pressure where it is broken into a fine mist and enters the respiratory tract with the oxygen.

Psychology. The patient receiving oxygen therapy and the patient in the mechanical respirator need to be continually reassured by the nurse.

Transparent canopies should be provided for the patient in the oxygen tent, since they help to lessen the feeling of restriction and isolation. The tent is not soundproof, so nurses and attendants need to remember that the patient can hear all that is said in the room.

Diversional activities are important in determining the mental attitude of the patient receiving inhalation therapy.

Sociology. Oxygen equipment is available from the home service division of oxygen supply companies on request of the attending physician.

Patients receiving inhalation therapy, especially if acutely ill, should have only a limited number of visitors, usually only a few members of the immediate family.

Situation Type Problems

1. Steam inhalations had been ordered for a patient with upper respiratory infection, and the head nurse asked a student to set up a croup tent so the inhalations could be given without disturbing the other patient in the two-bed room.

The student nurse used extra wool blankets which were in the room to form the inner part of the croup tent, covering the outer part with two sheets.

The head nurse, greatly disturbed because the woolen blankets had been used, told the student that steam from the inhalator would cause the blankets to shrink and that "any person" should know not to use woolen material for that purpose.

The student said that the textbook had said to use woolen blankets. The head nurse then stated that the student should have learned not to accept such statements from textbooks, and instructed the student to make the croup tent of sheets only. What would you have done?

2. A patient who had been in an oxygen tent for several days was improved enough to have use of the tent discontinued. The doctor suggested that the tank of oxygen and all equipment be left in the room for 24 hours, in event it should be needed again.

A student nurse found the patient smoking a cigarette and reminded him of the fire hazard with oxygen in the room. The patient said there was no danger so long as the oxygen was not being used. The student nurse was inclined to agree with the patient, but the head nurse told her to tell the patient that so long as the tank remained in the room he was not to smoke. The student was instructed to remove matches and cigarettes from the room. The patient became angry and demanded that the oxygen tank be removed. What would you have done?

Suggested Reference Reading

"The nurse in penicillin aerosol therapy," H. Heffeman; American Journal of Nursing, December, 1947.
"Inhalation therapy in pediatrics," E. W. Black; American Journal of Diseases of Children, August, 1948.
"Acute upper respiratory infections," William S. Jordan; American Journal of Nursing, January, 1950
"The patient in a chest respirator," Audrey M. McCluskey; American Journal of Nursing, April, 1951
"The patient in a respirator," Carmela Di Piano Parisi; American Journal of Nursing, June, 1951.
"Are you sure you have a cold?" Paul Osmum; American Journal of Nursing, February, 1952.
"The positive-pressure respirator dome," Alex J. Steigman and Pauline Hatfield Rumph; American Journal of Nursing, March, 1952.
"Newer methods of artificial respiration," Archer S. Gordon; American Journal of Nursing, March, 1952.
"Providing oxygen therapy in disasters," Benjamin de S. Barnes; American Journal of Nursing, April, 1952.
"Oxygen therapy," J. Mostyn Davis; Modern Hospital, March, 1953.

CHAPTER 36

Aspiration of Body Cavities

TOPICAL OUTLINE

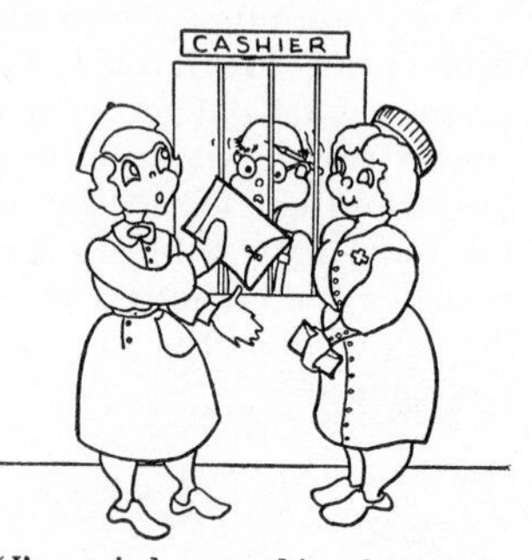

"I've tried everything but aspiration—last month I asked for a bigger pay envelope, guess I should have asked for more pay."

Aspiration is defined as the removal of fluid from a body cavity by insertion of a needle or trocar to permit drainage. Body cavities normally contain sufficient fluid to protect the organs contained within them. In certain diseases the amount of fluid is increased so extensively that symptoms of pressure or tension appear and there may be an interference with respiration, circulation, or other vital body functions. To relieve these symptoms, excess fluid must be removed.

If the abnormal accumulation of fluid is caused by inflammation it is termed an *exudate.* Such fluid is produced by the lining of the cavity and may be serous (watery and thin) or purulent (thick, made up of pus, blood, fibrin, and organisms causing the infection). An exudate has a high specific gravity, contains white blood cells, and will coagulate when exposed to air. Fluid that escapes from the blood and lymph vessels and is not associated with inflammation (caused by impaired circulation or renal damage) is termed a *transudate.* A transudate is usually sterile, has a low specific gravity and white cell count, and does not coagulate. It may be clear or slightly cloudy, and is usually pale or greenish yellow in color.

CAUSES OF ACCUMULATION OF FLUID IN BODY CAVITIES

Pathologic accumulation of fluid in a body cavity may result from inflammation of the serous membrane lining the cavity, the secretion of excessive fluid being nature's way of keeping the inflamed membranes separated from other areas not yet affected.

Excessive fluid may be caused by obstruction of a blood or lymph vessel by a tumorous growth, or by its invasion of the cavity with resultant inflammation.

Conditions affecting the circulation (heart and kidney diseases) may cause fluid to escape from the vessel walls into body tissues or body cavities.

ASPIRATION, AN ASEPTIC PROCEDURE

Body cavities that require aspiration are, of course, those which have no outside opening. Such cavities are lined with serous membrane and have very little or no immunity to infection. It is therefore necessary that all equipment be sterilized before it is used.

The skin should be prepared as for any surgical procedure. The doctor should scrub and wear sterile rubber gloves. The operative field should be properly cleansed and an antiseptic correctly applied. Sterile towels or a suitable sterile sheet should be used to drape the operative area.

DUTIES OF THE NURSE

Although aspiration of a body cavity is done by the doctor, the nurse is expected to be familiar with requirements of the procedure and to help in various ways to insure satisfactory results of the treatment from the standpoint of the patient.

Before the scheduled aspiration the doctor should explain to the patient the nature of the treatment and the reasons for believing that it will be of benefit to him. This explanation may be supplemented by additional information from the nurse, who can reassure the patient by explaining just how he can cooperate to secure best results from the procedure. She should mention the importance of overcoming fear and apprehension so his body will be relaxed. She can caution him not to move about in bed and to maintain the desired position throughout the procedure.

If the procedure involves pain or discomfort the nurse should prepare the patient by mentioning such facts to him. Her assurance that whatever pain he may experience will be of short duration, and that measures are taken to control discomfort, may help to relieve mental anxiety which the patient naturally experiences.

In addition to assembling all the necessary equipment, reassuring the patient, and placing him in the required position, the nurse will be expected to apply antiseptic solutions to the skin, drape the opera-

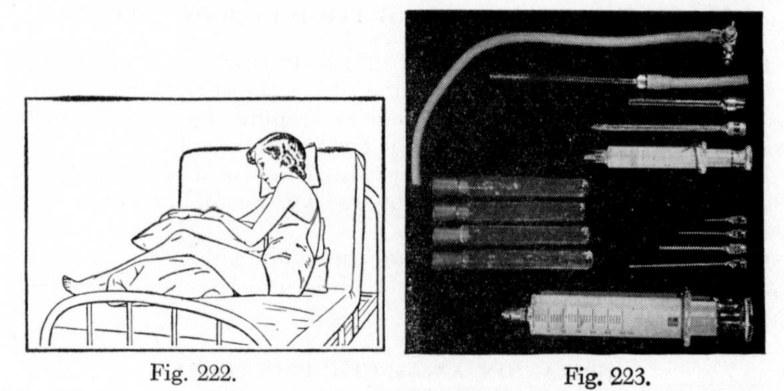

Fig. 222. Fig. 223.

Fig. 222. Correct position for thoracentesis. (M. C. Winters, Protective Body Mechanics in Daily Life and in Nursing.)

Fig. 223. Tray for thoracentesis. (Nursing Service Department, New England Center Hospital, Boston, Massachusetts.)

tive area, and assist the doctor in the collection of fluid specimens if examination of the fluid is needed for diagnosis.

While assisting the doctor the nurse must be conscious of her duties to the patient, encouraging him to stay quietly in the rather uncomfortable position, carefully observing his reaction to the treatment to detect symptoms of possible complications, and lending psychologic support through the comforting reassurance of her presence and her interest in his welfare.

Her care of the patient after the treatment has been concluded should include careful watching for undesirable effects, instructions relative to restricted activity, and intelligent, meaningful answers to his questions regarding the success or benefit of the procedure.

Specimens should be labeled and sent to the laboratory, and important data with reference to the procedure should be recorded on the chart. In all aspiration procedures notation must be made as to the exact amount of fluid withdrawn, and the character, color, and consistency of the fluid.

THORACENTESIS

Thoracentesis is the removal of fluid from the chest or pleural cavity, to determine the cause of pleurisy or of an excess accumulation of fluid (by study of a small quantity of it in the laboratory for diagnostic purposes); to relieve the patient of pain, dyspnea, and other symptoms produced by the accumulation of fluid; to promote absorption of fluid and to instill a drug such as penicillin for its direct local effect on the causative organism.

Fluid will not flow, by gravity, from the pleural cavity, since

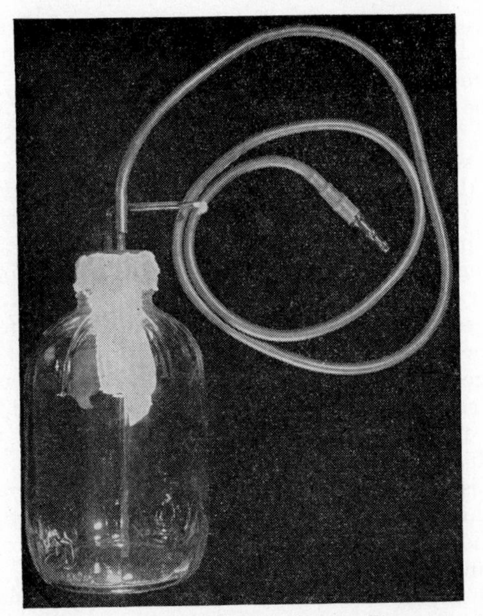

Fig. 224. Chest suction set— single. (Nursing Service Department, New England Center Hospital, Boston, Massachusetts.)

pressure in that cavity is subatmospheric, and it is necessary to use a suction apparatus to withdraw the fluid. The doctor will decide whether he wishes to use a needle and syringe or suction pump and bottle for the procedure.

So the fluid will collect in the lower part of the cavity the patient is asked to assume a sitting position. The patient too ill to sit up may recline on his unaffected side, resting against the backrest in a sitting position. The nurse should make certain that the patient is well supported and that he is comfortable in the elevated position required for the treatment.

Equipment necessary for the procedure includes the rubber sheets to protect the bed, an additional supply of rubber protected pillows, sterile gown, gloves and powder for the doctor, and sterile towels or fenestrated sheet for draping. For administration of the local anesthetic, a hypodermic syringe with hypodermic and intramuscular needles will be needed, as well as the anesthetic solution.

Aspirating needles of various size must be provided, and a trocar, a sharp pointed scalpel, a large syringe (20–30 cc. size), a large collection bottle and rubber cork with two holes to which rubber tubing is attached. One end of the rubber tubing fits the aspirating needle and the other is attached to the suction pump which creates a vacuum in the bottle into which fluid will be withdrawn from the chest. A stopcock to control the flow of fluid and the suction apparatus should be placed on each piece of rubber tubing.

A sterile medicine glass with solution of sterile water or normal saline will be needed to use in testing the apparatus. When the end of the tubing to be attached to the aspirating needle is placed in the medicine glass of solution and the stopcock opened, water should be drawn from the glass to the collecting bottle, demonstrating that the apparatus is properly set up and ready for withdrawing fluid from the chest cavity.

If the syringe method is to be used a 50-cc. Luer syringe, three-way stopcock, piece of rubber tubing sufficiently long to reach from the aspirating needle to the collecting bottle, and a graduate container for measuring the fluid will be needed.

The syringe method is not very satisfactory since it is slow and requires greater effort on the part of the doctor who must detach, empty and readjust the syringe without undue movement of the aspirating needle which would cause pain to the patient.

If a drug is to be instilled into the pleural cavity after fluid has been withdrawn, an additional sterile syringe and needle will be needed. If the drug is to be diluted a second sterile medicine glass should be provided.

Equipment should also include a sterile hypodermic syringe and needle and a stimulant which might be needed for use in treating complications that may occur during the procedure.

About half an hour before thoracentesis a narcotic is usually given the patient to lessen pain and discomfort and to prevent shock.

While the doctor is scrubbing his hands the nurse should assist the patient to the required sitting position and see that he is made comfortable. The arm of the affected side should be held forward with the hand resting on the opposite shoulder. The position must be such that there is no strain or exertion required in maintaining it.

Top covers on the bed should be draped securely around the patient's hips and buttocks, and arms and chest should be covered with a bath blanket. If the feet are resting on a chair to help support the patient in a sitting position, feet and legs should be covered with a blanket. The rubber treatment sheet should be adjusted so the bed is fully protected.

The tray containing equipment for skin preparation and the tray used for the procedure should be placed within easy reach of the doctor. He should then be assisted into sterile gown and gloves. The nurse may prepare the skin, using equipment and antiseptic provided for that purpose. If the skin is prepared by the doctor, it should be done before he is gowned and gloved for the sterile procedure. After sterile drapes are applied, the doctor may proceed with injection of the local anesthetic agent.

As soon as the surface area has been anesthetized the intramuscular needle is used to inject the anesthetic agent into deeper tissues of the area. While the anesthetic is taking effect, the suction apparatus may

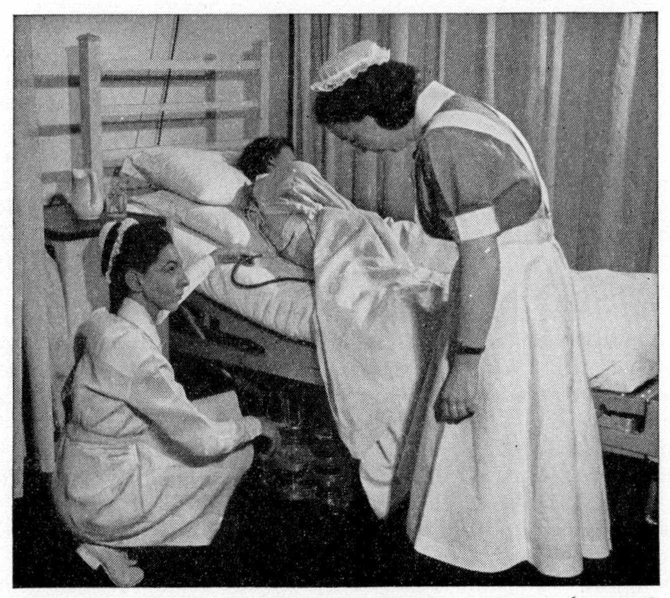

Fig. 225. Learning to adjust the chest suction apparatus. (Massachusetts General Hospital School of Nursing, Boston, Massachusetts.)

be tested to see that it functions properly. The doctor may attach the aspirating needle to the large syringe and insert the needle into the scapular or midaxillary line. In inserting the needle, the plunger of the syringe is pulled back frequently until the appearance of fluid in the syringe indicates that the needle has penetrated the pleural cavity.

Sufficient fluid is withdrawn into the syringe to be used for specimens. The syringe is then detached from the aspirating needle (the open end of the needle being covered by the doctor's thumb to prevent entrance of air into the pleural cavity), and the suction apparatus, by means of the rubber tubing with metal adapter, is attached to the aspirating needle. The stopcock is opened and fluid is withdrawn into the collecting bottle until the desired amount has been obtained. The doctor determines, by condition of the patient, the amount of fluid to be removed. Initial treatments produce 500–1000 cc., and after frequent aspiration as much as 3000 cc. may be withdrawn.

If the patient feels faint, begins to cough and expectorate, or complains of severe pain and discomfort, the treatment should be discontinued. As soon as the fluid is removed, if a drug is to be instilled, it should be injected slowly into the cavity by a syringe attached to the aspirating needle. The procedure is then terminated by withdrawal of the aspirating needle and application of a sterile dressing over the puncture wound.

The nurse should observe the patient carefully throughout the treatment for symptoms of complications which may arise, although the patient should never be made aware of the fact that her concern and watchfulness is more than routine observation to insure his comfort and relief following the operative procedure.

Complications which may occur as a result of thoracentesis include hemorrhage, due to the inadvertent puncturing of a blood vessel, and collapse of the lung, caused by air entering the pleural cavity. Either of these complications would require termination of the procedure and administration of a narcotic or sedative to keep the patient at rest. Pleural shock is a rare complication that has been known to occur, and the nurse must realize the possibility and be prepared to give the indicated treatment. It is thought to be caused by irritation of the pleura from the aspirating needle, resulting in a sudden rapid fall of blood pressure. The immediate injection of 1:1000 solution of Adrenalin helps overcome the unfavorable condition produced by pleural shock.

After completion of the procedure, the patient should be made comfortable; he should be kept warm and dry and encouraged to rest and sleep while he is closely watched for several hours. The usual benefits derived from the treatment are relief from pain and lessened difficulty in breathing.

The fluid withdrawn during the procedure should be placed in test tubes or in a specimen bottle, properly labeled, and sent to the laboratory for examination.

ARTIFICIAL PNEUMOTHORAX

Pneumothorax is the term used to designate collapse of a lung. When this condition is brought about intentionally by the introduction of air or nitrogen gas into the pleural cavity the partial or complete collapse of the lung which results is termed *artificial pneumothorax*. This treatment is used when infection, such as pulmonary tuberculosis, is limited to one lung or when there is a large lesion or cavity in the lung.

Collapse of the lung provides complete rest for the affected area and enables the damaged tissue to begin regenerative processes. It may be necessary to repeat the procedure at frequent intervals to maintain the desired amount of collapse. If the patient finds it inconvenient to report for treatment at frequent intervals oleothorax may be performed, with injection of sterile cottonseed oil instead of air, as it is absorbed much more slowly and keeps the lung collapsed for a longer time.

ASPIRATION OF THE PERICARDIUM

Pericardial aspiration is the removal of fluid from the membranous sac (pericardium) enveloping the heart. This procedure is rarely undertaken, except in extreme necessity, because of its hazards for the patient. It is usually done for diagnostic purposes, as in the case of suspected purulent pericarditis, and as a therapeutic measure for acute cardiac compression.

Equipment used for aspiration of the pericardium is essentially the same as that for thoracentesis. Usually the amount of fluid withdrawn is so slight that the aspiration can be performed satisfactorily with a large syringe and an aspirating needle.

The patient, who is invariably showing symptoms of dyspnea, should be placed on his back then elevated by means of the backrest to a sitting position. To relieve pain a preoperative narcotic may be administered. Oxygen should be available for use if necessary during the treatment. Pillows should be used to provide maximum comfort for the patient, and if he is aware of his surroundings the nurse should reassure him as to the benefit to be derived from the treatment. The procedure should be explained to him and every effort made to relieve mental stress as well as physical discomfort.

Pericardial aspiration is performed in much the same manner as that of thoracentesis with the anterior chest of the patient prepared for the site of operation. The prescribed dosage of a cardiac stimulant should be measured into a hypodermic syringe and kept ready for use in event it is needed. After the procedure has been completed the patient should be closely watched for some time. Care of the specimen is the same as for thoracentesis.

ASPIRATION OF A JOINT

Arthrotomy is the removal of fluid from a joint. Although it is usually done for diagnostic purposes only, it is sometimes performed to relieve pain caused by pressure of fluid within the joint space.

The most desirable position in which to place the patient for arthrotomy will depend on his general physical condition and on location of the joint to be aspirated.

The equipment needed and the procedure to be followed is the same as that used for aspiration of the chest for diagnostic purposes. The amount of fluid to be removed can usually be withdrawn satisfactorily by syringe and aspirating needle.

If the knee joint is aspirated an elastic pressure bandage should be applied over the sterile dressing to hold the dressing in place and prevent reaccumulation of fluid in the joint space.

ABDOMINAL PARACENTESIS

An excessive collection of fluid in the abdominal or peritoneal cavity is termed *ascites*. The fluid may be removed by means of a trocar and cannula in an operative procedure referred to as abdominal paracentesis. It is performed usually to relieve the patient of discomfort caused by pressure created by the excess amount of fluid. Ascitic

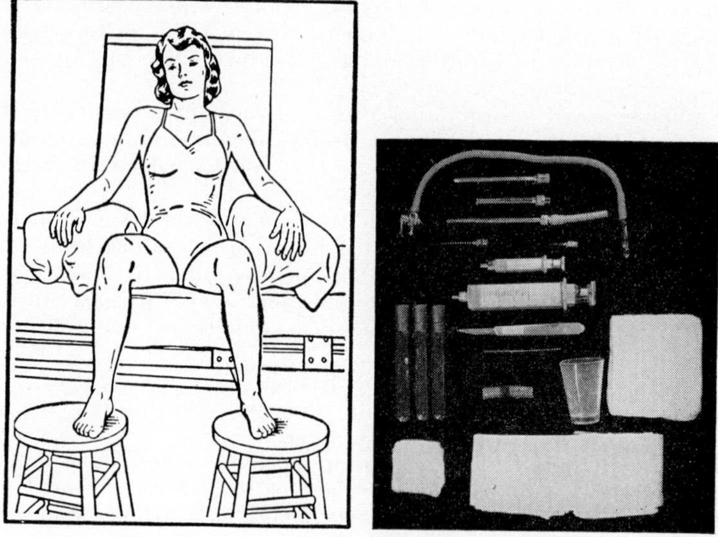

Fig. 226. Fig. 227.

Fig. 226. For paracentesis the patient should be placed in a sitting position. (M. C. Winters, Protective Body Mechanics in Daily Life and in Nursing.)
Fig. 227. Tray for paracentesis. (Nursing Service Department, New England Center Hospital, Boston, Massachusetts.)

fluid may be removed for diagnostic purposes, although this is seldom the primary reason for abdominal paracentesis.

The equipment needed will include the articles and antiseptic for cleansing and disinfecting the skin; sterile gown and gloves for the doctor; rubber treatment sheet to protect the patient's clothing; sterile towels or sheet and towel clips for draping; sterile hypodermic syringe with hypodermic and intramuscular needles; 1 per cent Novocain for use as a local anesthetic agent; a pointed scalpel, trocar and cannula, and rubber tubing properly equipped with an adapter. The sterile dressing and tubes or bottles for specimens should be ready for use when needed.

Large bottles or pails in which the fluid may be collected should also be provided. The amount of fluid usually withdrawn ranges from 2000 to 4000 cc., but if the procedure is postponed until a large amount of fluid has accumulated as much as 10–12 quarts may be obtained.

If the incision is to be closed after the procedure a needle holder, forceps, scissors, skin needle, and silk sutures will be needed.

An abdominal binder with a hole in the front of it should be ready for use when intra-abdominal pressure is great and the amount of fluid to be removed may exceed 3 quarts.

The patient should void before the procedure is started since there is danger of puncturing a distended urinary bladder in paracentesis. If the patient is unable to void, that fact should be reported to the doctor who may order catheterization as part of the preoperative preparation. If an excessive amount of fluid is to be removed the abdominal binder should be applied, the hole in the binder being placed over the site of operation. To offset pressure changes resulting from removal of large quantities of fluid which may produce symptoms of collapse, the binder can be tightened as the fluid is withdrawn, keeping pressure on the abdominal organs somewhat stabilized. Pressure from the binder will, to some extent, lessen the otherwise rapid reduction of pressure from the withdrawal of fluid, which could cause an unpleasant sensation of weakness and exhaustion.

For abdominal paracentesis the patient should be placed in a sitting position, preferably in an arm chair with feet resting on the floor, or seated on the edge of the bed, legs separated, with each foot resting on a stool or on the rung of a chair. A bath blanket should be draped about the patient's chest, back, and shoulders to protect him from drafts.

The procedure should be explained to the patient to insure his complete cooperation.

With the patient seated in a chair a protective rubber sheet should be arranged over his lap in such a way that it will not interfere with the placing of a large pail or bottle between his feet to receive the flow of fluid.

A low stool should be placed in front of the patient so the doctor may be seated to perform the procedure. The skin is prepared, drapes arranged, and local anesthesia injected as in other aspiration procedures. The doctor then makes the incision and inserts the trocar and cannula. When the trocar is removed, the fluid gushes from the cannula, and through the tubing attached to it by the adapter then flows into the pail. By compressing the tubing the rate of flow can be regulated. Fluid should be drained from the abdominal cavity rather slowly to avoid shock and discomfort to the patient. If no undesirable reaction appears, the entire amount of accumulated fluid may be withdrawn.

When the paracentesis is completed the cannula is removed and the incision is closed with one or more sutures. The sterile dressing is applied and an abdominal binder fastened securely in place.

If the incision is not sutured, a large absorbent dressing should be placed over the wound and the abdominal binder fastened in place, to support the abdomen until the intra-abdominal organs have adjusted to the change in pressure caused by withdrawal of the fluid.

The patient should be encouraged to rest for a few hours after the treatment and should be closely observed during that time. Specimens should be correctly labeled and sent to the laboratory.

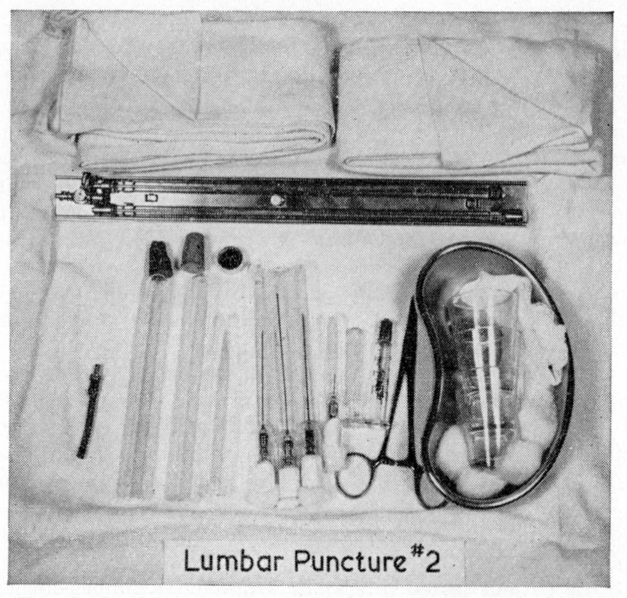

Fig. 228. Tray for lumbar puncture. (Central Supply, Hospital for Sick Children, Toronto, Canada.)

LUMBAR PUNCTURE

Lumbar puncture is the insertion of a hollow needle into the subarachnoid space for removal of spinal fluid from the spinal canal. This may be done to relieve pain and discomfort caused by pressure, for diagnostic purposes, to obtain a reading of spinal fluid pressure in order to know the intracranial tension, to determine the presence of an obstruction in circulation of the cerebrospinal fluid, or for such purposes as introduction of a drug to produce spinal anesthesia, introduction of air, oxygen, or an opaque dye to permit roentgen visualization of the brain or cord, or introduction of a drug, such as penicillin, for treatment of an infection of the central nervous system. When the needle is inserted into the subarachnoid space at the base of the brain, the procedure is termed cisternal puncture.

Equipment needed for lumbar puncture includes the articles and antiseptic solution used in cleansing and disinfecting the skin; the rubber treatment sheet to protect the bed; sterile towels or sheet for draping; sterile gown and gloves for the doctor; 1 per cent Novocain to be used for local anesthesia; syringe and needles for injecting the anesthetic agent; puncture needles (these needles are 19 or 20 gauge and are approximately 3½ inches long); a spinal fluid manometer (a device made up of a hollow glass cylinder graduated in millimeters of water or mercury, to be attached with a metal adapter to the lumbar puncture needle for registering the pressure as the spinal fluid flows into it); the sterile dressing to be placed over the puncture wound after the procedure is completed; and the collecting tubes for specimens.

Sight of the tray with these articles of equipment may cause the patient to be apprehensive or worried and the nurse will need to reassure him by again mentioning benefits to be derived from the treatment.

To insure adequate separation of the spinous processes and to widen the intervertebral space so the needle may readily be inserted the patient must be placed in proper position. For lumbar puncture the patient should be in a recumbent position, lying on one side with head and shoulders bent forward and downward and knees drawn up toward the chest. The curved back should extend along the edge of the bed, thus presenting a desirable working area for the doctor. A reasonable adult patient may maintain the proper position by clasping his hands together under his knees. An irresponsible adult or a child should be placed in the proper position and a rolled sheet or other restraint tied around the back of his neck and under his knees to help maintain the position.

The skin preparation, draping, and injection of local anesthetic is the same as for other aspiration procedures.

The doctor inserts the puncture needle, and when the subarachnoid space has been entered the stylet is withdrawn from the needle; if no fluid appears, the stylet is reinserted, the needle pushed gently forward, and the stylet again withdrawn. If there is still no fluid, the needle should be withdrawn and another puncture site chosen.

When fluid begins to drop from the needle, the first manometric pressure reading should be taken. Other readings will be taken according to the wishes of the doctor.

If compression of the jugular veins is necessary for pressure readings the doctor will instruct the nurse as to her part in the procedure. Pressure on the jugular veins increases intracranial tension by cutting off venous return from the brain and thus increasing cerebral venous pressure. Normally strain following jugular pressure produces an immediate rise in spinal fluid pressure followed by rapid return to the initial pressure as soon as jugular pressure is released. If pressure on the jugular vein fails to produce an immediate rise in spinal fluid pressure or if, after a rise, the return to the initial pressure is delayed, the presence of an obstruction in the circulation of the cerebrospinal fluid is made apparent.

After manometric pressure readings are completed specimens are collected.

If a drug is to be instilled an additional amount of spinal fluid should be withdrawn (the total amount of fluid withdrawn should equal the amount of fluid or drug to be instilled) and the drug injected. The drug should be in sterile liquid form and should be permitted to flow, by gravity, into the subarachnoid space.

During the procedure the nurse should closely observe the patient for signs of pallor, nausea, or dizziness. Any change in color, pulse, respiration, or mental attitude should be reported immediately to the doctor. The doctor should prescribe the amount of activity to be allowed, the position in bed to be maintained, and the length of time the patient must be kept quiet. The nurse should explain the doctor's instructions in regard to curtailed activity and position to the patient, and make sure that he is comfortable. Specimens should be labeled and sent to the laboratory.

Care of Equipment after Use

All equipment used for aspiration of any body cavity should be removed to the utility room, thoroughly cleaned, reassembled, tested and sent to central supply to be prepared for sterilization and use again.

Summary of Important Factors

Body cavities normally contain sufficient fluid to protect the organs they contain. In some disease conditions the amount of fluid is abnormally increased and must be removed.

Causes of fluid accumulation include inflammation, tumorous growths, and impairment of circulation.

Aspiration is done as an aseptic procedure; duties of the nurse include reassuring the patient, assembling needed equipment, placing patient in proper position, preparation of the skin, assisting the doctor, care of specimens, after-care of equipment used, and close observation of the patient during and after treatment.

Thoracentesis, removal of fluid from the chest, is done for diagnostic purposes, to relieve pain and dyspnea, or to instill a drug.

It is necessary to use suction to withdraw fluid from the chest. The doctor determines by the condition of the patient the amount of fluid to be withdrawn.

The treatment should be discontinued if the patient feels faint, coughs, expectorates, or complains of pain. Possible complications are hemorrhage, collapse of lung, or pleural shock.

Specimens should be correctly labeled and sent to the laboratory.

Patient should be closely watched for evidence of complications.

Artificial pneumothorax, intentional collapse of a lung, to provide complete rest for that organ.

Aspiration of pericardium, removal of fluid from pericardial sac enveloping the heart, is done usually for diagnostic purposes.

Aspiration of a joint, arthrotomy, is removal of fluid from a joint.

Abdominal paracentesis, removal of fluid from the abdominal cavity, is usually done to relieve discomfort. 2000–4000 cc. may be withdrawn.

Patient should be placed in a sitting position, and an abdominal binder should be used for support during and after treatment. The incision may be sutured or left free to drain.

Lumbar Puncture, removal of fluid from spinal canal; done to relieve pain or discomfort, for diagnostic purposes, to determine spinal fluid pressure, or to introduce a drug into the subarachnoid space.

The patient must be placed in proper position for the procedure. If a drug is to be instilled, the total amount of fluid withdrawn should equal the amount of drug to be used. A sudden change in the patient's condition requires that the procedure be discontinued. The care of the specimen and the after-care of the patient are essentially the same as for other aspiration procedures.

Factors To Teach the Patient

That his cooperation is necessary in maintaining correct position throughout the procedure so that best results will be obtained.

That pain and discomfort caused by the treatment may prevent greater pain and more discomfort later in the progress of the disease.

That doctors and nurses will be as gentle as possible and cause only a minimum amount of pain during the procedure.

That he must refrain from involuntary movement when the needle or trocar is introduced, since such movement may cause unnecessary pain or trauma.

That he must follow instructions in regard to activity after treatment, whether he is to remain in a horizontal position in bed or to walk about if he so desires.

That every effort is being made to insure his safety and comfort if complications should occur.

That the procedure is important for diagnosis or for continued treatment of the disease condition for which he is hospitalized.

Scientific Principles

Anatomy and Physiology. The size of the various body cavities determines the amount of serous fluid they normally contain.

Spinal fluid serves chiefly as a buffer or protective medium for the central nervous system.

Chemistry. Fluid associated with inflammation, termed an exudate, is usually of high specific gravity and white cell content; it varies in consistency from watery to purulent. If the inflammation is caused by infection bacteria may be present in the fluid.

Fluid not associated with inflammation, termed a transudate, is usually of low specific gravity and white cell content; it is usually a sterile fluid, either clear or slightly cloudy.

Microbiology. In handling test tubes or other collecting equipment for body fluids care must be taken not to contaminate the inside;

contamination of the outside of collecting equipment by fluid being withdrawn from the body cavity should also be avoided. Serous membranes are highly susceptible to bacteria, so procedures involving removal of serous fluids should be done with aseptic technique. The doctor should wear sterile gloves, instruments should be sterile, and sterile drapes should be used.

Many bacteria are found on the skin. A needle introduced through the skin for removal of fluid from a cavity must be sterile, and the skin should be treated with an antiseptic solution before the needle is inserted.

Cold inhibits the growth of bacteria, so fluids removed for diagnostic purposes should be kept at low temperature.

Pharmacology. In aspiration of body cavities, procaine is used to anesthetize the site of puncture.

Drugs, such as penicillin, that are not absorbed by spinal fluid from the blood, must be injected directly into the subarachnoid space.

Physics. In pneumothorax, limiting the activity of the lung, the transfer area for oxygen and carbon dioxide is greatly decreased.

Withdrawal of fluid from body cavities is dependent on differences in pressure. All confined body fluids, except fluid in the pleural cavity, are under greater pressure than atmospheric pressure, so the fluid flows out when a needle or trocar is introduced. A syringe or suction device is needed to withdraw fluid from the pleural cavity.

Pressure within a body cavity can be measured in millimeters of mercury or in centimeters of water. Measurements can be converted from water to mercury or vice versa as mercury is 13 times heavier than water.

Psychology. The nurse may need to give additional explanation of the procedure to the patient even though the reasons for and nature of the treatment have been explained by the doctor. Cooperation of the patient will be needed and he should be instructed as to what he is expected to do, as maintaining correct position and remaining immobile during the treatment. If the treatment is apt to be painful, the patient should be so informed, although reassurance should be given that every effort will be made to reduce his pain or discomfort.

By remaining close to the patient during the treatment the nurse can help him maintain the correct position and her presence helps to reassure him.

Privacy should be provided the patient who is undergoing an aspirating procedure.

Sociology. Specimens may be sent through the mail to local or state departments of health.

Situation Type Problems

1. A young man who was to undergo a lumbar puncture as part of the diagnostic procedures being done for him was very apprehensive

about the treatment. He expressed fear at the pain he would experience and requested that the procedure be postponed. The graduate nurse assigned to his care told him he "shouldn't be such a baby" and that "the treatment won't hurt you, anyway."

The patient asked a student nurse caring for the patient in an adjoining bed if she had ever assisted with such a treatment and if it had been painful for the patient. The student was explaining the procedure to the patient, indicating how it would be of benefit to him and offering reassurance that care would be taken to minimize pain and discomfort during the treatment. The graduate nurse returned to the ward in time to hear the concluding part of the explanation. She reprimanded the student for "interfering" and for "coddling" the patient. What would you have done?

2. A student nurse assisting with abdominal paracentesis called the doctor's attention to the fact that he had contaminated the rubber gloves he wore by handling an unsterile piece of equipment. The doctor changed gloves without comment, but complained of the nurse's inefficiency in assembling proper equipment for the procedure, said that she had placed the patient in an improper position, objected to the antiseptic prepared for use in cleansing the skin (although he had used it numerous times for other such treatments without objection), and finally reported to the head nurse that the student was not to be assigned to assist him again with any similar treatment. What would you have done?

Suggested Reference Reading

"A paracentesis drape," Elizabeth Reynolds, R.N. and Elizabeth Nielson, R.N.; American Journal of Nursing, March, 1949.

"Blood donor sets for thoracentesis," What's New, March, 1952.

"Hazards of lumbar puncture," Robert D. Dripps and Leroy D. Vandam; Digest of Treatments, April, 1952.

PART VI

Procedures for Advanced Clinical Study

CHAPTER 37

Spiritual Needs of the Patient

TOPICAL OUTLINE

EMOTIONS INDICATING SPIRITUAL NEEDS
- Apprehension—Fear—Loneliness
- Anxiety and Worry
- Feelings of Guilt and Hostility

SIGNS OF SPIRITUAL NEEDS

HOW TO MEET SPIRITUAL NEEDS
- By Listening
- By Reassurance
- By Emotional Adjustment to Disability
- By Books, Visitors, and Other Means
- By a Call from a Clergyman
- By Use of the Bible and by Prayer

RELIGIOUS MINISTRATIONS OF EACH FAITH
- The Protestant Patient
- Other Denominations and Faiths
- The Jewish Patient
- The Roman Catholic Patient

RELIGIOUS HOLIDAYS AND HOLY DAYS

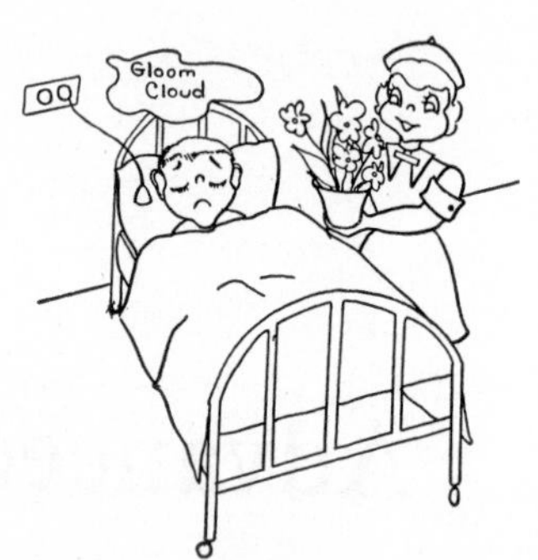

The patient who looks as though he cannot smile is the one most in need of the smile you can give him.

Because sickness and death have much in them that is primitive in nature, patients may frequently ask fundamental questions pertaining to both. Persons who have given little or no thought to religion while well and active may become much concerned in time of illness, and may turn to the nurse with doubts and conflicts and the need for reassurance and for spiritual help.

The patient who faces a crisis, such as impending operation, or expectation of becoming critically ill, does not need intellectual answers to some of his religious doubts or questionings so much as he may need a sense of understanding and assistance from the nurse in supplying spiritual needs and advising him of various religious resources that are available. Some patients may have developed an attitude toward religion which precludes help from a clergyman. The doctor may have little or no opportunity to offer spiritual aid, since the time he can spend with the patient is limited. The nurse, however, remains with

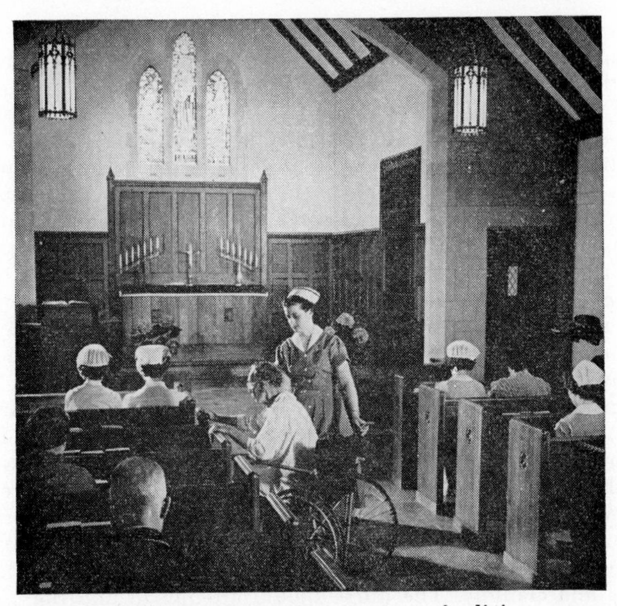

Fig. 229. Nurses as well as patients take advantage of religious resources of the hospital. (Wesley Hospital School of Nursing, Witchita, Kansas.)

the patient to perform essential nursing care and may offer, through her own faith and understanding, strength and encouragement to the patient.

In the course of routine duties the nurse will need to cooperate with ministers of religion who will visit patients of their church. She should be aware of her responsibilities in certain religious rites which may be required for patients in her care, and she will find constant renewal of her own faith and belief in observance of religious practices.

If the nurse understands the very close relationship between religion and the emotions she will be better able to understand the needs of the patient. By observing the emotional manifestations of the patient she may be able to accurately determine the form of spiritual ministration which will be of most benefit to him.

EMOTIONS INDICATING SPIRITUAL NEEDS

Apprehension. The patient hospitalized for the first time may be apprehensive about the strangeness of the surroundings, the very different daily routine, and the kind of care and attention he will receive.

Fear. The hospitalized patient may find many things to fear in his immediate situation. He may be afraid that the surgical procedure will endanger his life. He may be fearful of the anesthetic agent, dreading the experience of going to sleep under anesthesia and thinking of the possibility of not waking from that sleep, and the thought of dying may produce real terror.

If the patient is afraid of pain and of physical discomfort which may follow an operation he may be greatly reassured by a thoughtful nurse who takes time to explain to him that pain and discomfort can be controlled through the judicious use of morphine or other opiates.

The patient may be unduly modest and fearful of being embarrassed during the physical examination. If, at some time during his life, he had a venereal disease, he will fear that the fact will become generally known to hospital personnel. Such patients need to be reminded that doctors and nurses are usually impersonal in their reactions and view each patient objectively rather than emotionally

The patient may fear that he will be disabled because of illness or surgery. He may fear loss of sight or hearing, disfigurement of face or body, or impairment of body function. If such fears are expressed the nurse should understand the significance of the emotional reaction and do what she can to reassure the patient.

Fear and apprehension may be recognized by physical signs such as restlessness, tenseness of facial expression, dry mouth, and hands that are cold and clammy. The nurse should attempt to find the cause of the fear and then help the patient to overcome it.

Loneliness. Loneliness is one of the emotional factors which, at various times during an illness, will be felt by all patients. The sudden change from the familiar surroundings of home to the totally unfamiliar environment of the hospital adds to the feeling of strangeness, helplessness, and loneliness of the patient. Quite often hospital restrictions in regard to visiting hours and the necessity for friends and relatives to continue their own daily routine with only occasional visits to the hospital increases the loneliness of the patient. Loneliness, in turn, can lead to increased awareness of pain and discomfort, and cause the patient to change from an attitude of cooperation and hopefulness to one of discouragement and despair. The lonely patient is apt to be a "difficult" patient who finds fault with treatments being given, with food served at mealtime, and with the nursing care he receives. He is also a demanding patient, making numerous requests that are often unnecessary and therefore irritating to the nurse.

Understanding of the patient's need for companionship and an effort by the nurse to see him frequently throughout the day or to provide an occasional visitor in the person of another patient may relieve the feeling of loneliness and improve the mental and physical condition of the patient.

The nurse who avoids the unpleasant or disagreeable patient, who goes into his room only when summoned and then approaches the bedside with obvious reluctance and stays for only the few minutes needed to supply physical needs has little understanding of the emo-

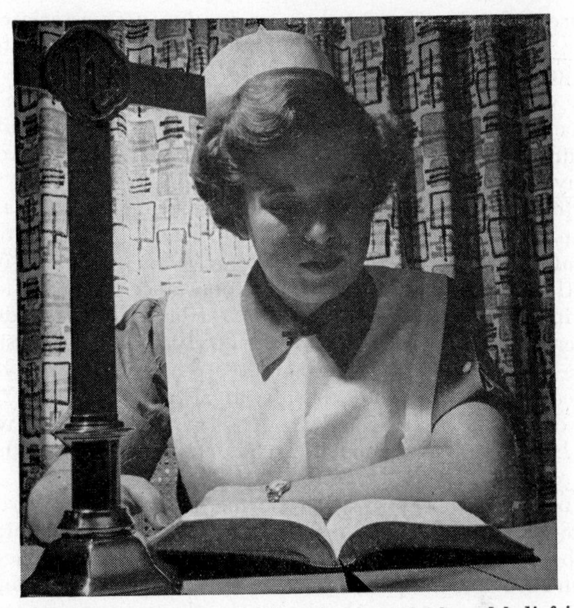

Fig. 230. The nurse may need to call on her own faith and belief in order to understand and help the patient. (Presbyterian Hospital School of Nursing, Chicago, Illinois.)

tional stress which is causing the patient to be disagreeable and uncooperative. His need of her time and attention may be greater than that of an acutely ill patient, even though his physical condition does not necessitate continuous nursing care.

The convalescent patient may be lonely because of the different situations imposed by convalescence and because as his physical condition improves he requires less medical attention and less nursing care, and sees doctors and nurses less often. His friends and relatives who came often during the critical stage of his illness spend less time with him. The nurse should understand this inevitable occurrence and should encourage the patient to become interested in various means of recreation, such as reading, radio, or television, or finding new companions among the other patients in the clinical service department.

Anxiety and Worry. Anxiety is closely related to apprehension and fear. Patients often tend to become unduly concerned about themselves. They are anxious about the outcome of their present illness. They worry about the effect of their illness on the financial budget. Absence from their job may cause great concern, not only because of loss of pay but because of the very real possibility that the job itself may be lost to them.

They quite often worry about other patients in the ward, or show great concern for family members or for business associates. Their anxiety, may be without foundation and cause, but can interfere with recovery just as effectively as if wholly justified.

Feelings of Guilt and Hostility. It is not unusual for a patient to relate his current illness and pain to some real or imagined offense of the past and to interpret the condition as a punishment. An offense which may have been of little concern to the person against whom it was directed, such as the theft of a small sum of money or a lie told to an employer, may seem of major importance to the patient and cause great mental stress because of the feelings of guilt which have resulted. If the matter seems of major importance to the patient, it *is* of major importance, and the nurse should be prepared to deal with the problem as part of the total responsibility in giving nursing care.

Patients with feelings of guilt are tense and anxious. They may question each procedure and consider it a potential cause for more pain and discomfort. They lack the sense of humor which would do much to help them overcome their tendency to increase their own mental stresses.

Illness requiring hospitalization can be, and often is, a frustrating experience for the patient. The mounting doctor and hospital bills, anxiety about the outcome of the illness, and pain and physical weakness all tend to make the patient resentful, irritable, and uncooperative. The nurse who understands the reason for the patient's attitude, even though it be one of animosity directed toward herself, must call on her own spiritual resources to refrain from reacting toward the patient with the same degree of hostility. To counter hostility with sympathetic understanding is the first step toward bringing needed spiritual help to the patient.

SIGNS OF SPIRITUAL NEEDS

The observant and interested nurse will soon learn to recognize physical signs which indicate that the patient needs and would probably welcome spiritual help.

The apprehensive or fearful patient may show the mental stress he is undergoing by facial expression, restlessness, and other physical signs. Help may be given him by a clergyman of his church, a friend, or a relative. Quite often a patient convalescing from a surgical procedure may bring peace of mind to the patient facing that crisis.

The patient who is lonely may indicate the need for companionship or for a person interested in his welfare through comments that show discouragement and despair, such as "What's the use?" or "Why bother?" Frequent tears or moods of depression, even disobeyance of routine regulations in the ward, may indicate that the patient feels alone and friendless. The nurse should see such patients frequently and encourage family and friends to visit them often.

The nurse who maintains an attitude of cheerfulness and obvious

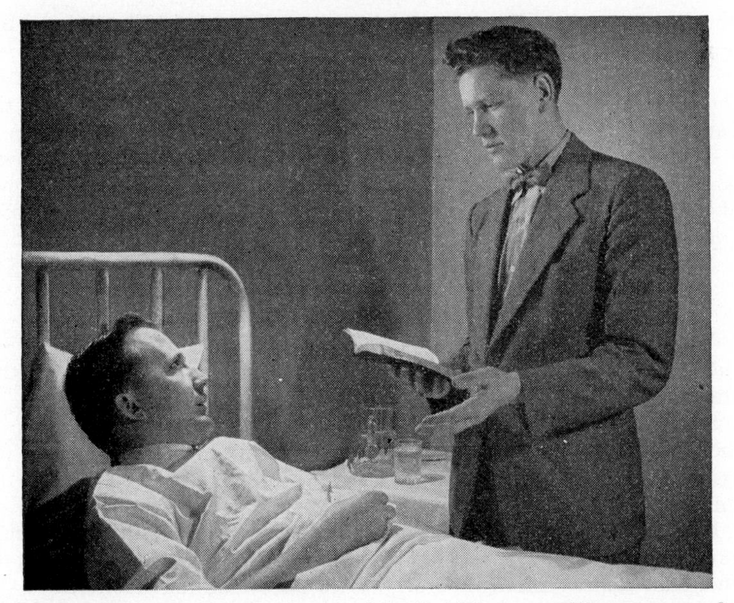

Fig. 231. The patient may ask for spiritual aid in many different ways that are readily apparent to the understanding nurse. (Moody Bible Institute, Chicago, Illinois.)

good will toward the patient who is unpleasant or abusive has learned well one of the basic requirements in answering spiritual needs of the patient. The patient with feelings of guilt may display resentment and aggressiveness. He is apt to be hypercritical and complaining. The statement "I don't know why this had to happen to me!" or similar remarks are a strong indication of feelings of guilt.

Other signs of the spiritual needs of patients may be found in their remarks and questions. The patient who asks the nurse for a Bible, uses religious terms in speaking, and asks about the practice of ministers or priests who come to the hospital to call on members of their congregation may be indicating a wish for spiritual help. The nurse may encourage the patient by offering to get in touch with his clergyman, or, if he isn't a member of a local church, by suggesting that he might enjoy meeting a clergyman who is frequently in the hospital. She may advise the patient that a hospital Chaplain is available and would enjoy seeing him.

The patient who expresses strong resentment toward the church, the minister, and religion in general may be indicating a desire to receive spiritual help. The nurse should never attempt to argue with a patient in regard to religious beliefs or practices, but a challenging statement from the patient opens the way for her to state "I think you would enjoy discussing that with (Reverend, Chaplain, Mr.) Smith. He was expressing some interesting views on that same subject recently, and I'm sure he would be pleased to hear your opinions on the matter." Here also, an offer to have the clergyman call on the patient may be made. The patient who is to face a major operation at a set time and says to the nurse, "Think of me at 9 o'clock tomorrow," is probably really asking for her prayers at that time. The response of the nurse who understands may give the patient the renewed faith and strength which is needed.

HOW TO MEET SPIRITUAL NEEDS

When the nurse is able to recognize emotional factors and to see their relationship to religious problems of the patient, she is better able to provide the spiritual help that is needed.

She should know the religious resources within the hospital and the community and the person or persons to whom she can appeal for assistance when needed. The nurse herself may supply some of the spiritual needs of her patients by various means available to her.

By Listening. The patient under stress, if encouraged to talk, may gain some measure of relief since talking is an activity and to talk about an apprehension or worry is to *do* something about it.

There is a difference between encouraging talk and probing into the depths of a patient's thoughts. The nurse lacks the skill and understanding needed to benefit the patient who may be under extreme emotional tension and should not attempt such probing. By listening to the patient the nurse helps him realize that others are interested in his welfare and in being of help to him, if possible.

Patients who are not used to praying, or who are not members of a church, may be reluctant to consult a clergyman. The nurse may, merely by letting them talk to her, help relieve their mind of worry and fear and guilt. In listening to a patient the nurse should be non-judicial in her attitude. She should not show shock or disapproval. Even if the patient's opinions are not in agreement with her own she should not pass judgment on him or on his beliefs. The nurse should be sincere in her expression of interest in the patient. Motivated by a real desire to be helpful, she will have no difficulty in finding the right words to comfort and encourage. If she does not like a patient she cannot be helpful to that patient spiritually, no matter how carefully she may listen to what he has to say.

By Reassurance. Most patients respect, admire, and like nurses in general, so they accept each nurse as a person whom they can trust when they must be dependent on her services. The nurse who has authority with the patient can effectively reassure that patient unless stress is so great that stronger measures must be taken. Through reassurance, the nurse attempts to put the patient's mind at ease. Although the reassurance is expressed in words, the emotional rela-

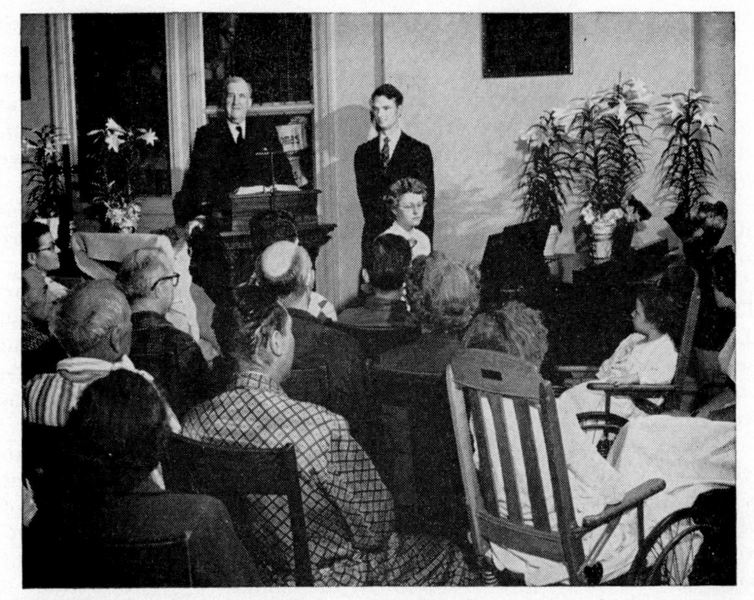

Fig. 232. Attendance at Chapel services may be a source of encouragement and spiritual help to the patient. (Presbyterian Hospital School of Nursing, Chicago, Illinois.)

tionship between nurse and patient may be the major factor in determining its effectiveness.

By Emotional Adjustment to Disability. That which many patients fear may come to pass, and disability may result from illness or injury. It then becomes necessary for the patient to make the emotional adjustment to the impairment or handicap that is sustained.

To adjust satisfactorily, the patient must learn to accept his disability. The nurse quite often is called on to remind the patient that there is a vast difference between *acceptance*, which is compounded of reconstruction and adaptation, and *resignation*, which consists of lying down, quitting, giving up. Through resignation the patient can achieve little more than mere existence as a helpless, hopeless being. Through acceptance he can change, adapt, and learn so that his life once more becomes interesting, meaningful, and worth while. Acceptance and reconstruction may require weeks or months of effort by the patient. His satisfaction in adjusting to the disability may exceed only slightly that felt by the nurse who plays an important part in helping him to adapt to the new physical condition.

By Books, Visitors, and Other Means. The Bible should be available to all patients; even patients who may not ask for it will appreciate the thoughtfulness which prompts a nurse to place it within easy reach. Other books may bring the quietness and serenity needed by patients who have been physically, mentally, and spiritually disturbed. There is something very soothing and restful about a book which brings pleasure when the patient is reading and waits near at hand for hours or days with no indication of becoming impatient, until needed again. Books may quiet the patient's fears and relieve loneliness or boredom.

Visitors are usually relatives or friends, although visits from complete strangers are not unusual and may bring comfort and pleasure to the patient.

Flowers are an important source of spiritual aid for the patient. They serve as messengers of hope and cheer from persons who wish the patient well. They brighten the immediate surroundings and help to keep the patient in an optimistic state of mind. Their fragrance and beauty can be enjoyed by nurses and other hospital personnel, as well as by the patient to whom they are sent.

Mail is as important to the hospital patient as it is to the man in service, and for the same reason. It is a reminder that the recipient is not forgotten at home and that he is still important in the lives of people who mean much to him. Delightful "speedy-recovery" and "get-well-quick" cards are frequently an important part of the decor of patient rooms in hospitals throughout the country.

A sense of humor will help the patient through many trying situations. If he is able to complain about the food in a manner similar to that of the wit who proclaimed "The butter is so strong it can walk over and say 'hello' to the coffee, but the coffee is too weak to answer" instead of voicing a surly complaint to the nurse who serves the food (but has no part in the preparation of it), the atmosphere of the room or ward is one of pleasant good humor and the point is still well made in regard to the food.

The nurse who possesses a sense of humor can boost morale for an entire department of patients. They look forward to the time each day when she will appear on duty and are benefited in many ways just by her presence and her way of counteracting the depression or discouragement which may have affected all or most of them.

By a Call from a Clergyman. A large number of patients who have no definite church affiliation will depend on the physician and the nurse to meet their spiritual as well as physical and mental needs. Doctors are sometimes embarrassed by the use of the vocabulary of religion, yet every doctor who is sincerely interested in the welfare of his patient must minister to spiritual as well as physical needs.

To be helpful to the patient in the matter of religious needs, the nurse should look at the chart to find if he is Protestant, Catholic, or Jewish, and should learn if he has been visited by his minister, priest, or rabbi. If the patient has not been visited, the nurse should ask if the church authority knows of the patient's admission to the hospital. If

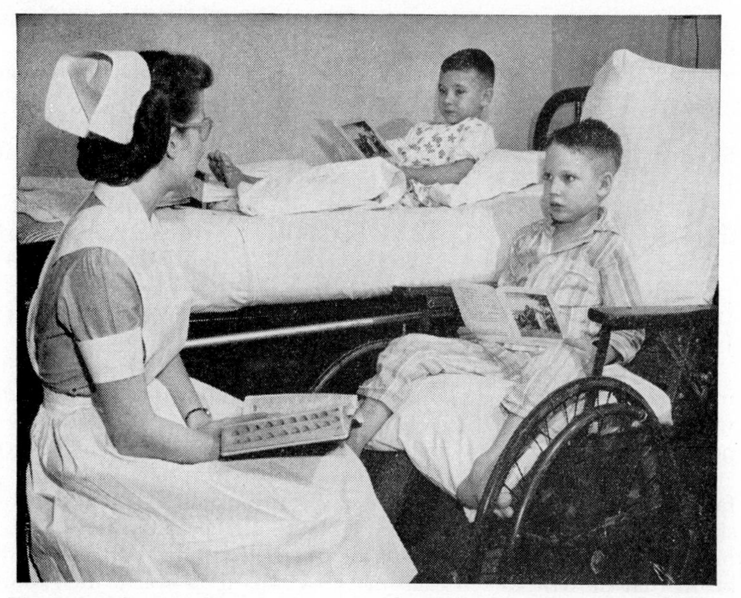

Fig. 233. When small patients are unable to go to Sunday School the nurse may bring Sunday School to them. (Alabama Baptist Hospital School of Nursing, Birmingham, Alabama.)

the patient does not wish to see the minister from his own church, he may request that a minister from another church be asked to call.

If the patient has no church affiliation and no clergyman is calling on him, the nurse should not attempt to take the place of a clergyman but should assume responsibilities in the spiritual realm comparable to those she may have in the medical field. In medicine, the nurse will not attempt to take the place of a doctor, but if she is unable to secure a doctor and the physical need of a patient is urgent she is obligated to do the very best she can for the patient until the doctor arrives. If unable to secure the services of a clergyman for the patient in need of spiritual help, she should do the best she can to meet that need. The manner in which the nurse responds to the signs that spiritual aid is desired may determine the patient's reaction. If she merely asks, "Would you like to see Rev. Smith?" the answer is almost invariably "No." However, if she introduces the clergyman with "Here is someone I want you to meet" or remarks to the patient, "Rev. Smith is visiting the patient in the next room, shall I ask him to stop by just to say 'hello'?" the patient will usually respond in the affirmative and be deeply grateful to the nurse.

By Use of the Bible and by Prayer. The Bible has long been the chief source of religious inspiration for Protestants. Regular readers of the Bible will need little assistance in finding selections which they wish to read. Under certain conditions, the nurse may need to suggest passages which may be most helpful to the patient.

For the patient who is restless, apprehensive, or discouraged, the following selections may effectively meet the need: Psalms 23, 91, and 121; Matthew 6, verses 25–34; and John 14, verses 1–4, and 27.

The person suffering from feelings of guilt may find comfort in the following: Psalms 23, and 121; Matthew 5, verses 21–24, 7, verses 7–8, and 18, verses 21–35; Luke 15, verses 1–7; and John 6, verse 35.

The dying patient may find strength and peace in: Psalms 23, and 121; Matthew 5, verses 1–16; Mark 4, verses 26–32; John 14, verses 1–7; and Revelation 21, verses 1–4.

Prayer has always been the chief instrument of religion. It is the means by which the patient turns his mind from himself to seek the will, mind, and strength of God. If the patient has a real desire to believe in prayer there will be an increase in belief through prayer.

The nurse should not be distressed if a patient professes to have no faith in prayer, in medical science, or in anything. Even the most skeptical person has faith in many things: that the sun will rise tomorrow, that Spring will come after a severe winter, that plants will grow, that he will waken each morning. His presence in the hospital indicates that he has some faith in doctors and nurses and in their ability to help him in his physical needs.

Patients who have not made prayer a part of their daily life may hesitate to pray in illness just because they have failed to pray in health. The nurse should be quick to assure them that the benefit to be derived from prayer is as available to them as to the deeply religious patient. The nurse should have memorized a few prayers which could be used for the patient if the request is made by him. A few such prayers are included here.

The Hail Mary

Hail, Mary, full of grace, the Lord is with thee;
Blessed art thou among women,
And blessed is the fruit of thy womb, Jesus.
Holy Mary, Mother of God, pray for us sinners,
Now and at the hour of our death. AMEN

The Lord's Prayer

Our Father, Who art in heaven,
Hallowed be Thy name; Thy kingdom come,
Thy will be done on earth as it is in heaven.
Give us this day our daily bread,
And forgive us our debts
As we forgive our debtors,

And lead us not into temptation,
But deliver us from evil:
For Thine is the kingdom, and the power, and the glory,
Forever. AMEN

Psalm XXIII

The Lord is my shepherd; I shall not want
He maketh me to lie down in green pastures;
He leadeth me beside still waters,
He restoreth my soul.
He guideth me in straight paths for His name's sake.
Yea, though I walk through the valley of the shadow of death,
I will fear no evil,
For Thou art with me.
Thy rod and Thy staff, they comfort me.
Thou preparest a table before me in the presence of mine enemies;
Thou hast anointed my head with oil, my cup runneth over.
Surely goodness and mercy shall follow me all the days of my life;
And I shall dwell in the house of the Lord forever. AMEN

RELIGIOUS MINISTRATIONS OF EACH FAITH

To meet the spiritual needs of the patient adequately the nurse needs some understanding of the requirements of the different religious faiths. She should feel it her responsibility to help the patient secure all the resources of his particular religion, regardless of her own belief or religious training. No attempt has been made to present detailed information on the various rites and practices of a particular faith. The following, however, should be helpful to the nurse who needs to understand the ministrations of the minister, priest, and rabbi in meeting the needs of patients.

The Protestant Patient. The Protestant denominations include Methodists, Baptists, Presbyterians, Episcopalians, Congregationalists, Reformed, etc. Some members of the various denominations adhere strictly to the customs and rituals of their own group; to others the theological differences among the denominations mean very little. Usually any Protestant minister is acceptable to a patient belonging to any one of the Protestant denominations, and in case of emergency the nurse should call the first Protestant minister who can be reached. For the Protestant patient with deep-rooted convictions his wishes in the matter of choice of ministers should be followed.

Although Protestants are not required to keep rules of fasting and abstinence, many of them do so as part of their own devotional pattern of living. The nurse should be considerate of the patient's wishes, if it is possible to do so without interfering with hospital routine.

General Rules To Be Observed for the Protestant Patient. The hospital chaplain should be notified when the patient is admitted, when a patient is to have surgery, and if he is in a critical condition. Privacy should be provided when the chaplain or minister is with the patient. The clergyman should be called while the patient is still conscious.

Where a chapel is maintained in the hospital convalescent patients and members of the medical and nursing staffs may attend religious services.

Other Denominations and Faiths. Denominations difficult to classify are such groups as Friends or Quakers, Jehovah's Witnesses, and Seventh Day Adventists. Some do not believe in an ordained ministry and a clergyman does not serve in the capacity of a clergyman, although he may be of great service as a counselor or friend. The Seventh Day Adventists keep the Sabbath on Saturday and do not eat pork. It would be impossible to point out all the individual differences, so the nurse is advised to consult the patient's wishes and comply with his requests as much as possible.

There are a number of other churches which are not Protestant and are not Roman Catholic. These comprise three groups: the Eastern Orthodox churches, the non-orthodox eastern churches, and the Western Catholic but non-Roman churches. Members of these various groups should be served by a priest from their own group. A Protestant minister should not be called when sacraments are to be administered. Clergy of all churches in these three groups are known as priests and should be addressed as "Father."

The Jewish Patient. Religious practices or rites which the nurse should understand in caring for the Jewish patient include: dietary laws or regulations, observance of the Sabbath and of Holy days, the rite of circumcision, and care of the deceased.

Patients of the Jewish faith may belong to the Orthodox, Conservative, or Reform group. The non-orthodox or Reformed Jew differs little, in his spiritual needs while in the hospital, from the Protestant who seems not to be deeply religious. The Orthodox Jew is usually non-committal in regard to religious customs and rituals, but will be deeply appreciative of an attitude of respect toward his religious beliefs.

If a Jewish patient has requested that a rabbi be summoned to visit him, the nurse should know to which group the patient belongs and then request that the rabbi of that same group be summoned. If such a rabbi is not available, the nurse may need to refer the request to a local Jewish community center where a rabbi may be contacted.

Dietary Laws or Regulations. Jewish dietary laws permit the eating of the flesh of only those animals that are ruminants and have divided hooves, as cows, sheep, and goats. Among the fowl they may choose chiefly those that are not birds of prey, as chickens, ducks, and turkey. The animals must be slaughtered, dressed, and prepared in a certain prescribed manner which is termed "kosher" or permissible.

Dairy products, fats, oils, and shortenings are kosher if they are derived from the animals mentioned above or from plants or vegetables. No dairy products, with the exception of eggs, should be eaten with or immediately after meat. Meat may be eaten, however, immediately after dairy products have been eaten. Fish that have both fins and scales, such as carp, salmon, and whitefish, are kosher (sanctioned by Jewish law) and need not be killed or dressed in a specially prescribed manner. Fish may be prepared with non-meat shortening and may be eaten with dairy products.

The nurse should avoid, when possible, the serving of pork or pork products to the Jewish patient. Whenever possible, dairy products and vegetables should be substituted for meat in the diet for the patient of Jewish faith. The Jewish patient should understand that he is permitted by Jewish law to deviate from the food restrictions when failure to follow the diet prescribed by his physician would endanger his health. If problems arise with reference to dietary or other religious laws, the nurse should confer with the rabbi on the best method of handling such problems.

Utensils used in preparing and serving non-kosher food should be cleansed in a prescribed manner before being used to prepare or serve kosher food.

The Rite of Circumcision. Circumcision is a religious rite of great importance to members of the Jewish faith. The ceremony and circumcision occurs on the eighth day after the birth of a male child unless for reasons of health the rite must be postponed. Circumcision is performed according to prescribed ritual by a specially trained religious official known as a "Mohel." The nurse may need to consult with the doctor and the rabbi to learn how to prepare for the ritual. A quorum of ten Jewish men, including the male members of the family, should be present during the circumcision ceremony. A room where privacy can be had by the family should be provided for the event. After the circumcision rite a reception and social ceremony is usually held for family and friends. If the Protestant nurse is asked to partake of food and wine at the reception she can hardly refuse without seeming to be prudish and intolerant.

Care of the Deceased. When a Jewish patient has expired and there are no relatives or friends to arrange for burial, the hospital authorities should ask a Jewish organization to arrange for burial in a Jewish cemetery. According to traditional interpretation, autopsies and transplantation of an organ or part are not permitted unless the deceased had given consent before his death.

The Roman Catholic Patient. The nurse who is caring for a patient of the Catholic faith, regardless of her own religious belief, should know the basic factors in the doctrinal background of the Roman Catholic religion. She may be required to assist Catholic chaplains or priests and will be better able to do so if she has some understanding of their beliefs.

The Roman Catholic belief, very briefly stated, is that Jesus Christ was born into the world, lived, suffered, and died for man, who is

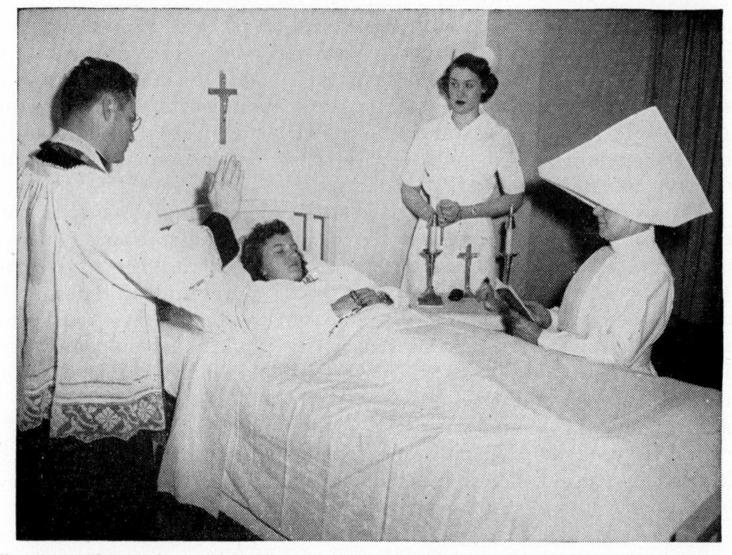

Fig. 234. The Roman Catholic patient is visited by a priest. (St. Vincent's College of Nursing, Los Angeles, California.)

often spiritually sick. He left behind Him the sacraments which are spiritual aids for the soul.

A sacrament contains the power of making the sick soul well, it can clear the soul of sin, and make it spiritually well and spiritually strengthened. Seven sacraments were instituted by Christ: Baptism, Confirmation, Penance, Holy Eucharist, Extreme Unction, Holy Orders, and Matrimony, and they are conferred in His name and by His authority. The sacraments commonly administered in the hospital are Baptism, Penance, Holy Communion, and Extreme Unction. Articles that may be needed include a crucifix, two candles (blessed for the purpose for which they are to be used), holy water, a spoon, and a glass of water. The articles may be obtained or replaced from the nearest Catholic church and should be kept in a safe place for use when needed.

Baptism is usually performed by the priest. If there is danger of death and no priest or other Catholic person is available the doctor or nurse may baptize the patient. Water from spring, pump, or hydrant is poured on the forehead of the patient so that it flows backward, and the person pouring the water should say aloud "I baptize thee in the name of the Father and of the Son and of the Holy Ghost." The exact words as stated above must be used, and a small portion of water must be poured over the head precisely as the words "Father," "Son," and "Holy Ghost" are uttered. In event the child is born seemingly dead,

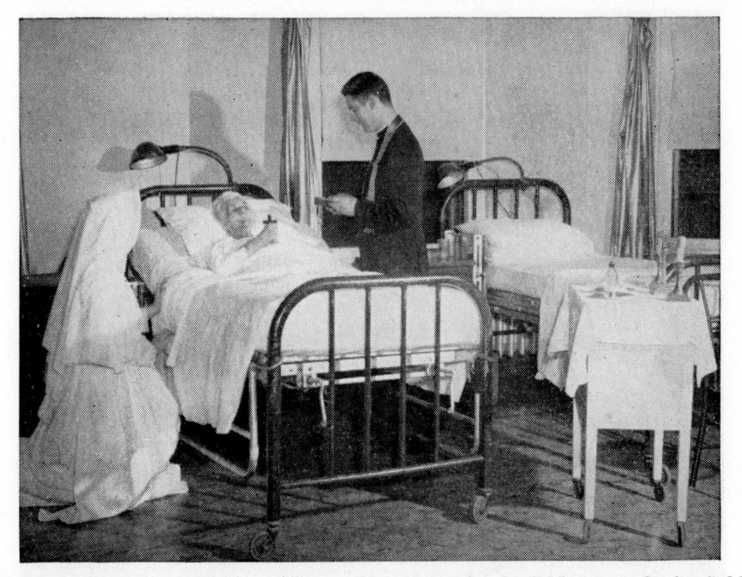

Fig. 235. Holy Communion. (Mercy Hospital School of Nursing, Springfield, Massachusetts.)

the baptism may be conditional, the same formula being used but with the prefix "If thou are living . . . "

Confession should be heard by the priest, who is left alone with the patient, and the nurse should see that their privacy is not interrupted. The priest will bring with him the stole needed for this particular ministry.

Holy Communion. A small table covered with a clean white cloth, three clean white napkins, a glass of water, and a spoon will be needed. A crucifix, two candles, and a bottle of holy water should be placed on the table. A corporal, a finger cloth, and a pall may be placed there for use if needed. Fasting may be necessary for a short time preceding the service and should be observed according to current practice and the physical condition of the patient.

Extreme Unction. In this ritual parts of the body are anointed with oil by the priest as special prayers are said. It is generally used as the patient approaches death. It can be administered only once during a given illness. In many instances improvement seems to occur from the time this sacrament was administered to the patient. The priest will bring his own materials for this rite, although a small table, covered with a white cloth, and a small amount of cotton should be provided. The bed covers should be loosened at the foot of the bed so the feet may be anointed.

If a patient brought to the hospital in a dying condition, as from

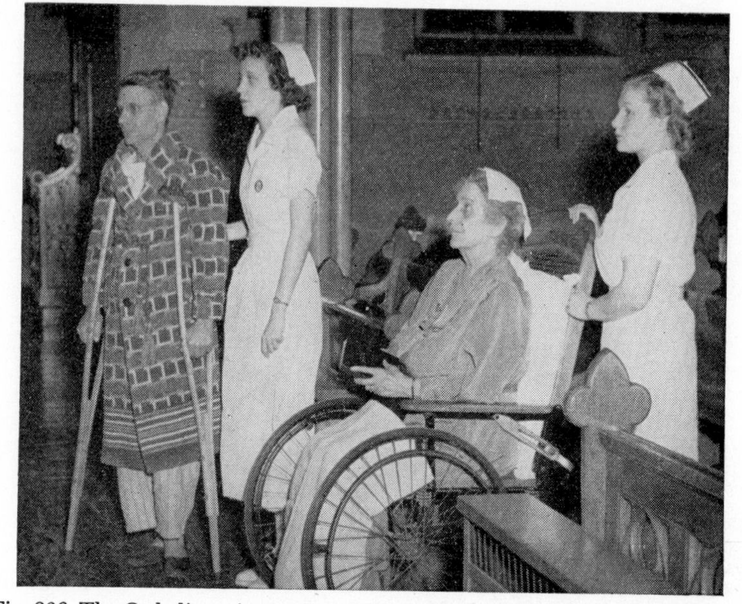

Fig. 236. The Catholic patient enjoys frequent visits to the Chapel. (St. Elizabeth Hospital School of Nursing, Lafayette, Indiana.)

a serious accident, has a rosary, medal, or crucifix on his person, a priest should be called so Extreme Unction can be administered. This sacrament may be administered when the patient is unconscious or within 30 minutes after death has occurred. The Catholic patient believes that a person must be free of sin in order to enter Heaven, and thus receiving the sacraments is necessary for cleansing of the soul.

Most Roman Catholic patients are familiar with the requirements of their church pertaining to illness. They know that patients are not expected to observe laws of fasting, attend Mass, or fulfill other obligations if doing so will jeopardize their health or interfere with treatment. They know that a priest may be summoned at any time he is needed and that he will administer the rites of the church if they are seriously ill. The nurse should feel obligated to notify the priest in each of the following situations: when a Catholic patient is admitted to the hospital, when he or his relatives asks that a priest be summoned, when he is to undergo surgery, is critically ill, or if death should occur without the sacraments having been administered.

If possible, the priest should be called while the patient is still conscious. When notifying the priest the nurse should inform him whether the patient is aware of his surroundings and is able to swallow.

Before the priest arrives the nurse should place screens around the bed so that the patient may have privacy, see that a glass of water and a glass drinking tube are on the bedside table, request visitors to withdraw from the room or unit during the priest's visit, and ask other patients in the ward to refrain from making unnecessary noise while the priest is attending the patient.

RELIGIOUS HOLIDAYS AND HOLY DAYS

Christian and Secular Holidays. The dates given may vary somewhat from year to year, but will indicate the approximate time at which the holiday occurs.

New Year's Day—January 1. A legal holiday in all states. It originated in Roman times, when sacrifices were offered to Janus, the two-faced Roman deity who looked back on the past and forward to the future.

Epiphany—January 6. The twelfth day after Christmas, to commemorate the manifestation of Jesus as the son of God. It is usually celebrated for three days preceding Lent.

Shrove Tuesday—March 1. Occurs the day before Ash Wednesday. The day is referred to as Mardi Gras (Fat Tuesday).

Ash Wednesday—March 2. The first day of Lent, which lasts for forty days. It is a day of public penance and the Catholic worshiper wears a cross on his forehead marked with ashes by the priest's thumb.

St. Patrick's Day—March 17. St. Patrick is the patron saint of Ireland and he is honored in America as well as in his native land.

Palm Sunday—April 10. Observed the Sunday before Easter to commemorate the entry of Jesus into Jerusalem.

Good Friday—April 15. The Friday before Easter Sunday, observed by all branches of the Christian Church in commemoration of the Crucifixion.

Easter Sunday—April 17. To commemorate the resurrection of Jesus.

Ascension Day—May 26. Ascension is believed to have taken place in the presence of the apostles forty days after the resurrection of Jesus.

Memorial Day—May 30. A legal holiday devoted to honoring the memory of the dead of all wars.

Pentecost—June 5. To commemorate the descent of the Holy Ghost upon the apostles fifty days after the resurrection.

Thanksgiving—November 24. A national holiday by Act of Congress in 1941. Most persons believe the holiday dates back to the day of thanks ordered by Governor Bradford of the Plymouth colony in 1621, but days of thanks stem from ancient times.

First Sunday in Advent—November 27. The season in which the faithful must prepare themselves for the advent of the Savior on Christmas.

Christmas—December 25 (Feast of the Nativity). The most important holiday of the Christian year, celebrating the anniversary of the birth of Jesus.

Observance of the Sabbath and Holy Days. Persons of Jewish faith believe that procedures which can be postponed until a later time should not be performed on the Sabbath or on Jewish Holy days. The Jewish Sabbath begins after sundown Friday and ends after sunset on Saturday. Holy days celebrated by those of Hebrew faith:

Purim (usually occurs in February) Haaman was Minister of State to the King of Persia. This is to celebrate nullification of Haaman's decree ordering destruction of all Jews.

Passover (the holiday celebrated at Easter time) Based upon the exodus of Jews from Egypt.

Shavouth (Hebrew Pentecost) Occurs fifty days after the Passover, about June 3. A feast of dedication and celebration of receipt of the Torah on Mt. Sinai.

Rosh Hashanah (Jewish New Year) Occurs in the Fall, September 24. It opens the ten days of penitence which close with Yom Kippur.

Yom Kippur (October 3) This is a day of atonement and requires fasting for the entire day. The holiest day of the Jewish year.

Sukkoth (October 8) Symbolizes the gathering of the harvest. It is similar to the Thanksgiving holiday in November and has much the same significance.

Hanukkah (December 16) Festival of Lights. To celebrate the purification of the Temple of Jerusalem. Only one cruet of oil was found and miraculously it burned eight days so the holiday is celebrated for eight days.

Since the above holidays do not occur on the same dates each year the dates given represent approximate time only. A Jewish calendar would need to be consulted for definite dates.

Summary of Important Factors

The nurse, regardless of her own religious beliefs, should cooperate with ministers of all faiths to help meet the spiritual needs of patients.

A close relationship exists between emotions and religion.

The disagreeable patient may be that way because of loneliness and may need the attention and care of the nurse more than others.

If a patient has guilt feelings that distress him, even though the offense be a minor one, the matter is of major importance to him.

Hostility or animosity of the patient should not be countered with hostility from the nurse.

Patients who show signs of such emotions as fear, worry, hostility, or guilt, and who ask questions about religious resources at the hospital may be indicating the desire for spiritual help.

Spiritual needs of the patient may be met by allowing him to talk, by reassuring him, and by helping him adjust emotionally to disability.

Need for spiritual help should be referred to a clergyman when his services are available.

The Bible should be placed within easy reach of the patient, even though he may not have requested it.

Prayer is the chief instrument of religion.

Usually the minister of any Protestant faith is acceptable to any Protestant patient.

Privacy should be provided for the patient and the clergyman who calls on him. The nurse should know the requirements for different religious rites and should supply all such requirements when necessary.

Religious dietary regulations should be observed when possible.

The nurse should know the circumstances under which a priest should be notified and should feel obligated to carry out this responsibility.

Factors To Teach the Patient

That many fears are based on hearsay rather than fact: that patients usually do *not* talk when recovering from anesthesia, that pain and discomfort can be controlled by opiates, that illness need not result in physical disability.

New friends among other patients, radio and television, books, or interesting hobbies can be substituted for visits from family and friends during convalescence.

Anxiety and worry can retard physical improvement and are often without foundation or real cause.

Feelings of hostility may be caused by frustrations of hospitalization and are quite understandable to the nurse.

That spiritual needs can be met in whatever way seems most desirable to him.

Expressing an emotional problem to a clergyman, doctor, or nurse may be a means of solving the problem.

Renewed strength and courage are usually forthcoming when pain or discomfort reaches the point where further endurance seems doubtful.

The difference between resignation and acceptance when facing physical disability, and how to adjust emotionally to disability.

The Bible and other books may bring to the patient the quiet and peace he needs and desires.

Enjoyment of visitors, mail, and flowers can supply physical, mental, and spiritual needs.

A sense of humor, which helps overcome discouragement and depression caused by illness, can be developed.

Visits from clergymen are routine and can be arranged for any patient regardless of his beliefs or church affiliation.

Certain passages from the Bible may be particularly appropriate and helpful to the patient with certain definite emotions or feelings.

Because prayer was not a part of his daily routine in health, a patient need not hesitate to pray in illness.

Suggested Reference Reading

"Religion in nursing practice," Helen Cromwell; American Journal of Nursing, December, 1949.
"The patient's spiritual needs," Hyla S. Watters, M.D., Rabbi Henry A. Schorr, Rev. Richard A. Nagle, and Rev. Benjamin R. Priest; American Journal of Nursing, February, 1950.
"Why I believe in God," A. J. Cronin; Reader's Digest, September, 1950.
"What prayer can do," Fulton Oursler; Reader's Digest, January, 1951.
"Ministers are human too," Margaret Blair Johnstone; Coronet, December, 1951.
"Triumph through faith," Jane Froman; Coronet, February, 1952.

CHAPTER 38

Care of the Dying Patient

TOPICAL OUTLINE

The routine nursing care is essentially the same for the patient who responds favorably to treatment and for the patient who does not respond to medical or surgical treatment in the desired manner. The patient who is critically ill will require additional medical attention and more frequent ministrations by the nurse.

When it is not in the physician's power to prevent death, it becomes his sacred duty, and that of the nurse who works with him, to make dying as easy as possible for the patient. The aim of the nurse attending a dying patient should be to keep him as physically comfortable as possible and, by her own calm and assured manner, provide strength and encouragement for him at a time when both are greatly needed. She will recognize the importance of relieving mental worry and fear, as well as of performing routine nursing procedures skillfully.

TO PROVIDE A SUITABLE ENVIRONMENT

Because the dying patient requires close observation and almost constant nursing care, he should be placed in a private room located near the nurses' station and treatment rooms. If he must remain in a ward where other patients are receiving care he should be placed where the usual ward activities will not disturb him. Many hospitals make a practice of transferring the dying patient to a private room, even though he may have previously been admitted to a semi-private room or ward.

The room should be quiet, well ventilated, cheerful, and pleasing in appearance. Sunlight should *not* be excluded from the room. The practice of drawing shades at the window and making the room dark and gloomy should be strenuously opposed. Numerous seriously ill patients complain of, and dread, the increasing darkness which comes with failing sight; many have expressed a desire for more light in the room. Glare from direct sunlight or a brightly lighted lamp should be avoided, but the room should be light and cheery during the patient's waking hours.

Air in the room should be kept fresh and the temperature should be maintained at 70–74° F. The environmental needs of the critically ill may vary somewhat, so the nurse will regulate the temperature and ventilation of the room, the amount of light admitted, and the degree of quiet maintained, according to the needs of each patient.

Supplies and equipment, especially the mechanical devices used in giving oxygen inhalations, blood transfusion, Wangensteen suction, and similar treatments, should be kept out of sight when not in actual use. Drugs or solutions with a penetrating or unpleasant odor should not be left in the room. If an offensive odor is present despite meticulous cleanliness and careful disposal of dressings and discharge, a room deodorant (liquid, spray, or an electrical device) should be used.

The dying patient should not be left alone. When the patient remains in a critical condition for a long period of time, members of his family may be permitted to accept the responsibility of staying at his bedside for long intervals. The nurse, however, should be nearby, and should see the patient frequently, closely observing any change in his condition.

TO GIVE ROUTINE CARE

In addition to performing routine nursing duties for the patient, the nurse must be alert for symptoms which indicate the unmistakable and progressive process of dying. She is also required to adapt routine procedures to fit the need of the patient, deciding to perform certain procedures more frequently and to omit others entirely. Although personal cleanliness is important in the care of all patients, rest is sometimes even more important, and it may be wise to postpone or omit the daily bath.

Special care of the skin may be needed, and a judicious use of massage for bony prominences to prevent occurrence of a pressure sore. Changing the patient's position frequently and keeping the bed dry and free of wrinkles will also help to prevent decubiti.

The position of the patient may add to his comfort or cause unnecessary suffering, depending on the knowledge and understanding of the nurse. The dying patient is usually seen lying flat on his back, and many persons assume that this position is most desirable and proper. Actually the very ill patient may too often be found in the dorsal position, not because it is the most comfortable, but because he is unable to move or to ask for a change in position. The best position, and the one likely to offer the greatest comfort, is that of lying on the back, with head slightly elevated and supported by a pillow, and with a second pillow rolled and placed beneath the knees to support the legs in a slightly flexed position. Any position maintained for too long a period of time will become uncomfortable, so frequent change of position is indicated. Even a very slight change, such as moving the head from one side to another, will give relief from discomfort. At frequent intervals the patient should be turned slightly to one side or the other, supported with pillows. This position permits the tongue to drop to the side of the mouth, allowing free passage of inspired air and relieving the stertorous breathing which annoys the patient and distresses his family.

Some patients with respiratory embarrassment may be relieved by being placed in a partial sitting position, supported by properly placed pillows. In the sitting position the arms should always rest on pillows to prevent their hanging heavily from the shoulders or weighing heavily on the abdomen.

The diet of the critically ill patient should consist almost entirely of fluids and should be given in small amounts at frequent intervals. Fluids may be given with a special feeder, teaspoon, or medicine dropper, and should be continued until motion and sensation are lost in the lower extremities and normal functioning of the stomach and intestines is improbable. The progressive process of death seems to begin with the lower extremities and travel upward, and the nurse should know that to continue to give nourishment after the digestive processes have failed may cause abdominal distention or the aspiration of fluid into the trachea with subsequent embarrassment to respiration. So long as the patient is able to swallow he should be given water or very weak tea. The fluids should be given in very small amounts, sufficient to relieve thirst and the dry, parched condition of the mouth and throat, yet not enough to cause distention.

In direct relationship to the amount of nourishment given the patient is the need to provide for adequate elimination. The nurse should keep an accurate record of intake and output and should offer the bedpan or urinal to the patient several times each day. If the patient is unable to void, the physician should be notified so catheterization may be ordered. If a retention catheter is used for the incontinent patient, it must drain properly and be changed daily. Bed linen should be changed immediately and the patient's back washed thoroughly with soap and water if involuntary urination occurs.

If the patient is able to take food as well as fluids the nurse will need to keep the doctor informed of the frequency and adequacy of bowel movements. The giving of a laxative or enema will depend on the written order of the attending physician.

In caring for the mouth, when the patient is no longer able to take fluid, the use of cotton swabs and a mouth wash or antiseptic solution may be required. Special care should be given often enough to keep the mouth clean and moist. Equal parts of mineral oil and lemon juice applied to the tongue, palate, and sides of the mouth help keep it in good condition. Cold cream applied to the lips will prevent chafing and the formation of unsightly incrustation. For excessive secretion from the mouth repeated use of the suction machine may be indicated.

The inner part of the nostrils should be kept clean and free from crust formation by regular use of cotton applicators moistened with mineral oil.

If the eyes contain secretions which are annoying to the patient and unsightly for those about him, occasional irrigations with warm boric acid solution will be helpful. Mineral oil applied to the eyelids will prevent accumulation of the discharge. If the eyes remain open and become dry because of lack of secretion, sterile mineral oil dropped gently into the eye will relieve the condition and prevent irritation.

SIGNS AND SYMPTOMS OF IMMINENT DEATH

The appearance of the dying patient is indicative of the physical changes occurring as the vital functions of the body are lessened and eventually stopped altogether. These bodily changes develop gradually, except in rare instances when death comes suddenly and without the usual preliminary manifestations. Although they may differ in each patient, the following signs and symptoms of impending death are usually apparent.

The patient's face shows a characteristic pallor and the presence of mental strain is evidenced by pinched features and an expression of anxiety. The eyes seem to stare fixedly into space, showing no response to variations of light and dark or to a movement of hands across the line of vision. The mouth may remain partially open except when the patient may attempt to respond to questioning.

As the lower part of the body is affected first, the diminished peripheral circulation in the legs may cause them to feel cold and clammy, yet the general body temperature maintains an elevation of several degrees above normal. Even though the lower part of the body may be covered with cold perspiration, the patient does not complain of being cold, and if the general temperature of the body is high he may feel uncomfortably warm. When the lower extremities become cold, light covering is all that should be provided. The use of heavy blankets, hot water bottles, and other means of applying external heat does little to warm the patient and will usually serve only to increase his restlessness.

Respiration may become increasingly slow and difficult. The accumulation of mucus in the bronchi and throat, with consequent interference to inspiration gives rise to the distressing sounds termed by the laity "the death rattle." Cheyne-Stokes respiration, identified by its distinctive alternating periods of apnea and of increasingly noisy and deep inspiration (with the periods of apnea becoming gradually longer in duration) is very often a part of the syndrome of approaching death.

At this stage of terminal illness the patient may be in a comatose condition, may experience alternate periods of consciousness and unconsciousness, or may be fully aware at all times of his immediate surroundings.

His attempts to talk or to make known his wishes may result in incoherent or irrational statements. Failure to make himself understood may cause increased restlessness and result in crying, moaning, and other indications of mental distress. Most doctors leave standing orders for the administration of narcotics or sedatives and the understanding nurse will not permit the patient to become so restless that he shows evidence of mounting disquietude.

It is generally conceded that patients who seem to be totally unconscious may retain sensory impressions, and that the sense of hearing is probably still acute when other senses may have ceased to function. For this reason, care must be exercised not to permit discussion of the physical condition of the patient in his hearing. Critically ill patients who have made an unexpected recovery are often able to repeat parts of conversations carried on in their presence when they were thought to be totally unconscious and unable to hear. Because it is impossible to determine accurately the ability of the dying patient to hear or understand, everyone who speaks while in the room should do so in their natural tone of voice and should say only those things which they would want the patient to hear.

Relatives should be instructed not to whisper or talk in subdued tones in the presence of the dying patient. He may be greatly disturbed by sounds that are indistinct or by conversation that is not clearly audible.

In addition to symptoms already described, imminent death produces a change in heart activity. The pulse may increase in rate but show increasing weakness and irregularity. Just before death occurs respirations cease and the pulse becomes imperceptible. The exact time of death is recorded as that time when the sound of the heart beat (through a stethoscope applied directly above the apex of the heart) is no longer evident. Although occurrence of one or several of the above signs and symptoms is usually indicative of approaching death, it does not necessarily mean that death is inevitable. Until the physician concedes that the only possible outcome for the patient is death, treatments and nursing care designed to save his life should be continued.

SPIRITUAL NEEDS OF THE DYING PATIENT

To be cognizant of the needs of the dying patient and to meet those needs fully the nurse must be aware that spiritual counsel may be far more important than physical or mental care. The ways of meeting spiritual needs have been discussed fully in Chapter 37.

MAKING A WILL

The making of a will is usually the responsibility of legal advisors or persons familiar with legal requirements, but it is not uncommon for the nurse to be asked to assist with such a document.

To be of real help to the patient in such matters she must know the basic parts of a will, the method of making a simple will, and the fundamental legal requirements which must be met if the will is to be valid. She should know the usual causes for wills being judged invalid, and the proper procedure for executing a will. In general, the nurse should know that any person, married or single, who is of legal age and sound mind, can make a will, that most wills made before a person marries become invalid after marriage; that a will should be changed when a child is born or adopted, when a beneficiary dies, or when a chosen executor dies or moves to a place where it would be inconvenient or impossible for him to serve as executor.

She should know that wills are considered invalid by the probate courts if they are improperly witnessed, if the person making the will is not considered to have been of sound mind, and if witnesses of the will were named as beneficiaries or are married to persons named as beneficiaries of the will. The fundamental parts of a will include the following.

The Introductory Statement. A statement, denoting that the patient is of "sound mind" and that the document being written is his last will and testament. The date should be included here.

Provision for an Executor. A member of the family or a close friend of the patient may be designated as executor of the will.

Disposition of the Property. Mention should be made of all the patient's legal heirs and stated amounts that are to be left to them. If the person making the will wishes to disinherit a near relative it is necessary that that relative be named so that his existence is recognized. He can be left one dollar or a worthless trinket to show that he has not been accidentally forgotten as a member of the family. Various other persons and organizations may also be left parts of the estate or property. In some states not more than half an estate can be left to charities if there is a surviving spouse or children.

The Signature. The will must be signed in the presence of witnesses. If the patient is too weak to sign a person not named as beneficiary may assist by guiding his hand while he attempts to make the signature.

Attestation Clause. The signatures of three witnesses is necessary. All three should have witnessed the signing of the will and should witness each other's signatures. The address of each witness should be given. A person named as a beneficiary in the will should not act as a witness to the will.

The nurse should refuse to assist with the making of a will or to act as a witness to the signing of it if there is any doubt in her mind as to the patient's mental competency.

The following is a copy of a simple, though valid, will which may be used if the nurse finds it necessary to help in the making of a will when other help may not be available.

LAST WILL AND TESTAMENT

(date) ______

Be it known hereby that I (name of person making the will), of the city or town of ______ in the County of ______ and State of ______, being of sound mind and memory, do hereby voluntarily make, publish and declare this to be my last will and testament, hereby revoking any and all other wills heretofore made by me.

I hereby nominate and appoint (name) of (address) ______ to be the Executor of this, my last will.

It is my desire and order that the above named Executor be allowed to act (with-without) bond.

After payment of my just debts, funeral charges and expenses of administration I dispose of my estate as follows:

In witness whereof I hereunto subscribe my name and affix my seal this ______ day of (month) in the year one thousand nine hundred and (year) at (city or town, (state).

(signature) ______

The above named (testator) has declared this to be (his, her) last will and testament and has requested us to sign as witnesses. We believe said testator to be of sound mind. In our presence said testator has signed, sealed, published and declared, and we, in said testator's presence, and in the presence of each other, subscribe our names as witnesses.

1. (name), (address)
2. (name), (address)
3. (name), (address)

DYING DECLARATIONS

All nurses during the course of their specialized education should be informed that statements made by a dying patient, if he realizes he is dying, are accepted in court as valid testimony. As a rule, such statements are made to nurses in an emergency when the patient's condition changes suddenly and there is no time to call a doctor or lawyer to receive the testimony. The nurse thus made witness to a dying declaration should write out the statement at the earliest possible time, writing it word for word as it was given by the patient. No nurse should trust to memory a statement that may be of vital importance to relatives of the patient or to someone whom the patient may have wronged. After a short time that which a person hears is largely forgotten, and so important a declaration should be written immediately so none of its content will be lost. A confession of a crime that was committed may be made in a dying declaration and may free an innocent person of charges or release him from confinement.

NURSE'S ATTITUDE TOWARD THE DYING PATIENT

To better understand the patient who is dying the nurse must have some understanding of death. Usually she is aware of the false conception which most people have of death. She knows that the average person believes such phrases as *pangs of death, the death struggle, agony of dying* accurately describe death.

To nearly everyone death is something to be greatly feared and to be avoided at any cost. Death is fearful primarily because it is unfamiliar, and we all tend to fear that which is unknown to us. The thought that "pain" and "death" are inseparable companions, that death cannot be experienced without pain and distress, is a common error. It is more true that "unconsciousness" and "death" bear a remarkably close relationship.

For the dying patient respiration becomes more and more feeble, gradually less air is being inhaled. The blood receives a lessening amount of oxygen, and circulation is impaired. As less blood reaches the brain the patient becomes less and less aware of his surroundings or of the experience he is undergoing. The amount of blood that does go to the brain is loaded with carbonic acid gas which acts as an anesthetic agent to produce unconsciousness, which is one of the most important symptoms of imminent death.

For the patient who is fully conscious the first indication that death is close at hand brings fear and dread. His first reaction may be one of panic, especially if he is in a dying condition when he is first aware of the fact that he is to die. When he turns to the nurse her calm manner, natural voice, and reassuring presence will help him overcome the mounting fear he may feel.

Many doctors advocate that the patient be told of the probability of death; some believe it is better not to inform the patient that his illness is in a terminal stage.

The doctor who feels that the patient should be told he will not recover usually prefers that a close relative or his minister be the one to tell the patient of his condition. The doctor knows that if he, in his official capacity as a member of the medical profession, imparts the knowledge that death is unavoidable, he leaves no room for doubt or hope in the patient's mind. If a relative or other lay person informs the patient he may be left the faint, but not impossible, hope that a mistake has been made and that death can be avoided. The time permitted by natural doubts as to the authenticity of the information he has received allows the patient to begin to get used to the idea or to comprehend its meaning for him.

When patients in terminal stages of an illness have not been told that they will live only a short time, they usually surmise that such is the case. They seem to know without being told. These patients are apt to question the nurse in regard to their condition. Inviting her by their questions to tell them that death is near and yet dreading to have her put the thought into words.

The nurse should understand that questions asked by the patient need to be given very careful thought. She should not answer halting questions as "Do they think I'm going to die?" with a blunt affirmative reply that robs the patient of all hope and may even produce shock.

Questions on prognosis or outcome of their illness that are asked by dying patients should be answered usually by counter questions from the nurse. The question "Do you think I won't get well?" or "Do the doctors think I'm going to die?" can best be answered by a question such as "Why should you ask such a question?" or "What makes you think you won't get well?" or the answer may need to be a statement which merely implies an answer, as mention of another patient, with the same disease, who recovered, or other patients who have been critically ill, yet did not die.

If the nurse can manage to say very little, yet encourage the patient to talk, there will be little need for her to answer specific questions.

Information regarding physical condition and probable outcome of his illness should be given the patient and his family by the doctor. The nurse may need to explain again to anxious relatives some of the statements made by the physician, but she should not add to that information or go into detail about phases of the illness which the doctor may not have discussed thoroughly.

By talking of his condition the patient may gain the relief and benefit that comes to all of us by finding a solution or a partial solution to a problem through discussion of it with another, or through merely acknowledging it to oneself. By listening sympathetically and unemotionally, the nurse may play an important part in helping the patient to understand the fact that death is not far away and to gain the strength needed to accept that fact.

NURSE'S ATTITUDE TOWARD RELATIVES

The nurse caring for a critically ill patient has an additional responsibility, that of being kind and considerate to close relatives of the patient or to any person to whom the patient may mean a great deal.

Hospitals usually provide a place of quiet and of privacy for the immediate family of a dying patient. Although several members of the family may be at the hospital, only one or two should be in the patient's room at one time.

The nurse caring for a dying patient should encourage members of the family who may wish to do so to assist in giving nursing care. It will probably be of no benefit to the patient if a wife or mother smooths the pillow for him, helps in changing his position or gently removes beads of perspiration from his forehead, but it will help in some measure to assuage the grief of the relative.

The nurse should see that very near relatives eat regularly and get the required amount of rest and sleep. She should discourage their attendance in the patient's room for prolonged periods and should recommend to others in the family that those most deeply involved emotionally be outdoors at intervals and, if possible, take an interest in the activities of others who may mean much to them.

Relatives or close friends who are with the patient at intervals may be deeply concerned if the patient is restless, if he moans or indicates by facial expression that he is in pain. The nurse should explain that the patient's reactions are automatic in nature and are not to be interpreted as manifestations of mental or physical distress. She should remind those most concerned that the patient receives medication which will prevent pain and discomfort and overcome anxiety or apprehension if he is conscious.

Relatives who may come from a distance to see the patient should be received first by the nurse who may need to explain the patient's condition and prepare the visitor for the change in the patient's appearance. The relative should be instructed not to distress the patient by a sudden and uncontrolled display of grief.

For the sympathetic and understanding nurse it is not easy to care for a dying patient and remain aloof from the emotional reaction of relatives who express their grief outwardly, yet her first responsibility is to the patient, and, whatever her own emotions may be, she must remain outwardly calm and unaffected.

If members of the family are present when death occurs, they may rely on the nurse to help make arrangements for care of the body and they look to her to give care and attention to a member of the family who may lose emotional control.

The patient's belongings and articles that might be of value should be given to a responsible member of the family, and the nurse should see that all such belongings and articles are listed and the signature of the person obtained so the hospital will be relieved of responsibility for such belongings.

CARE OF THE BODY AFTER DEATH

When death occurs in the hospital the doctor may be present or within the hospital so that he may be summoned immediately. To meet all legal requirements, it is necessary that a doctor pronounce the patient dead and certify as to the cause of death.

When death has occurred the nurse should lower the backrest if it has been slightly elevated, she should remove all pillows except one, and straighten the limbs so that the body is in correct alignment. The eyes of the patient should be closed, and if dentures have been removed, as is usual for the dying patient, they should be replaced and the mouth closed. If the eyes are wide open they should be closed by grasping the lashes and gently bringing the upper lid down over the eyeball. The eyelids should not be touched because pressure on the lids may give them an unnatural appearance and prevent closure.

By cupping her hand and applying some pressure to the chin the nurse is able to close the mouth of the patient and to see that it remains closed. If the patient had been restless, the nurse should comb his hair and do whatever is needed to give him the appearance of being in natural sleep, for the family who will wish to see him. All medications and equipment used in treatments should be removed from view. Window shades should be drawn to a few inches below the middle sash and the window should be opened a few inches.

No other action should be taken until the doctor has certified that the patient is legally dead.

If the patient is at home there may be some delay before the doctor arrives, and the nurse may need to give some care to the body, but it is still essential that the patient be pronounced dead by a physician. It is illegal for the undertaker to take the body and prepare it for burial before a doctor has pronounced the patient dead.

If members of the family were not present at the hospital when death occurred and there arrival may be delayed, the patient should be cared for as outlined above, and a screen should be placed between the bed and the door. All lights except one at the bedside should be turned off and the door to the room should be closed.

If the doctor wishes to perform an autopsy he will have asked permission of a responsible relative before death occurs or will request permission for autopsy at the time of the patient's death. The nurse should not assume the responsibility of asking the family to grant permission for an autopsy. If she is asked by the family to express her opinion in regard to the matter she may point out to them the benefit that may result to other members of the family through an autopsy, but should not try to influence them in their decision.

Immediately after death, if relatives are present, they should be permitted to see the patient once more, if they so desire. They should not be given the impression that it is necessary for them to hurry through this last time spent with him, neither should they be permitted to prolong their stay in the room beyond a reasonable length of time. The nurse may control the length of time given them by quietly suggesting to one who may not be so deeply affected as others that he be responsible for reminding them that they should leave the room to attend to other matters requiring their attention and to permit the nurse to continue her care of the patient.

If clothing and articles of value belonging to the patient have not already been given to a responsible member of the family, the nurse should ask that one remain to take charge of them. She should also ask the family's wishes in regard to removal of a wedding ring, if one is worn by the patient. All jewelry, money, eyeglasses, letters, keys, religious emblems, and fresh flowers or plants should be sent home with members of the family.

If earrings that cannot be removed are worn and if a wedding ring is to be left in place, these facts should be noted on the signed list of the items taken by the family. The wedding ring should be tied in place with a strip of 1-inch bandage so it will not be lost.

Before the body is sent to the morgue, the nurse should remove all soiled dressings and drainage tubes, and cover any incision or wound with a clean dressing held securely in place with adhesive tape. If the patient perspired freely or had not recently been bathed, a complete bath should be given. A perineal pad should be placed in position and held in place by a muslin square folded into a triangle and pinned on as a diaper, or by a T-binder made of 3-inch gauze bandage.

Some hospitals require that wrists and ankles be left free of restricting bandages; others request that the hands be crossed at the wrist and the wrists tied together with bandage. Ankles, too, are securely fastened together with bandage. Some institutions require that a rolled towel be placed firmly under the chin to prevent the mouth from sagging open. The nurse should know the requirements of the hospital in which she is working and comply with them.

A mortuary gown should be placed on the body, and identifying tags should be tied on the wrist and on the outer covering of the body. The identifying tag should bear the full name of the patient, room number, date and time of death, and name of doctor.

The body is wrapped in a shroud, a large piece of muslin which covers it completely, an identifying tag is pinned to the hood of the shroud and the body is then placed on a stretcher to be moved to the morgue. The body should be securely fastened to the stretcher and completely covered.

The body should be removed in an unobtrusive manner so other patients will not be aware that a death has occurred. Doors to patient rooms may be closed before the stretcher is wheeled through the corridor. Ambulatory patients should be asked to retire to their own rooms or to a sun porch or waiting room for the short time required to transport the body through the hallway. The freight elevator should be used to take the body to the floor where the morgue is located. If passengers are on the elevator, they should be delivered to their respective floors and the elevator should return, empty, to take on the stretcher bearing the body.

The nurse who attended the patient is responsible for all of his belongings that might have been left behind. They should be carefully wrapped and labeled and turned in to the administration office. Forms reporting the death of the patient should be filled out and delivered to the proper offices. The patient's chart should be completed and sent to the medical records office. Orders for treatments and diet should be discontinued. All equipment used in treatment of the patient should be returned to its proper place, and the housekeeping department should be notified so the room may be cleaned and prepared for another patient as discussed in Chapter 4.

PUBLIC HEALTH REGULATIONS

Report of the death (a death certificate) must be sent to the local health department. The certificate is made out by the physician, undertaker, and, if autopsy is performed, the pathologist.

State laws govern the disposition of all bodies, whether claimed immediately by the family or unidentified. Permission for autopsies must be granted by nearest of kin or by a custodial friend before an autopsy can be performed. Permission for autopsy on an unidentified body must be obtained from the local health department. The health department is responsible for trying to determine the identity of the body and for making arrangements for burial. If there is a question as to cause of death and if a coroner's inquest is required, an autopsy can be legally performed without obtaining permission.

Health departments also have special regulations concerning the care of bodies of persons who die of certain communicable diseases. In some states undertakers are not permitted to hold or to expose bodies of persons who died of cholera, bubonic plague, smallpox, and similar communicable diseases. Such bodies must be sealed immediately in a coffin, and funeral services are strictly private, with only members of the immediate family in attendance.

Care of Equipment after Use

All equipment used in special treatments given the patient should be cared for as outlined in the chapters dealing with those particular treatments.

The shroud and other articles used from the mortuary pack are discarded by the undertaker and must be replaced so that the pack is complete and ready for use again when needed.

The stretcher used in transferring the body to the morgue should be stripped of linen and washed with a disinfectant solution. It should be made up with clean linen and left in its usual storage place, ready for use again.

Summary of Important Factors

When death cannot be prevented it becomes imperative that the doctor and nurse do all in their power to make dying less difficult for the patient.

The dying patient should be in a private room that is quiet and attractive. Sunlight should not be excluded from the room; unpleasant odors should be eliminated; and supplies, equipment, and drugs, when not in use, should be kept out of sight.

The dying patient should never be left alone. Special care should be given to skin, mouth, eyes, and to the position of the body. Diet and elimination should receive careful attention from the nurse.

Signs and symptoms of imminent death include marked pallor of the face, expression of anxiety, coldness of the extremities, difficult respiration (Cheyne-Stokes respiration), restlessness or coma, and rapid, irregular, and weak pulse.

Attention should be given to the spiritual needs of the patient.

The basic parts of a simple yet valid will should be known so the nurse can help with this procedure if it is necessary. The nurse should not witness or help make a will for a patient who may not be mentally competent. Dying declarations are accepted as valid testimony in court and should be immediately recorded, word for word.

The request for permission to perform an autopsy should be made by the doctor.

All articles of value belonging to the patient should be signed for and taken by a responsible member of the family.

The body must bear proper identification tags, and should be transferred to the morgue without other patients knowing a death has occurred, if possible.

The body cannot be removed by an undertaker before certification of death has been made by the physician.

Factors To Teach Relatives and Friends of the Patient

That uncontrolled display of grief may cause great distress to the dying patient.

That nothing should be said within the patient's hearing which they would not wish to say directly to the patient.

That moans and groans or restless movements on the part of the patient do not mean that he is experiencing physical pain.

That all conversation in the patient's room should be in a natural tone of voice.

That window shades should not be drawn, but the room should be kept light and cheerful.

That relatives who have not seen the patient for a long time should be prepared for marked change in his physical appearance.

That only one or two should remain in the patient's room at any one time.

Scientific Principles

Anatomy and Physiology. Death may occur suddenly or require a prolonged period of several days, with progressive failure of vital body functions.

Circulation is slowed and respirations become increasingly shallow.

Cessation of breathing indicates the occurrence of death, although the heart may continue to beat for a very short time.

The mental condition of the patient may vary from complete consciousness to coma.

With inability to swallow, mucus collects in the throat; air passing through the secretions there causes the characteristic sound termed "death rattle."

Sphincter muscles may relax, causing incontinence of bladder and rectum.

Because of anemia and loss of muscle tone, the face may appear ashen, eyes may be sunken and glazed, nostrils pinched, and the expression is one of anxiety.

After death the body cools and rigor mortis, a stiffening of the muscles, occurs. Rigor mortis disappears after one to six days, and the muscles assume a softened, flabby consistency.

Postmortem hypostasis refers to the dark red or blue discoloration of the skin where pressure is exerted on it.

Chemistry. Lack of oxygen is the ultimate cause of death.

Muscle tissue immediately after death becomes rigid because of the coagulation of glycogen and the formation of lactic acid. Soluble proteins are temporarily converted into an insoluble form. When the acidity has been destroyed by slow oxidation, the reverse chemical change causes muscles to acquire their former texture.

Microbiology. Embalming fluids act as a germicide and penetrate all the body tissues. In cases of communicable disease state laws may require that the casket be sealed and the funeral and burial be private, to prevent spread of the disease.

Pharmacology. For the dying patient, morphine or other opiates are ordered in sufficient quantities to relieve all pain and discomfort. Atropine may be given to help reduce the secretion of mucus in the throat. Morphine may be effective in stopping a strangling cough, even though it may not check the rapid increase in respiration rate.

Physics. Loss of muscle tone makes it impossible for the patient to maintain his position in bed, so supports are needed.

Secretions collecting in the mouth and throat may be removed more easily by aid of gravity if the patient's head is turned to one side.

After death, if head and shoulders are elevated on a pillow, blood, because of gravity, will not collect in the face, causing discoloration there.

Psychology. In the very early stages of dying the patient may be subjected to intense physical pain and to mental suffering at the knowledge that he is forced to leave loved ones. To most patients, death does not hold much terror since they are too ill, too tired, and too weakened to be alert to what is happening. The nurse who understands the value of quiet, cheerful and light surroundings will be able to do much to make the patient's last hours serene and peaceful.

Sociology. As vital body functions are impaired by approaching death the patient becomes more and more dependent on the nurse to supply physical needs and guard against mental strain and fear.

Public health regulations pertaining to disposal of the body must be observed.

If the patient had a communicable disease, other members of the family may be under surveillance and required to have diagnostic tests, such as chest x-ray.

The nurse must offer reassurance by remaining close to the patient, leaving for a short time only when a relative or friend is there to take her place.

Relatives are notified by hospital authorities when the patient is placed on the "critical" list. The nurse should be sympathetic and kind, but must remain calm and unemotional. She should keep the relatives informed of changes in the patient's condition.

The nurse should assist in carrying out expressed desires of the patient as making a will, attending to a business matter, receiving religious consolation, or the last ries of his church.

For the Catholic patient, the priest must be called so that the sacrament of Extreme Unction may be administered.

The nurse's poise and manner may calm the fearful patient and serve as an example to relatives who may display uncontrolled emotion.

If death occurs shortly after the patient is admitted, or if there is a possibility that the death is a result of criminal action, the coroner must be notified. An investigation may be deemed necessary to determine the exact cause of death.

Situation Type Problems

1. A student nurse reported on duty at 3:00 P.M. and was assigned to remain with a dying patient. When she went to the room she found window shades had been drawn to exclude the sunlight.

The patient's wife, sister, and two brothers were seated in the room and were speaking in whispers to each other. The eyes of the patient were open, although he seemed unaware of what went on about him and made no movement, other than a rather nervous, aimless moving of his hands on the top covers.

As the student placed her fingers in position on the radial artery to count the pulse rate, the sister of the patient approached the bed and, standing beside her, asked in a tone of voice clearly audible to all in the room, "Don't you think he looks much worse now than he did at noon? It can't be much longer now, do you think?"

What would you have done?

2. The doctor attending a patient who was critically ill seemed most anxious that permission for autopsy be granted. He discussed the matter with members of the immediate family, who refused consent.

The doctor informed the nurse caring for the patient that an autopsy would help to confirm the tentative diagnosis that had been made and might provide information which would be helpful in preventing similar illness in other members of the family.

The older brother of the patient, who was "nearest of kin," explained to the nurse that his reason for refusing permission for an autopsy was based on the fact that the patient had always had a great fear of being subjected to a surgical procedure and that he felt an autopsy would be very like a surgical procedure. What would you have done?

Suggested Reference Reading

"Management of the comatose patient," R. Meyers and M. E. Meyers; American Practitioner, October, 1950.

"The tranquillity of death," J. D. Ratcliff; Reader's Digest, February, 1950.

"Care of patient after death," Ruth E. Hunter and Dorothy Eaton; American Journal of Nursing, November, 1950.

CHAPTER 39

Prevention and Control of Communicable Diseases

TOPICAL OUTLINE

A communicable disease is one which can be transmitted directly or indirectly, from one person to another. Several of the communicable diseases are caused by specific bacteria, but the greater number are believed to be caused by some form of virus.

MOST COMMON COMMUNICABLE DISEASES

Among the most common communicable diseases are: the common cold, pneumonia, conjunctivitis, gonorrhea, leprosy, erysipelas, chicken pox, measles, diphtheria, mumps, poliomyelitis, meningococcus meningitis, malaria, influenza, tuberculosis, trachoma, syphilis, puerperal sepsis, impetigo, smallpox, scarlet fever, Vincent's angina, whooping cough, epidemic encephalitis, typhoid, and yellow fever.

MODE OF TRANSMISSION OF PATHOGENIC MICROORGANISMS

Since communicable diseases are spread by transmission of pathogenic organisms from the body of the patient to that of another, the nurse should know the various routes by which the causative organisms may leave the body of the infected person and enter the body of another. Only with this knowledge can the nurse adequately protect herself and others through appropriate measures of prevention.

Most causative organisms of communicable diseases are transmitted by direct contact (directly from the host to the exposed person). Organisms capable of remaining alive for a time outside the body may be transferred indirectly, through articles that have been in contact with the patient and are then handled by the other individual. Organisms may also be transmitted through a *carrier*, a person who harbors and disseminates the causative organisms, yet shows no symptoms of having the disease. Organisms which remain suspended in the air and retain their virulence for long periods, termed air-borne, furnish still another mode of transmission of communicable diseases.

The various channels through which organisms may leave the body of an infected person or enter the body of a well person include:

By Nose and Throat. Most communicable diseases of the respiratory system and many so-called children's diseases are spread by discharges from the lungs, nose, throat, and mouth. In caring for patients with respiratory diseases the nurse should wear a mask to protect her own nose and throat and to lessen the danger of direct contact with the causative organisms.

Through Eyes, Vagina, or Urethra. The mucous membrane of the eye and of the vagina and urethra is susceptible to infection by various forms of bacteria, and infections of the genitourinary tract are often transmitted to the conjunctiva of the eye.

Through the Gastrointestinal Tract. Organisms which are found in discharges from the alimentary canal ordinarily must enter through the mouth to produce the disease in a healthy person.

Through the Skin. Although normally the skin is a means of defense against disease, a break in the skin surface may become the portal of entry for pathogenic organisms. The bite of an insect or material from an infected person coming in contact with such a break in the skin may serve to transmit disease.

The causative organisms of some diseases may enter the body through more than one of these portals, and may be discharged through several different routes. Care of patients infected with such diseases must be planned so that all necessary precautions are taken. The mode of transmission of the causative organism determines the precautionary measures required to protect others from the disease.

MEASURES FOR PREVENTION AND CONTROL OF COMMUNICABLE DISEASES

Many different measures are used to prevent and control the spread of disease, but relatively few are new in theory or in practice. The Bible contains references to such measures as quarantine, proper disposal of waste, and the enforcement of laws related to sanitation of entire communities and of individual dwelling places.

Measures currently used to help in the prevention and control of disease include public hygiene and sanitation, increased resistence to infection, daily practice of good personal hygiene, isolation of the infected individual, quarantine of the individual and of the family, disinfection and sterilization, and general health education.

Public Hygiene and Sanitation. The first line of defense in prevention and control of infection and disease is that of community hygiene and sanitation. Federal and local governments have set up regulations governing the purification of food and water supplies and regulating the disposal of garbage and sewage to insure protection of the general population.

Communities provide facilities for the purification of water by filtration or chlorination. Milk made available to the public must be pasteurized so it is free of contamination. Various national laws (Pure Food and Drug Law) have been enacted to insure that food is made safe for consumption through accepted methods of care and preservation.

Garbage and sewage disposal, control of insects, and extermination of animal pests which carry disease organisms are community measures which prevent the spread of disease within the community.

Increased Resistance to Infection. By increasing body resistance to infection or to organisms known to cause disease, the individual may help to prevent infection and disease. This may be done by injection of antibodies effective against the organism causing the disease which have been produced in the bodies of others, or by injection of the causative organism itself in a dose calculated to stimulate the production of defensive antibodies but not sufficient to cause the disease.

The effectiveness of vaccine in combating communicable disease has been demonstrated and many states require by law the inoculation of all school children against certain diseases, such as smallpox. Inoculation is defined as, "the introduction of the virus of a disease into the body of an individual." Its purpose is to produce a mild form of the disease so the individual will develop antibodies, blood substances, which combat the causative organisms of the disease, should the person come in contact with them.

Vaccines and sera (discussed also in Chapter 33) are commonly used in communities where the health and welfare of the population is of concern to public leaders and officials. Vaccination, especially during periods of greater danger of exposure, is a most effective means of increasing body resistance to disease.

Personal Hygiene. The regular observance of simple, yet effective, measures of personal hygiene will greatly decrease the danger of infection and disease, since bacteria are known to thrive and grow best in an environment of dirt and filth.

To increase resistance to infection the body should be kept clean, and the skin and mucous membranes should be kept functioning normally. A daily routine which should be practiced by the nurse and used by her in teaching prevention of disease would include the following basic requirements of good personal hygiene:

A daily bath, with use of generous amounts of soap and warm water.

Frequent, thorough washing of the hands at intervals during the day. Washing the hands in soap and water always before eating, and after defecation and voiding.

A sufficient amount of rest and sleep, with avoidance of mental stress and worry. At least one hour each day spent outdoors where exercise may be obtained in fresh air and sunshine. An adequate, well balanced diet, and establishment of proper habits of elimination.

Keeping hands and articles that may be unclean away from mouth, nose, eyes, ears, and genitals. Never putting fingers, pens, pencils, pins, corks, ear pieces of spectacle frames, or other articles that may carry disease-producing organisms into the mouth.

Avoiding use of common eating or drinking articles, and toilet facilities which are not adequately cleaned and disinfected.

Refusing to share with other persons towels, combs, razors, drinking cups, handkerchiefs, and other articles which may serve as a means of transferring infection.

Avoiding close contact with spray from nose or mouth of other persons.

Isolation. If transfer of infection and disease is to be prevented or controlled all individuals known to be affected by or to be harboring or producing the pathogenic organisms must be separated from others. This separation of the patient or affected person from others in such a way as to prevent transference of the disease is termed *isolation*.

The length of time the affected person must be isolated depends on the incubation period of the disease, the length of time the disease is infectious or transmissible, whether the person becomes a carrier, and the time of isolation that may have been established through medical treatment of the disease in the past. Patients who understand the possibility of endangering others, so long as the organisms are present in an active state, are usually eager to cooperate in observing regulations providing for satisfactory isolation technique.

Quarantine. Restriction of the activity of the affected person and of persons known to have been in contact with him is termed *quarantine*, and is another measure used to prevent and control the spread of communicable diseases.

If the patient is removed to a hospital, the family and those who have been in contact with him may be released from quarantine after proper precautionary measures, such as disinfection or fumigation, have been taken. In some instances, the quarantine remains in effect until the end of the incubation period, to determine if others of the family may have contracted the disease.

When the patient remains at home for treatment, an adult member of the family should be made responsible for his care and all other family members should remain outside the isolated unit or room occupied by the patient. Children are especially susceptible to disease and should be kept away from any possible direct or indirect contact with the patient.

The length of time the quarantine must be in effect depends on one or more of several factors. These include the disease which the patient has contracted; the incubation period of the disease; the length of time the patient remains a source of infection to others; if the patient becomes a *carrier*, if the infection is transmitted to other members of the family; laboratory findings to determine whether the disease is in an active or communicable stage.

Disinfection and Sterilization. The chief method of destroying pathogenic organisms is through some process of disinfection, accomplished by either chemical or physical means.

If disinfection is done by chemical means the agent chosen depends on whether or not it comes in contact with the patient. If used to disinfect the skin or other parts of the body, the chemical agent must be in a strength not injurious to body tissues. For such purposes safe concentrations of alcohol, Argyrol, Hexylresorcinol, Mercurochrome, Merthiolate, iodine, or potassium permanganate are usually used. For disinfecting body discharges or articles such as linen, instruments, etc., which have come in contact with the patient, chlorinated lime, bichloride of mercury, formaldehyde or Lysol of rather strong concentration may be used.

Disinfection by chemical means is effective only when the strength or concentration of the solution used and the length of time the infected article or material remains submerged in the solution is sufficient to destroy all organisms.

Disinfection by means of gas or vapor is termed *fumigation.* This method is used for clothing or books and to disinfect rooms or entire dwellings where there has been a patient with communicable disease. The articles being disinfected by fumigation must be exposed to action of the gas or vapor within a well closed container for at least 12 hours. Formaldehyde is the agent most commonly used for fumigation.

If disinfection is done by physical means it may be achieved through the use of soap and water, sunlight, and various extremes of heat and cold.

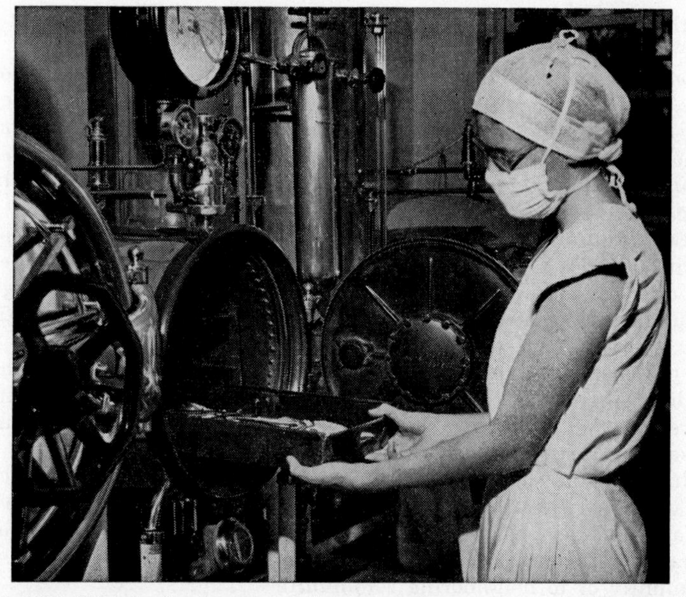

Fig. 237. Disinfection by means of steam under pressure requires use of the autoclave. (San Diego County General Hospital School of Nursing, San Diego, California.)

Burning is the most effective method of destroying pathogenic organisms and is used whenever possible. Contaminated paper articles, such as dishes, towels, handkerchief tissues, magazines, and soiled dressings or bandages, waste solid food, and cheap toys are burned. Contaminated articles which cannot or should not be destroyed must be disinfected by some other means.

Submerging contaminated articles such as dishes, silver, linen, syringes, needles, instruments that do not have a cutting edge, and rubber goods in boiling water for 10–20 minutes will destroy all pathogenic organisms except the spore-forming variety.

To disinfect mattresses, if a special autoclave is not available, exposure to bright sunlight for several hours is usually the method employed. Sunlight is considered an effective means for disinfecting books, furniture, rugs, and many other articles which may be difficult to handle and cannot be destroyed.

Articles not destroyed or harmed by dry heat may be baked in an oven 450° F. for at least one hour.

To destroy spore-forming bacteria or to sterilize, as well as disinfect, such articles as rubber goods, linens, instruments, and solutions steam under pressure is the method used. The article or solution is subjected to varying degrees of steam pressure in a sterilizer or autoclave for the length of time necessary to destroy all living organisms that might be present.

Concurrent disinfection is employed in caring for a patient in isolation. This includes disinfection of all excreta and discharges immediately after the infective material leaves the body of the patient; and immediate disinfection of all articles used in caring for the patient. *Terminal disinfection* is that done at the end of the disease, or when the patient has been released from isolation.

Health Education. The control of communicable disease in a community depends a great deal on the extent to which individual members of the community have been educated in regard to the dangers of communicable diseases and the most effective means of combating them.

If the people do not understand the danger to themselves and their children in unsafe water, milk, and food supplies, they show little interest in, and are often unwilling to abide by, regulations governing the safe production and distribution of such supplies.

Although state laws require practicing physicians to report to city or state authorities all cases of contagious diseases, unless the people cooperate, and persons infected are willing to submit to isolation and quarantine, a contagious disease may rapidly spread to others in the community or to neighboring communities.

Control measures, such as proper disposal of sewage, destruction of breeding places of insects or animals known to be sources of contamination, and early recognition of symptoms, with intelligent use of preventive measures, all depend on adequate instruction in personal and public hygiene for all members of a community. Only through cooperative effort on the part of all persons can there be effective prevention and control of infection or disease.

Summary of Important Factors

Terminology relative to the most common communicable diseases should be known to the nurse.

Channels through which pathogenic microorganisms enter and leave the body include nose, throat, eyes, vagina, urethra, gastrointestinal tract, and skin.

Increased body resistance is gained through the use of vaccines and sera as well as through use of precautionary measures.

Each community must assume much of the responsibility for having safe food, milk, and water supplies, and for proper disposal of garbage and sewage.

Daily personal hygiene measures, especially frequent washing of the hands, are safeguards against disease.

Isolation and quarantine are essential if communicable disease is to be controlled.

Disinfection and sterilization may be accomplished through the use of various physical and chemical agents.

The nurse is responsible for much of the teaching of health which is essential in the prevention and control of communicable diseases.

Factors To Teach the Patient

The danger to the individual and to the community if regulations pertaining to public hygiene and sanitation are inadequate or not properly enforced.

Precautions to observe in prevention of infection or disease.

The basic principles of good personal hygiene.

The benefit to the patient and to his family derived through cooperation in regard to isolation and quarantine.

The dangers involved in failure to report and get medical treatment for a communicable disease.

Methods of disinfection which may be carried out by persons caring for an isolated patient in the home.

The value of inoculation as a preventive measure against communicable diseases.

Scientific Principles

Anatomy and Physiology. Communicable diseases may be transmitted through direct contact or by indirect means, as through food, water, or air, and the handling of contaminated articles.

Pathogenic organisms may enter through the mouth or nose or through a break in the skin.

Instruction in sanitary measures and in personal hygiene helps to prevent the spread of communicable diseases.

Chemistry. Instruments should be dried before being put away to prevent oxidation and rusting.

Microbiology. Pathogenic microorganisms are found in the air and for that reason all isolated units should be kept clean and free from dust.

Isolation of the patient with a communicable disease is necessary to prevent spread of the disease.

Disinfection by means of physical or chemical agents must be both concurrent and terminal if it is to be really effective.

Ultraviolet rays may help prevent or overcome air-borne infections.

The hands of the nurse are kept relatively free of pathogenic microorganisms by careful washing in soap and water each time she leaves an isolation unit.

Pharmacology. Rinsing the hands with antiseptic solution helps to remove harmful bacteria.

Use of Lysol, hydrogen peroxide, phenol, and other germicides reduces the danger of spread of communicable diseases.

Various vaccines and sera are used to produce specific immunity to certain communicable diseases.

Physics. Areas occupied in hospitals by patients with communicable diseases are planned so that each patient unit provides larger floor space with better ventilation.

The cubical system of isolation serves to lessen the hazard of air-borne infections.

Psychology. The nurse must avoid close contact with the isolated patient to protect herself from the disease and to prevent transfer of the disease to other patients.

The patient should be told the reason for isolation technique and be instructed in various ways in which he can cooperate to prevent further spread of the disease.

The isolated patient is much alone since visitors are restricted, and for that reason recreational or diversional activities are an important part of his care. The nurse should visit the patient often to overcome any feeling he may have that he is neglected or that his family, friends, or the hospital personnel are indifferent.

Sociology. The isolation unit of the general hospital is usually in a separate building or in part of the building far removed form other patients.

The attitude of the patient toward the restrictions in family and social relationships is largely influenced by the nurse and the way in which she explains those restrictions.

The nurse plays an important part in health education to promote local and state control of infection and disease.

Each nurse should know the various community organizations set up to help with health and social problems, and should know the proper organization to help the patient. Some of the official health agencies are: The United States Public Health Service; The Children's Bureau; Bureau of Employment Security; Food and Drug Administration; Office of Vocational Rehabilitation; bureaus for the blind, the deaf, the aged. Some of the voluntary or nonofficial agencies are: American Cancer Society; National Tuberculosis Association; American Heart Association; Visiting Nurse Society; National Committee for Mental Hygiene.

Situation Type Problems

1. A case of smallpox was discovered in a small urban community and provision was made to vaccinate all grade-school children. The school nurse, informed that a certain child in the fourth grade refused to be vaccinated, on questioning the child learned that the parents were opposed to vaccination and had instructed the pupil *not* to be vaccinated with the other school children. The nurse visited the home to talk with the parents and was ordered by the irate father to leave the house. The father stated, "This vaccination hullabaloo is all a racket, the

doctors are in league with school officials to do vaccinations just so they can collect fees from parents. *I* was never vaccinated, and *I* never had smallpox. No kid of mine is going to be a party to this form of graft." What would you have done?

2. A patient who had just been admitted to a six-bed ward for men informed the student nurse performing the admission procedure that, "Dr. Graham thinks I have trenchmouth, so he told me I had better come in to the hospital and have it checked."

The doctor's orders were for general routine care; no diagnosis was given, and there was no indication that the patient might have a communicable disease. Precautionary or isolation measures had not been ordered or observed. What would you have done?

Suggested Reference Reading

"How polio is spread," Elizabeth Flagg; American Journal of Nursing, January, 1950.

"Typhoid fever," Kirk T. Mosley; American Journal of Nursing, February, 1952.

"Fluoridation—mass control for dental caries," H. Trendley Dean; American Journal of Nursing, February, 1952.

"The importance of vaccination," Arthur S. Brackett; American Journal of Nursing, July, 1952.

"T.B. control in the general hospital," Jean South and Frank T. Jones; American Journal of Nursing, September, 1952.

"When it's catching," Elizabeth Flagg; Today's Health, November, 1952.

"Some factors in tuberculosis control," Robert J. Anderson; American Journal of Nursing, January, 1953.

CHAPTER 40

Care of Patient with a Communicable Disease

TOPICAL OUTLINE

THE ISOLATED UNIT

The isolated unit is the room or cubicle within a ward where the patient in isolation is given care and attention. The unit comprises the immediate surroundings of the patient and all the supplies and equipment used in those surroundings to give medical and nursing care. When it is at all possible, a private room with running water should be provided for the isolated patient. In a ward, if only one unit is isolated, another unit should not be closer than six feet to the contaminated area.

The area (including furnishings, equipment, and supplies) inside the isolated unit is considered to be *contaminated*. Even the patient is "contaminated," since microorganisms may be transmitted by direct contact with him. The area outside the isolated unit is considered *clean* or free from pathogenic microorganisms. To illustrate the very marked distinction between clean and contaminated areas, the

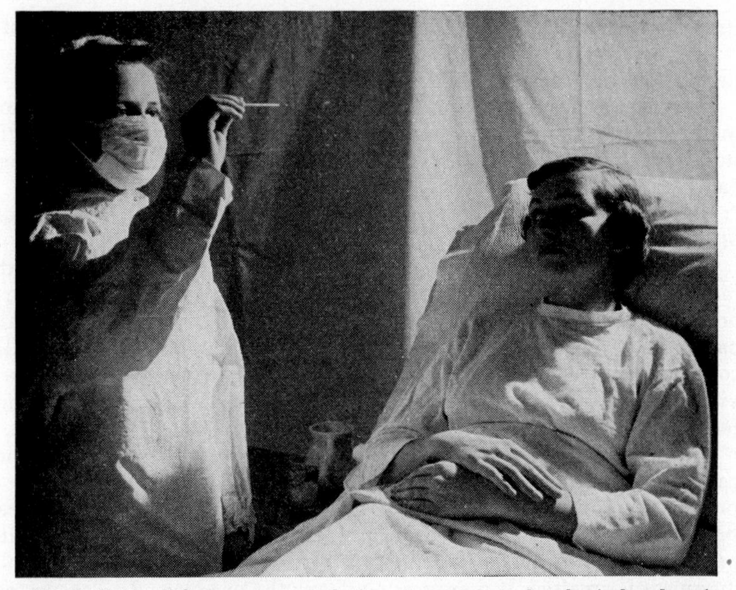

Fig. 238. Individual thermometer technique is necessary for the isolated patient. (Massachusetts General Hospital School of Nursing, Boston, Massachusetts.)

outside of the door to an isolated room is considered "clean," whereas the inside of the same door is "contaminated." The knob on the outside of the door may be touched with clean hands without danger of contamination; the knob on the inside of the door is a source of contamination and should not be touched by "clean" hands.

Preparation of the Unit for a Patient. Whether the patient is to be isolated in a private room or in a ward unit, the preparation for receiving him is essentially the same. The room (or unit) should have all unnecessary furniture and equipment removed. Heavy drapes should be replaced with washable curtains. Rugs should be removed, and the floor should be left bare to facilitate daily cleaning. Upholstered pieces of furniture should be replaced with pieces that can be cleaned by washing with a disinfectant solution. Cloth dresser and table covers should be removed and paper or plastic ones substituted.

The isolated room or unit should be well ventilated and should receive plenty of sunshine. Screens should be provided for the windows and the doors to prevent insects from entering the room. This is particularly important if the patient has malaria.

Besides the bed, bedside table, tray table, footstool, screen, and straight chair which are standard furnishings for any patient unit, the isolated unit will need a wastebasket lined with several thicknesses of newspaper, a standard, a laundry hamper, and one or two additional straight chairs. If there is not an adjoining bathroom, or running water, a table on which to set up handwashing facilities for persons caring for the patient will be needed.

Individual equipment which should be placed in the room or unit includes a thermometer in its holder, and water glass and pitcher, the standard equipment for the bedside table, and a supply of paper bags, paper tissues, and old newspapers.

Articles used to clean the room each day (broom, dust mop) should be kept in the room and used only for that particular unit.

Equipment needed in the isolated unit will vary, depending on the facilities provided by the hospital, the current isolation procedures practiced in the hospital, and the kind of communicable disease the patient has. If the patient has typhoid fever, dysentery, or a similar condition and does not have the facilities of a private bathroom, provision will need to be made for disinfection and storage of urine and feces.

Many general hospitals which do not knowingly accept isolation cases may be required to set up an isolated unit rather hurriedly to provide for care of a patient placed on "precaution." Precaution measures are needed for the protection of nurses and other hospital personnel who may come in contact with the patient while a definite diagnosis is awaited. If diagnosis confirms the presence of a "suspected" communicable disease, other patients and personnel will not have been needlessly exposed. If final diagnosis is a disease not considered communicable, the precautionary measures may be discontinued.

Several devices have been assembled which provide for the equipment needed to set up a unit for isolation. One such apparatus contains, ready for immediate use, gowns and masks, green soap solution, two solution basins, paper towels, and a waste receptacle, assembled on a mobile frame which provides hooks for hanging the gown and also serves as a standard. The apparatus may be wheeled to a room or unit and isolation technique may be placed in operation in a very shirt time without unnecessary confusion or inconvenience.

Daily Care of the Unit. Equipment used in cleaning the isolated room or unit should remain in the contaminated area and not be used elsewhere. A clean floor mop, one with detachable mop head, should be used each morning to clear the floor of dust and lint. No oil should be used on the mop. If it is dampened slightly the floor can be cleaned without setting an undue amount of dust in circulation in the air. The mop should be freed of dirt and lint after use and at frequent intervals should be removed from the frame and sent with other contaminated laundry to be washed and sterilized.

Each morning all furniture in the room should be dusted with a slightly damp cloth. The cloth should be sent with other linens to be washed and sterilized. Windows should be kept clean and window ledges and table tops should be cleaned every day. Paper covers used on dresser, tables, and work areas or other surfaces should be replaced with clean ones each day or several times during a day, if necessary, for cleanliness.

The room should be kept free of old newspapers, magazines, and other articles which need to be destroyed after use so the surroundings are kept neat and attractive. Flowers that are no longer fresh should be discarded after asking permission from the patient to dispose of them.

Candy, fruit, and other perishable foods should be brought into the isolated room only in limited quantities. The patient should be given such foods in an amount that is in accordance with his dietary regime. He should be instructed not to offer food which has been in the contaminated area to nurses or other hospital personnel or to visitors who may be permitted in the isolated unit.

Care of Unit after Dismissal of the Patient. After dismissal of a patient with a communicable disease the room or unit must be subjected to terminal disinfection, to destroy all disease-producing microorganisms that may be present. All newspapers, magazines, books, plants, flowers, food, and other articles left by the patient should be burned.

Rubber goods, such as hot water bottle or ice bag, should be fully immersed in a disinfecting solution, as Lysol 2 per cent, for half an hour, then washed and rinsed well to remove all disinfecting solution. Surgical instruments used in the unit should be washed and autoclaved. Instruments with sharp edges, as knives and scissors, should be immersed in a chemical disinfecting solution for 15–20 minutes. Sterilization by steam under pressure is likely to dull the sharp edge of the instrument.

All linen, including clean linen which may have been brought to the unit for later use, should be placed in the linen bag marked "Isolation" and sent to the laundry to be sterilized and then washed. Curtains should be removed from the window and sent to the laundry to be similarly treated. Wool blankets should be fumigated then sent to be dry cleaned before use by another patient.

All metal equipment, such as wash basin, emesis basin, bedpan, urinal, and soap dish should be washed, then placed in the large utensil sterilizer for the time required to kill all microorganisms. Smaller equipment, such as glass tumbler, container for thermometer, dishes, pitcher, and similar articles, should be boiled.

If irradiation is available as a means of disinfecting the room, the mattress and pillows should be placed so that as much surface area as possible is exposed to the light rays. After one hour of irradiation, mattress and pillows should be turned so that the under surfaces are then exposed to the rays of light. For rooms in which a tuberculosis patient has been given care, the time of irradiation should be doubled. The person operating the irradiation lamp and entering the room to turn mattress and pillows should wear protective goggles while in the room. All other persons should be kept from the room during the irradiation procedure. Where irradiation is not available, mattress and pillows should be placed in a special autoclave for disinfection or should be allowed to remain in bright sunshine for at least six hours.

The furnishings and floor of the unit should be washed with strong Lysol solution. The person responsible for this should wear rubber gloves to protect her hands from the strong solution. In some instances it may be necessary to wash the walls of the room. After all phases of terminal disinfection have been completed for the room or unit, it should be thoroughly aired for at least 24 hours, so it will be safe and pleasant for the next occupant.

THE NURSE AND COMMUNICABLE DISEASES

The nurse in a general hospital may be in contact each day with patients who are in the incubation period of development of a communicable disease. She attends patients with undiagnosed and unrecognized communicable diseases and is closely associated with people who are carriers of disease-producing microorganisms.

To protect herself and to safeguard other patients, she must observe principles of aseptic technique in practically all nursing procedures. She should wash her hands carefully after caring for one patient before going to another. She should thoroughly disinfect a thermometer used for one patient before using it for another. She should sterilize instruments and equipment after use so they are aseptically clean for use again. Application of such principles in the daily care of all patients makes it relatively easy for her to acquire the additional skills or technique required in giving nursing care to the patient in isolation, the patient with a known communicable disease.

Protective Measures for the Nurse. Various measures have been devised to protect the health of the nurse in daily contact with patients on the communicable disease service or at work in the "contagious" hospital. The causative organisms of communicable disease are virulent in nature, and it is vitally important that the nurse's health be safeguarded by the following practices: If Schick and Dick tests show susceptibility to diphtheria and scarlet fever she should be immunized by being given diphtheria toxoid or scarlet fever toxin. She must have had a successful smallpox vaccination and have been given a series of three typhoid injections within the preceding two years. She should be artificially immunized against tetanus. She should have a complete physical examination before assignment to the communicable disease service, including x-ray of the chest, and special attention to teeth, tonsils, and sinuses.

Personal Hygiene as an Added Protection. In addition to the above precautionary measures, the nurse should observe good personal hygiene practices. To resist infection and to overcome the hazards of close contact with patients in isolation, she should:

1. Take a daily bath and shampoo her hair at least once each week.
2. Get sufficient rest and sleep (eight hours of sleep is needed for most young adults).
3. Eat well balanced meals, including fresh fruit and vegetables.
4. Drink plenty of water.
5. Develop good habits of elimination.
6. Observe fundamental principles of good oral hygiene.
7. Set aside some time each day for recreation, preferably some form of outdoor activity.
8. Keep her hands in good condition. Since pathogenic microorganisms may gain entry through a break in the skin, special care should be given the hands. Frequent washing of the hands in strong antiseptic solution is necessary in caring for the isolated patient, and hand lotion should be used consistently to overcome the drying effect of such frequent handwashing. Care must be taken to avoid minor cuts or lacerations. Even the accidental pricking of a finger with a safety pin may permit entry of the causative organisms of a communicable disease.
9. Guard against infection that enters the body through the mouth. The nurse's hands should be thoroughly washed before she goes to the dining room for her meals. She should be cautious about accepting from patients any articles of food that may have been contaminated through handling by the patient. Under no circumstances should the nurse assigned to the communicable disease service continue the undesirable habit of biting her fingernails. Besides being an undignified and unclean habit, it is hazardous for any person who helps care for the sick or injured, and is especially dangerous for the person who helps care for patients with a communicable disease.
10. Use precautionary measures to protect the eyes. While caring for the isolated patient, the nurse must refrain from touching her eyes. Eye infections are always serious and may cause impaired vision.

    In some instances, as in the care of a patient with gonorrheal infection, it may be necessary for the nurse to protect her eyes by wearing goggles while performing certain nursing duties.
11. Protect the hair from contamination. A cap or head tie may be required when caring for some patients with communicable diseases. It is especially important to make use of such a protective device if the nurse caring for a child with measles or chicken pox may be in contact with other children.
12. Wear a uniform that is sensible. A uniform with short sleeves and one that is 10–12 inches from the floor is better for work on the communicable disease service. The short sleeves will not interfere with the handwashing technique and the skirt, well above floor level, is less likely to become contaminated.
13. Omit wearing of jewelry. Rings and other jewelry should not be worn in the isolated unit. Rings are a harboring place for microorganisms and cannot be easily cleaned or disinfected; the wrist watch interferes with adequate and proper washing of the hands and wrists.

THE COMMUNICABLE DISEASE PATIENT

The patient who is placed on "precaution" or assigned to a room or bed on the communicable disease service requires special attention from the nurse and members of the medical staff. Besides performing procedures with special technique, the nurse should help promote a

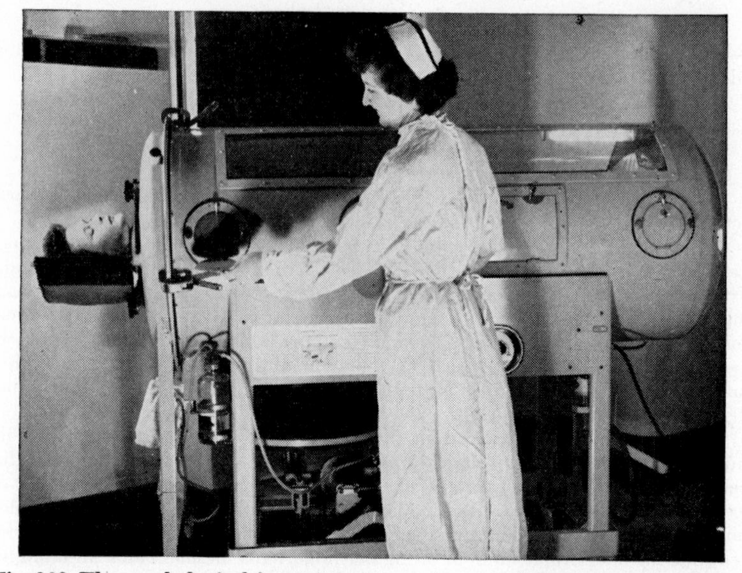

Fig. 239. The psychological factor is important in care of the patient in a respirator. (Joseph Lawrence Hospital School of Nursing, New London, Connecticut.)

desirable mental attitude and inform the patient fully of the part he must play in following isolation restrictions.

The Adult Patient. The care of the communicable disease patient is essentially the same as that given all other patients, with two possible exceptions. First, the special technique required in giving care to the isolated patient must be strictly observed to prevent spread of the communicable disease. Isolation technique, to be effective, must be observed by all who serve the patient. Each procedure has been worked out carefully so that the nurse and other hospital personnel are safeguarded, other patients are protected, and the patient with the disease is not reinfected.

The second difference is a psychological one. The emotional reaction of the isolated patient may be one of tension and anxiety because of the "precautions" taken in caring for him. Without completely understanding the need for all special procedures, such as frequent handwashing, he may resent being alone much of the time, may feel that he is being neglected by friends at a time when he needs them most, and is very apt to be uncooperative in carrying out his responsibilities in relation to isolation technique. The psychological reaction of any patient is a very important factor in his recovery, and for the isolated patient this factor may assume undue proportions.

The nurse will need sensitivity, tact, and understanding to establish the good relationship which is necessary if she is to receive the cooperation of the isolated patient. Because he is much alone, the nurse should encourage him to find entertainment and relaxation in books, magazines, newspapers, puzzles, radio, and television. He should understand restrictions placed on visitors, and should not expect to see more than a few, or expect them to remain for long in his room. If the patient understands the reason for his isolation, he will wish to do all that he can to cooperate in carrying out the regulations made to protect his family and friends and to further his own recovery from the disease.

The isolated patient who is hospitalized for the first time may tend to feel fear and apprehension because he is seemingly rejected by family and friends, as well as by hospital personnel. When the nurse washes her hands in a disinfectant solution each time she touches the patient or renders nursing service, there is an implied rejection in the act. The patient needs to understand that isolation procedures are of an impersonal nature and done routinely to help him get well and to prevent others from becoming ill of the same disease.

If at all possible, a telephone should be available at the bedside of the isolated patient. By this means he can keep in touch with family and friends without danger of exposing them to the communicable disease.

The Child Patient. Since most communicable disease patients are children, the nurse assigned to communicable service should have had previous experience in pediatrics.

The isolation technique with which procedures are performed for children are the same as for the adult patient, although the psychological reaction of the child may be quite different from that of the adult. The nurse should understand that all children need continual reassurance that they are loved and wanted, and that such reassurance may be even more essential to the child who is "shut away" or isolated from others without fully understanding the reason.

Any child who must leave home and family to enter a hospital suffers profound emotional upset, and the youngster who is put into a strange room and bed and left much alone may suffer mental strain that will affect personality as well as health. The nurse must replace the mother in giving care and attention to the child and should do her utmost to give, also, part of the understanding and sympathy and warmth which mothers express so freely to their children.

All children should be treated with respect and consideration. Procedures should be explained to them in simple terms, and care must be taken that isolated children are kept busy with interesting and varying activities so that being alone does not mean they must also be lonely. The understanding nurse will make a special effort to keep the child busy during the day and to see that the bedtime routine is similar to that which the child has been accustomed to at home. A youngster used to the comforting presence of a favorite soft and cuddling toy, as a teddy bear or rag doll, should not be deprived of that toy when confined to bed in a hospital. If the toy is not at hand, one may be quickly improvised from a bath towel or similar article.

The child in isolation, the same as any other child, is interested in play and in group activity as soon as the acute stage of the illness is over. For such children, games and books are available. Television and radio programs help keep them entertained, and in a relatively short time the isolated child may be happily adjusted to the situation and environment which at first was frightening and strange.

Recreational Facilities. Facilities or provision made for entertainment of the isolated patient are usually the same as those for other patients, but the demand is greater and the supply must therefore be increased. Books provided for such patients should be inexpensive copies when possible, as they must be burned when they are no longer useful to the patient. Magazines and newspapers supplied to the patient in isolation cannot be given later to other patients, but must be burned after they have been read.

Hobbies, such as painting, drawing, or needlework, and even various handicrafts may be pursued or even learned in the isolation department, but all objects made in the unit will need to be subjected to terminal disinfection before they can be taken from the communicable disease service. Cut flowers and plants may be of special benefit to the isolated patient, quite often serving as the only tangible link with home and friends. They should be destroyed when the patient is taken out of isolation.

Radio and television provide many hours of enjoyment to the isolated patient and enable him to keep up on local and national affairs. Mail, whether in the form of cards, letters, or small gifts, furnishes a welcome diversion for any patient. For the patient in isolation, mail is of special benefit since it is a way in which friends may make their presence felt, even though they are not permitted to appear in person.

Visitors. Usually visitors are not permitted to enter the unit of patients with communicable diseases. Children are especially susceptible to such diseases and should not visit patients in isolation. If a member of the family is allowed to visit the patient, he should wear a gown while he is in the unit. The following instructions, given orally or in written form, should be helpful to visitors permitted within isolated units.

Because your relative has become ill with a disease that may be transferred to other persons, he (she) has been placed in isolation. You can help prevent the spread of this communicable disease and protect yourself from it, by observing the following regulations.

1. Visit the patient only infrequently and remain several feet distant from the bed.
2. Explain to his (her) friends that no visitors are permitted except members of the immediate family. Ask them not to call at the hospital.
3. Wear an isolation gown (obtained from nurse at desk) while you are in the patient's room.

4. Do not touch the patient or handle articles in the room.

5. Remove the gown and wash your hands thoroughly when ready to leave the room.

6. Do not take articles from the room when leaving. Germs are carried through newspapers, magazines, books, clothing, fruit, flowers, etc.

7. Do not visit other patients in the hospital after leaving the room of an isolated patient.

8. If you are returning home where there are young children, take a bath and change clothes before coming in contact with them. Young children are especially susceptible to communicable diseases.

9. If there is cause to believe that you or other members of your family have been exposed to the communicable disease, consult your family physician as to preventive measures necessary to protect yourself and family.

10. Do not bring to the patient articles that cannot be destroyed or properly disinfected when he is released from isolation.

ISOLATION TECHNIQUE

The special technique developed for use in caring for an isolated patient, to prevent spread of a communicable disease, achieves two purposes: preventing direct contact with the patient, and destroying pathogenic organisms which by indirect contact may cause others to become infected. No attempt will be made to give in detail the special technique to be used for all the various nursing procedures, but important factors in those most commonly performed will be briefly outlined.

Mask Technique. A mask worn by the nurse caring for a patient who has been isolated because of a respiratory infection serves as a protection only if it is properly used. Masks are usually made of gauze, muslin, or some form of transparent plastic. Masks should be worn when patients are uncooperative, too ill to cooperate, mentally deranged, or when the nurse's face will come in close contact with the patient. The mask should be impervious to the microorganism causing the disease and should be large enough to completely cover the nose and mouth. The hands of the nurse should not touch the mask after it has been tied in place. If it becomes moist from exhaled air (after being worn for approximately one hour), it is no longer useful in screening out organisms and should be replaced with a clean one. It should be discarded or washed and autoclaved immediately after use; the mask should never be worn outside the isolated unit.

Gown Technique. The gown is worn in isolation to prevent contamination of person and clothing of anyone who enters the isolated room or comes in contact with the patient. The gown is made of heavy muslin, with a snug-fitting neck band, stockinette cuffs (usually on long sleeves), and two waist-band ties which can be tied to hold the gown in place. The gown should be long enough to cover the nurse's uniform completely. Clean gowns should be available for doctors and nurses whenever needed.

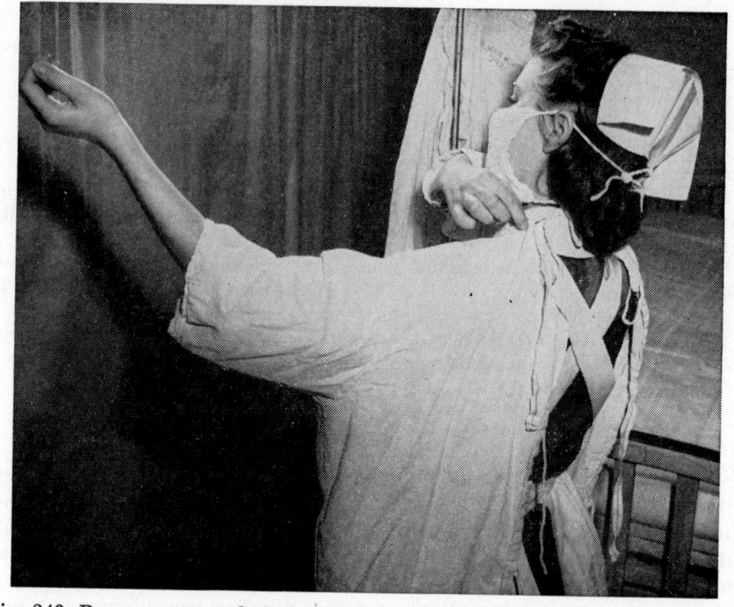

Fig. 240. Proper gown technique protects the nurse who works in an isolation unit. (Michael Reese Hospital School of Nursing, Chicago, Illinois.)

If it is possible to obtain a clean gown each time protection of the uniform is needed, gown technique is simplified. The nurse need only put on the clean gown outside the isolated unit and when ready to leave the unit she can remove the gown and place it in the laundry hamper with other contaminated linens. When the supply of gowns is limited, it is necessary to use the same gown a number of times before it is placed with other contaminated linen to be disinfected. In that event it must be carefully removed so that its inner surface and the neckband are not contaminated. It is then hung on a standard placed conveniently near the door of the isolated unit. The gown is hung so that the inner surface is not exposed to view or to contamination. The nurse or attendant should always remove wrist watch and wedding band (if worn) before putting on the isolation gown.

The outer surface of the gown should not be touched as the gown is removed from the standard. The gown is put on while the wearer's hands are clean, and the neckband is fastened with clean hands. The nurse's hands become contaminated when the waist-bands (which are contaminated by contact with the outer surface of the gown) are brought into position to hold the open edges of the gown together at the back.

When the gown is to be removed, the waist-bands must be untied,

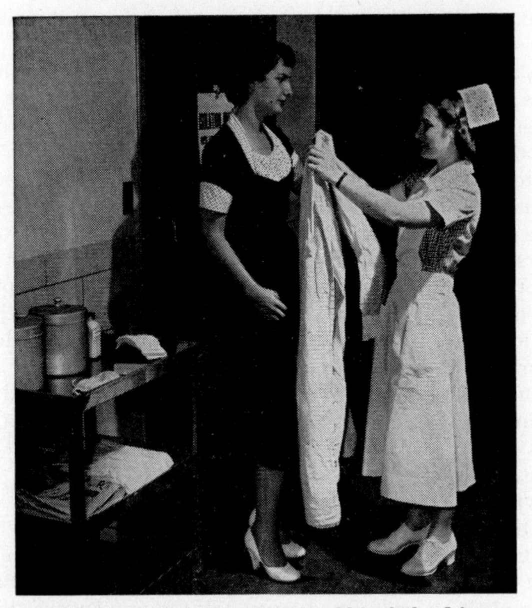

Fig. 241. The visitor to an isolation unit should be helped into a gown and instructed on protective measures. (Delaware Hospital School of Nursing, Wilmington, Delaware.)

the hands must be washed, then the neckband untied with clean hands. The sleeves may be removed by placing one hand within the cuff of the opposite sleeve and pulling the sleeve down over that hand. The other sleeve is then removed by the covered hand. The gown is removed, folded in half lengthwise, and hung by the neckband so that the inner surface is concealed and the open edges of the gown face the door to the room. If the inside of the gown should inadvertently be contaminated, the gown should be discarded and a clean one brought into the room to replace it.

When caring for several patients who have the same disease, the nurse need not change the gown when going from one patient to another. The gown used in an isolated room or unit should never be worn outside the unit. Under no circumstances should a nurse wear a contaminated gown at the bedside of a patient who does not have the same communicable disease.

General Instructions. All articles that will be needed for the treatment or nursing procedure should be taken into the isolated unit before beginning patient care. If additional articles are needed, the patient's signal light should be used to summon another nurse or attendant to ask that additional articles be brought to the unit.

Hands should be washed carefully after completing each service to the patient, and kept in good condition (free from abrasions) by the liberal use of hand cream or lotions.

Faucets, sinks, and light switches are considered contaminated. If it becomes necessary to touch them after the hands are "clean," a clean paper towel may be used to prevent contact of the clean hands with the contaminated article.

All visitors, before entering the isolated unit, should be given detailed instructions on the wearing of the gown and how best to protect themselves and others from possible contamination.

The nurse may enter an isolated unit to deliver mail or to place an article on table or dresser without putting on the gown, provided she does not come in contact with the patient or touch anything in the unit. If she enters the unit to perform a nursing procedure, even a very minor one, the gown should be worn.

The door of an isolated room should be clearly labeled with signs of "Isolation Unit" and "No Visitors," to protect hospital personnel and others who might enter the unit without knowing that the patient has been isolated.

Concurrent Disinfection. Isolation technique cannot be effective to the point that all microorganisms will be destroyed, but the number and vitality of microorganisms capable of spreading the disease to others can be greatly reduced. Measures used in carrying out concurrent disinfection are aimed primarily at preventing the spread of the disease. Procedures included in concurrent disinfection include those discussed in the following paragraphs.

Handwashing. If running water is available for the isolated unit, hands should be washed with soap under running water, dried with a clean paper towel, and the towel then used to protect the "clean hands" as the faucet is turned off.

If running water is not available, handwashing facilities should be set up on a table inside the isolated unit. The table should be covered with newspapers, and a basin of soap solution or disinfectant solution and a basin of clear water should be placed on it. Clean paper towels should be placed on or near the table, and a paper-lined wastebasket should be near at hand. The nurse or attendant should wash her hands in the soap or disinfectant solution, rinse them in clear water, and dry them with a paper towel which is then discarded into the wastebasket. Solutions in each basin should be changed frequently during the day. Since strong soap or disinfectant solution may be irritating to the skin, a hand cream or lotion should be used to keep the skin of the hands in good condition.

Care of Linen. A linen hamper is part of the necessary equipment in the isolated unit, and is used as a container to receive all linen or cloth articles used in caring for the patient. Each day the laundry bag in which the contaminated linen has been collected should be removed from the hamper frame and placed, by the nurse working in the isolated unit, inside a clean laundry bag, held by a nurse outside the unit. The top of the clean laundry bag is then folded inward and fastened without contamination of the nurse's hands or of the outside of the laundry bag. The clean laundry bag should not be more than two-thirds full when it is tightly closed and sent to the laundry.

Hospital laundry is routinely disinfected, so no special technique is used for linen from the isolated unit. Laundry bags containing contaminated linen should be clearly labeled, however, so workers in the laundry will use caution in handling the linen, omitting the usual sorting process, and thus protecting themselves from needless exposure to the disease.

Serving the Tray. The tray with salt and pepper shakers is kept in the isolated unit. Tray covers and napkins are of paper and are discarded after use. Food and dishes with needed silver is brought to the entrance of the isolated unit by a nurse or attendant. The contaminated nurse, inside the unit, brings the tray from the unit to the entrance and holds it in position to receive the contents of the other tray. The clean nurse, handling clean dishes from the clean tray, transfers them to the contaminated tray without touching the tray or the hands of the nurse who is holding it. The tray is then served to the patient by the contaminated nurse inside the unit.

Care of Dishes. After the patient has eaten, the tray should be removed from the isolated unit and placed on newspapers on the work table in the utility room while the dishes are being cared for. The tray should then be cleaned and returned to the unit. The contaminated newspapers should be burned. All food remaining on the tray should be discarded into a waxed paper bag and burned with other waste from the unit. Liquid waste is emptied into the toilet or added to waste pails containing a disinfectant solution. Dishes should be boiled for 15 minutes or placed immediately in the dish sterilizer so that all microorganisms are destroyed. Dishes that have been sterilized may be returned to supply cupboards and placed once more in general use.

The Bath Procedure. All articles needed for giving the bath, including clean linen and a supply of paper bags, cleansing tissue, and newspapers, should be taken into the unit and placed on a clean newspaper. The gown should be put on by the nurse and the bath procedure done as for other patients. Soiled linen should be placed in the linen hamper, and after the patient has been made comfortable, the room should be cleaned and all waste discarded. The unit should be left in order and, if the patient is able to read or be entertained, magazines, writing materials, or needlework should be made available. Fresh water should be placed at the bedside and the radio or television should be within easy reach.

Giving Bedpan or Urinal. The nurse must wear the gown while giving the bedpan or urinal to the patient in isolation. If toilet facilities are not available in the isolated unit, the bedpan or urinal, when being removed, should be placed on a newspaper near the door of the unit. The nurse should then wash her hands and remove the gown. As she leaves the room she carries the bedpan or urinal in one hand, and empties the contents into the hopper, using the clean hand to turn on faucets and to handle the brush for cleaning the utensil. She then returns it to the bedside table and again washes her hands before leaving the isolated unit. If disinfection is required the contents of the bedpan or urinal are added to a strong solution of disinfectant, such as chlorinated lime, and allowed to stand for 6–12 hours before it is emptied into the toilet or hopper.

Giving Oral Medications. Pills, tablets, or capsules for patients in isolation should be carried to the patient in paper containers. Liquid medicine should be measured in the glass medicine glass, then poured into a paper cup to be given to the patient. All medications are kept outside the unit, where they are measured and prepared, and then carried to the patient on a small medicine tray. The nurse should place the tray on a clean newspaper or paper towel in the unit and remove the paper cup or containers without touching the tray. After the medicine has been given and the nurse has washed her hands, she should pick up the clean tray, without touching the paper beneath it, and take it from the unit.

Giving Hypodermic Injections. The hypodermic is prepared outside the

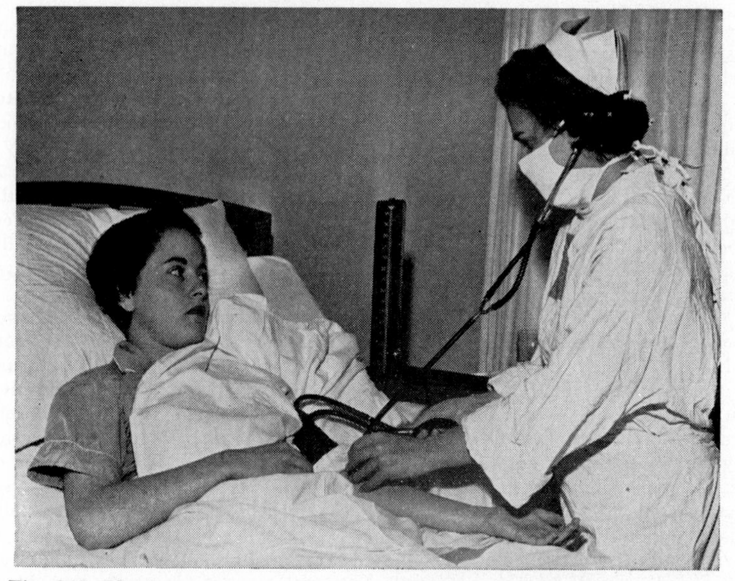

Fig. 242. Blood pressure may be taken for the isolated patient without contamination of the sphygmomanometer. (Bridgeport Hospital School of Nursing, Bridgeport, Connecticut.)

unit, then carried to the patient's bedside on a clean tray which is placed on a clean newspaper or paper towel. The nurse then puts on the gown and administers the hypodermic, placing the empty syringe and needle again on the tray. After washing her hands and removing the gown, she carries the tray with the contaminated needle and syringe to the utility room, rinses them in soap and water, and places all three articles in the small sterilizer to be sterilized.

Taking Temperature, Pulse, Respiration, and Blood Pressure. The wrist watch, placed on a clean paper towel, is carried to the isolated unit and put on the bedside table so the second hand can be seen when standing in position to take pulse and respiration. The nurse puts on the gown, removes the thermometer from its container, dries it with cotton pledget or cleansing tissue, and places it in the patient's mouth. The pulse and respiration are counted without lifting or touching the watch.

The thermometer is removed, read, cleansed, and returned to its container. The nurse washes her hands and removes the gown, then picks up the watch without touching the towel it is lying on and carries it from the unit. The nurse must remember the reading of the thermometer and the correct count for pulse and respiration so she can record it accurately after she leaves the unit.

For taking blood pressure, the stethoscope and sphygmomanometer should be placed on several layers of clean newspaper on the bedside table. The nurse then puts on the isolation gown. A clean patient gown is used to drape an area on the bed with the farther sleeve placed over the near arm of the patient. A clean towel is placed over the hand and forearm. After the procedure is completed, the manometer, cuff, and stethoscope are still free of contamination and can be taken from the unit. The gown and towel used for draping should be discarded with soiled linen in the unit.

Refilling Hot Water Bottle. A pitcher of hot water (of correct temperature) is brought to the isolated unit and placed on clean newspaper or paper towel. The nurse puts on the gown, empties the hot water bottle, then, holding the empty hot water bottle in left hand, takes clean paper towel from handwashing table, touching only the top surface of the towel. The handle of the clean pitcher is grasped, the clean or under surface of the paper towel touching the pitcher handle. Hot water is poured into the hot water bottle, being careful not to touch the top of the hot water bottle with the rim or lip of the pitcher. Pitcher is returned to the clean paper towel, the paper towel used to lift it being discarded. The hot water bottle is placed for the patient, the hands are washed and the gown is removed. The pitcher is picked up without touching the towel it was placed on, and taken from the unit.

Refilling Ice Caps. Ice is brought into the unit in a clean basin and transferred to the wash basin in the unit, without contaminating the clean basin.

Care of Equipment Used in Treatments. All equipment that has been contaminated and can be boiled (as syringes, needles, rubber goods, enamel ware, and glassware) is boiled for 10 to 15 minutes. Equipment which cannot be boiled (as sharp instruments or other special examining articles) should be immersed in disinfectant solution for 15 to 20 minutes. Articles such as flashlights, razors, hand mirrors, metal or wooden toys, should be washed with soap and water, cleansed with a disinfectant solution, then rinsed well and dried. Blankets and pillows should be placed outdoors in air and sunshine for 6 to 12 hours, or subjected to irradiation for at least 1 hour.

Care of Secretions and Discharges. Cleansing tissues used by the patient for excessive secretion of sputum, nasal discharge, or discharge from the eyes are collected in paper bags and burned. Soiled dressings are wrapped securely in several thicknesses of newspaper and discarded into the incinerator.

Collection of Specimens. Specimens of urine or feces are placed in clean containers properly labeled, identified as isolated specimens, and sent to the laboratory in the usual manner. Sputum cups handled by the patient should be placed in clean containers, labeled to indicate that the patient is in isolation, and sent to the laboratory.

Signing a Legal Document. If it is necessary for the patient to sign a legal document, it should be placed between two paper towels so that the line for signature is exposed to view. The patient may sign by placing the hand which holds the pen on the paper towel which covers the document below the line for signature. Lifting the document from between the paper towels with clean hands, it may be taken from the unit by the nurse and it will not have been contaminated.

Care of Outgoing Mail. The patient should be instructed to write cards or letters in pencil so they may be autoclaved without danger of the written words becoming illegible. The letters (unsealed and unstamped) or cards should be placed in a clean paper bag. The bag is placed in the autoclave. After autoclaving is completed, the letters are sealed, stamps are affixed, and the mail can then be placed with other outgoing mail.

Terminal Disinfection. When isolation technique is no longer required, the patient must undergo terminal disinfection before he can be transferred to a clean unit or dismissed from the hospital.

A shampoo and complete bath should be given the patient and he should be dressed in clean clothes. The clothes should not be brought into the isolated unit if it is possible for the patient, after the shampoo and bath, to be covered with a clean robe or sheet and taken to a clean dressing room. If the patient must dress in the isolated room, care must be taken so that the clothing he will wear does not come in contact with any of the contaminated furnishings or articles in the unit. The room is cared for as discussed earlier in this chapter.

CARE OF THE COMMUNICABLE DISEASE PATIENT AT HOME

When one member of a family becomes ill with a communicable disease and is cared for at home, there is a very good chance that other members of the family may also contract the disease. The experience of having the common cold go from one member of the family to another is not at all unusual. If proper precautionary measures are taken in caring for the first person who becomes ill, the secondary cases may be avoided. By observing the basic principles of isolation technique the person caring for the patient may prevent spread of the disease through the entire family.

The following general rules will be helpful in dealing with communicable disease in the family.

At the first sign of illness, seek medical help. Early treatment may prevent the illness from becoming serious. Understand that even minor communicable diseases may be serious if complications appear; early treatment helps to avoid such complications.

Know the early signs of a communicable disease, such as abdominal pain, fever, headache, nausea, and symptoms of the common cold.

Keep the sick child away from other members of the family until a definite diagnosis has been made.

If the disease is communicable and immunization is possible, other members of the family should be immunized against the disease.

To avoid exposure to communicable diseases, keep children away from movies and other public places where they might come in contact with children who may have a communicable disease.

The Isolated Room. The patient with a communicable disease who remains at home for treatment and care should be in a room which can be isolated from other rooms in the house. The room should be located away from the living room or kitchen where traffic by family members is most heavy. If an adjoining bathroom can be used only for the patient, nursing care will be greatly facilitated. The room should be sunny and well ventilated. During the summer months it is essential that the room be screened from flies and insects. If no wire screens are available, a temporary screen of gauze or mosquito netting may be used.

The room should be prepared in the same way as that described for the hospital patient. All rugs, draperies, and upholstered furniture should be removed. All unnecessary furniture or articles which cannot be readily cleaned should be taken from the room. So that the room is cheerful and attractive, washable curtains may be hung at the window, or inexpensive paper drapes can be used and destroyed at the time of terminal disinfection.

Precautions for the Nurse or Attendant. The nurse or person caring for the patient should be the only person permitted in the isolated room, and she should avoid close contact with other members of the family.

Certain precautions will help her to protect herself and to safeguard others. She should be immune to the disease, having a natural immunity or having been immunized. She should avoid taking her personal clothing and possessions into the isolated room, and should not bring contaminated articles from the room. Cover-all gowns or aprons should be worn while she is giving care to the patient.

If hospital equipment needed to set up isolation technique is not available, she should improvise equipment so that suitable technique may be followed. Handwashing facilities should be set up and each time she is in direct contact with the patient or with articles in the room, the hands should be washed in soap and water.

Daily Care of the Patient. In caring for the patient the nurse or attendant will need to assume responsibility for keeping the room clean. A damp cloth should be used to remove dust from furniture and from the floor. Care must be taken to avoid causing free circulation of dust in the room, since many communicable disease germs are air borne.

Articles brought into the sickroom should be considered contaminated and should remain in the room as long as the patient remains in isolation. Thermometers should be washed after each use and kept in a container of 70 per cent alcohol so they are adequately disinfected. Hot water bottles, enema cans, and tubes, and other equipment should be kept in the room, then properly disinfected when no longer needed. Bedpans and urinals should be washed after use and disinfected.

Bath water and other fluid wastes may be emptied into the toilet for disposal. Linens used on the bed or articles of clothing should be boiled for at least 15 minutes or allowed to soak in a disinfectant solution for 1 hour. When the patient is able to be accorded bathroom privileges, concurrent disinfection of the bathroom must be part of the daily routine. The toilet and lavatory bowl should be washed with a strong disinfectant solution each time they are used by the patient.

Dishes used in serving food to the patient should not be used by other members of the family. Glassware, silver, and other utensils should be set aside for the patient's use and should be sterilized before being returned to general usage. Dishes should be boiled each time and returned to the room for use when the next meal is to be served.

Disposal of Discharges. Paper napkins, cleansing tissues, or absorbent material such as cotton should be in easy reach of the patient at all times, to receive discharges from the nose and throat. A paper bag pinned on the side of the mattress makes an appropriate receptacle; as it is filled it can be burned and another put in its place. Discharges from eyes, ears, skin lesions, and glands may be disposed of in the same manner.

Terminal Disinfection. When the patient has recovered from the disease and there is no longer need for isolation from other family members, the room should be disinfected in much the same way as terminal disinfection is done in the hospital. Furniture, walls, and floor should be washed with a disinfectant solution. The mattress and pillows should be placed out of doors where they can be exposed to strong sunlight for approximately 48 hours. All bed linen and clothing used by the patient should be boiled. Toys that cannot be boiled or properly disinfected and books that are of no great value should be burned. Before being allowed to come in close contact with other members of the family, the patient should be given a complete bath and shampoo, and should be dressed in clothing which has not been contaminated by previous use or by coming in contact with articles in the isolated room.

Regulations set up by the Department of Health in the community in regard to termination of isolation or of quarantine should be closely followed in terminal disinfection for each communicable disease patient cared for at home.

Care of Equipment after Use

Care of equipment used for the isolated patient is discussed in the appropriate paragraphs under concurrent and terminal disinfection.

Summary of Important Factors

The meaning of the terms "clean" and "contaminated," with reference to the isolated unit.

Adequate concurrent disinfection makes terminal disinfection a less difficult procedure.

Sharp instruments should be disinfected by immersion in a disinfecting solution. A cutting edge is made dull if instruments are autoclaved.

Adequate protective health measures should be required for all personnel on the communicable disease service. Good personal hygiene practices protect the nurse against communicable diseases.

The psychological factor in the care of the isolated patient is most important from the standpoint of recovery.

Most isolated patients are children, and the nurse assigned to their care should have experience in pediatrics.

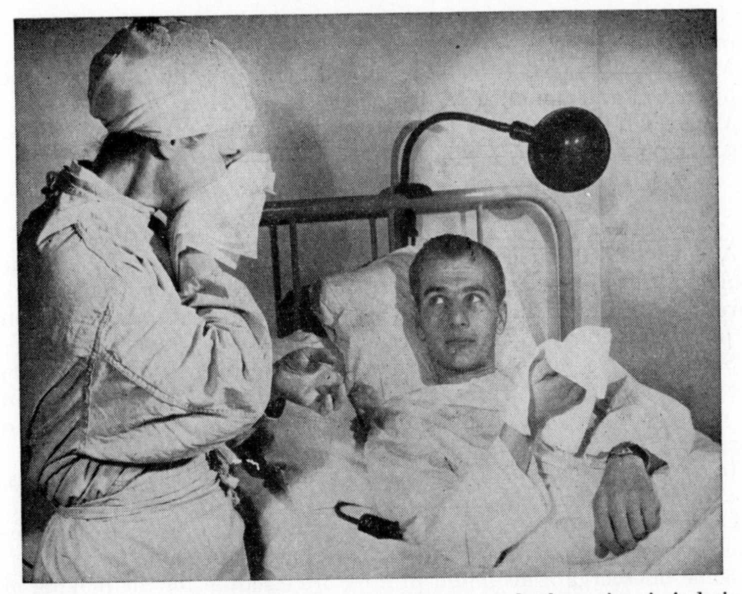

Fig. 243. Protection of others is an important factor taught the patient in isolation. (Veterans Administration, Washington, D.C.)

A soft, cuddly toy animal or substitute should be provided each hospitalized child at bedtime.

The patient in isolation should be provided various means of entertainment, such as magazines, radio, television, and puzzles.

Regulation and instruction of visitors are important aspects of the nurse's obligation to the isolated patient.

Terminal disinfection is necessary for the patient, as well as for the room or unit in which he was isolated.

Care of the communicable disease patient at home is similar to that given in the hospital, even though equipment must be improvised, and other members of the family must be protected from spread of the disease.

Factors To Teach the Patient

The meaning of the terms "clean" and "contaminated," or "unclean," with reference to isolation, so he will not feel insulted if the nurse or doctor uses the term "unclean" in speaking of him.

The various ways in which he may cooperate to help prevent the spread of his disease.

The importance of substituting an interest, hobby, work project, or form of entertainment for the visitors which are not permitted to come into the isolated unit.

Methods of protection for himself and family should they again be subjected to a communicable disease.

Where to find help from agencies of city, county, state, or national organizations concerned with public health and welfare.

Scientific Principles

Anatomy and Physiology. It is impossible to completely disinfect the hands, although washing them thoroughly in soap and water, with careful cleansing of the nails, will remove or destroy the major portion of pathogenic microorganisms that are present.

Since disinfectant solutions and frequent washings are irritating to the hands, a soothing cream or lotion should be used to keep the skin in good condition. The danger of infection is greatly increased when the hands are chapped or roughened and the skin is broken.

In general, organisms enter the body through three main channels, the respiratory tract, the gastrointestinal tract, and the skin.

Chemistry. Penicillin, a substance of value in treating diseases caused by gram-positive organisms, is formed by a mold.

Some microorganisms found in milk are essential for the making of certain dairy products, such as cheese. The chemical reaction or fermentative action of certain organisms is necessary for the making of beer, wine, and other alcoholic substances.

Instruments are dried thoroughly before being put away, to prevent oxidation or the formation of rust.

Microbiology. Dust in the air may carry a large number of bacteria, some of which are pathogenic.

Isolation units are set up or the cubical system of isolation used to prevent transfer of air-borne bacteria. The air of a room cannot be disinfected by strong-smelling solutions left in open containers. Ultraviolet rays can be successfully used to help overcome transfer of infections which are air-borne.

The number and virulence of the causative organisms of a communicable disease which enter the body determines the seriousness of the disease that may result.

Microorganisms that cause communicable diseases are parasitic in nature, existing on living tissue and thriving when given food, warmth, and moisture.

Spore-bearing microorganisms can be destroyed only by fractional sterilization.

Pharmacology. Vaccines are antigens (bacteria, viruses, toxins) which have been modified so that they will not produce disease, but still possess the ability to stimulate the production of antibodies. Active immunity is produced by vaccines.

Immune serum (from an animal or human immunized against a

specific disease) possesses antibodies that are specific for that disease. Antibacterial serum is a form of immune serum containing protective substances against certain bacterial antigens.

Antitoxins are protective antibodies which unite with soluble toxins to destroy their harmful effects.

Physics. In sterilizing articles in the autoclave, the heat must be distributed throughout the article or package. Air inside the autoclave must circulate to conduct the heat; for this reason the autoclave must be only loosely packed, and hollow instruments, as well as needles, must be open.

Psychology. Because the patient in isolation is not permitted to receive visitors, he is alone much more than is the ordinary patient. Besides being lonely, he may be depressed by the fact that his disease is one which relatives and friends would avoid, if possible. His mental outlook will be greatly influenced by the manner and attitude of the nurse assigned to care for him while he is on the isolation service. She should be cheerful and friendly, explain the necessity for special techniques used in his care, and provide various means of entertainment for him so time will pass more quickly. The patient's interests should be known and an attempt made to enlarge them. If he has no particular hobby or leisure time activity, the nurse may be instrumental in persuading him to develop one that will afford him many hours of interest and enjoyment.

Sociology. The nurse should be acquainted with official and unofficial health agencies concerned with the prevention and treatment of communicable diseases. The Federal Security Agency, of which the U. S. Public Health Service is a division, aims to prevent disease and to help control communicable disease.

Each state, most counties, and cities have their own health departments to bring health services closer to the public by providing special clinics for diagnosis, prevention, and treatment of disease.

Unofficial health agencies include the American Public Health Association, National Tuberculosis Association, National Foundation for Poliomyelitis, American Red Cross, and life insurance and pharmaceutical companies which also aid in public health work. The nurse should refer the isolated patient to the proper agency for care that may be needed after he is dismissed from the hospital.

Situation Type Problem

1. A student nurse assigned to duty on the communicable disease service discovered a visitor on the department who seemed to be visting not just one, but several patients. The nurse explained to the woman that visiting in that particular department of the hospital was not permitted and told her, also, of the requirement that any one entering an isolated room or unit must first put on the protective isolation gown.

The woman drew herself to full height and in a haughty manner informed the student that she happened to be a member of the Women's Board of the hospital, that her family had donated large sums of money to the institution, and that she was permitted to go anywhere in the hospital that she wished. What would you have done?

Suggested Reference Reading

"Nursing care of the patient with tularemia," S. G. Tillman; American Journal of Nursing, June, 1948.

"Newer drugs in the treatment of communicable disease," Franklin H. Top; American Journal of Nursing, November, 1949.

"Aseptic technique in the care of tuberculous patients," W. H. Oatway; American Journal of Nursing, March, 1950.

"Tuberculosis nursing affiliation," Louise Cady and M. H. Douglas; American Journal of Nursing, April, 1951.

"Hospitalization of patients having communicable disease," American Journal of Nursing, May, 1952.

"All-paper service for food," Ann Lucille Laird; American Journal of Nursing, September, 1952.

"An isolation unit on wheels," Wilbur A. Krell; Hospitals, January, 1952.

CHAPTER 41

The Chronically Ill—The Aged

TOPICAL OUTLINE

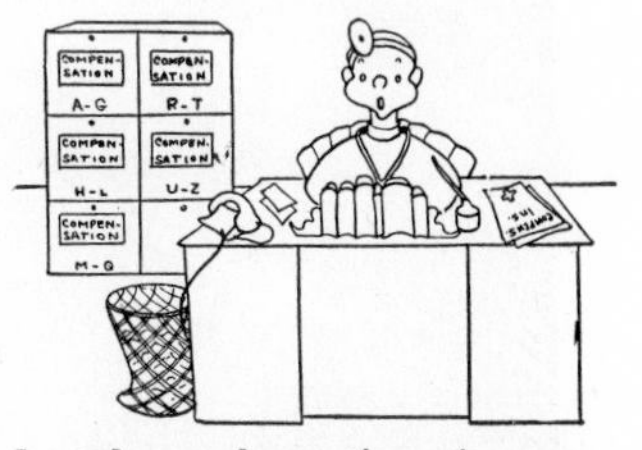

It takes a long time for some people to recover from an illness —if compensation sets in!

The Chronically Ill

With increasing awareness of the needs of the chronically ill and acceptance of the fact that they are a problem of the community rather than of the individual family, chronic illness now receives the same consideration that has long been given to diseases classified as acute or severe in nature.

A chronic disease is any disease that is mild in nature, slow in its course, and long continued. It includes those diseases requiring medical or surgical care for periods of six months or longer. It represents changes that take place in the structure of the body as a result of some abnormality of the body's functioning.

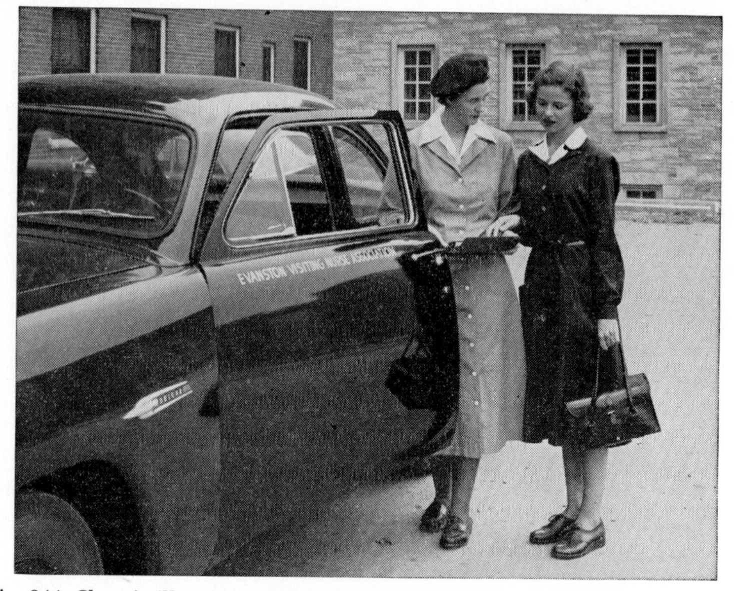

Fig. 244. Chronic illness is a community problem. (Evanston Hospital School of Nursing, Evanston, Illinois.)

The chronically ill patient, because of the duration of the disease, may be weakened in body, in mind, and in spirit. Interaction between body and mind is such that disease of the body may cause a definite mental condition, and abnormality of mental activity may cause an organic disturbance which will interfere with normal body functioning.

Many persons affected by a chronic illness recover and are able to resume normal activities. The treatment and nursing care is specific for each disease, and no attempt will be made to discuss it here except in general terms as related to all chronic illnesses.

Heart disease and cancer rank as the first and second causes of death. Other chronic diseases that may affect millions of persons are nephritis, tuberculosis, arthritis, multiple sclerosis, diseases of the central nervous system, chorea, diabetes, mental illness, epilepsy, gastric and duodenal ulcers, anemia, asthma, and bronchitis.

INCIDENCE OF CHRONIC ILLNESS

With the increase in the life span of the individual there has been a corresponding increase in chronic diseases. It has been estimated that over 50 per cent of persons 65 years of age or older have some form of chronic illness or a disability which requires long continued treatment and nursing care.

Chronic illness is not limited, however, to elderly persons. Many of the younger age group are subject to chronic diseases. About 16 per cent of patients with chronic illness are under 25 years of age and approximately 50 per cent are under 45. Many young persons are afflicted with such chronic diseases as rheumatic heart disease, epilepsy, and multiple sclerosis. Even cancer, which was long considered a disease of the old, affects large numbers of those of the younger age groups.

Chronic disabilities affect countless young men who suffered illness or injury during World War II and the Korean conflict. Such patients are apt to be chronically ill for the rest of their lives.

The number of persons with mental illness has also increased materially, and most mental illnesses are of a chronic nature, requiring long periods of treatment and care to effect recovery.

There is also a possibility that the incidence of chronic illness may again be increased if large numbers of persons are subjected to atomic attack.

FACILITIES FOR CARE OF THE CHRONICALLY ILL

With the increase in the number of persons with some form of chronic illness there is increased need for facilities for their care. Some patients with chronic illnesses need to be cared for in a hospital for all or part of the illness, although such care is very expensive because of the long-continued course of the disease. Most hospitals care for only a limited number of patients with chronic illnesses, since the beds are more urgently needed for surgical cases, for those acutely ill, and for the injured.

Large numbers of patients with a chronic illness do not really need hospital care, and the cost of such care is prohibitive because of the long duration of the disease.

Convalescent homes, nursing homes, or homes for the aged care for large numbers of patients who are chronically ill, yet it is not unusual for a home for the aged to refuse admittance to all aged persons who are not in good condition, physically and mentally.

The young patient who is chronically ill may find it difficult to adjust to the convalescent or nursing home, since most of the patients there are in the older age group.

The cost of caring for a patient in a nursing home, although less than that required for hospitalization, is often a burden to those who must bear the expense. Nursing homes are of different types and range from very good to very bad in the kind of service given. They often set up their own standards, since they are not controlled in all areas.

Some children with chronic illness are cared for in foster homes or

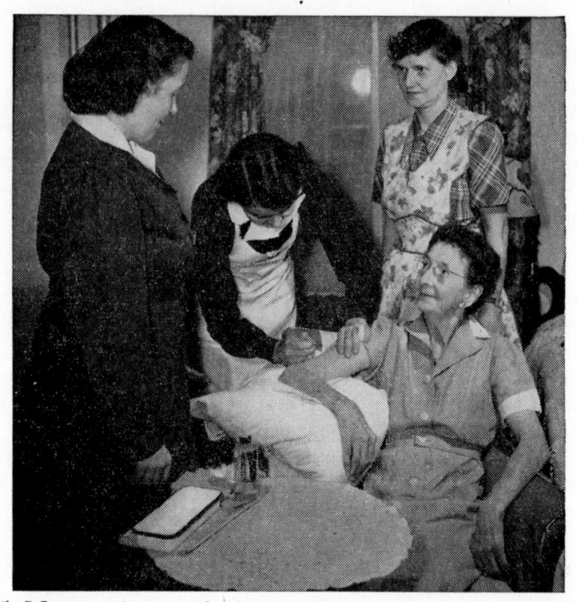

Fig. 245. Many patients with chronic illness prefer to be cared for in their own home. (Massachusetts General Hospital School of Nursing, Boston, Massachusetts.)

in boarding homes and receive benefit by the care given them. Such care should be under close supervision of a doctor, and at least part time nursing care should be made available to the patient.

Patients usually prefer to remain in familiar surroundings and are happier when cared for in their own homes. In many homes all members are employed. The chronically ill patient from such a home may be forced to enter an institution, since there is no one at home to give him needed care. If the chronically ill patient is extremely upsetting to members of the family, causes great disruption in the management of the home, or exposes other family members to possible illness it may be necessary for him to be cared for outside the home.

Those cared for at home should have the services of various agencies made available to them. For such patients nursing service is available through the local health department. Other services which are being provided for the chronically ill include housekeeping, case work, physical and occupational therapy, and financial aid.

NURSING CARE OF THE CHRONICALLY ILL

The patient who has been ill for weeks or months and has had much pain is not likely to maintain a cheerful attitude during the prolonged course of the disease. He may be bored and dissatisfied with the monotonous daily routine in the hospital or nursing home. He may be easily discouraged and depressed. As day after day goes by and his general condition remains the same, the hope of ultimate recovery may give way to a mental state that retards recovery. Financial and family worries become more burdensome as expenses increase and the weeks away from gainful employment grow in number. The nurse caring for such a patient will need to help him overcome despondency and develop an attitude of hope and encouragement, so medications and treatments will be effective in improving his physical condition.

She will soon be aware that patients with a chronic illness are extremely sensitive. They are easily offended and can be extremely difficult, especially about cooperating in various procedures, if their wishes or whims are not promptly responded to by those in attendance.

A major factor in improvement of the patient is his attitude toward the illness or disability. This may be determined, to some extent, by the attitude of others, especially of his family, friends, and prospective employers.

A person with a chronic disability finds it difficult to obtain employment even though it is generally known that such persons may do efficient work and are not in any way endangering their own health or that of their co-workers.

During the past few years a number of organizations have made it possible for the chronically ill and the disabled to become self-supporting by giving them jobs which do not require physical stamina and which may be performed in a sitting position at desk or table. The Bulova school for watch making takes for training only disabled veterans of World War II and the Korean War. Other similar industries are granting more and more such opportunities for the physically handicapped and the chronically ill.

Persons with chronic illness or disability may be indifferent in regard to personal appearance and general rules of good personal hygiene. With tactfulness and perseverance the nurse may be able to correct poor hygiene practices and instill in the patient a pride in being clean, neat, and well groomed.

The chronically ill patient, because each day tends to become a monotonous repetition of the preceding day, may become self centered and jealous of attention given other patients, and may grow more and more demanding as time goes on, with little or no improvement in his physical condition. The nurse must exercise good judgment and patience in dealing with him and in attempting to create an atmosphere of cheerfulness and optimism which will boost his morale and give him a brighter outlook. She must constantly reassure him that he is making progress, that he is receiving excellent medical care, and that he should plan for the day when he will once again resume the activities of normal living.

Comfort Measures. Keeping the chronically ill patient comfortable

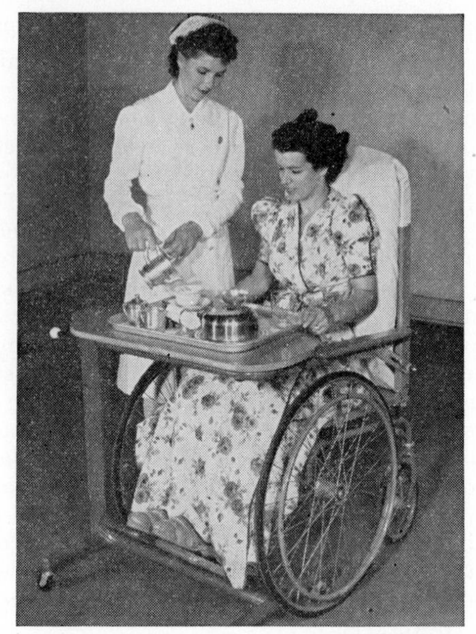

Fig. 246. Diet is of great importance in the care of the chronically ill. (Hill-Rom Co., Batesville, Indiana.)

is an important part of nursing care. The room should be kept clean, neat, and attractive. Bright drapes, plenty of sunlight, and fresh flowers or plants will make the room cheerful and pleasant and will help keep the patient in an optimistic frame of mind.

The room should be well ventilated, without exposing the patient to drafts. A common controversy in a ward where several patients are housed concerns the benefits to be derived from fresh air or the ill effects of "night air." The nurse may need to exercise tact and diplomacy to regulate the length of time and extent to which windows are opened so that all patients in the ward are satisfied, or at least so that no one patient is too dissatisfied.

Bed linens should be kept clean and the foundation sheet should be kept tightly in place and free of wrinkles. The bed should also be kept dry and free of crumbs. An air mattress and plenty of additional pillows may be needed to cushion areas where pressure is felt and pressure sores are apt to develop. The hazard of decubitus ulcers is always present when the patient must remain in bed for long periods of time. Prevention of a pressure sore is accomplished more readily than is successful treatment after the tissues have broken down.

Providing recreational facilities and helping the patient to find or develop new interests will also add to his general comfort and feeling of well being.

Diet. Because of the long duration of the illness and the patient's tendency to be discouraged or depressed, loss of appetite may become a problem. Every effort should be made to provide nourishing food that is well cooked and served attractively.

The patient should be encouraged to aid in the choice of foods to be served unless the diet is necessarily restricted. Relatives or friends of the patient should be permitted to bring certain favorite dishes from home if they wish to do so.

As a rule, eating between meals should be discouraged, although in some illnesses nourishment between meals is ordered as a part of the treatment.

The observant nurse will soon notice the relationship between loss of appetite or lack of interest in food and the patient's mental attitude. Encouragement and hope for recovery should be extended so that loss of appetite may be overcome and the dietary problem can be solved.

Exercise. For the chronically ill patient who must remain in bed, exercise is limited but should not be entirely eliminated from the daily routine. He should be turned frequently from side to side and should have his position in bed changed at intervals, to reduce fatigue.

Posture in bed should be as nearly like correct standing posture as possible. The feet should extend upward (with support, if necessary) at right angles to the leg, the head should be in correct alignment with the body. Knees should be slightly flexed to prevent strain on the leg muscles. Care should be taken to prevent such deformities as wrist drop or foot drop, even though the patient is confined to bed for months. For the very weak patient passive exercise may be needed until he is stronger physically. For the patient able to move or turn with help, use of an overhead trapeze may be beneficial, enabling him to move himself with greater ease and giving him the satisfaction of being somewhat independent.

It is generally agreed that patients improve more rapidly when they are not confined to bed all the time. For that reason, even the very weak or very helpless patient may be carried from bed to wheelchair or chair and permitted to remain up for short intervals during the day. Patients who are able to be up and around are encouraged to remain out of bed, because being ambulatory contributes to a better mental outlook, as well as greater physical improvement.

Rest and Sleep. Relaxation, rest, and sleep are essential in the successful treatment of chronic illness. Merely lying in bed does not bring relaxation and rest. If the patient is worried and apprehensive, if his mind is in a state of turmoil, and if muscles are tensed as though set for defense against possible pain or discomfort the body may soon feel the same fatigue that is produced by manual labor or vigorous physical exercise.

The nurse may need to encourage the patient to adopt a simple daily routine which will help to bring complete muscular relaxation and promote greater peace of mind.

With complete physical relaxation, the mind should be freed of its constant play of thoughts. By concentrating on a single mental image or scene, as the quiet view of a large lake or a peaceful forest, the patient may be able to exclude other thoughts and be able to relax in mind as well as in body.

Rest and sleep are necessary if the patient is to overcome the cause of chronic illness. Bedtime for all patients with chronic illness should be not later than 9:00 P.M., and 8 to 10 hours of sleep each night should be the minimum. In addition to sleep at night, the patient should sleep at least 2 hours each day. The best time for sleep during the day is soon after the mid-day meal. With practice, even the patient who "can never sleep during the day" will soon become accustomed to the afternoon rest period and will be able to sleep each afternoon. The patient should be informed, too, that even if sleep does not come right away there is no harm in lying awake so long as he doesn't worry about not being able to sleep. If he lies quietly in bed the body is at rest the same as if he were sleeping.

For patients who find it difficult to sleep several methods of encouraging sleep may be suggested. Light reading helps to free the mind of worries or personal problems and helps the body to relax. A good rule to observe and one which helps to induce sleep is "Never attempt to solve a problem after dark." A small amount of food or nourishment at bedtime may help; warm milk and a light sandwich often has the same effect as a sedative for the patient who is somewhat tense or restless.

Sleeping pills or sedatives should not be used unless specifically ordered by the physician. With proper attention to preparation for sleep and sincere effort by the patient to develop the habit of sleeping at night and during the afternoon, sufficient rest and sleep will be obtained.

Diversion. Some institutions caring for the chronically ill have a special department of recreational and occupational therapy. For ambulatory patients who remain in the institution for long periods of time there is little or no problem related to diversional activities. For the chronically ill who must remain in bed or who may be cared for outside the hospital, much of the responsibility for providing recreation or opportunity for diversion rests with the nurse and her co-workers. The recreational needs of the patient who is chronically ill are usually much greater than for the acutely ill patient, and the problem of keeping morale high and mental outlook bright may be a major factor in treatment.

Various means of diversion are available to patients, and the sincerely interested nurse will encourage any one or more of the available activities. When choosing diversion or recreational activities for the patient, certain factors, such as age, sex, natural ability and interests, and the patient's general condition, must be given consideration.

Age. For the average adult patient age is not as important a factor as for the child. Great differences exist in children of different age groups, and a play activity suitable for one child may not be at all suitable for another.

Patient Interests. Interests of the patient must be considered if he is to be stimulated to active participation in a recreational activity. If he is really interested in the activity selected he will receive greater satisfaction from it.

Play or Work Activity. Whether the diversion is a play or work activity is also important. If the selection is based on a need, as for self-support after recovering from the chronic illness, the incentive to learn the work or trade will be greatly strengthened.

Cost. Many activities may provide recreation for the bed patient at little or no expense. The financial status of the patient may be a determining factor in the choice of diversion.

Natural Ability. No person will long remain interested in an occupation or undertaking which is so difficult for him that his efforts result in failure, or in one that is too simple for his ability. The chronically ill patient will become discouraged and depressed if in his chosen diversion he cannot accomplish what he set out to do.

Sex. Sex is a factor to be considered in choice of diversion, even though many activities are of equal interest to both sexes. Men are more apt to be interested in leather work, carpentry, etc., while women prefer such activities as sewing, knitting, and weaving.

General Condition. Finally, the general condition of the patient, both physical and mental, will help determine the most suitable diversion. The patient in a weakened physical condition may be restricted to the position of listener or onlooker. An ambulatory patient or one making definite progress toward regaining health may actively engage in many forms of recreational activities.

The diversion for the discontented or discouraged patient must be chosen wisely if it is to be of value to him. An unwise choice may lead to even greater discontent, and improvement in physical condition may be retarded.

Nature of Diversion. The list of diversions from which to choose is an ever-growing one, and varies widely. It may be wholly for recreation or it may become the foundation on which a new trade or new occupation is built.

Numerous patients find that they will be required to change their occupation when they have recovered. While confined to bed they may begin to learn a new trade. They may learn by self-education, they may choose to enroll in a correspondence school, or they may learn from a fellow patient or through the occupational therapy department. Sedentary occupations, as jewelry repair, leather work, or sewing may occupy many hours of their time while they are ill and become a source of income and their life's work after they have recovered.

Radio and television offer entertainment and educational advantages

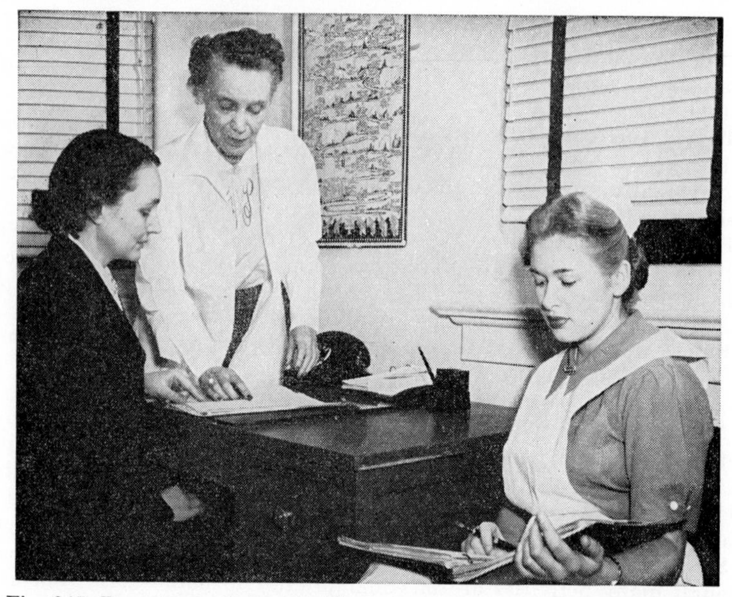

Fig. 247. Prevention of chronic illness is one of the chief responsibilities of the Public Health Service. (Evanston Hospital School of Nursing, Evanston, Illinois.)

for the patient confined to bed. Even if the patient is restricted in physical activity he may, through these media, learn to enjoy and appreciate all kinds of music, and through music may come to know the leading composers and the outstanding performers on stage, radio, and screen.

The patient who has read widely and is at home in the world of books should not be shut out of that world if his illness prevents him from seeing and thus from reading. Books should be read to him. If the nurse is too busy to take time to read to him, she should find another patient or a friend who will read for the patient.

Mail is an important diversion for all patients. The "Get well" cards, the note of greeting, the newsy letters, all serve to reassure the patient and to remind him that he is still an important part of the family circle and of the community from which he comes.

Friends who are sometimes at a loss as to what they can do should be reminded that few gifts or remembrances bring more pleasure to the patient than does a subscription to his home town newspaper. Other newspapers may be larger and better, but none will ever be more carefully read and re-read than the little hometown paper in the hands of a patient away from home.

Chess, checkers, and other games and puzzles furnish welcome diversion, and collections of all types of items may be given consideration. Model making, soap carving, whittling, sewing, knitting, weaving, and rug making are other activities that may appeal to many patients.

Large numbers of persons have felt the desire to express themselves through the medium of writing. The chronically ill patient with such a desire may relieve the monotony of enforced idleness by writing. He may write and send letters to all parts of the world; he may write magazine articles, fiction, poetry, or merely a few notations each day in a diary.

It takes great courage to remain in bed day after day for weeks, or months, or years, and a patient may become easily upset by things that would not ordinarily bother him. Given something interesting to do and allowed to work toward a brighter future, the chronically ill will return to health much more quickly than if left to their own resources.

PREVENTION OF CHRONIC ILLNESS

The prevention of chronic illness is dependent on several factors: (1) the control of causative agents and improvement of the body's resistance to disease; (2) the kind of treatment and care given individuals now suffering from some form of chronic illness; (3) accurate and early diagnosis, with early institution of treatment; (4) periodic examinations to facilitate early diagnosis; (5) removal of foci of infection; (6) opportunities for recreation and rehabilitation with improvement in treatment and nursing care; (7) close adherence to rules of good personal hygiene.

By observing the above suggestions, as well as the general rules of health, and by refraining from overeating, overworking, lack of sleep, constant worry and excessive use of stimulants, an individual is more likely to escape the development of any one of the conditions classified as chronic illness.

The Aged

All living things must grow old, and members of the human race are no exception to that general rule. The process of aging creates new problems which require scientific study and research. All other age periods, including infancy, childhood, adolescence, and maturity, have been studied, have benefited by medical research and by care and attention to physical and psychological needs. The diseases and disabilities of the aged have only recently begun to receive the attention of medical schools and of social, educational, and governmental organizations.

The older members of society in this country are not cared for and respected as in other countries such as China, Sweden, and Norway.

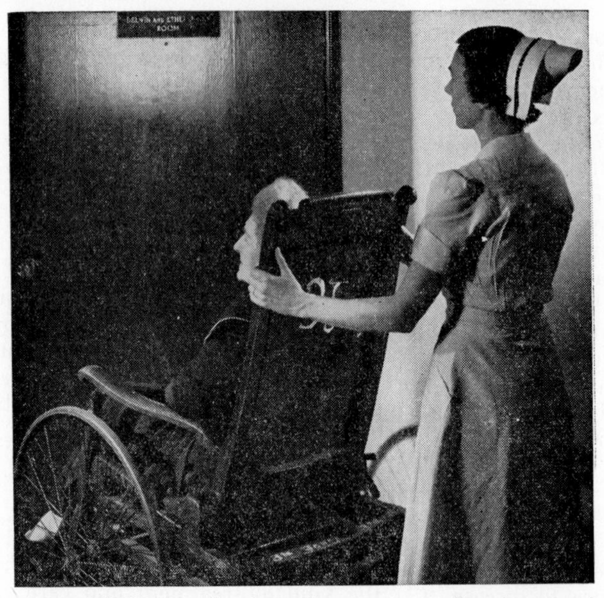

Fig. 248. Increased life span has brought a corresponding increase in chronic illness. (Presbyterian Hospital, Chicago, Illinois.)

The material increase in the number of older people in our population has made it imperative that the needs and problems of that older age group be studied and provision be made for their security and happiness.

INCREASED LIFE SPAN

The number of older people in this country has increased at a remarkable rate in the last 10 or 12 years. Before that time the increase was gradual. In 1940 approximately 7 per cent of the population were 65 years of age or older. It is estimated that by 1980 about 12 per cent of the population will be 65 years or over. This remarkable increase in the length of life is due largely to: lowered infant mortality rate, better child care, control of communicable diseases, decrease in the number of young people coming to the United States from other countries, and medical research which has led to more effective medical and surgical treatment.

Although the life span has been lengthened there has been little progress in the control and treatment of chronic diseases which commonly occur in old age. In enabling persons to live for more years only half the ultimate aim has been achieved: those additional years must be healthy, happy, and productive years, and not merely a few years of meaningless survival.

GERIATRICS

The word "geriatrics" is Greek in origin and means care of the aged. From the nursing standpoint, geriatrics means the prevention, treatment, and care of disease conditions affecting persons in the older age group. The study of the process of aging is termed *gerontology*. Aging is a process that takes place from the time of conception to the time of death, although it is popularly considered the process of gradual change and deterioration which characterizes the person after age 45. Generally a person of 65 or more is considered aged, or old. At that time usually certain characteristic results of the aging process have appeared. No definite age has been established as indicative of maturity, since some persons are mature at 18 and others are still immature at 38; the age at which one is old is also indefinite, some are old, mentally and physically, at 35 and others are still young at 65.

It is difficult to ascertain the real biological age of a person since the various organs of the body do not age at the same rate. The heart may be old or "worn out" while other organs are still functioning normally. The greatest tragedy is this unequal aging of various parts of the body. The biological age is the real indication of whether a person is old; the chronological age merely indicates the passage of a certain number of years.

Senescence is the term applied to the appearance of changes characteristic of age. *Senility* denotes advanced deterioration in both mental and physical faculties, occurring usually with age.

SIGNS OF AGING

Certain signs indicate that normal aging is taking place in the individual. The age at which these signs appear may vary widely. In many instances the physiological (or biological) age is not at all the same as the chronological age. For that reason, the practice of compulsory retirement for persons of a stated chronological age is fallacious and wasteful of valuable physical and mental assets, possessed by persons who have lived long and profited by their experiences.

Signs of normal aging include changes in visual acuity; increased susceptibility to cold because of circulatory changes; graying or loss of hair; changes in texture and appearance of the skin; increased fatigue, often without more than usual activity; delay in recovery from injury, illness, or infection; increased tooth decay, with subsequent loss of teeth; digestive disturbances, with the necessity to eat only easily digested foods; normal changes in functioning of the

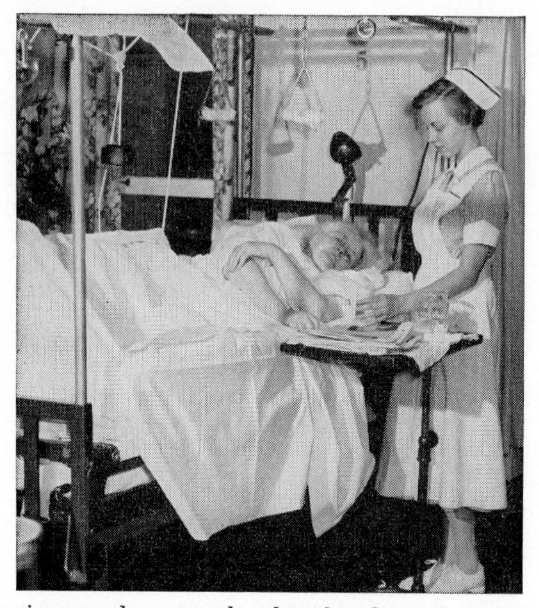

Fig. 249. Nursing procedures must be adapted to the needs of the aged patient. (Grant Hospital School of Nursing, Chicago, Illinois.)

reproductive system; changes in the skeletomuscular system which results in the characteristic appearance of the aged person.

The nurse who is helping in the care of aged patients must recognize that the changes occurring with age make it necessary to adapt nursing procedures to the needs of the patient. She should also be aware of the fact that she, too, is undergoing the changes of aging and should plan intelligently for the time when her own needs and desires will be those of the aged person.

BASIC NEEDS OF THE AGED

Large numbers of older people are restless, unhappy, and uncertain. Their basic needs are those of any person. The old do not become old over night, and during the years that the aging is in process the basic needs remain the same.

Basic needs of the aged, as for all other persons, are the need to love and to be loved; the need of companionship; the need for recognition; the need for personal achievement; the need for economic security; the need for an occupation.

The needs of the older age group have been defined in the simple quotation, "Someone to care, something to do, and somewhere to live." Of these three, the need for someone to care is probably the most important. Evidence that economic security is less important than emotional security is manifest by the large numbers of persons who are very old, very wealthy, and, in many instances, very unhappy.

Old age is a period when friends are lost and disappear from the scene one by one. The person left more and more alone experiences a feeling of desolation which can grow into panic as companionship is denied to him more and more. In many cases the older person, lacking means of self support, must leave friends of many years to move to a strange city or location to live with a son or daughter. Older persons find it more difficult to adjust to a new location. They may feel unnecessary and unwanted. They are unable to visit old friends or to see and talk with persons of their own age group. They are often lonely and unhappy. The son or daughter, in a different social economic situation, finds it difficult to understand why "Mother" or "Father" is not satisfied, with a nice place to live and not being required to work. The older person usually is not allowed to help around the house and is given no responsibility. Such a situation only adds to the feeling of uselessness and to the concern about being a "burden."

Another factor which adds to the unpleasantness of the older person's lot is the present-day trend of living in small apartments in urban areas. Rambling old houses with many rooms have given way to the modern two- or three-room apartment. An older person in a small apartment where there are children is constantly aware of the fact that he is an extra burden, someone who is in the way, another mouth to feed, and quite often the cause of quarrels or of difficulty between the younger persons.

The need to love and to be loved is one of the most essential of the basic needs. Each person, young or old, must have at least one person to whom they are really important, and one who is of great importance to them. In the very young, the important person is the mother or the person who provides the care and attention needed by the helpless infant. In the young adult sex is a vital part of the need to love and to be loved, and sex activity becomes the means of expressing that love. For the older person, deep affection and tenderness may gradually replace the sexual manifestation of love. If the love is real and lasting, a decrease in sex activity need not mean a decrease in love. The old are inclined to return to the earlier and more simple expressions of love, such as exchange of a smile or a look of understanding, the touch of a hand, an act of thoughtfulness or consideration. They tend to become less interested in the world about them and to rely on each other for companionship and for reassurance. An older person deprived of the companionship of a well-loved partner may grow more and more dependent on the assurance of God's love and may find satisfaction and contentment in religion.

The old have need of personal achievement which is often difficult for them to meet since few jobs are available to them. In the city it is usually the young who go to work, since only the young find employment readily. Even if a job is found by the older person, transportation may be too difficult for him and the job is given to another.

The retirement of employees merely because they are 65 years of age is an unfair and unsound practice. The usefulness of the employee, rather than chronological age, should determine the time of retirement. The incompetent should be eliminated long before the age of 65.

The policy of forced retirement at a certain chronological age, and the reluctance of employers to give jobs to the old, deprives them of the stabilizing influence or security of an established daily routine. Without the stimulus of work and the need to conform to a daily working schedule, the old spend the daytime hours in aimless activity and unsatisfactory measures for killing time. Their life is without purpose and may readily become burdensome to themselves unless they can work to feel personal achievement or have memories of achievements in the past.

Older people who still have the companionship of some one in their own age group may learn to depend on the other for interests and for ways of occupying their time. The old person who is single is apt to become bitter and resentful, unless he has developed a substitute for the companionship and interests of family which has been denied him.

COMMON PROBLEMS OF THE AGED PATIENT

To give better nursing care to the elderly patient, the nurse must be aware of some of the problems confronting him and must realize that such problems can affect his mental attitude or outlook and be directly responsible for his physical actions.

Many problems of the aged relate to the lack of financial security. A few have made financial provision for old age, some have hospital or health insurance, some receive small pensions from the state, but many are dependent on their families for their entire support. Those who are dependent on others for support often feel they are an unwanted burden. That feeling is intensified when they must be given hospital and medical care, and the cost of that care increases by many times the total expense of providing for them which must be borne by the family. It is not surprising that under such conditions the aged patient is often despondent, takes little or no interest in his surroundings, and expresses the desire to be relieved of his unpleasant situation by death.

Social insecurity is another problem of many aged persons. Those who live alone may become more and more lonely and neglected, as their old friends die or move away to be cared for in distant places by their own families. Those who make their homes with their children are often unable to adjust to the changed surroundings and the constant reminder that their presence creates a problem for the young adults. Old people who live in nursing homes are often there against

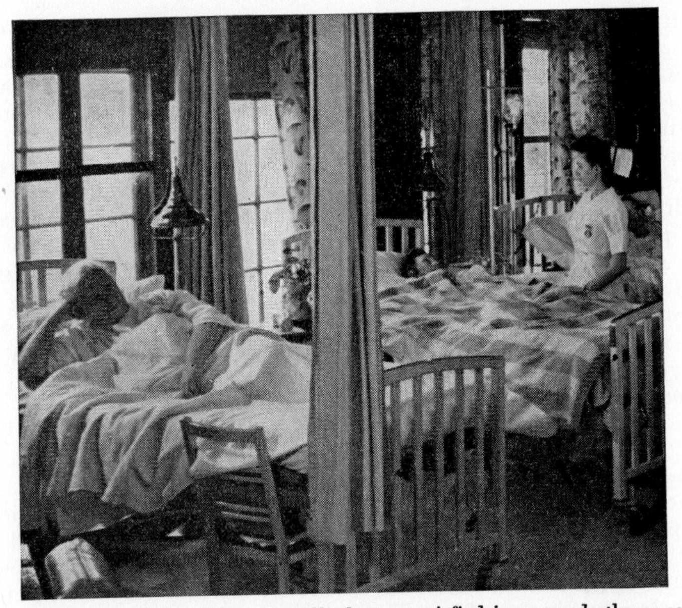

Fig. 250. The aged patient is usually better satisfied in a ward; the presence of other patients is reassuring. (Ravenswood Hospital School of Nursing, Chicago, Illinois.)

their wishes. They worry about the expense incurred by the family, and know that the only alternative is to live at their children's home where there is no room for them and no desire to have them present.

Another problem of the aged relates to their need for psychological security. The age of mental maturity is reached at about 40 by the average person, and with added interests and activities may continue to develop slowly for the next 25 years. The best mental period is normally between 40 and 65. Sometimes learning ability and imagination remain at a high level throughout the entire life span. The actual period of senility or severe old age is the time of general reduction of mental efficiency.

Many persons beyond the age of 65 have had only an elementary school education, and their interests have been entirely within the boundaries of a small rural area. Their work activities may have been limited to the daily routine of housework or of farm labor. When they are no longer able to perform tasks of manual labor they can only sit idle and wait helplessly for the passing of the remainder of the time left to them. Added to their inability to continue activities which they have had during the years are other difficulties such as hearing defects, impaired vision, and partial loss of memory. Although the nurse may feel that some form of recreation is needed for such patients, she should know that it is futile to attempt to interest them in a hobby or to try to teach them a simple form of craftsmanship. After old age has arrived, there is little or nothing that can be done to provide an interest or activity which will relieve the monotony of the existence of the aged person.

Spiritual comfort often becomes a primary need for the older patient, and the nurse should be quick to honor any request made for such comfort. She should see that the priest, rabbi, or clergyman of the patient's church knows of the patient's admission to the hospital and of the patient's desire to see and talk with him. If the patient has derived pleasure from reading the Bible and because of failing eyesight is no longer able to read, arrangements may be made for someone to read to him. If the nurse is too busy to read to the patient, she can usually find a reader among members of the patient's family or among the convalescent patients on the clinical department.

ROUTINE NURSING CARE OF THE AGED

Routine care for the aged each day consists of careful attention to all phases of personal hygiene and to the basic needs of the aged.

It is not necessary for a daily bath to be a part of the regular routine for the aged. With their lessened activity, the skin may be kept clean with less frequent bathing. The aging process and the inelasticity of the skin does predispose to the development of decubiti if the patient is allowed to lie immobile for long periods of time. Skin surfaces where pressure is exerted should be massaged frequently. Alcohol should not be used, since it is drying to the skin; mineral oil or lanolin creams will help keep the skin supple and in good condition.

Some nurses may unknowingly tend to neglect the aged patient, by providing only for physical needs. The patient may be kept clean and well groomed, the bed linens may be changed each day, food may be given to the patient unable to feed himself, elimination may be checked daily, and medications and treatments given on time, yet the mental or spiritual needs may be given little or no attention.

Although the elderly patient may not see or hear as well as formerly, he may still enjoy recreational diversion depending on sight and hearing. For such patients the careful selection of radio and television programs may be important in providing entertainment and answering the need for mental and spiritual stimulation. So long as the sense of sight or of hearing is present, the patient need not depend entirely on others for recreation. He may derive pleasure from reading or being read to, from musical programs, from simple games, and especially from visitors and from mail received from family and friends.

The senses of smell and taste are usually the most acute and may be retained by the patient to a very old age. Old people need nourishing food, although the quantity they eat is usually less than that taken by the younger adult. It is unwise to try to change the established food habits of an older person. Loss of appetite is a common occurrence among the aged, and patients should not be coaxed or forced to eat other than foods deemed essential to health. Malnutrition is not uncommon among the aged, but it usually results from poor oral hygiene and defective teeth.

Few elderly people are overweight, since obesity contributes to causes of early death and very fat persons seldom live to be elderly. Old people may overeat, however, although usually it is because of emotional problems rather than a desire for food. In some instances food acts as a sedative for the old, and the patient may overeat in order to receive the sedative effect of the food.

Since the sense of smell is retained by the aged patient the nurse should make an effort to have food of a pleasant aroma on the tray at mealtime. A bright flower on the tray helps to make the meal pleasant, too.

In addition to being malnourished, older patients may show signs of dehydration. In such cases proper fluid balance becomes the responsibility of the nurse. She will need to be very patient and tactful in urging the intake of fluids. Old people with urinary frequency or discomfort are reluctant to take fluids by mouth, their body does not readily absorb fluids into the tissues, and they fear other means of administering the fluid which they need.

Older patients may be very noncommittal in regard to past experiences or to present situations. They should not be forced to talk, even to respond to questions, if they appear to wish not to do so. Continued silence which may seem to be contrariness on their part may often be their only means of reacting to a frustrating situation.

The number of hours of sleep needed is decreased as chronological age increases. Old people seldom sleep soundly throughout the night. Intermittent periods of sleep is common and seems not to interfere with general well being. They may doze at intervals during the day, so that the total hours of sleep is approximately that of the average adult. Aged individuals often read at night or get up to wander about the house. They may even prepare and eat a meal at night and fail to understand that such action appears somewhat peculiar to others. The nurse should make no concentrated effort to alter the sleeping habits of an aged patient, although she may be partially successful in providing interesting activities to keep them awake during the day so that they may sleep for longer periods at night.

A common cause for controversy and unhappiness for old people is attempt by a nurse or other person to change their lifelong habits in daily living. The older person has developed definite likes and dislikes and even though they may differ widely from present-day trends or methods, efforts at correcting or changing them should be avoided. The very old lady who has worn woolen bed socks for years will not understand that such articles of clothing are not necessary in modern rooms where the temperature is thermostatically controlled and is not affected by the sub-zero temperature outside.

The old person should have personal freedom so long as his safety is not jeopardized. The belief of family or friends that the old are incapable of caring for themselves and the attempt to "take charge of them" causes discontent and unhappiness. Even for the old person who is ill, unnecessary adjustments should not be forced on him, and change in the daily routine should be made only when it becomes absolutely essential.

The older patient retains his sense of touch and is better satisfied when doing something with his hands. Weaving, knitting, whittling, or the making of very simple objects gives him the needed thrill of accomplishment and keeps him busy at intervals during the day. In encouraging the aged to use their hands, the nurse should remember that old hands and eyes tire quickly. The patient should not be urged to spend prolonged periods at such activity, and should not be pushed to complete an article he may be making.

Patients who may not have learned to use their hands for even simple tasks will derive satisfaction merely from handling an object that may be moved about in their hands. A soft rubber ball or small sponge will be useful in helping to give the exercise or movement needed by the fingers which tend to become stiff if they are not used at all.

The surroundings or environment for the aged patient should be attractive and cheerful. Even if the patient's sight is failing, the room should be made pleasant with bright drapes and colorful furnishings. Window blinds should be up to permit plenty of sunshine in the room. Flowers should be tastefully arranged and given daily care. The room may be brightened, too, by a display of the "get-well" cards which are usually received by all patients.

Most people over 60 years of age require glasses for reading. Care should be taken that glasses are within easy reach, and that they are kept clean. When not in use, the glasses should be put away. Loss of glasses which cannot be quickly and easily replaced has caused many hours of enforced idleness to patients in the hospital. Reading is a source of comfort and relaxation to the elderly patient who has, over a period of years, developed an enjoyment of reading. Such a patient who is in a private room in the hospital should be permitted to turn on the light and read at intervals during the night if he wishes to do so.

The aged, because of impaired circulation, are more sensitive to temperature changes. They should be clothed in bright, warm gowns and bed-jackets. Warm nightshirts should be used for aged men.

It is not unusual for older people to lose interest in their appearance and to neglect such basic factors of personal hygiene as proper care of hair, teeth, and nails. An understanding nurse will help the patient to regain the desire to appear at his or her best. The older woman

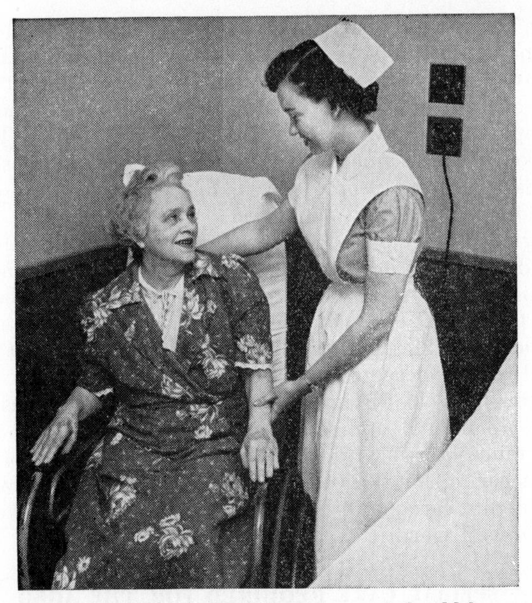

Fig. 251. Because of impaired circulation the aged should be warmly clothed even during summer months. (Alabama Baptist Hospital School of Nursing, Birmingham, Alabama.)

who has her hair gently brushed and arranged in an attractive and simple style with a small ribbon or flower fastened in place and who may have been persuaded to wear soft curlers during the night is usually pleased and proud of her improved appearance. The hair should be kept clean but should be washed only about every three or four weeks. There is no reason why the older woman patient should not be given a permanent wave. She should be encouraged to care for her own hair and should be praised for any attempt she may make to keep it attractively combed and arranged.

One of the trying aspects of growing old for women may be the appearance of coarse and bristly hairs of the eyebrows and of stray hairs on the face, especially on the chin. Plucking of stray hairs may be done quickly and effectively by the nurse and will help to improve the patient's morale. Hairs growing from moles should not be plucked but may be snipped off close to the surface of the mole by a pair of very sharp scissors.

Old people are sensitive about the fact that the senses may not be as acute as in former years. The nurse should always speak to them in a natural tone of voice. Even patients who are partially deaf should not be shouted at or addressed in a different manner than that used for other patients. And the nurse should know never to hurry or appear to be in a hurry when caring for an aged person. Care hastily given will emphasize to the patient the thought which causes them greatest concern and unhappiness, the thought that they are in the way, a nuisance, a burden, that they are unneeded, unloved, and unwanted.

Old people need to avoid haste in their own activities. The old man should take twice the amount of time for shaving that was required in earlier years. All old people should dress slowly, walk slowly, and adopt a slower pace for all activities.

Although frequent periods of rest are necessary for the aged, too much waiting on by others and prolonged periods of inactivity may be harmful both physically and mentally. Permission to be out of bed indicates to the patient that the doctor is confident of ultimate recovery, and the value of early ambulation for any patient is now generally and readily accepted.

No matter how old the individual, so long as he retains capacity to participate in mental and social experiences life is still meaningful and very much worth while for him. The nurse must bear in mind always, in caring for the old, that for them time is slowly running out. Considerate care and a little extra attention will make them happier and is well worth the effort required.

SPECIAL CARE REQUIRED FOR THE AGED

As a rule the aged are better satisfied when cared for in their own homes. When they must be hospitalized the nurse should help them adjust to hospital routines by allowing them to maintain their own pattern of daily routine whenever possible.

Special care should be taken to prevent accidents or injury to the aged patient by judicious use of side rails on the bed and by almost constant supervision by nurse or attendant. If the patient is permitted out of bed, floors in the room should not be waxed and rugs should be placed so there is no danger of falling or tripping over them. The use of heating and electrical appliances should be adequately supervised.

Special care is needed for the incontinent patient. A condition of incontinency means that the patient is often wet and uncomfortable. It may mean the presence of an embarrassing ammoniacal odor in the room. It is a predisposing cause to the development of a decubitus ulcer and may produce in the patient a tendency to retreat from all social contacts. When indicated, the use of an indwelling catheter may be the means of overcoming many of the difficulties caused by incontinence.

Special care of emergency situations is also part of caring for the aged. The nurse must know what is expected of her, and what she is permitted to do in case of sudden heart failure or other conditions of an emergency nature.

As a final suggestion to be made to those responsible for the care of an aged person, the use of pets should not be overlooked. An elderly person caring for a pet kitten, canary, or goldfish derives satisfaction and comfort from the knowledge that he is essential to the welfare of the pet. Even the old who cannot see or hear may derive satisfaction from holding or stroking a small kitten. Such activity is limited but even limited activity is better for them than no activity at all.

THE ELDERLY SURGICAL PATIENT

Surgery which is most commonly required for elderly patients includes gastrointestinal surgery (consisting principally of tumor resections); genitourinary surgery (usually made necessary because of prostatic hypertrophy); cardiovascular procedures (usually related to leg ulcers and amputations); eye surgery (resulting from cataracts and glaucoma), and procedures necessary for correction of neurological, gynecological, or thoracic conditions.

Care given to elderly patients following surgical treatment is essentially the same as that for other adult patients. The aged patient may be confused and disoriented for a longer period of time and will need to be carefully watched to prevent him from removing surgical dressings or taking an intravenous needle from his arm or from removing drainage tubes that may have been put in place during the operation.

The giving of morphine as a postoperative narcotic for the older patient will need to be closely supervised. Respiration rate should always be carefully checked before morphine is given. If the rate of respiration is 12 or lower there is danger in giving morphine, which is a respiratory depressant. The elderly patient who often wakes and ordinarily begins his day early in the morning should be cared for as early as possible, and the nurse should make a special effort to see him frequently throughout the day.

PREPARATION FOR OLD AGE

The nurse who is in daily contact with aged patients and aware of the many problems confronting most of them not only should do her utmost to improve the mental outlook of the patient but should plan her own life so that she lives fully in the present and prepares for her own old age in the future.

Several ways of insuring a happier old age for herself would be: to take stock of herself, to consider her assets and liabilities and to discover that which is needed if she is to provide for her own basic needs in the future. She, too, will need financial security, companionship, and a sense of having made a worth-while contribution to the world. She, too, will need "someone to care, something to do, and somewhere to live."

In preparing for her own future she should plan to do work that is enjoyable and satisfying and of which she can be proud in later years; to strive for economic security by following a budget providing for wise spending and saving; to cultivate new friends and keep in touch with those of long standing; to develop a variety of interests so that advancing age need not be a time of idleness and boredom. Old people can maintain an active interest in widely divergent fields. Though active participation in sports may not be possible in later years, the interest need not be diminished when the change from active to passive participation in the sport must take place.

The nurse should know that persons who are most active and whose days are spent in vigorous pursuit of their chosen profession or occupation to the exclusion of all outside interests are those most apt to be unable to adjust satisfactorily to enforced retirement and inactivity when they are classied as "old." She should find an interest or hobby that may be carried on alone, to be prepared for the eventuality of being thrown upon her own resources. She should learn to enjoy something which does not require the use of the eyes, and to develop an interest in at least one activity which is not dependent on hearing. She should cultivate a hobby requiring group activity so she will not be denied needed association with others.

In this age of so-called "shortage of nurses," the nurse may find little time for cultivation of a hobby or of interests which require group activity, but she should be the first to recognize that it is essential for her to develop interests and make friends as a means of insurance against loneliness and discontent in old age.

Care of Equipment after Use

Equipment used in the care of the chronically ill and the aged is cared for in the same manner as that described in preceding chapters where the specific procedures are discussed in detail.

Summary of Important Factors

THE CHRONICALLY ILL

Patients with a chronic disease are a problem of the community rather than of the individual family.

Chronic illness is mild in nature, slow in its course, and long continued. Two chronic diseases, heart disease and carcinoma, rank first and second in cause of deaths.

Most patients with chronic illness are cared for in nursing homes or in their own home.

A major factor in improvement of the physical condition is the patient's attitude toward his illness, and the attitude taken by his family and friends.

Loss of appetite is frequently the result of a depressed mental attitude.

Exercise should be planned according to the patient's ability to participate. More sleep is required by those chronically ill than is needed by the average person. Need for diversion is greater for the patient with a chronic disease.

The prevention of chronic illness depends primarily on observance of good personal hygiene and early diagnosis and treatment of disease.

THE AGED

Increase in the life span has increased the number of aged people and of problems related to the older age group.

Organs of the body do not age simultaneously, and for that reason the biological age of the person is more accurate than the chronological.

Basic needs of the aged include: to love and be loved, companionship, recognition, personal achievement, economic security, and some work to do.

The actual period of senility is the time when mental efficiency is reduced.

No attempt should be made to change the lifelong habits of the aged patient unless they interfere with the treatment being given.

Slight activity for the aged is preferable to no activity at all. Pets may be a source of companionship and will help the older person to feel important through being needed.

The nurse should begin now to prepare for her own old age.

Factors To Teach the Patient

THE CHRONICALLY ILL

Various agencies are set up to help solve problems related to family, finance, employment, etc., brought about by chronic illness.

Recovery may be helped or hindered by mental attitude.

The importance of being ambulatory or of moving and turning in bed as a means of physical exercise.

Diet, rest, sleep, and recreation are important in recovery.

How to relax physically and how to free the mind of fear, worry, and depression. "Never attempt to solve a problem after dark."

That rest, without sleep, is beneficial to the body and will aid recovery.

A diversional activity can be interesting and may sometimes become the foundation for means of livelihood after recovery.

Recreational activities may promote physical improvement, spiritual satisfaction, financial reward, and a better mental attitude.

THE AGED

The need for great care in avoiding illness or injury since recovery is slow. The need to avoid haste—to hurry has adverse effects on their physical condition and makes them more susceptible to accidental injury.

Decrease in sexual activity need not mean decrease in love and affection.

Light work or an avocation will add interest and purpose to life.

Their services are needed and their lives can still be usefull.

The importance of diet in maintaining a good physical condition.

Situation Type Problems

1. A young man who had been hospitalized for treatment of a chronic disorder was forced to remain in bed all the time. He had formerly been employed as a railroad switchman and found it very difficult to adjust to the inactivity of complete bed rest.

A nurse assigned to care for him made several attempts to interest him in some form of light recreational activity. He seemed to appreciate her efforts in his behalf, but took little or no interest in the various suggestions made by her. He spent long periods each day gazing into space or pretending sleep by lying with eyes closed. He had a radio at his bedside, but seldom turned it on or showed interest in the programs.

The only reading material that he seemed to enjoy was a small collection of comic books which had been brought to him by a friend. The nurse told him that comic books were for children and implied that only the "not very bright" children enjoyed reading them. She brought the patient some really good books to read, choosing for him a book of plays by Shakespeare and a well written though lengthy volume on the subject of Music Appreciation.

The young man glanced through the books then carefully placed them at the back of the bedside table. He did not continue to read the comic books, but spent even more time in complete inactivity. What would you have done?

2. A private duty nurse who had been called to help care for a 92-year-old male patient reported for duty at 3 P.M. She found the patient very uncooperative and in a belligerent frame of mind. He had been in the hospital for three days and all efforts to remove a suit of long underwear which he was wearing on admission had failed. The patient was certain he would have pneumonia if the underwear was taken from him.

The nurse tried to convince him that he would be sufficiently warm without the underwear and that it was essential to remove it so he could be given a bath. She, too, failed in her attempt to persuade the patient to be separated from the "red flannels."

At bedtime the patient was given a sedative and was soon sleeping soundly. The nurse decided it might be possible to remove the underwear while the patient was asleep and at once set to work to do just that. She had succeeded in removing both arms from the sleeves and was turning the patient in order to pull the underwear down from back and shoulders when the patient showed signs of waking. He was very drowsy and somewhat confused mentally. He did not resist efforts to remove the underwear, but seemed greatly concerned because the nurse was "up" so late at night. He seemed to have the mistaken idea that she was his wife Martha (the patient's wife had died several years before). He addressed her as "Martha," and complained that she would "take cold from being up at night after the fires were out." He insisted that she come to bed immediately and, taking hold of her hand and arm, tried to pull her down beside him on the bed.

The nurse was highly insulted by the patient's actions. She reported to the nurse in charge that the patient had been offensive, had made "advances" to her, and had bruised her arm. She refused to go back into the patient's room again. What would you have done?

Suggested Reference Reading

"Winning the war on arthritis," Madelyn Wood; Coronet, December, 1949.
"How to guess your age," Corey Ford; Reader's Digest, February, 1950.
"Old age is your business," Max Jacobson; Reader's Digest, November, 1950.
"They retired—and got busy," William S. Dutton; Reader's Digest, October, 1951.
"Life begins at any time," Peter J. Steinchrohn; Coronet, January, 1952.
"After a long illness," Bruce Barton; Reader's Digest, April, 1952.

CHAPTER 42

Radiation

TOPICAL OUTLINE

VARIOUS FORMS OF RADIATION
NURSING MEASURES IN RADIOTHERAPY
RADIATION INJURIES
ATOMIC ENERGY
THE NURSE AND AN ATOMIC ATTACK
THE NURSE IN THE FEDERAL CIVIL DEFENSE PROGRAM

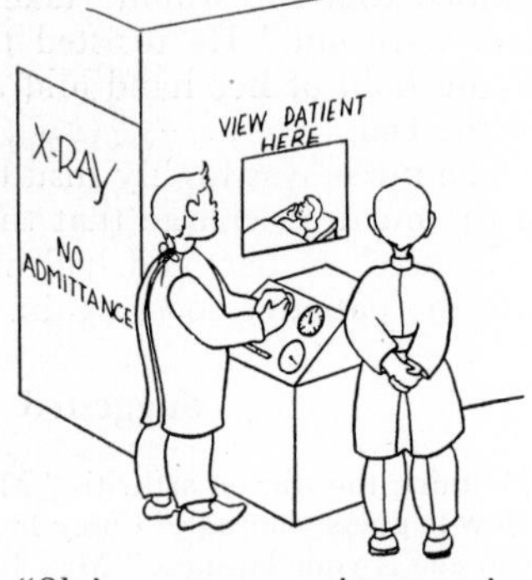

"She's pretty as a picture—nice frame too!"

Radiation includes light rays, heat rays, x-rays, and the energy emitted by radium and radioactive isotopes. All of these forms may be used in treatment of various conditions.

Infrared radiation is treatment by means of the infrared lamp to produce erythema of the skin. The apparatus consists of generator and reflector. The treatment may be given once or twice each day for a period of 30–40 minutes. The lamp should be placed about 2 feet from the skin area to be treated, and the rays should strike the skin at right angles.

Ultraviolet radiation is produced by a mercury vapor lamp. The initial dose is given with only 1 minute of exposure. In succeeding doses the time is increased by 1 minute until maximum time has been reached. An eye shade is necessary since ultraviolet rays cause conjunctivitis. The lamp should be placed about 3 feet from the area being exposed, and the treatment is given by a physiotherapist.

Diathermy is the production of heat in the tissues by means of a high frequency current. The heat penetrates all tissues without being intense enough to be destructive.

Patients receiving treatment with x-ray, radium, radon, or radio-

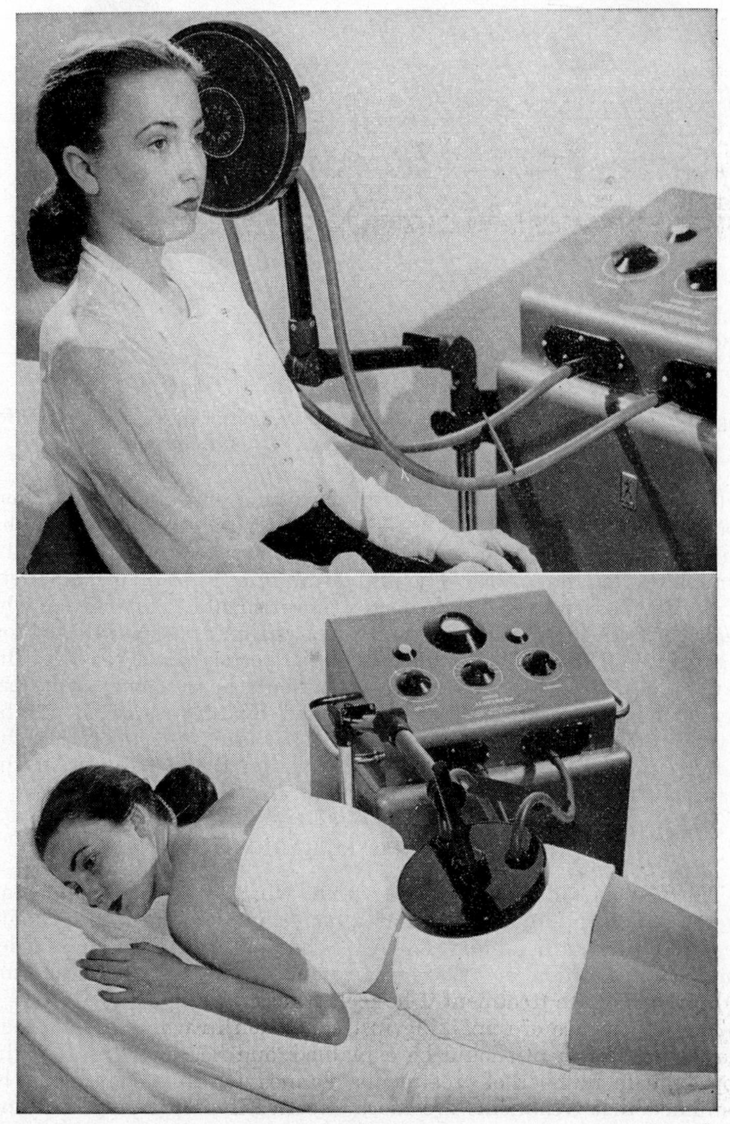

Fig. 252. The diathermy unit with treatment drum in use for head and low back treatment. (A. S. Aloe Co., St. Louis, Missouri.)

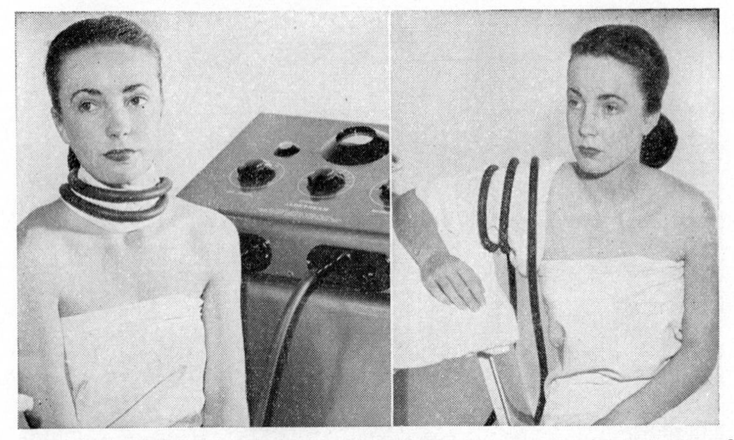

Fig. 253. The diathermy unit with cable for treatment of throat and neck or for shoulder treatment. (A. S. Aloe Co., St. Louis, Missouri.)

active isotopes require special nursing measures and intelligent understanding of their emotional reaction. Most patients will benefit by having an opportunity to talk about their physical condition and the kind of therapy prescribed. The responsibility of informing the patient of the diagnosis rests with the doctor, and it should be the doctor who decides whether or not the patient is to be given accurate information regarding his physical condition. After the doctor has talked with the patient, a complete report of that talk should be attached to the patient's hospital record. Terminology used by the doctor should be given on the report, so interns and nurses who have contact with the patient can be consistent in the information they give and in the way in which questions from the patient are answered.

NURSING MEASURES IN RADIOTHERAPY

The nurse should reassure the patient who is just beginning x-ray therapy and explain to him that treatments are not painful. He should be told that even though he is alone in the treatment room he is under constant observation, and that he can signal for the technician to come to him during the treatment if he feels it necessary to do so.

The importance of remaining in the position in which he has been placed for treatment should be explained, and he should be told the approximate number of treatments planned for him. He should be reminded that treatments are more effective if properly spaced, and that it is important to him to be present for each treatment at the time specified.

If the patient develops radiation sickness or a skin reaction, the doctor should discuss the matter with him and explain that the dosage needed to treat affected body tissues is such that it is not unusual to have some degree of undesirable reaction. The nurse can reassure the patient by explaining that radiotherapy is used frequently and that it has become the accepted means of treatment for a wide variety of conditions. She should refrain from using the term "cancer" when talking with the patient, even though he may have been told of the diagnosis. If the patient does not know definitely that his condition has been diagnosed as being malignant, the nurse should not reveal that information.

Whether radiotherapy is being given for a malignant condition or not, three factors should be considered in relation to nursing care of the patient: maintaining accurate dosage, proper care of the involved area, treatment of radiation sickness, and maintaining good physical and mental condition.

Maintaining Accurate Dosage. The dosage of radiation should be given to the involved area only, and other parts of the body should be protected from exposure. Colored markings can be used to outline the skin surface that will be affected in the treatment of underlying organs. The nurse should make sure that such markings are not removed from the skin before the series of treatments has been completed.

In radium therapy the nurse should see that the radium is removed at the exact time indicated by the doctor. An overdose to the area being treated may cause destruction of tissue. While caring for the patient with radium the nurse should watch carefully for signs that the radium applicator has shifted in position. If it occurs unnoticed, the area being treated may receive a lessened amount of radiation and adjacent areas may be overexposed. Care should be taken to see that structures near the treated area do not become distended and thus receive a larger dose of radiation than can be safely given. Doses of radioactive isotopes are calculated and administered by the doctor. Patients receiving radioactive iodine are placed on a diet low in iodine. The nurse should see that the special diet is adhered to, so the body will utilize the iodine that is radioactive.

In working with radium the nurse should observe certain precautionary measures. Care should be taken to protect against loss of radium. Radium is very expensive even in minute amounts, and there is danger of persons accidentally coming in contact with radium that has been lost.

Radium should be kept in a thick, lead-lined container under lock and key when not in use.

In cleansing a radium applicator it should be washed in a basin to avoid danger of losing it down the drain of an open sink.

Patients receiving radium therapy should not be permitted bathroom privileges because of the danger of losing the radium.

All dressings, linen, and equipment used for a patient being treated with radium should be carefully examined before being taken from the unit, or room, to make sure that they contain no radium.

The nurse should not handle radium except with forceps, and should work rapidly so that she is not unduly exposed to radiation. Whenever possible, the radium should be held at arm's length.

Radon seeds are tiny gold tubes into which has been sealed the gas given off by radium. The seeds should be handled with the same precautions observed in handling radium. Radon seeds soon lose their radioactivity, since most of the emanations are gone from them within 30 days. When no longer effective, the seeds should be returned to the company from which they were obtained.

Proper Care of the Involved Area. The part being treated should be kept clean and free from irritation. As the tumor cells are being destroyed, normal cells are also subjected to injury by radiation and care must be taken to avoid infection or other undesirable effect on normal cells.

In treatment of the skin the following precautions are indicated: Solutions, powders, or ointments which contain heavy elements, as zinc, bismuth, magnesium, should not be used on the affected area, since they tend to increase the radiation dose.

The areas should be kept dry to avoid water or aqueous solution coming in direct contact with the area. Sponge baths should be given during the time treatment is being given, and for a few weeks after treatment. Adhesive tape should not be used on the affected skin areas because of the zinc contained in it. Loose clothing should be worn to avoid irritation of the area. The area should be protected from extremes of heat and cold, and from the sun, diathermy, and other physical phenomena.

When the mouth is involved, the teeth should be examined and given corrective treatment as required. The patient should be encouraged to keep his mouth clean and to brush his teeth at least three times daily. Smoking should be discouraged because of the irritation produced by heat and smoke.

Patients receiving radiotherapy for treatment of a uterine condition should be given vaginal irrigations for cleanliness and for relief of vaginal discharge.

Radiation of parts of the intestinal tract usually precludes the giving of medications which contain metals, as milk of magnesia, since they tend to increase radiation dosage.

Treatment of Radiation Sickness. Radiation sickness may be experienced in varying degrees by patients undergoing radiation therapy. Symptoms are nausea, loss of appetite, general malaise, and a tendency to become tired very easily. Treatment usually consists of intravenous glucose or saline, liver extract, and some form of vitamin therapy. Withholding food for several hours before and after exposure to radiation may help prevent nausea and discomfort. Symptoms such as vomiting, diarrhea, pain, or bleeding should be treated as the need arises.

Maintaining Good Physical and Mental Condition. To help build up a weakened physical condition and to promote a desirable mental attitude on the part of the patient is of major importance in the nursing care of patients receiving radiation therapy.

Rest and sleep at night, approximately eight hours, should be supplemented with rest periods during the day. The diet should be high in protein and carbohydrate to repair damaged tissue and to maintain or increase weight. Small frequent servings of food may be more acceptable to the patient than the regular three meals per day. Patients who find it difficult to eat or digest foods contained in the average diet may be given soft or liquid foods. Strained baby foods available commercially can be used for such patients.

The desirable mental attitude can be obtained only through careful attention to the patient's surroundings, his room or unit being kept neat, attractive, and pleasant, and through diversional activities to keep him busy and interested. Friends and relatives can be encouraged to make frequent visits and to continually assure the patient of their interest in his welfare.

The nurse should be informed in regard to the subject of radiation in order to answer questions which will be asked of her. Her care of the patient and her response to his emotional reaction may be a determining factor in the benefits received by treatment, and the degree to which he is made comfortable and satisfied during hospitalization. Although she must emphasize the benefits of radiation for the patient, she must be aware of the dangers involved in radiation therapy.

No attempt is made here to explain in detail the extensive list of conditions under which radioactivity can be injurious or harmful. The sole purpose of the following is to summarize, for the student nurse, essential factors which she should know to understand the work being done in radiation and to be able to assume the responsibility placed on her in helping with that work.

Radiant energy is a primal energy that exists throughout the universe. It is produced in a natural state by certain metallic ores, such as uranium, thorium, and radium. It is produced in a form known as x-ray by the action of high voltage discharges striking a metal target in an evacuated tube; and it is released as radioactive waves and particles in the explosion of an atomic bomb. Although the various sources of radiant energy may have similar biological effects, all interfering with normal structure and functioning of tissues, and injuring living cells, they produce different clinical effects.

RADIATION INJURIES

Most important in the study or handling of radiant energy is awareness of the hazards involved and avoidance of unnecessary exposure. The greatest protection against unavoidable exposure should also be studied.

Everyone who may come in contact with any of these forms of

radiation should be concerned with the problem of protection against undue exposure to them.

All types of radioactive energy are termed "ionizing radiation." In general, they may be classified according to the radioactive substances they contain, as alpha particles, beta particles, gamma waves, and neutrons.

Exposure to radiation in small amounts given frequently over a prolonged time is cumulative in action. Tissues may be damaged by multiple minute exposures or by large doses or exposures to x-ray. By the very nature of its action, radiation is capable of producing injury in those who work with it and are thereby constantly exposed to it, even though exposure may be in minute amounts. The effects of repeated small doses are insidious and, therefore, must be guarded against by strict adherence to procedure techniques that are scientifically controlled. Known hazards to personnel handling roentgen ray equipment have led to construction of large, well shielded x-ray rooms and in the use of lead gloves and lead aprons. Similar precautions are observed by personnel using any kind of radiation.

The most common ill effects of radiation include:

Radiodermatitis. Radiation may cause an acute or chronic inflammatory condition of the skin. The first symptom, erythema, may appear a few days after administration of a sufficient single dose or days later, after administration of repeated small doses. Erythema with desquamation may be the sole effect of slight tissue damage. The more severe injury or dermatitis may be characterized by appearance of vesicles and by subsequent excoriation and weeping surface. When the injury is severe, the patient experiences pain and itching. Areas of necrosis develop, and subcutaneous and deeper tissues are involved. If hairy surfaces of skin are involved, permanent baldness may result.

Cancer of the Skin. Exposure to x-ray and radium has induced cancer of the skin in many research workers in the specialty, especially in the early or pioneer years when the need for protection for workers was not known.

Growth Retardation and Bone Lesions. The growing fetus may be injured by irradiation of the mother's pelvis, especially during the early months of pregnancy. Serious deformity of the skeletal and nervous systems of the unborn child may result from therapeutic or diagnostic radiology of the mother.

Serious bone conditions may result, too, from intensive irradiation for malignant disease of neighboring structures. Treatment of pelvic or oral lesions may induce obliterative arteritis in bony tissue.

Malignant tumors of bone have resulted from industrial radium poisoning and from prolonged use of irradiation in the treatment of bone cyst or of benign giant cell tumor.

Intestinal Lesions. Persons exposed to heavy total body irradiation are subject to injury to the lining of the intestinal tract, from pharynx to the large intestine.

As a result of treatment of a primary lesion, such as carcinoma of the uterus or cervix, injury to the intestinal mucosa may appear years later. Damage to the intestinal tract is characterized by hemorrhage, ulceration, and the appearance of strictures due to scar formation. Surgical resection is usually required for relief if the condition persists and interferes with normal functioning. Medical treatment by antibiotic therapy is sometimes effective.

Radiation Injuries as an Occupational Hazard. In certain occupations radioactive materials and x-rays are used, and the amount of exposure to which employees are subjected must be strictly controlled. Special hazards exist, too, in plants having to do with atomic energy and nuclear fission. In refineries and physics laboratories, where radium is handled, employees are exposed to the same kind of industrial hazards.

The most important problem in all such establishments where radioactive materials are handled, stored, processed, or transported is protection of the worker. Devices have been invented which permit remote handling of the substances, and the use of adequate shields helps provide the needed protection. In plants where radioactive wastes are produced, their safe disposal is a problem requiring the services and ingenuity of the expert radiological engineer.

Precautions Against Radiation Injury. When it was learned that doctors and technicians working with radiation materials were unwittingly exposed to harmful effects, a means of protection was deemed essential.

From this need a new science was developed, that of radiation safety engineering. Members of this new group were given the task of making diagnostic and therapeutic radiology a safe procedure. They also were asked to solve control problems pertaining to therapeutic use of radioactive isotopes. Patients being treated with radioactive materials are a source of radioactive energy and of potential danger to themselves, other patients, and members of the hospital staff.

Specific recommendations for the protection of radiological personnel are now made by the International Commission on X-Ray and Radium Protection.

Radium Protection. The commission established a tolerance dose or maximum permissible exposure on a routine day-by-day basis for the life of the worker. The tolerance dose was expressed in terms of measurable units and a specific biological standard. The tolerance dose is 0.2 r per day; the erythema dose of radiation is 600 r.

The tolerance dose was defined as "The safe upper limit of radiation dosage which will produce no permanent physiological changes in the average individual."

Evidence obtained by animal experimentation indicates that radioactive substances can produce the following harmful effects: injuries that are superficial in nature and effect; general systemic effects, as related to the blood and blood-forming organs; malignant tumors;

cataracts; obesity; impaired fertility; reduction of the span of life; and genetic effects.

Research in regard to the effects of radiation on man is still in such an early stage that it cannot be stated definitely that the effects on man will be essentially the same as those noted in animal experimentation.

ATOMIC ENERGY

To most persons throughout the world who are living in the age of "atomic energy," the term is only vaguely defined. It calls forth a feeling of apprehension and discomfort, since the possibilities of the destructive power of one small atom bomb is almost unbelievable. The bomb exploded in the air, over the Japanese city of Hiroshima in 1945, killed 78,000 people.

The average adult knows that the release of atomic energy by explosion is highly destructive. When released through a slower and controlled process, atomic energy can be constructive and accomplish many wonderful things: It can produce heat and power for homes and industry, and provide effective treatment for disease, improvement in agriculture, and advances in industry. Each branch of science will benefit by the use of atomic energy.

Atomic Energy Defined.* Atomic (nuclear energy) energy is defined as "the force locked up in the center of the atom." The atom is too small to be seen, even with electronic microscopes, but all matter is composed of atoms. Atoms are made up of three basic particles: electrons, protons, and neutrons. Electrons form the outer shell of the atom, and carry negative charges. Protons, in the nucleus of the atom, carry positive charges of electricity. There is one proton in the nucleus for each electron of the outer edge of the atom. The number of protons determines the kind of atom it is. Neutrons, contained in the nucleus, carry no electrical charge. The protons and neutrons of the nucleus of an atom are held together by nuclear energy.

At the present time 98 elements have been discovered in nature or created in the laboratory. Each element has an atomic number (ranging from 1 to 98), which is the number of protons in the nucleus of an atom of the particular element. Elements combine to form compounds; compounds (materials made of more than one element) can be any conceivable article in the world.

Scientists created the atomic unit of weight in order to determine the weight of a proton or neutron.

The atomic unit of weight is approximately the same as the weight of one neutron or one proton, and is one-sixteenth the weight of an oxygen atom. The weight of an atom of an element is about the same as the total number of neutrons and protons in its nucleus.

All the atoms of a specific element have the same number of pro-

*From "Primer of Atomic Energy," by John Lewellen. (Science Research Associates, Inc., Chicago, Ill.)

tons, but the number of neutrons may vary, creating atoms of different weights. An isotope, formed in an element, is made up of all the atoms having the same weight. There may be several isotopes within an element. In the study of nuclear energy this fact is important, since the weight of an atom determines how easily it may be split.

Splitting Atoms. The word "atom" is derived from the Greek and means "something that cannot be divided." Until recently, scientists were of the opinion that atoms were the smallest units of matter. Now it is known that the atom is made up of smaller particles and can be divided or split. Tiny protons or neutrons travelling at a fantastically high rate of speed will split atoms. In the laboratory, charged particles can be given the necessary high speed in a cyclotron, a machine that whirls them around within an electro-magnetic field that constantly increases their speed. Because the cyclotron can produce only minute quantities of materials and the atoms to split were so few in number it was necessary to devise a means for the splitting atoms to carry on a chain reaction.

In a chain reaction one atom splits into two parts which are about the same in size and new atoms of different elements are formed, unneeded neutrons in the new, smaller atoms fly off into space at 10,000 miles per second. If a flying neutron hits the nucleus of another atom, it splits, repeating the process above. When the number of neutrons produced is constant, a chain reaction occurs. This chain reaction is the basic principle of the atomic bomb and the atomic furnace.

Each time an atom splits part of the nuclear force which held its protons and neutrons together in the nucleus is released and a very small part of the original material (that part used to bind neutrons and protons together) is changed from matter to energy.

Atomic Weapons. In a chemical reaction, such as that which occurs in the explosion of T.N.T., whole atoms are merely shifted about. The nucleus of the atom remains undisturbed. In an atomic explosion, the nuclei split apart and tremendous energy is released as new, smaller atoms of a different material are formed. An atomic explosion produces a temperature 10,000 times that of the surface of the sun, and the first atomic bomb had a destructive force equal to 20,000 tons of T.N.T.

Radiation. When an atomic bomb is exploded it produces heat and an expansion of gases on a much greater scale than was ever before known. It also produces gamma rays (energy rays similar to x-rays), beta particles (high energy electrons), and alpha particles (heavy particles consisting of two protons and two neutrons). In large concentrations, all of these radiations are deadly. The gamma rays are the most dangerous, because of their power to penetrate. They pass through ordinary walls without difficulty.

The Hydrogen Bomb. Hydrogen atoms, heated to a very high temperature, fly around at great speed and smash into other nuclei with such force that they fuse or are joined together. When the nuclei join, part of the material turns into energy. The energy released is greater than that of the atomic bomb. The hydrogen bomb, pound for pound, would release about seven times as much energy as the atom bomb.

The hydrogen bomb can be made in any size and will not explode unless its temperature is raised to the necessary degree. Before the atom bomb was developed there was no way of achieving the high temperature needed to explode the hydrogen bomb. Now an atom bomb can be built into the center of the hydrogen bomb, to provide the millions of degrees of heat needed to "trigger" it.

Radiation Injuries to Victims of Atom Bomb Attacks. The injurious effects of total body radiation, as that experienced in the atom bomb attack, may be roughly classified as the immediate and acute post-irradiation effect, and the syndrome of delayed effects.

Acute Post-Irradiation Effects. Widespread tissue destruction is the immediate effect of total body radiation. A condition of shock, similar to that seen in severe burns, is evident, resulting from a disturbance of fluid balance and of adrenal function. Nausea and vomiting occur very rapidly, followed by fever and diarrhea. *Leukocytosis* (increase in number of white corpuscles in the blood) develops in a few hours and is followed in a few days by *leukopenia* (abnormal deficiency of white corpuscles in the blood) because of damage to the blood-forming cells.

Persons surviving the immediate effects may seem to recover from these symptoms but after about two weeks are subject to other adverse symptoms. They may experience increasing malaise, gradually rising temperature, loss of hair, pain in the pharynx, and appearance of ulcerative and hemorrhagic lesions of the skin, lips, mouth, and throat. The appearance of blood in the feces denotes the same ulcerative and hemorrhagic condition in the stomach and intestinal tract. The white cell count is markedly decreased, and severe anemia may exist. The patient is likely to die in one month after exposure. Those who survive are usually subjected to a prolonged period of weakness and debilitation, with a gradual return of the blood cell count to normal.

Delayed Effects of Irradiation. When the exposure to radiation is less severe the clinical symptoms vary. Some show no symptoms at all yet may have a resulting leukopenia. Others may experience general malaise, anorexia, diarrhea, and loss of hair. The symptoms are usually mild, and most patients recover completely.

Local Burns as a Radiation Injury. A common cause of disability among victims of an atomic explosion are local burns. They may be either the flash or flame type and are produced by the intense heat radiated from the bomb.

The local symptoms are numbness and tingling of the affected part, followed, very shortly, by marked redness of the skin. After a day or so blisters appear, and there is involvement of skin areas over the body. The lesions become open areas and exude large quantities of fluid. After several weeks the affected areas become less moist and finally progress to a condition of dry gangrene. Toxic systemic symptoms include those described in the paragraph on acute post-irradiation and delayed effects. Clothing protects to a slight extent against local burns from beta rays.

Treatment of Radiation Injuries. Because of the possibility of atomic attack in this country, much attention has been devoted to the treatment of radiation injuries, the casualties at Hiroshima and Nagasaki having been studied intensively. At the present time effective treatment is very limited and must be directed almost entirely to preventive measures.

Victims will need to be classified according to extent of exposure. Those close to the source of radiation who have been exposed to intense total body radiation will not survive. The damaging effects of radiation take place instantaneously at the time of exposure. Cells receiving sufficient radiation die immediately; other cells will be damaged so they die subsequently. Treatment is largely directed toward protecting the partially damaged cells from further injury and instituting corrective measures for conditions resulting from physiological disturbances such as edema, hemorrhage, ulceration, and secondary infection. Shock will be treated, as at the present time, with intravenous infusion and blood transfusion.

Burns. About the only treatment that may be instituted for burns is that of protective measures. Simple dressings may be applied. Pressure points or needle puncture wounds should be avoided; antibiotics may be administered and an attempt should be made to maintain normal fluid balance.

Systemic Symptoms. The patient who has been subjected to exposure to radiation should be treated for shock and given complete physical and mental rest; body heat should be conserved, and normal fluid balance should be maintained. An accurate record should be kept of intake and output, and, if necessary, fluids should be supplied parenterally. When fluid is lost through vomiting and diarrhea, glucose 5 per cent should be given to counteract dehydration.

Systemic treatment must also include measures to control hemorrhagic manifestations and prevent infection due to loss of resistance and exposure of denuded surfaces. Antibiotics are used to combat infection and damage to the intestinal tract.

Reconstructive Surgery. Tissue that has been damaged by radiation does not function as before and often becomes greatly deformed as a result of scar formation. Circulation to the affected tissue is usually impaired and fibrosis is evident, factors which make surgical reconstruction a difficult problem.

Inadequate nutrition and severe infection often contribute to the unsatisfactory results of attempted surgical treatment.

In severe deformity, reconstructive surgery may be indicated to make the deformity less pronounced.

Atomic Energy for Peacetime Use. The possibilities of benefits to be derived from nuclear fission devoted to peaceful purposes are as great as its potentialities for destruction. Atomic energy may eventually be used to develop power plants that can operate at a fuel cost much lower than that of coal or oil. The ashes of atomic fuel are radioactive and may be used to help combat disease, to further scientific research in diagnosis and treatment, and to promote industrial research.

THE NURSE AND AN ATOMIC ATTACK

The nurse should know the following which will be helpful to her in caring for herself and others in event of an atomic attack.

Persons under the atomic explosion or within ½ mile of the center of the explosion have very little chance of survival. Those ½–1 mile away have about a fifty-fifty chance of escaping death or injury. Those 1½–2 miles away may suffer only two or three casualties out of each 100 population. Those beyond 2 miles will probably not be harmed. Bombs larger than the atom bomb do not do a proportionately greater damage. Two atom bombs dropped relatively close together would do greater damage than one hydrogen bomb which might be twice as large.

Blast and Burns. Blast and heat are the biggest dangers in the explosion of a bomb. To protect yourself from blast, lie down flat in a shielded spot. Inside a building, lie close against a basement wall or under a desk or table. Outdoors, lie close to the base of a heavy building or jump into a ditch. To avoid temporary blindness, bury your face in your arms for at least 10–12 seconds.

Heat from the explosion (flash burns) may cause serious injury. Near the center of the explosion persons will suffer fatal burns; those 1 mile away may be seriously burned. Heat may be felt on bare face and hands at a distance of 4 or 5 miles. Solid material between the person and the explosion will provide protection from flash burns. At a distance, a hat, long sleeves, or even thin cotton clothing may prevent serious burns.

Radioactivity. Injury from radioactivity depends on the power of the rays and particles, duration of the exposure, and amount of body area exposed. Two types of radioactivity are (1) initial radioactivity, which occurs at the time of explosion and lasts only a moment; and (2) lingering radioactivity, which may remain for a few minutes or for weeks or months.

Initial Radioactivity. Injury range of a bomb exploded in the air is about 1 mile. Beyond a mile the effects of explosive radioactivity would be minor and temporary in nature. Less than two-thirds of a mile away those unprotected would probably suffer a fatal dose of radioactivity. Ground level or underwater bursts are less dangerous from the standpoint of initial radioactivity.

Radiation Sickness. Vomiting and diarrhea are the first symptoms of radiation sickness. The stronger the dose of radiation the sooner the symptoms appear. In severe radiation sickness the affected person would be very ill in about two weeks and would lose most of his hair. Even in severe radiation sickness there is about an even chance for recovery and for regrowth of hair.

Protective Measures Against Initial Radioactivity. A basement offers the best shelter against blast, heat, and radioactivity. Cyclone cellars offer good protection. Fireproof housekeeping may prevent fire after the explosion. Know the safest part of your home. Know how to turn off oil burners and electrical equipment. Close windows and doors if time permits. Keep emergency equipment and supplies on hand, including flashlight, radio, canned goods, and first aid equipment.

Lingering Radioactivity. Bombs exploded in the air leave no dangerous lingering radioactivity, most of which comes from bomb ashes and from unexploded atomic fuel. The radioactive particles act like dust and when present in quantity contaminate all persons and articles they contact.

In air bursts radioactive particles or dust is spread so widely that it is not apt to be harmful to persons on the ground, and radioactive clouds are not potential sources of danger since the radioactive materials are widely scattered before they fall to the ground.

Protective Measures Against Lingering Radioactivity. If caught out of doors at the time of explosion, cover yourself, if possible, to keep from being showered with radioactive waste materials.

Change all outer garments after leaving a contaminated area. Leave shoes outside when entering the house. Wash your body thoroughly in soap and warm water to remove radioactive dirt. Shampoo your hair for the same reason.

Keep windows and doors closed for several hours after an atomic bombing. In a heavily contaminated area, broken windows should be covered with blankets.

Close the dampers in fireplaces and flues, and shut off ventilating fans and air conditioners.

Discard all unpackaged foods. Wash the outside of cans before opening canned foods.

Boil water, unless there is official notification that it is safe for use. Boiling will not remove radioactivity but will kill microorganisms that may have come from damaged water mains.

Use the telephone only for emergency calls.

Keep the radio turned on for emergency instructions.

Keep your head—don't be the cause of a panic that can cost the lives of many who might otherwise have survived the blast, heat, and radioactivity loosed by an atomic explosion.

THE NURSE IN THE FEDERAL CIVIL DEFENSE PROGRAM

On January 12, 1951, the Federal Civil Defense Act became law, and the legal basis was formed for a national civil defense program. The main purpose of the program is to prepare for defense activities in event the United States is subjected to enemy attack.

The Federal Civil Defense Administration is an agency within the executive branch of the government. Its organization provides for ten essential services during emergency caused by enemy attack: rescue of the injured, police work, fire fighting, welfare work, health, warden duties, engineering, transportation, communications, and staff duties. Nine federal regional offices have been established to give assistance to state and local civil defense programs.

The nurse is a useful member of the department of the Health and Special Welfare Defense Division. This division is primarily responsible for the care of casualties and the maintenance and restoration of public health facilities. Various branches of the health and welfare office would include: health program planning, health supply requirements, ambulance and medical evacuation, first aid stations, hospital facilities, medical regulating service, blood and shock therapy, nutrition service, food sanitation service, chemical and biological warfare treatment, sewage and waste disposal, industrial health, dental service, mental health, communicable disease control, emergency housing and shelter sanitation, evacuation planning, and registration and information.

The department also recommends the organization and administrative policies for state and local civil defense health services. At the local level of the defense program the nursing service director should be responsible for planning and putting into effect the nursing service program in time of disaster.

In event of a war-time disaster the entire nurse group, active, inactive, and retired, may be pressed into service. In addition to the professional nurse group the non-professional group of practical nurses and nurse aides will also be expected to serve as a part of the nursing service teams, to assist in nursing duties in first aid stations, hospitals, and mass shelters which may be improvised to care for the injured and disabled.

A manual, "The Nurse in Civil Defense," released in June, 1952, by the Federal Civil Defense Administration, deals specifically with the important part to be played by the nurse in event of a war-caused disaster. Personnel needed to properly staff the first aid station unit would include doctors, dentists, nurses, administrative assistant, nurse aides, chaplain, first aid technicians, recording clerk, supply clerk, messengers, orderlies, and decontamination technicians. In addition, litter bearers, ambulance drivers, and other service groups would be needed for evacuation and field work. The senior nurse in the first aid station should be a public health nurse with experience in emergency nursing service.

Nursing in hospitals, those already in existence and those hastily improvised, should be under the supervision of the director of nursing service.

The nursing teams suggested for each department and the personnel required to staff the teams include: intravenous and blood therapy, one registered nurse, and three auxiliary workers; surgical dressings, one registered nurse, and two auxiliary workers; medications, one registered nurse, and two auxiliary workers; oxygen therapy, one registered nurse, and two auxiliary workers; routine patient care, auxiliary workers.

Nurses will be needed to help care for victims who may be housed in emergency shelters. If hundreds of homes are destroyed, lodgings must be provided by welfare services of the community, and members of health service organizations must work in cooperation with welfare agencies to care for the people. Nurses will also need to assume responsibility for helping combat the effects of atomic, biological, or chemical warfare, and will be expected to know the methods of treatment and nursing measures required in caring for casualties.

Care of Equipment after Use

The reflectors on infrared lamps must be kept cleaned and polished or the intensity of reflected rays will be decreased.

X-ray film should be stored away from the hospital or in fireproof vaults because of danger of fire.

Radium should be kept in lead-lined containers which can be locked in a cabinet or safe.

Radium should be handled with forceps and should be replaced in its container as soon as possible after use.

Summary of Important Factors

The distance of the heat lamps above the area being treated determines the intensity of the rays.

Eye shields should be worn when ultraviolet treatment is given.

The doctor should determine what information should be given the patient receiving treatment by x-ray or radium.

Radium is expensive and should be handled with great care.

Radium must always be removed at the exact time ordered by the doctor.

A patient with radium inserted should not be given bathroom privileges.

Radium should be handled with forceps.

The emotional factor is of great importance in caring for the radiation patient.

The nurse should know and observe precautions against radiation injury.

In the atom bomb energy is released when atoms are split.

In the hydrogen bomb energy is released when atoms fuse.

In an atomic attack: lie flat in a shielded spot, keep face buried in arms for 10-12 seconds to avoid temporary blindness, cover body, even with thin clothing, to prevent flash burns, turn off all electrical equipment, know how to protect yourself and others from lingering radioactivity.

Know the part the nurse will need to play in civil defense.

Factors To Teach the Patient

Eyes need to be protected when taking ultraviolet treatment.

Radiation therapy may be dangerous; even sun bathing may cause painful burns if exposure is prolonged.

In x-ray therapy it is necessary to remain in the same position during the treatment.

How to protect himself and family in an atomic attack.

Scientific Principles

Anatomy and Physiology. The only one of the various forms of radiation detectable by the body is heat waves.

Ultraviolet rays cause redness of the skin, and increase the number of red blood cells and hemoglobin content.

Diathermy increases temperature of body tissues and lowers blood pressure.

X-rays and radium radiation destroy tissue cells and induce local fibrosis to hamper the spread of a tumorous growth.

Radioactive isotopes produce ionization of protoplasm.

Chemistry. Ultraviolet lamps emit ozone, a dangerous gas, if the lamp is not enclosed in glass. Ozone has a toxic effect if the room is not well ventilated.

Microbiology. Bacteria may be killed by sunlight and by radiation.

Radium retards the growth of bacteria.

Seeds, needles, and tubes of radium may be boiled, or immersed in alcohol or bichloride of mercury to be sterilized.

Physics. Light or heat rays are most intense when striking the affected area at right angles.

Ultraviolet rays do not penetrate clothing. Infrared rays can penetrate clothing of normal weight. X-rays have very short wave lengths and are able to pass through body tissue.

Radium emits alpha, beta, and gamma rays.

Gamma rays penetrate into the deep structures of the body.

Radon is a gas produced when radium loses alpha rays.

In some instances radioactive isotopes have been used to administer localized internal radiation therapy.

Psychology. Ultraviolet rays stimulate the patient and help produce an optimistic state of mind.

Infrared rays relax, warm, and heal the patient.

Treatment with x-ray or radium may cause mental depression, and patients receiving such treatment require skill and understanding from the nurse.

Sociology. Specially trained technicians apply radiation therapy. Radium should be inserted and removed by the physician.

Rules for handling or working with x-rays and radium have been set up by the International Commission on X-Ray and Radium Protection.

Situation Type Problem

A member of the medical staff of a small community hospital who specialized in the field of gynecology owned several needles of radium which he reserved for use of his patients when radium insertion was required.

While performing surgery for a patient he needed the radium which was locked in a safe in his office. He asked the hospital to call his office nurse and ask that she send the radium to him by cab. The practice of having the radium transported from office to hospital by cab soon became routine, since it enabled the doctor to have the radium soon after he determined its need.

A nurse who had formerly been employed in the small hospital became interested in a rather heated discussion in the men's ward of a large city hospital where she was newly employed. The men were discussing the monetary value of radium and the extreme care with which it was handled because it was so expensive. The nurse received the undivided attention of the patients when she told them of the smaller institution in the nearby town where radium was transported to and from the hospital by cab drivers. She stated proudly that the practice had continued for several years and there had never been any question as to the safety of the radium.

One young man in the ward was impressed by the story and asked many questions about the exact method in which the radium was transported from the doctor's office to the hospital. The nurse admitted that the method used was possible because there was only one cab company in the town and the drivers were known to personnel in the doctor's office and to staff members at the hospital.

A few weeks later the nurse read in the small town's newspaper that the supply of radium owned by the doctor had been stolen. A young man had stolen one of the cabs, called at the doctor's office, stated that he was serving as relief driver of the cab, and asked for the radium. The office nurse had given the radium to him but he had failed to deliver it to the hospital. The abandoned cab had been found in a nearby town and no trace had been found of the "relief driver" or the radium. What would you have done?

Suggested Reference Reading

"X-ray in diagnosis," A. C. Galluccio; Hygeia, July, 1950.

"A hospital's defense against atomic attack," Elmina L. Snow; Hospitals, February, 1952.

"Rehearsal for atomic disaster," James B. Stapelton; Hospitals, October, 1952.
"Our preparation for a date with disaster," Beatrice A. McHarg; American Journal of Nursing, October, 1952.
"Working in a radioisotope clinic," Jane Perini; American Journal of Nursing, November, 1952.
"A re-evaluation of the radioisotope program," David A. Gee; Modern Hospital, January, 1953.
"Care of the normal skin," F. Torrey; American Journal of Nursing, April, 1953.
"Radiation hazards," Lee B. Fosdick; Nursing Outlook, July, 1953.
"Survival under atomic attack," National Security Resources Board Doc. 130, Civil Defense Office.

CHAPTER 43

Rehabilitation

TOPICAL OUTLINE

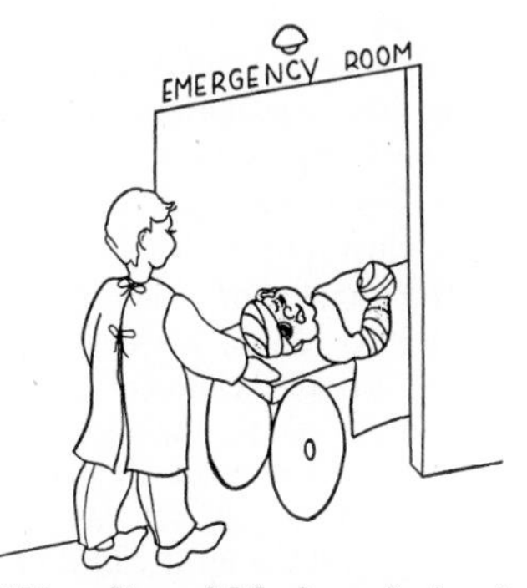

"My wife and I had words, but I didn't get to use mine!"

The increased life span for the individual, with subsequent increase in the age group of 65 years or more, has brought a marked increase in chronic diseases and disability. Victims of highway and industrial accidents, and of injuries sustained in war, increase the number of physically handicapped persons. The medical and allied professions have only recently recognized that **rehabilitation** may be the key to the solution of the medical-social-economic problem created by those who are disabled.

The student nurse of today is already learning to care for the patient as a whole instead of merely helping to cure a diseased part or treat an isolated physical condition. With rehabilitation as the ultimate goal of treatment and care, the nurse must be concerned with three phases of illness: the protective phase, with emphasis on prevention of or protection against disease; the definitive phase, when the disease is in progress; and the rehabilitative or final phase of disease, when the fullest possible measure of recovery is realized and the patient returns to a normal or nearly normal life.

One of the most interesting and dramatic histories of medical progress is that of the development of rehabilitation from primitive times,

Table 8. Dates of Significance in the History of Rehabilitation*

Year	Event	Person	Country
2380 B.C.	Earliest record of use of crutches		Egypt
400–300 B.C.	Use of exercise as means of treating disease	Hippocrates	Greece
1633	Founding of institutions for care of crippled children	Vincent de Paul	France
1798	First known use of occupational therapy in treating the mentally ill	Philippe Pineal	France
1854	Organization of professional nursing	Florence Nightingale	England
1873	First training school for nurses in U. S.	Bellevue Hospital	United States
1877	Founding of American Red Cross	Clara Barton	United States
1893	First school for vocational training of crippled children		United States
1908	First school for vocational training of disabled adult civilians	Paul Pastur	Belgium
1917	Establishment of American Red Cross Institute for disabled men		United States
1942	Beginning of convalescent training programs in Army Air Force Hospitals	Howard A. Rusk	United States
1946	Beginning of rehabilitation program in Veterans Hospitals	Donald A. Covalt	United States
1947	First medical rehabilitation service in a civilian hospital	Howard A. Rusk George G. Deaver	United States

* From "Rehabilitation Nursing," by Alice B. Morrissey; G. P. Putnam's Sons, New York City.

when the disabled were left to die, to the present, when medical rehabilitation is recognized as a fundamental part of the treatment and care, and the patient not only recovers from disease but is restored to his community with the desire and intent to be as active at work and at home as his capabilities will permit. Table 8 outlines briefly, in chronological order, various important events in the history of rehabilitation, giving the year, event, person responsible, and the country in which the event occurred.

Hospitals can no longer adequately meet the needs of their community by providing treatment and care for physical needs only. The patient's social, spiritual, psychological, and vocational needs must be served as well. To meet all the needs of the patient, hospital staffs now include, in addition to doctors and nurses, persons trained in psychiatry, psychology, physiotherapy, occupational therapy, social welfare work, vocational counseling, recreational activities, and Christian education or service. The need for a rehabilitation program in the general hospital is being recognized, and the rehabilitation unit is becoming part of the special services rendered by community hospitals throughout the country.

INCIDENCE OF MAJOR DISABILITIES

Physical disabilities may be classified in numerous ways, although the three main categories would be those related to the duration of disability (temporary or permanent), extent of disability (partial or complete), and cause of the disability (war injury, illness, or accidental injury).

It has been estimated that approximately one sixth of the total population of the United States have chronic disability of some type, and that each year accidents alone add about 350,000 to the total number. The three major causes of accidental injuries are accidents in the home, automobile and other motor vehicle accidents, and accidents in industry.

Disability caused by illness is due largely to such diseases as arthritis, blindness, cardiac conditions, cerebral palsy, deafness, and diabetes. Many persons are disabled or handicapped by: tuberculosis, poliomyelitis, multiple sclerosis, and orthopedic conditions causing impairment of normal function or of body activity.

The great number of physically handicapped persons serves to emphasize the need for rehabilitation programs which would provide the needed help for training the disabled to help themselves whenever that is possible.

ADJUSTMENT TO DISABILITY

In primitive times, when disabled persons were of no use to their tribe and became unwanted burdens to others, they were abandoned. At present, largely through the philosophy and practices of modern rehabilitation, the handicapped person is being educated to overcome the disability and to utilize remaining abilities to the greatest possible extent.

Every person, as an individual, represents a merging of many factors, physical, mental, spiritual, social, and vocational, into the total entity or personality. The different factors are closely related, but the conviction that a deformed or disabled body must house an equally disabled mind and spirit is erroneous and must be corrected if rehabilitation is to be effective.

The disabled patient must be taught to accept the physical handicap with its limitations on activity and behavior and to focus attention on abilities that are left, utilizing them to the fullest extent. If the disabled person is to face reality and accept the inevitable, he will do so through an inner quality, essentially spiritual, that enables him to integrate all the factors of his being, to gain a better insight into life by realization that he possesses mind and spirit as well as body, and

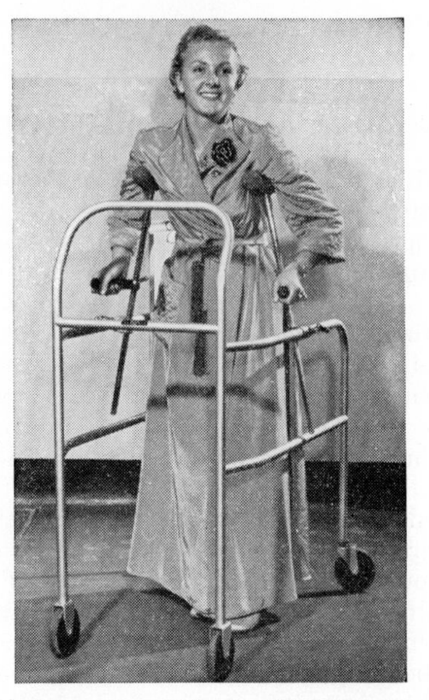

Fig. 254. The disabled person must be taught to overcome the disability and to utilize remaining abilities to the greatest possible extent. (Presbyterian Hospital School of Nursing, Chicago, Illinois.)

that others like him have found the courage and strength needed to rise above severe handicap by refusing to allow the spirit to be crushed or damaged.

The disabled who make satisfactory adjustment to their physical condition seem to have greater patience, tolerance, and understanding for others than do those who are sound in body. They do not indulge in petty bickering and in self-pity. They appear to realize, more poignantly than others, that there is a definite plan or purpose in life, and that their own difficult experience or suffering is part of the greater plan involving all mankind.

Although the disabled may be spiritually strong, they (like all others) want to be self-supporting and to possess some measure of economic security. Such factors are essential if the personality is to be integrated and a desirable adjustment made to the disabling physical condition. The needs and desires of the handicapped were adequately expressed by Michael Dowling, who at the age of 14 had lost both legs, his left arm and his right hand, when he talked in behalf of disabled veterans of World War I saying, "What the so-called cripple wants is not charity, but a chance."

Work therapy, then, becomes a very important part of any rehabili-

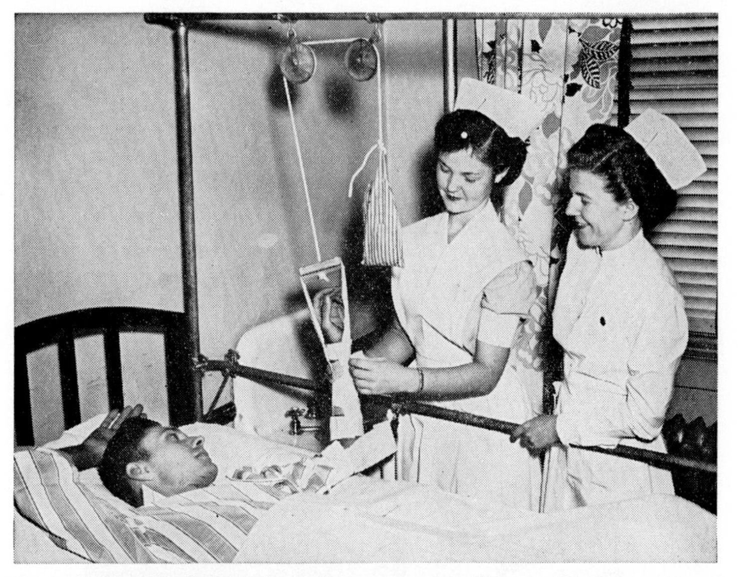

Fig. 255. The physical needs of the patient must be met first, then attention can be given to psychological, spiritual, and vocational needs. (Alabama Baptist Hospital School of Nursing, Birmingham, Alabama.)

tation program. Although the goal of rehabilitation is to restore the disabled to complete vocational and economic security, about 2 per cent of those disabled will not be helped and must remain non-productive.

Rehabilitation is accomplished by meeting the physical, psychological, and spiritual needs of the patient. The physical needs must be met first, a wholesome adjustment psychologically, a rich spiritual life, and help in achieving vocational and economic security will complete the successful rehabilitation of the individual.

THE NURSE IN REHABILITATION

In the past, and in some instances in the present, the tendency in medical and nursing care has been to treat the disease rather than the patient. If surgical treatment was needed and amputation of a part, as an arm or leg, was required to effect a cure, when the stump had healed the patient was sent home "cured." Little or no thought was given to the fact that, although his life had been saved, he had not been helped in making a satisfactory adjustment to his physical deformity, or in solving the many problems which he must face because of that deformity, and no attempt had been made to prepare him for

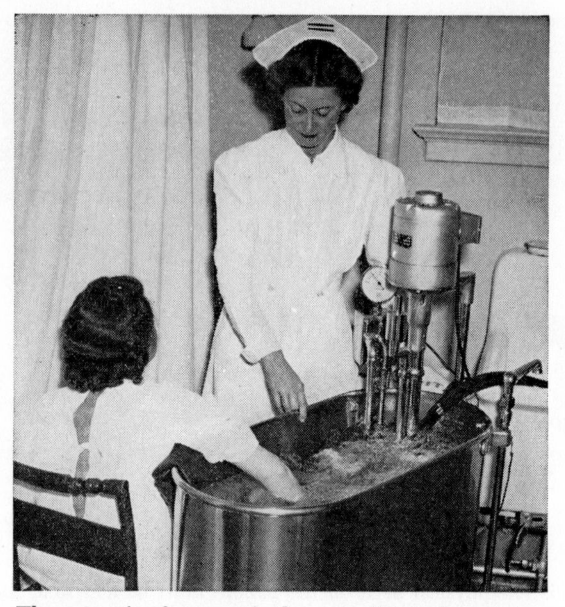

Fig. 256. The nurse is often required to coordinate the services of physical therapist, psychologist, social worker, and others concerned with rehabilitation. (Presbyterian Hospital, Chicago, Illinois.)

the change he must make in relation to occupation and to daily living. In the true sense he had not been cured, because the needs of the whole man had not been met.

Nursing care today requires more than concern with ills of the body and skill in procedures to meet physical needs. The nurse must know and practice certain specialized rehabilitation techniques, such as preventing physical deformities, teaching crutch walking, teaching self-care, and assisting with speech therapy. She must know and observe principles of psychotherapy in her relationship with patients, especially those who are disabled, and she must be able to render some service in the social, vocational, and recreational areas of rehabilitation. To meet such expanded obligations she must work cooperatively with physical and occupational therapists, with social, spiritual, and recreational workers, with volunteers and nurse aides, and with psychologists, as well as with the doctor and the dietitian. She will, in fact, need to assume the responsibility for coordinating the services of these other groups with those of the medical and nursing professions.

The tendency in many hospitals, where a shortage of nursing personnel exists, to reserve the time and attention of the nurse for the acutely ill patient and to delegate much of the nursing service for other patients to inadequately trained aides is unfortunate from the standpoint of rehabilitation. The patient may receive a diet that meets all the needs of the body, but when the tray is served by a kitchen helper who knocks once, enters the room without so much as looking at the patient, places the tray in front of him with the mumbled comment of "Breakfast" or "Lunch," and walks out, nothing has been done to make the patient feel that the hospital or the nursing staff are interested in his welfare or in him as a person. And when the convalescent or ambulatory patient is left to shift for himself, receiving little or no attention from the nursing staff, little is being accomplished in teaching the students of nursing that caring for physical needs of the patient is only part of their total responsibility in giving nursing care.

Principles of rehabilitation nursing should be applied to the care of all patients. In a general hospital the rehabilitation service requires different physical surroundings for the patient. Beds must be lower and have wheels and castors removed to be safe. The height of sinks, tables, mirrors, etc., may need to be changed. The time required for giving care to patients will need to be increased, since teaching the patient to do the things that will help make him independent is time consuming. Instruction that must be given by the nurse will include teaching the patient self-care activities, such as walking up and down steps, feeding himself, shaving, turning the pages of a book or magazine, and dressing or undressing. Correct methods and techniques must be taught the handicapped person, and in order to teach him effectively the nurse herself must have been taught. Each rehabilitation unit will require the services of a specially trained rehabilitation nurse, and the success of this newest concept of nursing will depend to a great extent on the willingness of all members of the nursing profession to accept the responsibilities it imposes.

Prevention of Physical Deformities. Nursing care of the disabled patient must include special nursing procedures for the prevention of physical deformities. This may be accomplished through correct posture in bed and corrective, remedial, or preventive exercise.

Re-education in Elimination. Because of the emotional factor involved in bladder and bowel incontinence (the patient may experience embarrassment, disgust, anxiety, and anger), the beginning of a rehabilitation program for patients with such disabilities must be on the psychological level. The patient's confidence and cooperation is needed if rehabilitation is to be effective.

Bladder irrigations and training in a systematic and regular schedule for emptying the bladder will eventually result in automatic bladder, one that has become accustomed to emptying itself at periodic intervals. A schedule can be worked out that can be relied on by the patient, who is thus relieved of much of the discomfort and embarrassment caused by incontinence.

Training in control of the bowel is also a matter of a planned schedule and regularity. Patience and persistence will usually bring satisfactory results. The prevention and treatment of decubitus ulcers must be part of the rehabilitation program, since many disabled persons are particularly prone to their development.

Teaching the Activities of Daily Living. The nurse who works with disabled people is inspired by the courage and determination with which the patients strive against great odds to become self-sufficient by learning to perform the simple tasks of daily living.

To serve such patients effectively, she must be prepared to teach the scientific techniques that have been devised for the handicapped. If she would understand the patient, she should put herself in the place of the patient. If she knows how much the patient desires to be able to perform simple tasks for himself, she will be better able to teach him to live and act normally within the limits of his disability.

To teach effectively, the nurse must refrain from "helping" the patient. She should instruct, then permit the patient to do the work without assistance. She must help to motivate the patient to a desire to learn and to act. An unwilling patient cannot be effectively instructed in self-care.

When properly taught, self-help procedures may be the means of changing the condition of a patient from helpless and complete dependence to one of almost normal usefulness. Helping to make possible the return to self-help and self-respect of a disabled person is a constant source of real satisfaction for the nurse in rehabilitation.

CRUTCHES—LEG BRACES—WHEELCHAIRS

By skillful instruction, hours of practice, and an earnest desire to be able to walk, patients who have lost the use of one or both lower limbs may become adept at walking with crutches.

For crutch walking, the patient must have confidence in his ability to handle the crutches and must be eager to learn the correct technique so he is less dependent on others. From a physical standpoint he must do exercises which teach muscle control and balance. Measurement for crutches must be accurate, and in using crutches the weight of the body must be supported by the hands rather than on the shoulder pieces of the crutches. The correct crutch gait will be determined by the kind and extent of the patient's disability.

A brace is a mechanical aid used to strengthen or support weakened muscles or limbs. All braces should be checked periodically for correct alignment, loose or missing parts, and the condition of straps and buckles. The patient who wears braces is subject to emotional problems connected with his handicap and will need help and encouragement to overcome the tendency to withdraw from all forms of social contact before he has made an adjustment to the new and necessary accessories.

The kind of wheelchair provided for the disabled person should be

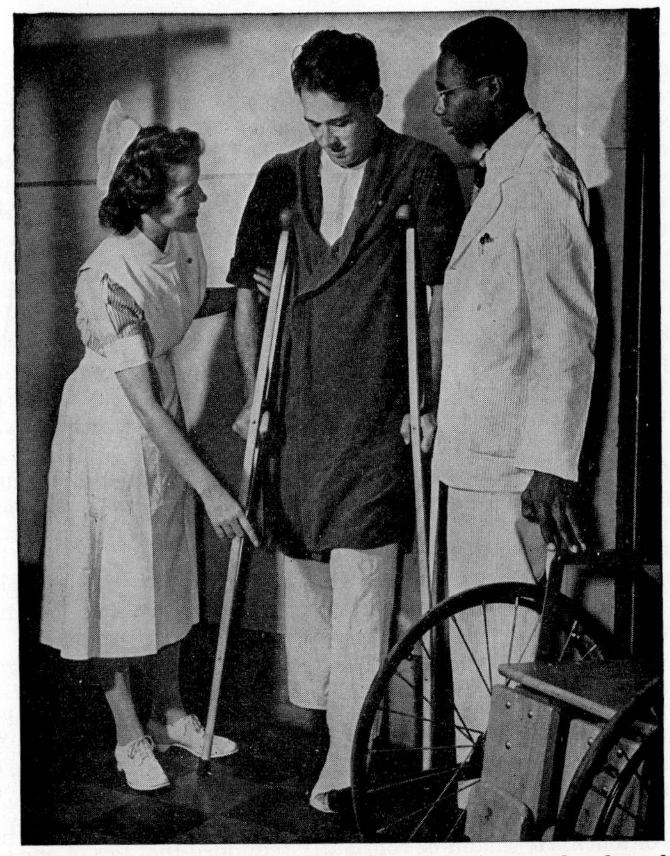

Fig. 257. The patient who learns to walk with crutches becomes less dependent on others. (Lenox Hill Hospital School of Nursing, New York, New York.)

adapted to his height, weight, and physical disability. In general, the large propelling wheels should be in the rear if the chair is to be used out of doors. If used indoors, the large wheels should be placed in front and the small wheels behind.

The wheels should be covered with solid rubber tires and the small wheels should swivel so the chair can be easily turned. The chair must be equipped with brakes to prevent rolling when it is stopped on an incline. Specially built wheelchairs are available for the amputee, the hemiplegic, the paraplegic, and the quadriplegic. When possible, each patient should care for his own chair by following directions given by the manufacturer.

SPEECH–SIGHT–HEARING

Because rehabilitation is concerned with the total person, speech therapy has become part of the rehabilitation process, and a trained speech therapist may be needed for complex speech disorders. The nurse needs to know the function of speech therapy and to work in cooperation with trained personnel in recognizing speech defects, reporting progress made in speech therapy, and becoming an understanding and appreciative audience for the patient to try out newly found skills or practice exercises for freeing speech of muscle tension.

Speech disorders stem from a variety of causes, such as cleft palate, neurotic hoarseness, cerebrovascular accidents, and brain tumors.

The goal of speech rehabilitation is for the patient to be able to communicate with those in his immediate environment. The nurse plays an important part in helping the patient to successfully accomplish the improved speech which the therapist has indicated is possible. Although each patient may require individual techniques, one thing is true of all patients in the speech rehabilitation program: If the patient feels that the nurse believes in him and has confidence in his ability to overcome the defect, he is able to rise above apparently insurmountable difficulties.

Patients handicapped by loss of vision experience severe psychological trauma. Those who are suddenly deprived of sight feel hopelessly isolated and helpless. The shock of being forced to live in a world of darkness may well lead to the urgent desire not to go on living at all. The nurse will need to use all her knowledge of psychology and to exert her full measure of tact and patience in helping the patient accept the physical impairment, and then begin the long and arduous task of learning to utilize the capabilities that are left.

The patient who is blind needs to learn to help himself in doing the daily tasks of living. He can learn to dress and undress, through the sense of touch. He should be constantly reminded that loss of one sense (sight) makes him increasingly aware of his surroundings through increased development of other senses, such as hearing and touch. He can learn to recognize faces by feeling them. During World War II blind workers were employed to sort delicate and precise parts of machinery used in radar equipment. Their skill, through the sense of touch, in detecting differences in thickness of only a few ten-thousandths of an inch was greater than that of workers who could see and were given expensive micrometers with which to measure the parts.

The nurse who is trained in caring for the blind will know the importance of sameness in the daily routine. Furniture in the room should remain in the same place. Doors should be consistently closed or just as consistently left wide open. Personal articles as comb, tooth brush, and razor should always be kept in the same place. Food should be served with coffee cup, napkin, sugar and salt containers, etc.,

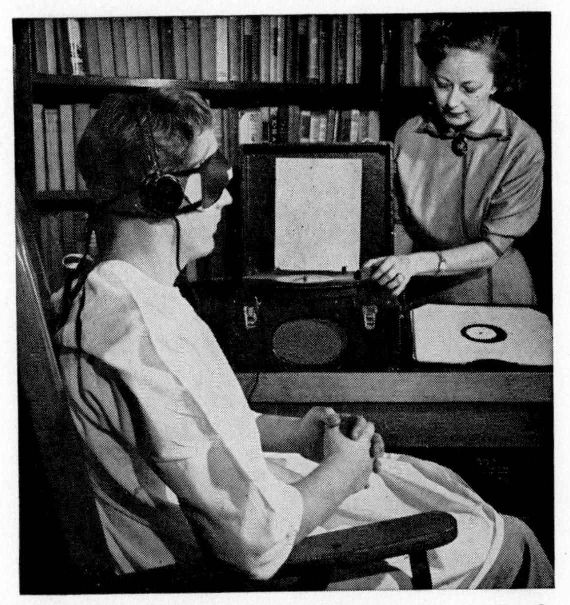

Fig. 258. Talking books provide entertainment for the blind. (Presbyterian Hospital, Chicago, Illinois.)

always in the same place on the tray. The patient should be told before the tray is served what kinds of food have been prepared. If he is instructed to think of the tray with dishes arranged in a relative position to figures on the face of a clock, he soon learns to feed himself. If told that the salad is in position of 8 o'clock, he knows exactly where to find it.

The nurse should always announce her presence when entering the room so as not to startle the patient, and she should always identify herself so he will not undergo the unpleasant experience of being aware of the presence of someone in the room without knowing who it might be.

As in the case of other disabled persons, the blind do not want pity or undue attention. They ask only that they be given an opportunity to learn to be self-sufficient and self-supporting.

Deafness, as stated in Chapter 30, is of two kinds: conduction or bone deafness, in which sound waves are unable to reach the inner ear, and perception or nerve deafness, in which the function of the auditory nerve is impaired. Congenital deafness may be due to various causes; usually the cause remains unknown and rehabilitation may be difficult to achieve.

The child who is unable to hear is deprived of emotional experiences and may be subject to behavior disorders or severe emotional re-

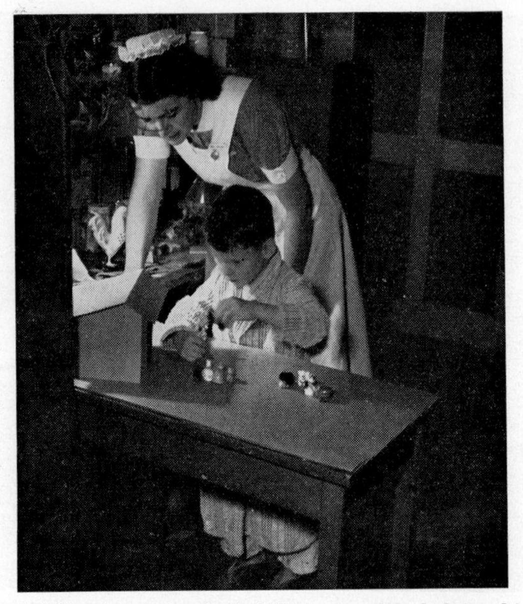

Fig. 259. Rehabilitation of the deaf child is aimed at helping him prepare to join those of his own age group when ready to start to school. (Massachusetts General Hospital School of Nursing, Boston, Massachusetts.)

actions. Without sound, many exciting adventures of daily life (the fire truck, clanging down the street with siren shrieking and bells ringing) become merely an objective experience (the fire truck is only a rapidly moving, red object). Usually, the child makes a better adjustment if cared for in an institution where needed facilities and trained personnel are available.

With a hearing loss of 40–70 per cent (determined by use of the audiometer), use of a hearing aid is indicated, as is training in lip reading and speech development. If hearing loss is greater than 70 per cent the hearing aid will be of little use, and emphasis should be placed on lip reading. It may be necessary for the child to receive special training in a school for the deaf.

Parents of the deaf child need help in adjusting to the child's handicap. This is usually achieved through group conferences, lectures, and informative printed material. They must understand the extent of the child's hearing loss and learn to care for him without being overprotective and too solicitious. They should be discouraged in the normal desire to take the child from doctor to doctor in a vain attempt to find some means of improving his hearing.

The rehabilitation of the deaf child is aimed at helping him to take his place with the normal public school group at the time he is of an age to start regular school training.

A patient who is almost totally deaf made the following suggestions to nurses who try, often unsuccessfully, to communicate with patients who cannot hear: Speak quietly and distinctly on the side of the "good" ear if hearing is impaired on one side only. Don't startle the deaf patient by tapping or punching him to draw his attention. He will notice if you merely raise your hand. See that the light is on your face as you talk to him so he can read your lips easily; don't turn your head aside when talking to him. Avoid word-by-word speech; speak in the normal manner. Don't shout. If the patient doesn't understand, use different words to express the same thought. Write out proper names and thoughts which he fails to understand.

THE AMPUTEE

The psychological adjustment required of the amputee may be such that he is overwhelmed at first and is subject to many kinds of fear: fear of being helpless, and fear of social and economic insecurity. If the amputation is not done as an emergency measure (in case of accidental injury), the patient may receive some preliminary psychological preparation from the doctor and the nurse. He may learn of plans for his rehabilitation for vocational replacement, and he may be advised of community resources which are available to him.

In the immediate postoperative period, the amputee needs to be kept active mentally and physically to overcome depression. Occupational and recreational activities should be introduced at this time. If he is to wear a prosthesis, exercises may be started to prevent contracture deformities, to help maintain joint movement, and to strengthen muscles of the stump.

After the stump has healed it must shrink considerably to change from the cylindrical to the cone-shaped form which is necessary for the wearing of a prosthesis. Two methods may be used to shrink the stump, bandaging with elastic bandage or applying a leather or canvas stump shrinker.

The amputee may be taught how to care for his own stump and to observe adequate stump hygiene. All amputees experience the condition of "phantom limb," feeling pain, itching, burning, and other sensations in the part that has been amputated. In some cases the symptoms persist for a long time, in most cases the condition clears gradually and permanently. The prosthesis is made of willow wood, metal fiber, or plastic. Mechanical hooks are the most serviceable type of prosthesis for hand and arm amputees, although plastic hands resembling human skin are preferable from the standpoint of appearance. Most amputees prefer to have both types, using the hooks for practical purposes and wearing the plastic hands for social occasions.

The amputee must be trained in the use of the artificial limb and the training period usually requires a relatively long period of time. After rehabilitation, the amputee stands a very good chance of finding desirable employment and of returning to a nearly normal life.

CAMPS FOR DISABLED CHILDREN

The disabled child is exposed to the dangers of isolation and of overprotection from parents because of his handicap. To become confident and self-sufficient he must mingle with others, especially with those of his own age. Camps to provide needed companionship and activities during vacation time are in existence throughout the country.

Guests at these particular camps may be disabled by causes ranging from cerebral palsy to congenital deformities, and they may be slightly handicapped or nearly completely helpless. Most camps are specially planned to facilitate activity for the handicapped. Ramps provide means of traveling from one level to another rather than stairs, doors swing easily at a light touch, and washbasins in the bathroom, as well as dresser drawers and closets, are made so they may be used easily by the patient in a wheelchair.

Cooperation is practiced in most activities. A child with an injured leg stands at bat in a ball game, and another boy with a deformed arm runs the bases for him.

Entertainment such as movies, hayrides, reading, music, dancing, and other activities fills the evening hours. Talent shows are frequently arranged, with the guests contributing to the entertainment. Such camps play an important role in helping rehabilitate the disabled child or adult.

HEMIPLEGIA–PARAPLEGIA–QUADRIPLEGIA

Hemiplegia is defined as "paralysis of one side of the body." It is not a disease, but the result of a disease condition, caused by damage to motor nerve cells in the brain. The chief causes are thrombosis, embolism, hemorrhage, tumors, trauma, inflammation and degenerative diseases. Rehabilitation of such patients requires special care to prevent pressure sores and deformity, to overcome speech difficulties, and to help the patient meet emotional problems which may cause extreme depression.

Exercise is an important part of the rehabilitation program and should be provided for the unaffected side, as well as for the paralyzed side. Loss of speech causes frustration for the patient, especially if there is no corresponding loss of mental capacity. Inability to use words is too often interpreted as a sign of mental deterioration. The nurse, through observation and reports, is often able to help the doctor and the psychologist, psychiatrist, and social worker determine the amount of brain damage and thus to decide whether rehabilitation for the patient is possible or feasible.

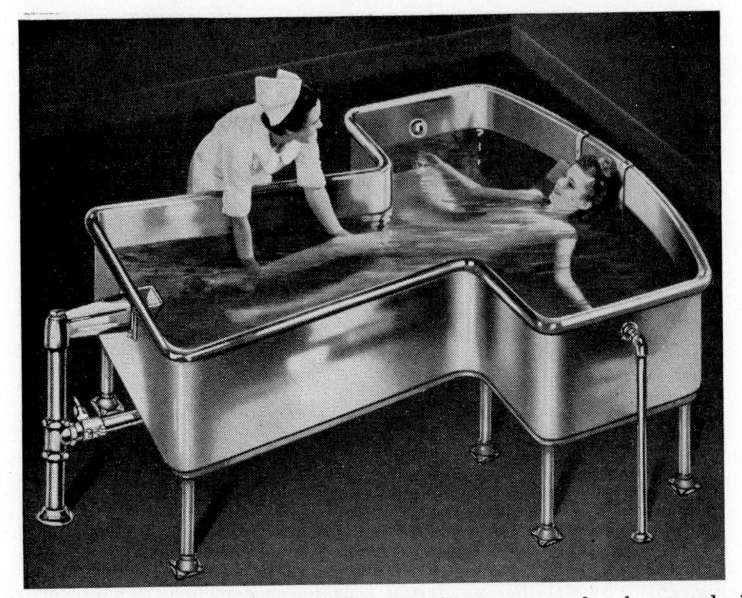

Fig. 260. Special equipment is needed to provide treatment for the paraplegic patient. (Crane Co., Chicago, Illinois.)

Paraplegia designates the condition in which the lower part of the body and the legs are paralyzed. The patient with lower limbs paralyzed has been given a motorized frame which enables him to move about without the help of nurse or attendant. Such a frame can be made from a discarded chain-drive tricycle, with the foot pedals removed and spool handles put in their place for hand manipulation.

The original front wheel assembly may be removed from the conventional Stryker frame and the new front assembly put in place. The patient, with full use of arms, hands, and shoulders, can "pedal" the frame about with his hands. In addition to exercising the muscles that are functioning, and improving the general physical condition, the patient is improved psychologically by having overcome part of the helplessness imposed by the injury or disease which caused the paralysis.

Quadriplegia is defined as paralysis of the upper part of the body, as well as the lower, that is, of all four extremities. The patient thus disabled must usually forego hope of ambulation. Both paraplegia and quadriplegia are considered permanent total disabilities, but rehabilitation is still possible and is achieved through the combined efforts of a rehabilitation team.

"By the side of the doctor and standing squarely in the center of the team around the patient is the nurse. . . . From the earliest age of

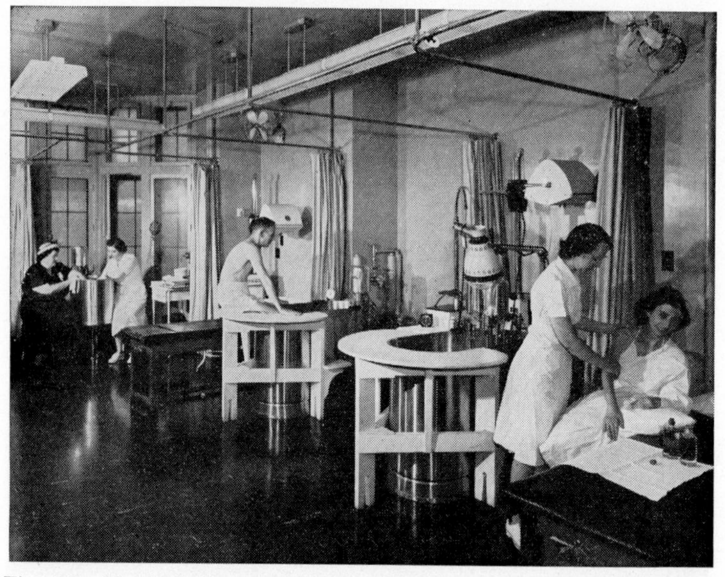

Fig. 261. Physical therapy during convalescence includes the use of such agents as light, heat, and massage. (Department of Medicine and Rehabilitation, University of Illinois, Chicago, Illinois.)

man, the nurse's place has been with the patient. In rehabilitation, the most recent specialized branch of medical care, the nurse must continue to play her ancient role. The spirit of nursing embodies love and service and, in rehabilitation nursing, the rich glow of that spirit is ever present. For the paralyzed patient, as well as for all other disabled people, the nurse can repeat inwardly with belief and confidence the words of a great Teacher, 'Blessed are ye that mourn, for ye shall be comforted.' "*

REHABILITATION UNITS IN THE GENERAL HOSPITAL

In the past, the doctor and the hospital staff were primarily concerned with medical or surgical treatment to correct or improve a physical handicap or disability. Inactivity was the lot of the convalescent patient who quite often left the hospital unable to return to his former job because of his physical condition and unprepared to seek or perform a different kind of work.

Today the concern is with rehabilitation of the patient. During the time of convalescence emphasis is placed on physical and occupational therapy, with such agents as light, electricity, heat, cold, mas-

* From "Rehabilitation Nursing," by Alice B. Morrissey; G. P. Putnam's Sons, New York City.

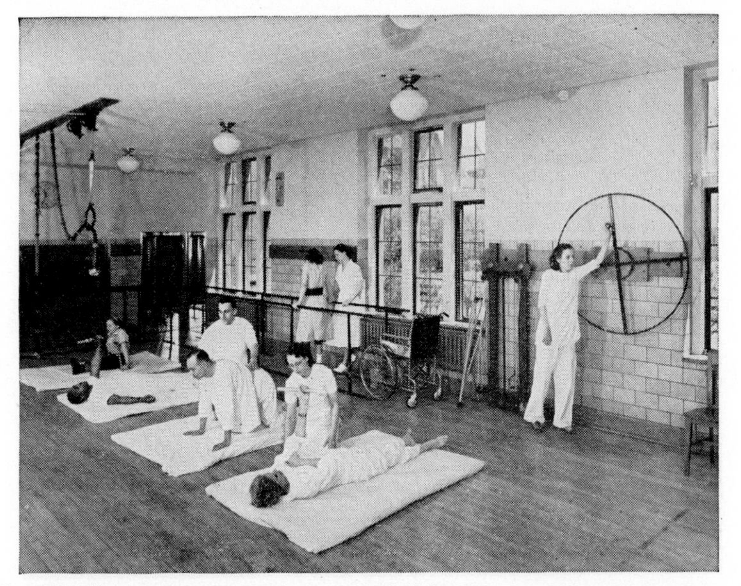

Fig. 262. Therapeutic exercise is part of rehabilitation for each patient. (Department of Medicine and Rehabilitation, University of Illinois, Chicago, Illinois.)

sage, and therapeutic exercise being used to improve the patient physically.

Vocational adjustment or rehabilitation is now being recognized as an essential factor in the total care and treatment being given.

Various phases of rehabilitation require certain types of equipment, depending on the patient's age, size, handicap, and choice of vocational activity to be pursued after leaving the hospital.

In the room for therapeutic exercise are facilities for step and curb climbing, for progressive heavy resistance, walking bars, and other articles needed for activities related to locomotion. Wall mirrors 6 feet high and 2 feet wide are needed in large numbers for work with ambulation training. Hubbard tanks and pools should be available for patients receiving hydrotherapy for neuromuscular disabilities.

Rehabilitation serves as a link between hospitalization and return to normal activity of home and community. It rebuilds morale as the body is being rebuilt and repaired. It provides encouragement and hope with incentive to continue the effort toward a more active, more worth-while life. The patient who is unable to return to his former work, through facilities of the rehabilitation department, may learn a different trade and prepare for a new job while recovering from physical disability.

Patients who have suffered permanent disabilities, as blindness,

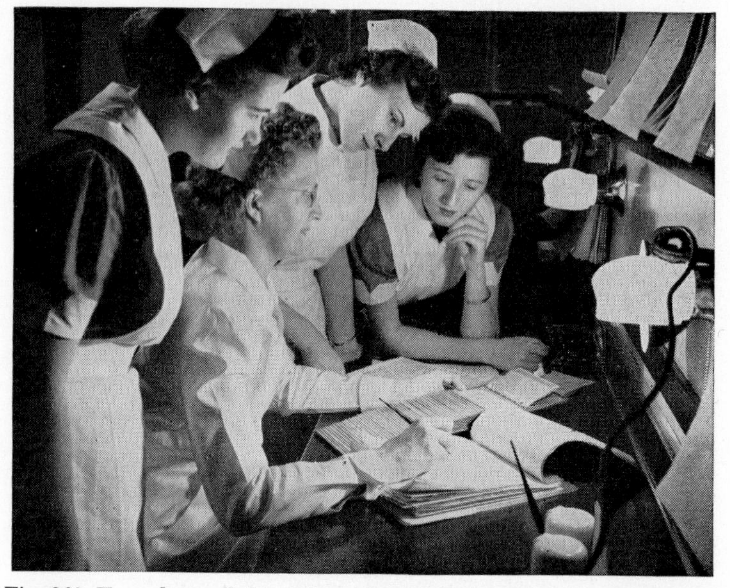

Fig. 263. To understand the patient as a whole the student is referred to the chart and other records to learn pertinent facts about the patient. (Maine Eye and Ear Infirmary School of Nursing, Portland, Maine.)

deafness, or paralysis, or who are handicapped by loss of a hand or leg may be functionally re-educated and trained for the building of a new life and adjustment to their changed condition.

Instead of accepting the role of a helpless invalid, many handicapped persons are learning to care for their personal needs, to walk or travel by ordinary means of locomotion, and, in many instances, to acquire new skills so that once more they are able to take their place in the world. From their beds and wheelchairs they are performing tasks that not only make them self-supporting, but give to them the self-confidence and will to succeed which is necessary if they are to remain worth-while and satisfied members of the community.

Care of Equipment after Use

The wheelchair should be dusted each day and should be thoroughly cleaned at least once each week, by brushing the upholstery and washing the metal parts in soap and water. Leather or fabric upholstery should be cleaned with a damp sponge

Once or twice each month certain parts of the chair should be oiled. The air pressure in the tires should be maintained at a level that will provide good service.

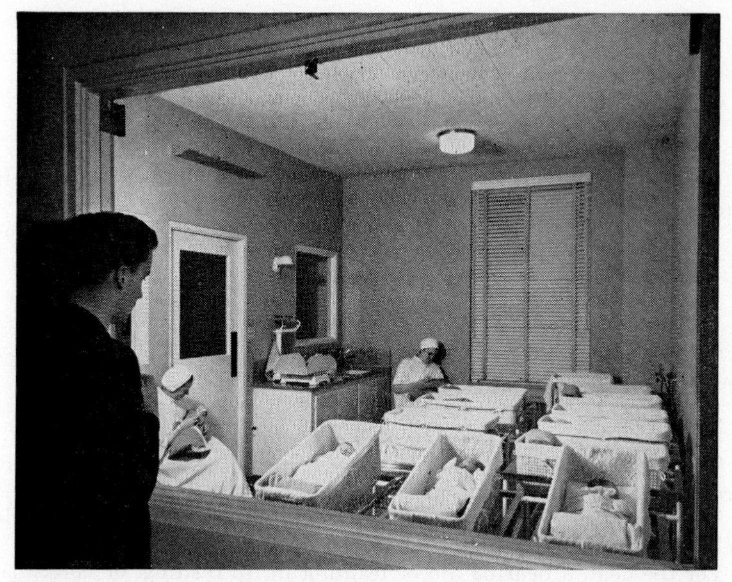

Fig. 264. The infant in the nursery must remain helpless and dependent until he grows older; the handicapped person may usually begin at once to learn to overcome helplessness and dependency. (Presbyterian Hospital School of Nursing, Chicago, Illinois.)

The wheels of the chair should be examined at intervals for loose bolts and nuts.

Summary of Important Factors

The patient must be treated as a whole with attention to psychological, spiritual, and vocational, as well as physical, factors.

About one sixth of the total population are disabled to some extent. The patient should be helped to understand and accept his handicap and then taught to utilize to the fullest extent abilities that remain.

The disabled are more understanding, more tolerant of others.

The disabled want to be self-sufficient, and self-supporting.

The nurse often is required to coordinate services of other trained personnel to accomplish rehabilitation for the patient.

Automatic bladder can be achieved through extensive training, and incontinence need not be a permanent physical condition for many.

Cooperation of the patient is needed to prevent deformities.

To teach effectively the nurse must refrain from "helping" the patient.

Crutch walking and wheelchair manipulation can become a fine art.

Speech rehabilitation may be necessary if the patient is to be able to communicate with those in his environment.

Loss of vision may cause severe psychological trauma.

Sameness is important in rehabilitation work with the blind.

A natural tone of voice should be used in speaking to the deaf.

The amputee should be taught to care for his own stump.

Caring for paralyzed patients offers much job satisfaction to the nurse.

The attitude of the nurse is a very important factor in the success of rehabilitation for the disabled patient.

Factors To Teach the Patient

To accept the physical handicap and then to learn to make the most of the abilities remaining.

Rehabilitation is possible even when the handicap is severe.

Incentive to learn makes learning less difficult.

Training and patience can overcome incontinence, thus relieving probable discomfort and embarrassment.

When deprived of one sense (such as sight) other senses can be developed to a much greater extent.

For the deaf, a hearing aid or training in lip reading, or both, may be necessary.

The amputee has a good chance of being gainfully employed after completing a rehabilitation program.

Phantom limb is usually a temporary condition; interests and activities will help to overcome the condition.

Social agencies are available to help the handicapped to solve problems and make a satisfactory adjustment to his disability.

Situation Type Problem

1. A patient who was totally deaf had been hospitalized for treatment of a minor physical condition not related to her deafness. She communicated with doctors and nurses by means of written notes, although she had learned to convey many thoughts by simple gestures. For instance, her way of saying "thank you" for nursing services was the simple gesture of throwing a kiss. Her semi-private room was one of the most pleasant and most cheerful on the department, and students often spent a longer time there than was actually required for procedures being done. The effect on patients who at different times shared the room and noted the handicapped patient's refusal to be depressed or disturbed by her physical defect was quite obvious. Complaints stemming from their own physical discomfort or mental attitude were heard less frequently and finally not at all. The head nurse at one time commented that "Exposure to the deaf patient's personality for a short time acted as a vaccination against too much self-concern by the other patients."

On the same department a young girl who had lost her right arm in an automobile accident had been in a private room for several weeks. She refused to accept her own personal handicap and to try to adjust to it. Most of her time was spent in outbursts of hysterical sobbing or in long periods of silent depression. Her parents were over-solicitous and had rejected the suggestion that the girl be placed in a room with other patients.

The student nurse who had tried unsuccessfully to divert the girl's attention from her physical condition took matters into her own hands one day. She was returning the girl, by wheelchair, to her room from one of her daily trips to the treatment room and without asking permission of either patient, wheeled the girl into the room occupied by the deaf woman. Mumbling a vague statement about a pressing duty to perform and her intent to return in a few minutes, she hastily left the room.

It was at least an hour later that she returned to find the girl busily engaged in a not very successful attempt to communicate with the other patient by writing a note with her left hand.

Visits to the deafened patient's room became a frequent occurrence for the girl whose mental attitude soon showed definite improvement. Then the parents of the girl became aware of her association with the other patient and they requested that the visits be discontinued, explaining to the nurse that they wouldn't permit their daughter to become a part of the group of handicapped who had to seek their own kind because they didn't or couldn't associate freely with so-called "normal" persons. What would you have done?

Suggested Reference Reading

"Rehabilitation care of patients," Alice B. Morrissey; American Journal of Nursing, July, 1949.

"New devices to help the blind," George Mann; Hygeia, July, 1949.

"The crippled are not beggars," C. J. Lampos; Hygeia, July, 1949.

"Nursing techniques in rehabilitation," Alice B. Morrissey; American Journal of Nursing, September, 1949.

"The major amputations," John R. Glover; American Journal of Nursing, September, 1950.

"Nursing care for the amputee," Mary E. Moskopp and Jane Sloan; American Journal of Nursing, September, 1950.

"Psychosocial and spiritual factors in rehabilitation." Alice B. Morrissey; American Journal of Nursing, December, 1950.

"A blind diabetic patient can learn to give insulin," Shirley Jo Eichel; American Journal of Nursing, June, 1951.

"Rehabilitation after laryngectomy," Warren H. Gardner; Public Health Nursing, November, 1951.

"Rehabilitation unit," Worley H. Kendall; Modern Hospital, March, 1952.

"Teaching aphasic patients to talk again," Elmer C. Baker and Martin Sokoloff; American Journal of Nursing, July, 1952.

"Motorizing the Stryker frame bolsters paralytic's morale," Ralph L. Perkins; Hospitals, December, 1952.

CHAPTER 44

Bandaging

TOPICAL OUTLINE

A man all wrapped up in himself usually makes a very small package.

A bandage is defined as "a piece of gauze or other material used to wrap, bind, support or immobilize a part." The art of applying a neat and effective bandage is learned through practice, and is an ability that may be utilized on many different occasions. Doctors who have not learned to apply bandages in a neat and systematic way view with added respect the nurse who is able to bandage any part of the body and do it well.

Patients are grateful when bandages they need to wear are kept clean and neat by being changed frequently by a skillful nurse. Friends and relatives, as well as the public in general, take for granted that the graduate, registered nurse is fully qualified to expertly apply any kind or type of bandage. With all of these factors kept in mind, the importance of learning the technique of bandaging becomes readily apparent.

THE PURPOSE OF BANDAGES

Bandages are used primarily in giving emergency or first aid treatment to the injured. When properly applied, so that pressure is exerted

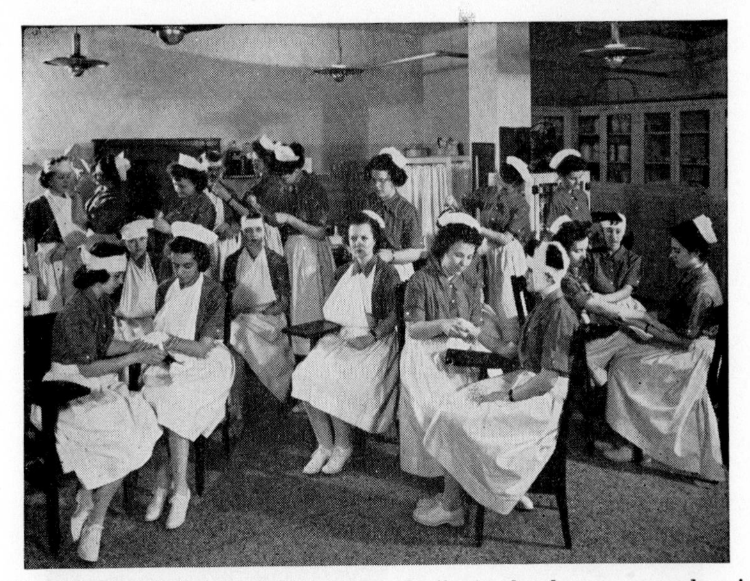

Fig. 265. The ability to apply a neat and effective bandage comes only with practice. (Presbyterian Hospital School of Nursing, Chicago, Illinois.)

on various parts, bleeding may be controlled. Bandages may also be used to immobilize a part, such as a limb or joint; they may serve as a sling or support for an injured part; they may be used to hold splints securely in place, and to prevent or reduce edema or swelling.

Bandages are used also to protect a surgical wound against infection; to hold surgical dressings or local applications of a medication in place; to help in the correction of a deformity, and to afford support to a weakened or affected part.

MATERIALS USED IN BANDAGES

Materials most commonly used for bandages are: gauze, muslin, canton flannel, flannel, elastic webbing, woven cotton, crepe paper, and crinoline impregnated with plaster of Paris.

Gauze is perhaps the material most often used for bandages. It is thin, light, soft, porous, and relatively cool. It is pliable and easily kept in place. It can be easily applied so that uniform pressure is maintained over the area covered.

Muslin is heavier and more firm than gauze. It is used when there is need to apply pressure, give firm support to a part, limit motion, or hold splints securely in position.

Canton flannel is very soft and is commonly used under splints or casts to protect the skin surface. It is pliable and can be used effectively to cover uneven surfaces. It is suitable for use in tailed bandages.

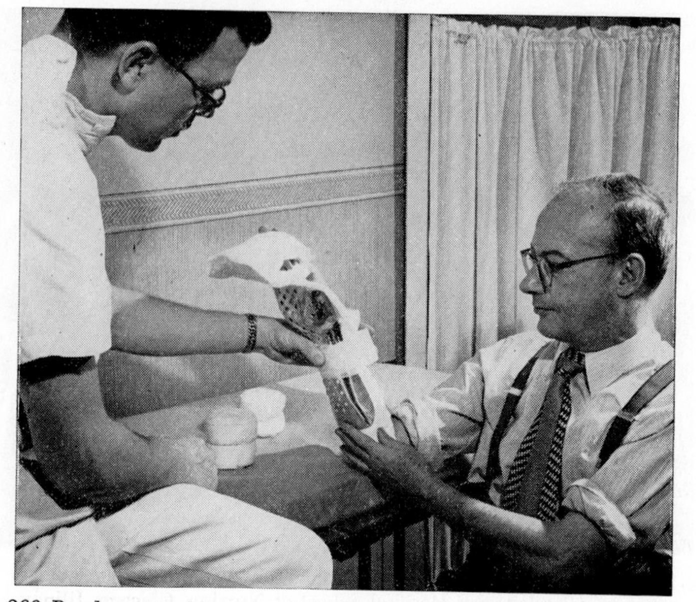

Fig. 266. Bandage may be used to hold a splint in place. (Presbyterian Hospital, Chicago, Illinois.)

Flannel, which absorbs moisture and supplies warmth, is used in bandaging painful joints and extremities in conditions such as rheumatism and gout.

Elastic webbing, made of an elastic network covered with silk or cotton, is used to give support and to apply pressure over varicose veins, and to help control hemorrhage.

Woven cotton bandage is made so that it is able to withstand stretching. It, too, is used to give support and apply even pressure to a part. It may be used for the same purposes as the elastic bandage and has the advantages of being lighter, less expensive, and readily washable.

Crepe paper is light, smooth, and easily adjusted. It is suitable for use in most instances where bandages are required, except possibly for holding in place dressings that are soon saturated with drainage or a fluid discharge.

Crinoline impregnated with plaster of Paris is used to immobilize a joint or part and to give firm support to the part of the body to which it is applied.

BANDAGES CLASSIFIED ACCORDING TO SHAPE

Bandages classified according to shape include: triangular, cravat, tailed, handkerchief, and roller.

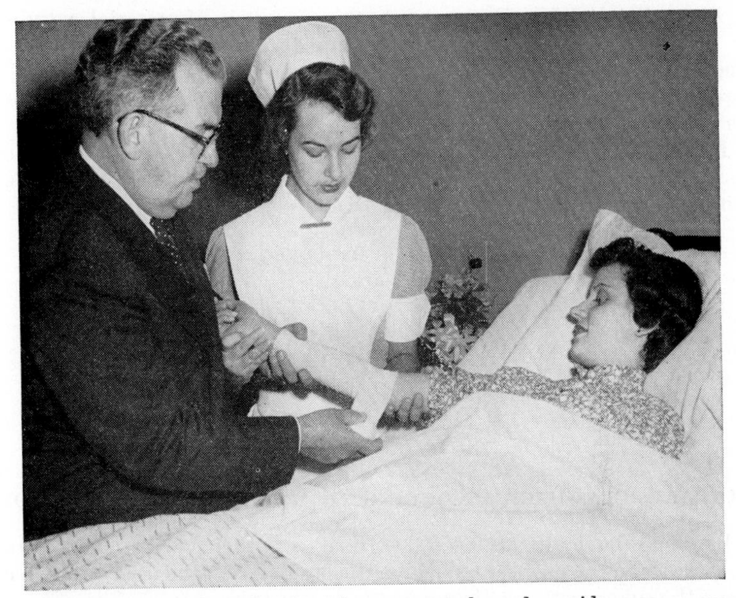

Fig. 267. Woven or elastic bandage is easy to apply and provides even pressure. (Missouri Baptist Hospital School of Nursing, St. Louis, Missouri.)

The triangular bandage is triangular in shape and is used to hold dressings in place on hand, arm, shoulder, foot, hip, breast, and buttocks. When used as a swinging bandage to support hand, forearm, or elbow it is termed a *sling*.

The cravat bandage is triangular in shape but is folded with the apex toward the base, then rolled or loosely folded until the bandage is of the desired width. It is used as a sling for the arm or wrist, as a tourniquet for extremities, and to hold dressings in place on the hand, forehead, axilla, groin, or back of the neck.

The tailed bandage is oblong with two or more tails attached lengthwise at each end. It is used to retain dressings in place on various parts of the body. It is used when dressings must be changed frequently and the affected part should be disturbed as little as possible. The body of the bandage is placed directly over the dressing, and the tails are used to fasten the bandage in position.

The handkerchief bandage is a square of thin pliable material large enough to be adjusted to fit different parts of the body. The ends of the bandage may be tied so that it remains in place on such parts as the head, hand, foot, knee, or elbow. This bandage is useful in first aid or emergency work where a temporary bandage is required, or it may be used successfully to hold in place dressings which require frequent changing.

The roller bandage is a simple continuous strip of material, varying in width and length, and tightly wound to form a compact roll. It is the most commonly used bandage, as it can be applied in several different ways, will fit any part of the body, and will answer any purpose for which a bandage is needed or used.

Roller bandages to be used on various parts of the body should be of the following widths and lengths (length is dependent on purpose of bandage, those given here are approximate only):

Part of body	Width of bandage	Length of bandage
finger	½–1 inch	1–3 yards
hand	1–2 inches	3 yards
arm	2–2½ inches	7–9 yards
foot	1½–3 inches	4 yards
leg	2–3 inches	9 yards
body	3–6 inches	10 yards
head	2 inches	6 yards

BANDAGES CLASSIFIED ACCORDING TO METHODS OF APPLICATION

Bandages have already been described as to their various shapes and purposes, and the purpose for which the bandage is to be used will determine the shape or type of bandage that is needed.

Since the roller bandage may be used for any purpose, the different methods of application to be classified are concerned with only the roller type bandage. The methods explained are those most commonly used, and from the seven methods described have grown numerous modifications or combinations of these few fundamental bandages. For purposes of classification the term "bandage," as used in the next few paragraphs, refers to the "roller bandage," which is the most commonly used type.

The circular bandage consists of a number of circular turns around a part. Each turn exactly covers the preceding turn and holds it securely in place. It is used to hold dressings in place on such parts as the forehead, neck, wrist, and ankle. One or two circular turns are made, when other methods of application are used, to anchor the initial end of the bandage or to keep it firmly in position.

The oblique bandage is a series of slanting (oblique) turns around a part, each turn higher than the previous one so that the turns are separated by an area of exposed skin surface and there is no overlapping of the edges of the bandage. It is used for holding dressings in place on a part where pressure is to be avoided. The bandage is light in weight and non-restrictive, yet serves adequately to retain the dressing in the desired position. The oblique bandage may be used to hold splints in place in emergency treatment.

The spiral bandage consists of a series of turns ascending a part, each turn higher than the preceding one and overlapping it approxi-

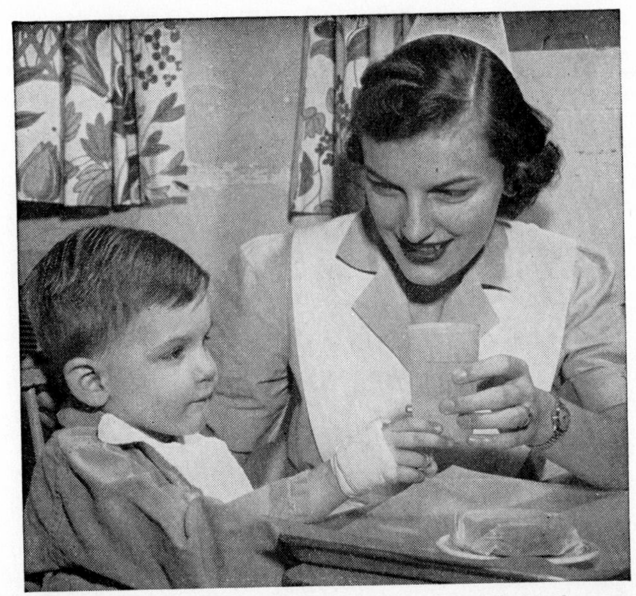

Fig. 268. The circular bandage is applied with a number of circular turns about the part. (University of Michigan School of Nursing, Ann Arbor, Michigan.)

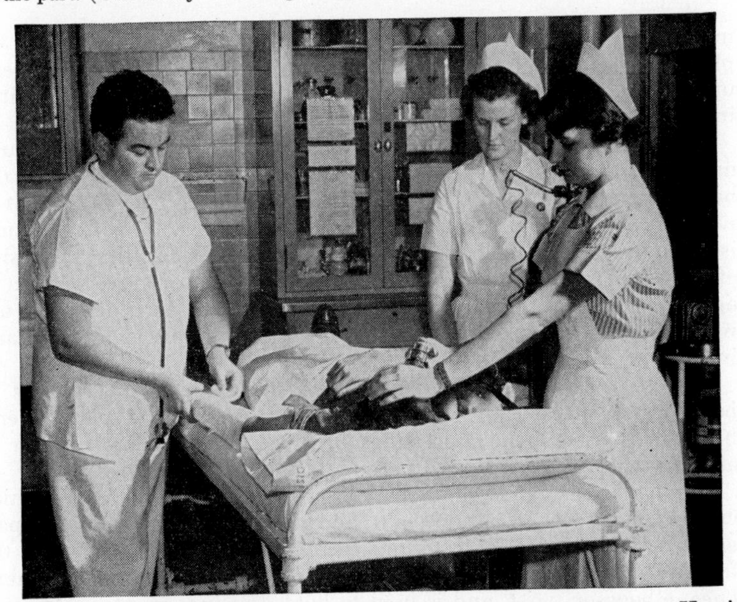

Fig. 269. The spiral bandage is used to hold splints in place. (Allentown Hospital School of Nursing, Allentown, Pennsylvania.)

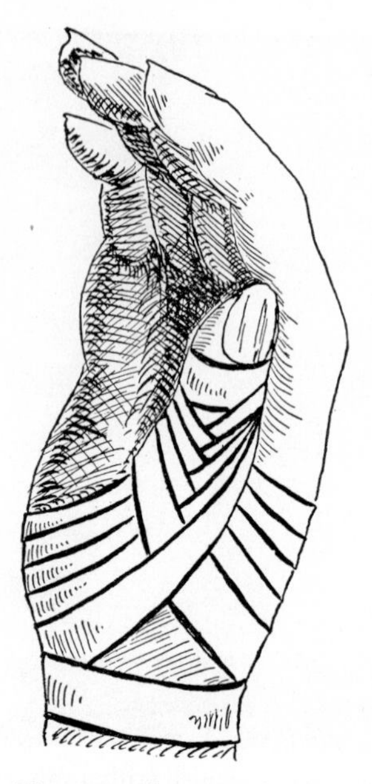

Fig. 270. The spica bandage.

mately one-half to two-thirds the width of the bandage. It is applied on parts that are of uniform circumference, as the fingers, upper arm, and trunk. It is used chiefly to hold dressings or splints in place.

The spiral reverse bandage is the spiral bandage with a reverse turn made each time the part is circled. By means of the reverse turns the bandage may be made to smoothly fit parts that are tapering or not of uniform circumference, such as the forearm or leg. The reverse turn is made by turning the bandage as it is being applied so that the inside of the bandage becomes the outside and at the next reverse turn is again the inside. As the turns are continued, each turn advances upward beyond the preceding turn, with the reverse angles uniform and in line.

Reverse turns of the bandage should not be made over joints or bony prominences, as they cause increased pressure. The spiral reverse bandage is used to hold dressings in place, to apply pressure, or to afford support to the affected part.

The figure-of-8 bandage consists of overlapping turns, each of which crosses the other at a mid-point and ascends or descends the part adjacent to a joint. Each complete turn of the bandage is made in the form of the figure 8. This bandage is applied to joints, as the ankle, knee, elbow, or wrist, and is used to hold dressings in place, to exert

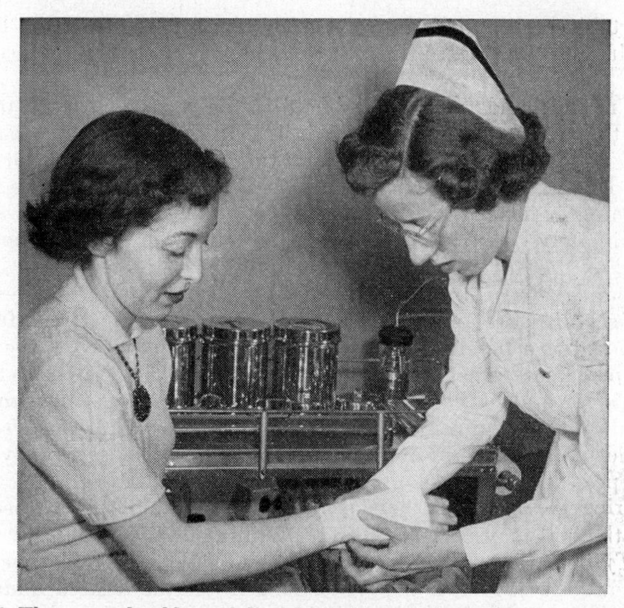

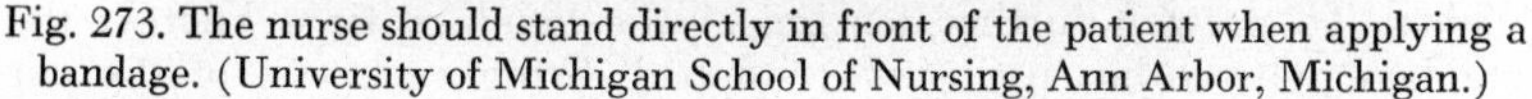
Fig. 273. The nurse should stand directly in front of the patient when applying a bandage. (University of Michigan School of Nursing, Ann Arbor, Michigan.)

A wet or damp bandage should not be applied to a part, since shrinkage as the bandage dries will increase the amount of pressure exerted by the bandage.

In applying the bandage care should be taken that the bandage is applied with even tension over the entire area, and that the bandage is neither too tight nor too loose. A too-tight bandage may interfere with circulation and cause death of the tissues in the part bandaged. A bandage applied too loosely is likely to become displaced or to be ineffective in holding a dressing in place. The degree of pressure which should be used in applying the bandage will depend on the condition of the affected part and the purpose for which the bandage is used.

Factors To Be Avoided in Applying a Bandage. Effort should be made when a bandage is being applied to avoids pads that are improperly placed so they do not offer protection; dressings that are poorly placed; uneven tension on the bandage as it is being applied; varying degrees of overlapping in the turns of the bandage; crosses or reverses that are uneven or made over inadequately covered joints or inflamed surfaces; use of excessive bandage so that the part is unnecessarily bulky; and incorrect fastening of the end of the bandage.

Directions for Applying the Roller Bandage. With the patient in a comfortable position, the nurse should stand directly in front of him or slightly to one side, so the part to be bandaged can be reached with ease.

The roll of bandage should be held in the right hand with the roll above the bandage as it is applied. The initial turn of the bandage should be held in place by two or three additional circular turns which exactly cover the first. The bandage roll is held close to the part being bandaged so that the unwound portion does not exceed approximately six inches in length. Even tension or pressure should be exerted on the full extent of the bandage as it is applied.

To bandage an extremity application is begun at the smallest part and the bandage applied upward over the increasing circumference. In bandaging a hand or foot the tips of the fingers or toes should be left exposed so the part may be closely observed for the characteristic bluish color and lowered temperature which indicates impairment of circulation and requires that the bandage be loosened or removed.

Avoid useless turns in applying a bandage, as they serve only to increase pressure and cause discomfort to the patient.

Securing the End of a Bandage. When the bandage has been applied, the end may be secured in a number of ways.

By Tying. When securing the end of a bandage by tying, the bandage should be cut down the center lengthwise the desired number of inches. To prevent further tearing of the bandage tie a knot at the bandage where the cutting was stopped. Bring each end of the cut bandage around the part from opposite sides and tie securely in place.

By Pinning. If a bandage is to be secured by pinning, a safety pin should be used, and the pin should be so placed that it will not cause discomfort to the patient by causing pressure against the affected part.

By Sewing. A bandage may be fastened by sewing when other means of securing the end might cause discomfort to the patient. Abdominal bands used in the nursery as part of the necessary clothing for the newborn baby are usually sewed in place to eliminate the use of safety pins or other methods of fastening.

By Strips of Adhesive Tape. Strips of adhesive tape may be used to fasten the end of a bandage or to hold spiral reverse turns in place. When used to fasten the bandage, the adhesive strips should be applied so as not to detract from its neat appearance.

Methods of Removing a Bandage. If a bandage is so fashioned that unwinding it would be painful to the patient, or is soiled so there is danger of contamination, it should be cut for removal. To remove a bandage by cutting, be sure to make the cut on the side opposite the injured or affected area. The bandage, cut for the entire extent, can be laid open and, if necessary, the separate pieces may be removed with forceps so contact with drainage or other material that may have soiled the bandage can be avoided.

If it is not necessary to cut the bandage for removal, it may be unfastened, the end held lightly in one hand and passed from hand to hand, gathering up the bandage as it is unwound.

If the bandage (cotton or other firm texture) is to be used again, it should be thoroughly washed and autoclaved, then rewound and stored in a clean place until needed.

SPECIAL BANDAGES FOR VARIOUS PARTS OF THE BODY

The gauntlet bandage, for the fingers, each finger is bandaged separately, with the bandage secured by circular turns around the wrist.

The demigauntlet bandage, for the back of the hand, each finger is left exposed and the back of the hand is covered. The bandage is secured by circular turns around the wrist.

The mitten bandage, a piece of gauze is placed between the fingers, then the bandage is applied to the entire hand. Hand and fingers are bandaged together; the thumb is left exposed or bandaged separately. The bandage is secured by circular turns around the wrist.

The Velpeau bandage, for the shoulder, used in treatment of fractures of the clavicle and scapula or in dislocation of the shoulder. Before applying the bandage the hand of the injured side is placed well up on the opposite shoulder. The bandage is applied so that turns are made first over the shoulder then around the chest and this repeated, with slight overlapping of each turn, until the vertical turns reach the base of the neck and the horizontal turns reach the wrist. The hand is left free, the arm being bandaged close to the patient's chest.

The Barton bandage is used to hold dressings on the chin and in treatment of fractures of the lower jaw. The turns are applied, each exactly covering the preceding one, alternately around the chin to encircle the upper part of the neck and around the chin upward to cross the top of the head and frame the face. Several thicknesses of bandage are needed to make the bandage secure. It is secured at the top of the head and adhesive strips should be used to secure it at the points where the turns cross at the sides of the chin and nape of the neck.

The monocular bandage is applied over one eye. Figure-of-8 turns are used, alternately encircling the forehead and obliquely covering the cheek, eye, and head, until the eye is sufficiently covered. The bandage is secured by circular turns around the head.

The binocular bandage is applied over both eyes. Double figure-of-8 turns are used, the lower edge of the first turns crossing at the bridge of the nose. The double figure-of-8 turns are continued until both eyes have been sufficiently covered. The bandage is completed by one or more circular turns.

The suspensory bandage is applied to retain dressings in place or to afford support to a pendulous part, such as the breast or scrotum.

ADHESIVE TAPE

Adhesive tape is a bandage of the roller type with a plaster base which causes it to adhere to the skin. It is flexible, yet affords strong support for any part to which it may be applied. It is available in waterproof form, which will not absorb perspiration or drainage.

Uses of Adhesive Tape. Adhesive tape is used extensively to secure or fasten the end of a bandage, to hold a dressing in place, to hold splints in proper position, to bind together the edges of a gaping wound, and to immobilize a part where complete rest is needed for relief of pain or for recovery.

Methods of Applying Adhesive Tape. Before adhesive tape is applied, the part to be covered should be washed, shaved, and dried. If all hair is removed from the skin surface, there is less irritation and less discomfort for the patient when the tape is removed. For drying the skin before applying adhesive tape, the area should be cleansed with benzine, which quickly evaporates, leaving the skin completely dry. If adhesive tape is to be applied over bony prominences, the part should first be well padded with a protective bandage. Adhesive tape should not be applied over raw surfaces of skin; the affected area should be protected with an appropriate dressing.

When applying adhesive tape, care should be taken that the tape is not too tight or permitted to completely encircle a part, thus interfering with normal circulation. Adhesive tape should be applied evenly so as to prevent wrinkling of the skin beneath the tape bandage.

Adhesive tape should not be used on patients who have extremely sensitive skins and are predisposed to development of inflammation or infection. If the skin beneath the adhesive tape shows signs of irritation or inflammation when the tape is removed, tape should not be reapplied to the same area.

Agents Used in Removing Adhesive Tape. The best agent for removing adhesive tape is one that contains an oily base which will dissolve the adhesive mass and leave no unsightly marks on the skin surface. Benzine, which is commonly used, not only dissolves the plaster base and cleanses the skin, but has an antiseptic action that is of benefit. Ether is sometimes used for removing adhesive tape, but evaporates very quickly and must be reapplied several times before it is effective. Carbon tetrachloride is non-inflammable and will effectively remove adhesive tape, but is somewhat irritating to the skin.

Method of Removing Adhesive Tape. Lift the end of the strip of adhesive away from the skin surface and apply a small amount of the solvent or agent which is to be used in removing the tape. Allow sufficient time for the agent to dissolve the plaster base, then gently remove the loosened strip.

To remove adhesive strips without the use of a solvent, fold the loosened end of the tape back upon itself, keeping the removed portion

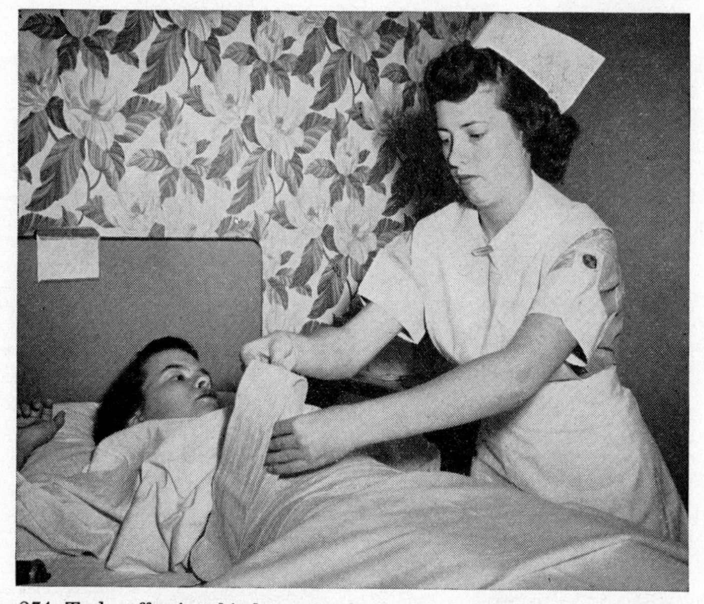

Fig. 274. To be effective, binders must be correctly applied. (Baylor University School of Nursing, Waco, Texas.)

directly above the strip still to be removed. Continue to remove the tape while gently pressing the skin down and away from it.

In removing adhesive tape long strips should be cut into shorter sections and removed piece by piece, working from the end of the tape toward the middle. When the adhesive tape has been removed, the entire area should be cleansed with the solvent, to remove all particles of the plaster base which may have adhered to the skin. The uncovered area is then washed with warm soap and water, and patted dry with a soft towel. Powder is applied to the area where the tape has been removed. If a portion of the uncovered skin surface is raw (upper layer of skin removed with the tape), a sterile dressing is applied to the affected area as a protection against possible contamination.

THE APPLICATION OF BINDERS

Binders are applied for the general purposes of keeping applications or dressings in place, to apply pressure to a part, and to give support to the patient where needed.

Various types of binders include the scultetus, the straight abdominal, the T, the double T, and the breast binder.

The scultetus binder, termed the many tailed binder because of its

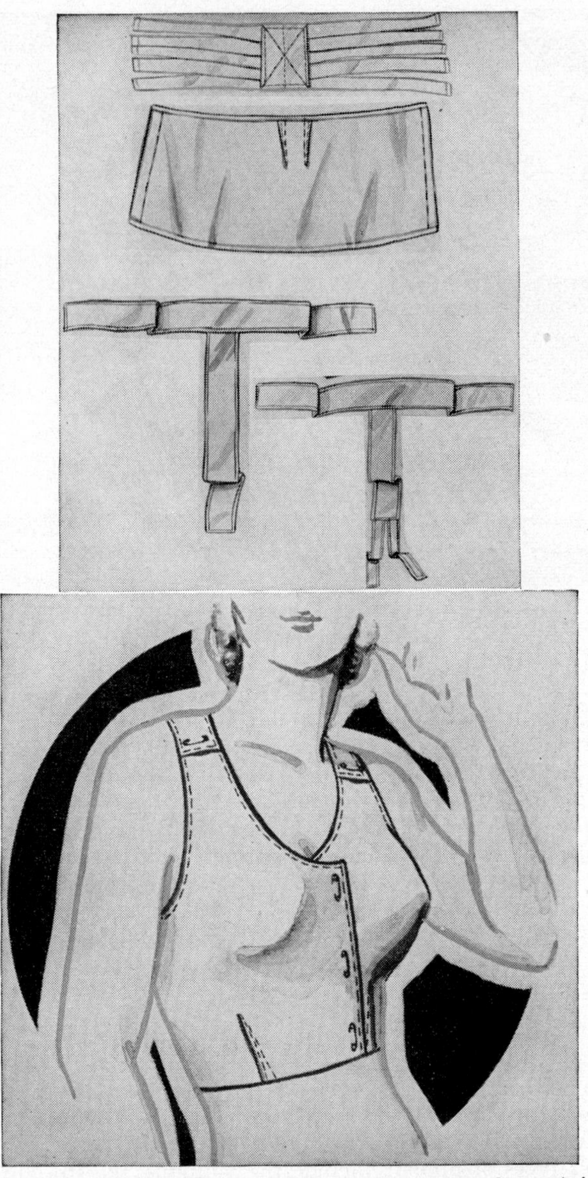

Fig. 275. Various binders (as shown in order from top to bottom) including scultetus, abdominal, T, double T, and breast binder. (Carolina Absorbent Cotton Co., Charlotte, North Carolina.)

shape, is used to hold dressings in place, to apply pressure, and to afford support. It is applied from below upward and is fastened with safety pins.

The straight abdominal binder is used for the same purpose as the scultetus binder. Darts should be pinned in the binder to make it snug fitting.

The T *binder* is used to hold perineal pads in place and to hold dressings for hemorrhoidectomy. When necessary a T binder made from gauze bandage can be used temporarily.

The double T *binder* is used for the male patient to hold perineal dressings in place.

The breast binder is used to give support to the breasts, to hold dressings in place, and to compress the breasts when it is necessary to dry the secretion of milk. Darts should be pinned to make the binder snug fitting. Breasts should be in proper position before the binder is applied.

Summary of Important Factors

Bandages are used chiefly to hold dressings in place, to protect wounds, and to afford support or immobilization.

Gauze, flannel, muslin, and elastic bandages are most commonly used.

Bandages are triangular, square, tailed, or roller in shape.

A roller bandage may be applied in any of the following ways: circular, oblique, spiral, spiral reverse, figure-of-8, spica, and recurrent. Use variations in methods of applying the bandage to fit the part being bandaged.

Have the part clean, dry, and the patient comfortable, before applying a bandage.

Pad all bony prominences before bandaging.

Never apply a bandage so two skin surfaces are in contact.

Do not apply a wet or damp bandage.

Apply the bandage with even tension.

Always leave finger tips and toes exposed to permit observation of any impairment of circulation.

Bandages may be secured by tying, pinning, sewing, or by use of adhesive strips.

A soiled bandage should be cut before it is removed, the cut being made away from the injured area.

Have the skin clean and dry before applying adhesive tape. Do not apply adhesive tape over raw surfaces of skin.

Benzine, cold cream, or ether may be used to remove adhesive tape. Hold the tape close to the patient and pull it back upon itself to remove.

Use precautions against fire if an inflammable agent is used in removing adhesive tape.

Factors To Teach the Patient

Not to remove a bandage that has been applied by a doctor or nurse unless specifically instructed to do so. To apply an outer bandage if necessary for a neat, clean appearance.

If the bandaged part becomes swollen and painful to call these facts to the attention of the nurse in charge.

To report to the doctor any bandage that is uncomfortably tight or interfering with normal circulation.

If a bandage becomes wet or damp it may shrink as it dries and require readjustment to avoid exertion of too much pressure.

Bandages can be fastened or secured so the end of the bandage does not cause uncomfortable pressure on the bandaged part. All such discomforts should be reported.

If removing a bandage by cutting, the cut should always be made some distance from the site of injury.

If the agent used to remove adhesive tape is inflammable, caution against possible fire must be observed.

Bandages should never be applied so that two surfaces of skin are in contact.

Scientific Principles

Anatomy and Physiology. Structures involved in injury to tissue depend on whether the wound is superficial or penetrates to greater depth.

Wounds heal rapidly if no infection is present.

The type bandage to use depends on the part to be bandaged.

The fingers and toes, when being bandaged, should have ends exposed, so interference with circulation caused by applying the bandage too tightly can be readily observed.

Chemistry. Benzine acts as a solvent for adhesive plaster and may be used to remove adhesive from the skin.

For slight cuts or small open areas on the skin alcohol (70 per cent) or other antiseptic solution should be applied before the part is bandaged.

Microbiology. Bandages are used to cover small dressings and to help protect a wound from contamination.

Contaminated bandages should be discarded into the incinerator to be burned.

Bandages which are made commercially and have their own protective outer covering, an adhesive inner coat, and a small dressing impregnated with an antiseptic, are more effective for fingers and for small skin areas than is the bandage applied by doctor or nurse.

Pharmacology. Antiseptics usually used for the skin are alcohol, iodine, and Mercurochrome.

Protective ointments, such as zinc oxide, may be covered by dressings held in place with a bandage.

Penicillin in powder form may be used in open wounds to prevent the growth of bacteria.

Physics. The tourniquet is a pressure bandage used to control bleeding.

Each succeeding turn of a circular bandage nearly doubles the pressure exerted by the bandage.

Gauze fibers absorb drainage by capillary attraction, yet gauze bandage contains so few fibers that it is not used primarily for its absorbent qualities.

When roller bandage is being applied the nurse should bear in mind that useless turns of the bandage increase the pressure which it exerts.

Friction between the bandage and the part being bandaged helps hold the bandage in place.

Bandages and binders when correctly applied afford support to the part.

Psychology. Bandages that are clean and neat are more acceptable to the patient and for that reason outer bandages should be changed frequently.

Soiled dressings and bandages should be removed from the sight of the patient as soon as possible after they have been changed.

A bandage that has been applied with the right amount of tension may become tight enough to cause discomfort if the bandaged part begins to swell. A too-tight bandage should be removed and reapplied so that less pressure is being exerted.

Sociology. All nurses, as well as doctors, are expected to be able to apply bandages neatly and effectively.

If bandages will be necessary for some time the nurse may need to teach a member of the patient's family how to apply the bandage properly.

If an elastic bandage can be used it may be more economical for the patient, since it can be washed and reapplied many times.

Members of all first aid groups should be well instructed in the dangers of a pressure bandage. Any bandage applied to control bleeding should be loosened about every 10 to 15 minutes to re-establish circulation to the part.

Situation Type Problems

1. After dressing the stump made by amputation of a limb the week before, Doctor Jones left written orders on the patient's chart that the bandage holding the dressing in place was *not* to be removed. Several hours later the bandage was badly soiled from drainage that had seeped through the dressings.

The nurse in charge attempted to call the doctor to ask that she or an intern be permitted to change the dressing. Doctor Jones' secretary reported that he had been called from the office by an emergency and would not return for several hours. The patient was insistent that the dressing be changed as she planned to be in a wheel chair on the sun porch during visiting hours. What would you have done?

2. Doctor Black applied a bandage to an injured leg in the out-patient department during the early morning clinic hours. At the time the bandage was being applied the patient complained that it felt "too tight." Doctor Black assured the patient that the bandage was not too tight and finished applying it, fastening it securely in position with several strips of adhesive tape.

The patient returned to the out-patient department early in the afternoon, complaining that the bandage was causing great discomfort. The patient's foot was badly swollen, and the toes showed blue discoloration. When the nurse reported to Doctor Black that the patient had returned and was complaining about the bandage, Doctor Black stated that he was busy with another patient and that "Mrs. Brown is a chronic complainer, anyway. Tell her to go home and stay off that leg, and the bandage will be all right." What would you have done?

3. Doctor Smith removed several strips of adhesive tape and a sterile dressing from an injured arm. After cleansing the wound he applied another sterile dressing to it. He then asked for benzine or another solvent to cleanse the arm of marks left by the adhesive. The benzine bottle had an insufficient amount of benzine in it. The only other solvent on the dressing cart was a bottle of ether. When he opened this bottle it was found that the ether had evaporated. He was very much annoyed, but avoided making any remarks that would reveal his annoyance to the patient. He asked the nurse for a length of adhesive, obviously intending to place it on the patient's arm without cleansing the arm. What would you have done?

Suggested References Reading

"Better bandages," The Trading Post, American Journal of Nursing, May, 1948.

"Nursing care for the amputee," M. E. Moskopp and Jane Sloan; American Journal of Nursing, September, 1950.

"Dressings for fingers and toes," Lorraine M. Wistein; American Journal of Nursing, March, 1951.

"Pelvic binder," Mary G. Patterson; American Journal of Nursing, April, 1951.

"Dyed bandages and casts for children," Paulette Drummonds; American Journal of Nursing, December, 1952.

Index

C

D

T

W

X

AMER. JOUR. Dec 1952

Sleep Tight — 1522

Feb 1954

What is sleep Pg 202

Diehl & Boynton - Health living for Nurses

136 - 140

Why Sleep - pamphlet

T.B - Sleep & Relaxation